MANUAL of PERIOPERATIVE CARE in ADULT CARDIAC SURGERY

Fifth Edition

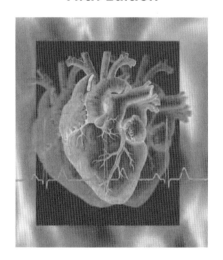

By

Robert M. Bojar, MD

Chief of Cardiothoracic Surgery
Saint Vincent Hospital
Worcester, Massachusetts, USA

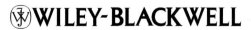
WILEY-BLACKWELL

A John Wiley & Sons, Ltd., Publication

This edition first published 2011 © 2011 by Robert M. Bojar

Blackwell Publishing was acquired by John Wiley & Sons in February 2007. Blackwell's publishing program has been merged with Wiley's global Scientific, Technical and Medical business to form Wiley-Blackwell.

Registered office: John Wiley Sons Ltd, The Atrium, Southern Gate, Chichester, West Sussex, PO19 8SQ, UK

Editorial offices: 9600 Garsington Road, Oxford, OX4 2DQ, UK
                        The Atrium, Southern Gate, Chichester, West Sussex, PO19 8SQ, UK
                        111 River Street, Hoboken, NJ 07030-5774, USA

For details of our global editorial offices, for customer services and for information about how to apply for permission to reuse the copyright material in this book please see our website at www.wiley.com/wiley-blackwell

The right of the author to be identified as the author of this work has been asserted in accordance with the UK Copyright, Designs and Patents Act 1988.

Library of Congress Cataloging-in-Publication Data

Bojar, Robert M., 1951-
  Manual of perioperative care in adult cardiac surgery / by Robert M. Bojar. – 5th ed.
      p. ; cm.
  Includes bibliographical references and index.
  ISBN 978-1-4443-3143-1
  1. Heart–Surgery–Handbooks, manuals, etc. 2. Therapeutics, Surgical–Handbooks, manuals, etc. I. Title.
  [DNLM: 1. Cardiac Surgical Procedures–Outlines. 2. Perioperative Care–methods–Outlines. WG 18.2 B685m 2011]
  RD598.B64 2011
  617'.412–dc22
                                                                                    2010010689

A catalogue record for this book is available from the British Library.

This book is published in the following electronic formats: ePDF 9781444325294; Wiley Online Library 9781444325287

Set in 9/11pt, Caslon by Thomson Digital, Noida, India

Printed and bound in Malaysia by Vivar Printing Sdn Bhd

1   2011

Dedication

To my parents, Leah and Samuel Bojar, who instilled in me a lifelong desire for learning, the importance of sharing knowledge, and a dedication to provide all patients with the best possible care.

Table of Contents

Preface

The future of cardiac surgery faces significant challenges with the widespread application of transcatheter technologies, including coronary stenting, percutaneous valves, endovascular approaches to thoracic aortic disease, and ablation of arrhythmias in the electrophysiology laboratory. Most of these technologies evolved from the concept that a less invasive approach to structural heart disease is preferred by patients to reduce trauma, minimize complications, expedite recovery, and improve the quality of life.

Although these approaches may be applicable to patients at both ends of the clinical spectrum, surgery will still remain the best approach for many patients – especially those with advanced cardiac disease and significant noncardiac issues. Although less invasive surgery is seeing wider applicability, most surgical procedures require use of cardiopulmonary bypass with its inherent morbidity. There is little doubt that surgical patient acuity continues to increase, and excellence in perioperative care will remain essential to optimizing surgical results, no matter which surgical technique is used. This has become especially important with the increasing demand for transparency, with the perception that outcomes are directly related to the quality of care. Thus, it has become essential that surgical programs maintain the highest level of care to remain competitive.

The 5th edition of the Manual has been completely updated to provide current approaches to patient care. The reference lists have also been extensively updated to direct the reader to some of the best resources available on most topics. I am hopeful that this 5th edition will provide a comprehensive up-to-date review that will assist healthcare providers in delivering the best possible care to their cardiac surgical patients.

Robert M. Bojar, MD
Worcester, MA
December 2010

Acknowledgments

Cardiac surgery requires meticulous attention to detail to ensure the best possible surgical result. Decision-making in the perioperative period involves close cooperation and communication among all members of the healthcare team, including cardiac surgeons, anesthesiologists, physician assistants, nurse practitioners, and critical care and floor nurses. Identifying problems and seeking consultations with experts in other fields is important to ensure optimal outcomes. I am greatly appreciative of the efforts of many individuals who set aside valuable time to review sections of the manuscript in their areas of expertise. I would like to acknowledge the assistance of David Liu, MD, Gary Noroian, MD, Timothy Hastings, CRNA, Bettina Alpert, CCP, Kathi O'Leary, CCP, and Wanda Reynolds, CCRT, for their review and comments. I am especially indebted to George Gordon, MD, whose vast knowledge of anesthesiology, echocardiography, pharmacology, and physiology allowed him to provide insight and suggestions on multiple areas of clinical management. Lastly, I am indebted to my Chief Physician Assistant, Theresa Phillips, PA, who helps coordinate the care my patients receive, and who reviewed many sections of the manuscript to ensure their accuracy.

Abbreviations used through this book are typeset and easy to read. However, many hospitals have lists of approved abbreviations designed to prevent medication errors, which are often caused by inability to interpret handwriting. It is therefore advisable that all orders be written according to individual hospital regulations to ensure that accurate medication doses and intervals are provided to patients.

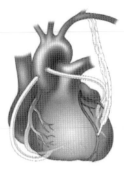

CHAPTER 1

Synopsis of Adult Cardiac Surgical Disease

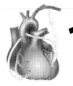

1 Synopsis of Adult Cardiac Surgical Disease

It is essential that all individuals involved in the assessment and management of patients with cardiac surgical disease have a basic understanding of the disease processes that are being treated. This chapter presents the spectrum of adult cardiac surgical disease that is encountered in most cardiac surgical practices. The pathophysiology, indications for surgery, specific preoperative considerations, and surgical options for various diseases are presented. Diagnostic techniques and general preoperative considerations are presented in the next two chapters. Issues related to cardiac anesthesia and postoperative care specific to most of the surgical procedures presented in this chapter are discussed in Chapters 4 and 8, respectively. The most current guidelines for the evaluation and management of patients with cardiac disease can be obtained from the American College of Cardiology website (www.acc.org).

I. Coronary Artery Disease

A. **Pathophysiology**. Coronary artery disease (CAD) results from progressive blockage of the coronary arteries by atherothrombotic disease. Significant risk factors include hypertension, dyslipidemia (especially high LDL and low HDL levels), diabetes mellitus, cigarette smoking, and obesity. Clinical syndromes result from an imbalance of oxygen supply and demand resulting in inadequate myocardial perfusion to meet metabolic demand (ischemia). Progressive compromise in luminal diameter producing supply/demand imbalance usually produces a pattern of chronic stable angina. Plaque rupture with superimposed thrombosis is responsible for most acute coronary syndromes (ACS), which include classic "unstable angina", non-ST-elevation myocardial infarctions (NSTEMI), and ST-elevation infarctions (STEMI). Interestingly, plaque rupture commonly occurs in coronary segments that are not severely stenotic. Endothelial dysfunction has become increasingly recognized as a contributing factor to worsening ischemic syndromes. Generalized systemic inflammation, indicated by elevated C-reactive protein levels, is usually noted in patients with ACS, and appears to be associated with adverse outcomes.[1]

B. **Management strategies**

1. Symptomatic coronary disease is initially treated with medical therapy, including aspirin, nitrates, and β-adrenergic blockers. Calcium channel blockers (CCBs) are considered if β-blockers are contraindicated. Statins should be given to control dyslipidemias and are effective for plaque stabilization. Angiotensin-converting

Manual of Perioperative Care in Adult Cardiac Surgery, 5th Edition. By Robert M. Bojar.
Published 2011 by Blackwell Publishing Ltd.

enzyme (ACE) inhibitors are used for control of hypertension, especially in patients with compromised left ventricular function. Clopidogrel generally does not provide benefit to patients with chronic stable angina, except in selected subsets, but is beneficial in patients with an ACS.[2-6]

2. STEMIs are preferentially treated by percutaneous coronary intervention (PCI) (angioplasty and stenting), although thrombolytic therapy may be considered when PCI cannot be performed within a few hours. Clinical benefit is time-related ("time is myocardium"), and the best results are obtained with "door to balloon" times less than 90 minutes. However, myocardial salvage may still occur if reperfusion can be accomplished within 6 hours of the onset of chest pain.[7,8]

3. Patients presenting with an ACS should be treated with aspirin and unfractionated or low-molecular-weight heparin (LMWH), as well as the standard therapy listed above (nitrates, β-blockers, statins).[9,10] Clopidogrel may provide clinical benefit to these patients if they are to be treated medically, and it may be given if an early invasive strategy is proposed. The 2007 ACC/AHA recommendations were that it should not be given if urgent surgery is considered likely, but this can be difficult to predict and therefore it is given routinely. Most studies have shown that 30-day outcomes are better in patients undergoing coronary artery bypass graft (CABG) surgery who initially received clopidogrel.[2-6] However, one study showed that there was no difference in outcomes whether clopidogrel was given or not if patients had surgery within 5 days, but outcome was better if it was initially given on presentation, then stopped for at least 5 days before surgery.[11] This study supports the ACC/AHA recommendation that clopidogrel be stopped at least 5 days before surgery except in urgent or emergent situations.[9] If prasugrel is given in anticipation of PCI, but CABG is recommended instead, it should be stopped at least 7 days prior to surgery.

4. In patients with continuing ischemia and high-risk features (crescendo angina over 48 hours, rest pain, ECG changes at rest, congestive heart failure [CHF], hemodynamic instability, or an elevated troponin level), platelet glycoprotein IIb/IIIa inhibitors, such as tirofiban or eptifibatide, may be added to the regimen with plans to proceed to an early invasive strategy of catheterization. At that time, the appropriate means of intervention (PCI vs. CABG) can be determined. If a IIb/IIIa inhibitor is used and a clopidogrel load is not given prior to PCI, it will provide antiplatelet activity until the initial dosing of clopidogrel achieves adequate platelet inhibition (a few hours after a 600 mg load). Numerous trials are evaluating the role of various platelet inhibitors and the use of bivalirudin rather than heparin during PCI.

C. **Selection of an interventional procedure**

1. An assessment of the patient's clinical presentation, the extent and nature of coronary disease, degree of inducible ischemia on stress testing, and status of ventricular function are taken into consideration when determining whether the patient is an appropriate candidate for an interventional procedure.[12] In patients with convincing evidence of an ACS, stress tests are not indicated prior to cardiac catheterization. The primary objective of any intervention is the relief of ischemia to prevent or minimize the extent of myocardial damage.

2. PCI has seen wide applicability beyond its proven benefit in early randomized trials, which generally had very selective inclusion criteria. It is often preferable to surgery in patients presenting with STEMIs or with ongoing ischemia with NSTEMIs because

it can more promptly salvage myocardium – unless the anatomy is such that CABG is preferable (see below). The benefits of PCI in patients with chronic stable angina are not as well defined.[13,14]

3. The indications for PCI in multivessel disease are controversial. Although several studies suggest that CABG improves long-term survival better than PCI, other trials indicate that survival is comparable, although more patients undergoing PCI require reintervention.[15-20] The rationale is that PCI only addresses focal lesions despite CAD being a multifocal disease, whereas CABG bypasses the entire proximal segment. Thus, repeat intervention, usually in sites other than the original stent location, is much more likely if PCI is utilized. Evidence-based guidelines have been established by major organizations to identify when PCI and/or CABG is indicated (Figures 1.1 and 1.2).[12] These guidelines will continue to evolve when the results of additional trials including multivessel and left main disease,[21-23] reoperative situations, varying patient subpopulations, and newer stent technologies become available. One approach to decision making is use of the SYNTAX score (accessible at www.syntaxscore.com), which assesses the extent and nature of coronary artery disease and provides comparative major adverse cardiac event (MACE) rates for PCI and CABG for multivessel as well as left main disease.[23-25] Use of such data can provide patients with adequate evidence-based clinical information to give informed consent for any interventional procedure.

4. Although drug-eluting stents (DES) are associated with a lower risk of restenosis than bare-metal stents (BMS), most studies have not shown a significant impact on the risk of myocardial infarction or death.[26] In fact, the risk of stent thrombosis is greater with DES, and this is accentuated in patients who are resistant to the antiplatelet effects of aspirin and/or clopidogrel.[27] Platelet function testing may be beneficial in determining which patients are resistant to their antiplatelet effects. To minimize the risk of stent thrombosis, it is recommended that patients receiving BMS take aspirin and clopidogrel for at least 1 month, and those receiving DES take these medications for at least 1 year.[28]

5. One should not consider either PCI or CABG an exclusive approach to a patient's coronary artery disease. For example, one hybrid approach is to perform a PCI of the culprit lesion in an unstable patient in the interest of myocardial salvage and then refer the patient for surgical revascularization of other lesions.[29] It has even been proposed that placing a left internal thoracic artery (LITA) to the left anterior descending artery (LAD) in a patient with three-vessel disease provides the essential long-term benefit of a CABG and converts the patient's anatomy to two-vessel disease which can be managed medically or with PCI.[30]

D. **Indications for surgery.** The justification for proceeding with an intervention is based primarily upon an assessment of whether the patient is at increased risk for an adverse cardiac event. Studies have shown that surgery is very effective in relieving angina, in many cases is able to delay infarction, and in most cases can improve survival compared with continued medical management. CABG can be deemed appropriate based on an assessment of the patient's symptom status, non-invasive imaging studies, and the degree of anatomic disease (Figure 1.1).[12] It should be considered when PCI is not feasible or when the short- and long-term benefits of CABG are superior to those of PCI (Figure 1.2).

Asymptomatic

Stress Test / Med. Rx					
High Risk / Max Rx	U	A	A	A	A
High Risk / No/min Rx	U	U	A	A	A
Int. Risk / Max Rx	U	U	U	U	A
Int. Risk / No/min Rx	I	I	U	U	A
Low Risk / Max Rx	I	I	U	U	U
Low Risk / No/min Rx	I	I	U	U	U
Coronary Anatomy	CTO of 1 vz.: no other disease	1-2 vz. disease; no Prox. LAD	1 vz. disease; of Prox. LAD	2 vz. disease with Prox. LAD	3 vz. disease; no Left Main

CCS Class I or II Angina

Stress Test / Med. Rx					
High Risk / Max Rx	A	A	A	A	A
High Risk / No/min Rx	U	A	A	A	A
Int. Risk / Max Rx	U	A	A	A	A
Int. Risk / No/min Rx	U	U	U	A	A
Low Risk / Max Rx	U	U	A	A	A
Low Risk / No/min Rx	I	I	U	U	U
Coronary Anatomy	CTO of 1 vz.: no other disease	1-2 vz. disease; no Prox. LAD	1 vz. disease; of Prox. LAD	2 vz. disease with Prox. LAD	3 vz. disease; no Left Main

CCS Class III or IV Angina

Stress Test / Med. Rx					
High Risk / Max Rx	A	A	A	A	A
High Risk / No/min Rx	A	A	A	A	A
Int. Risk / Max Rx	A	A	A	A	A
Int. Risk / No/min Rx	U	U	A	A	A
Low Risk / Max Rx	U	A	A	A	A
Low Risk / No/min Rx	I	U	A	A	A
Coronary Anatomy	CTO of 1 vz.: no other disease	1-2 vz. disease; no Prox. LAD	1 vz. disease; of Prox. LAD	2 vz. disease with Prox. LAD	3 vz. disease; no Left Main

	CABG			PCI		
	No diabetes and normal LVEF	Diabetes	Depressed LVEF	No diabetes and normal LVEF	Diabetes	Depressed LVEF
Two vessel coronary artery disease with proximal LAD stenosis	A	A	A	A	A	A
Three vessel coronary artery disease	A	A	A	U	U	U
Isolated left main stenosis	A	A	A	I	I	I
Laft main stenosis and additional coronary artery disease	A	A	A	I	I	I

Figure 1.2 • Recommended method of revascularization based on extent of coronary disease. A, appropriate; U, uncertain; I, inappropriate. (Reproduced with permission from Smith, *Ann Thorac Surg* 2009;87:1328–31.)[19]

1. **Clinical scenarios**. The patient with refractory angina or a large amount of myocardium in ischemic jeopardy has an indication for an intervention relatively independent of the extent of coronary involvement:

   a. Class III–IV chronic stable angina refractory to medical therapy

   b. Acute coronary syndromes, including unstable angina and NSTEMIs

   c. Acute ischemia or hemodynamic instability following attempted PCI, which may include dissection and compromised flow or coronary perforation with tamponade

   d. Acute evolving STEMI within 4–6 hours of the onset of chest pain or later if there is evidence of ongoing ischemia (early postinfarction ischemia)

   e. Markedly positive stress test prior to major intra-abdominal or vascular surgery – but not necessarily if the patient has chronic stable angina

   f. Ischemic pulmonary edema

2. **Anatomy**. A second group of patients includes those without disabling angina or refractory ischemia in whom the extent of coronary disease, the status of ventricular function, and the degree of inducible ischemia on stress testing are such that surgery may improve long-term survival. This is presumed to occur by preventing infarction and preserving ventricular function. Surgery is especially beneficial for patients with impaired ventricular function and inducible ischemia, in whom the medical prognosis is unfavorable. The following recommendations for surgery, based on the randomized controlled trials of primarily chronic stable angina in the early 1980's have been incorporated into the 2009 appropriateness criteria guidelines noted in Figure 1.2. For patients with ACS, they are all class I indications for surgery, and for patients

Figure 1.1 • Appropriateness ratings for coronary artery bypass grafting. The grid incorporates Canadian Cardiovascular Society (CCS) class, extent of coronary disease, and results of non-invasive testing in determining whether CABG is an appropriate procedure. A, appropriate; U, uncertain; I, inappropriate. (Reproduced with permission from Patel et al., *J Am Coll Cardiol* 2009;53:530–53.)[12]

with fewer symptoms or moderate degrees of ischemia, they are class IIa and IIb indications (see Appendix 1).

a. Left main stenosis >50%

b. Three-vessel disease with ejection fraction (EF) <50%

c. Three-vessel disease with EF >50% and significant inducible ischemia on stress testing

d. Two-vessel disease with involvement of proximal LAD and EF <50% or significant inducible ischemia on stress testing

e. One- and two-vessel disease not involving the LAD with extensive myocardium in jeopardy but lesions not amenable to PCI

Although surgery is appropriate in these patients, most patients with one- or two-vessel disease are preferentially treated by PCI. Furthermore, although the 2009 guidelines consider PCI for left main disease to be "inappropriate" and for three-vessel disease to be "uncertain", use of the SYNTAX score, the Mayo Clinic risk score, and other risk models for PCI may modify this approach.[23–25]

3. **Other conditions**. A third group of patients should undergo bypass surgery for coronary stenoses exceeding 50% when other open-heart procedures are indicated:

a. Valve operations, septal myectomy, etc.

b. Surgery for postinfarction mechanical defects (left ventricular aneurysm, ventricular septal rupture, acute mitral regurgitation)

c. Coronary artery anomalies with risk of sudden death (vessel passing between the aorta and pulmonary artery)

E. **Preoperative considerations**

1. Preoperative autologous blood donation has been considered to reduce the requirement for homologous transfusion. This may be feasible in patients with chronic stable angina, but not in those with acute coronary syndromes or left main disease. With the increasing safety of blood, the use of antifibrinolytic drugs, and the performance of off-pump surgery, this is no longer a common practice.[31]

2. **Anemia**. Preoperative blood transfusions should be considered in patients with an ACS and a hematocrit <28%. This may not only improve the ischemic syndrome but will minimize hemodilution during surgery. Low preoperative hematocrits may increase operative mortality following CABG, often because of an association with other adverse risk factors for mortality, and it is not known whether transfusions can reduce that risk.[32] Certainly, indiscriminate use of transfusions must be avoided because of their association with adverse outcomes following cardiac surgery.[33–35]

a. In addition to blood withdrawal for preoperative lab tests, it is not uncommon for the hematocrit to fall several points after a cardiac catheterization from both blood loss and hemodilution with hydration. One study showed that coronary angiography was associated with a fall in hemoglobin of 1.8 g/dL (equivalent to about a 5.4% fall in hematocrit).[36]

b. Hemodilution on cardiopulmonary bypass (CPB) to a hematocrit <20% may be associated with an increased risk of renal dysfunction, stroke, optic neuropathy, and death.[37–40] Low hematocrits lower oncotic pressure and viscosity, increase fluid requirements, which contributes to extracellular edema, and make it more difficult to maintain an adequate blood pressure during and after CPB. Patients with profound anemia tend to bleed and require more blood component transfusions. Thus, preoperative transfusions to an adequate level may be considered to reduce patient morbidity, possibly reduce the overall number of transfusions required intra- and postoperatively, and potentially decrease mortality.

3. **Ischemia.** Aggressive management of ongoing or potential ischemia is indicated in patients with critical coronary disease to reduce surgical risk. This may include adequate sedation and analgesia, antiischemic medications to control heart rate and blood pressure (intravenous nitrates and β-blockers), antiplatelet and anticoagulant medications (aspirin, clopidogrel, heparin, IIb/IIIa inhibitors), and/or placement of an intra-aortic balloon pump (IABP) for refractory ischemia. It cannot be over-emphasized that just because a patient has been catheterized and accepted for surgery does not mean that medical care should not be aggressive up to the time of surgery! If the patient has persistent ischemia despite all of these measures, emergency surgery is mandatory.

   a. All antianginal medications should be continued up to and including the morning of surgery. Studies have demonstrated the benefit of preoperative **β-blocker** therapy in lowering perioperative mortality in cardiac surgery patients.[41] Patients being admitted the morning of surgery should be reminded to take their medications before coming to the hospital.

   b. **Unfractionated heparin** (UFH) is often used in patients with acute coronary syndromes, left main coronary disease, or a preoperative IABP. The heparin should generally be continued up to the time of surgery. Central lines can usually be placed safely while the patient is heparinized. Patients receiving heparin should have their platelet count rechecked daily to be vigilant for the development of heparin-induced thrombocytopenia (HIT). Note that preoperative assessment for HIT antibodies is not indicated in the absence of a clinical indication.[42]

   c. **Low-molecular-weight heparin** (LMWH) is often used in patients presenting with an ACS and may be used in the cath lab as well. It must be stopped at least 18–24 hours prior to surgery to minimize the risk of perioperative bleeding. **Fondaparinux**, often used routinely for venous thromboembolism prophylaxis, has a half-life of 17–21 hours and must be stopped at least 48 hours prior to surgery.

   d. **Aspirin** is routinely used in patients with known coronary disease or given upon presentation to the hospital. Platelet function generally returns to normal within 3 days of cessation of aspirin, so it can be stopped at that time for truly elective cases.[43,44] Otherwise, aspirin 81 mg should be continued up to the time of surgery in patients with an ACS or critical coronary disease, since it may improve outcomes without a significant increase in the risk of bleeding.[44–47]

   e. Preoperative use of **clopidogrel** has generally been shown to significantly increase the risk of bleeding and reexploration for bleeding.[5,44,47,48] Thus, it has been recommended that it should be stopped 5–7 days before elective surgery, although stopping it for only 3 days may be acceptable prior to off-pump surgery.[49] **Prasugrel** is a more potent ADP inhibitor that can achieve 80% platelet inhibition within 30 minutes of administration. Because of its effectiveness and comparable half-life to clopidogrel, it may contribute to an even greater risk of perioperative bleeding and should be stopped at least 7 days prior to surgery, if possible.

    i. A loading dose of clopidogrel (300–600 mg) is frequently given to patients presenting with an ACS in the emergency room or in preparation for a PCI. Alternatively, a loading dose of prasugrel (60 mg) may be given in the cath lab. If PCI is not feasible or fails, the patient will then be at higher risk for bleeding following CABG.

    ii. In some cases, emergency stenting of a culprit lesion causing an evolving infarction may be performed with subsequent referral for urgent surgery to achieve complete revascularization. In this situation, it is preferable to use a IIb/IIIa inhibitor to minimize stent thrombosis as a bridge to surgery. It should be stopped 4 hours prior to surgery, so that by the time surgery starts, 80% of platelet activity will have recovered.

    iii. In patients with prior stenting (<1 month for a BMS and <1 year for a DES), there is an increased risk of stent thrombosis if clopidogrel is stopped.[28] Either surgery must be performed with the patient still taking clopidogrel or one might possibly stop the clopidogrel for only 3 days to have some residual protective antiplatelet activity, yet hopefully less intraoperative bleeding.

4. Other preoperative medications to be considered

    a. Amiodarone is beneficial in reducing the incidence of postoperative atrial fibrillation (AF). One respected randomized trial showed a benefit to giving 10 mg/kg daily starting 6 days prior to surgery, although a shorter course may be just as effective.[50]

    b. Statins have been demonstrated to reduce operative mortality, the risk of stroke, and the occurrence of AF when used in high doses (atorvastatin 40 mg).[51–53]

    c. Steroids have been evaluated as a means of reducing the systemic inflammatory response of surgery and have been shown to improve myocardial function and possibly reduce the incidence of AF.[54–57] However, improvement in pulmonary function has not been clearly shown, and steroids do worsen postoperative hyperglycemia. Since the benefits are controversial, steroids have not seen widespread usage.

F. Surgical procedures

1. **Traditional coronary artery bypass grafting** is performed through a median sternotomy incision with use of CPB. Myocardial preservation is usually provided by cardioplegic arrest. The procedure involves bypassing the coronary blockages with a variety of conduits. The left internal thoracic (or mammary) artery (ITA) is usually used as a pedicled graft to the LAD and is supplemented by either a second ITA graft or radial artery graft to the left system and/or saphenous vein grafts interposed between the aorta and the coronary arteries (Figure 1.3).

    a. The saphenous vein should be harvested endoscopically to minimize patient discomfort, reduce the incidence of leg edema and wound healing problems, and optimize cosmesis.[58] There are some concerns that endoscopic harvesting could produce endothelial damage that might compromise long-term patency and reduce long-term survival.[59,60]

    b. Use of additional arterial conduits (bilateral ITAs, radial artery) can be recommended to improve event-free survival,[61–63] although one study of statin use showed comparable survival of patients receiving one or two ITAs.[64] The radial artery can be harvested endoscopically using a tourniquet to minimize bleeding

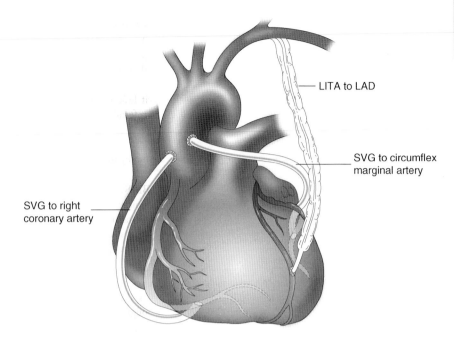

Figure 1.3 • Coronary artery bypass grafting. A left internal thoracic artery (LITA) has been placed to the left anterior descending artery (LAD) with aortocoronary saphenous vein grafts (SVG) to the circumflex marginal and right coronary arteries.

during the harvest with placement of a drain afterwards to prevent blood accumulation within the tract.[65–67] With radial artery grafting, a vasodilator is initiated during surgery to minimize spasm (either IV diltiazem 0.1 mg/kg/h (usually 5–10 mg/h) or IV nitroglycerin 10–20 μg/min (0.1–0.2 μg/kg/min).[68] This is continued in the ICU and then converted to either amlodipine 5 mg po qd or Imdur 20 mg po qd for several months. The benefit of such pharmacologic management to prevent spasm has been universally accepted, but not proven.

2. Concerns about the adverse effects of CPB spurred the development of **"off-pump" coronary surgery (OPCAB)**, during which complete revascularization should be achieved with the avoidance of CPB. Deep pericardial sutures and various retraction devices are used to position the heart for grafting without hemodynamic compromise. A stabilizing platform minimizes movement at the site of the arteriotomy (Figure 1.4). Intracoronary or aortocoronary shunting can minimize ischemia after an arteriotomy is performed.[69]

   a. Conversion to on-pump surgery may be necessary in the following circumstances:

      i. Coronary arteries are very small, severely diseased or intramyocardial.

      ii. LV function is very poor, or there is severe cardiomegaly or hypertrophy that precludes adequate cardiac translocation without hemodynamic compromise or arrhythmias.

      iii. The heart is extremely small and vertical in orientation.

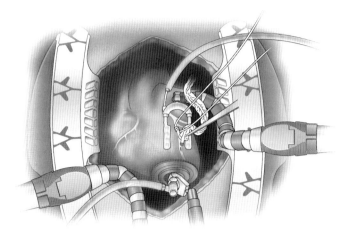

Figure 1.4 • Off-pump bypass grafting requires displacement of the heart using techniques to avoid hemodynamic compromise. These may include placement and elevation of deep pericardial sutures or the use of an apical suction device. A stabilizing device is used to minimize motion and a proximal vessel loop is placed to minimize bleeding at the site of the anastomosis.

> **iv.** Uncontrollable ischemia or arrhythmias develop with vessel occlusion that persists despite distal shunting.
>
> **v.** Intractable bleeding occurs that cannot be controlled with vessel loops or an intracoronary shunt.

b. OPCABs reduce transfusion requirements, and arguably lower mortality and reduce the risk of stroke, renal dysfunction, and atrial fibrillation.[70–73] Despite these potential advantages, enthusiasm for this technique is modest, and it is estimated that fewer than 20% of CABGs are performed off-pump. Many surgeons reserve its use for patients with limited disease. Its major advantage may be in the very high-risk patient with multiple comorbidities in whom it is critical to avoid CPB.

c. In some patients with severe ventricular dysfunction, the heart will not tolerate the manipulation required during off-pump surgery. In this circumstance, right ventricular assist devices can be used to improve hemodynamics. Alternatively, surgery can be done on-pump on an empty beating heart to avoid the period of cardioplegic arrest. This technique may be beneficial in patients with ascending aortic disease that prevents safe aortic cross-clamping, but does allow for safe cannulation and use of aortic punches, such as the HEARTSTRING proximal seal system (Maquet Cardiovascular), to perform the proximal anastomoses.

3. Minimally invasive direct coronary artery bypass (MIDCAB) involves bypassing the LAD with the LITA without use of CPB via a short left anterior thoracotomy incision.[74] An additional incision in the right chest can be used to bypass the right coronary artery. Combining a LITA to the LAD with stenting of other vessels ("hybrid" procedure) has also been described.[29,30]

4. **Robotic** or **totally endoscopic coronary artery bypass (TECAB)** can be used to minimize the extent of the surgical incisions and reduce trauma to the patient. Robotics can be used for both ITA takedown and grafting to selected vessels through small ports. These procedures can be done without CPB or using CPB with femoral cannulation. Generally, TECAB is used for limited grafting, but wider applicability is certainly feasible.[75]

5. **Transmyocardial revascularization (TMR)** is a technique in which laser channels are drilled in the heart with CO_2 or holmium-YAG lasers to improve myocardial perfusion. Although the channels occlude within a few days, the inflammatory reaction created induces neoangiogenesis that may be associated with upregulation of various growth factors, such as vascular endothelial growth factor. This procedure can be used as a sole procedure performed through a left thoracotomy for patients with inoperable CAD in regions of viable myocardium. Alternatively, it can be used as an adjunct to CABG in viable regions of the heart where bypass grafts cannot be placed.[76]

II. Left Ventricular Aneurysm

A. **Pathophysiology**. Occlusion of a major coronary artery may produce extensive transmural necrosis which converts muscle into thin scar tissue. This results in formation of a left ventricular aneurysm (LVA) which exhibits dyskinesia during ventricular systole. In contrast, early reperfusion of an occluded vessel may limit the extent of myocardial damage with preservation of epicardial viability, resulting in an area of akinesia. This will result in an ischemic cardiomyopathy with a dilated ventricle that remodels with altered spherical geometry but does not produce an aneurysm.

B. **Presentation**. The most common presentation of LVAs and ischemic cardiomyopathies is CHF due to systolic dysfunction. With LVAs, there is a reduction of stroke volume caused by geometric remodeling of the aneurysmal segment due to loss of contractile tissue and an increase in ventricular dimensions. Angina may also occur due to the increased systolic wall stress of a dilated ventricle and the presence of multivessel CAD. Systemic thromboembolism may result from thrombus formation within the dyskinetic or akinetic segment. Malignant ventricular arrhythmias or sudden death may result from the development of a macroreentry circuit at the border zone between scar tissue and viable myocardium.

C. **Indications for surgery**. Surgery is usually not indicated for the patient with an asymptomatic aneurysm because of its favorable natural history. This is in contrast to the unpredictable prognosis and absolute indication for surgery in a patient with a false aneurysm, which is caused by a contained rupture of the ventricular muscle. Surgery may be beneficial in the asymptomatic patient with an extremely large aneurysm or when extensive clot formation is present within the aneurysm. Surgery is most commonly indicated to improve symptoms and prolong survival when one of the four clinical syndromes noted above (angina, CHF, embolization, or arrhythmias) is present. Arrhythmias may be treated by a non-guided endocardial resection through the aneurysm with/without cryosurgery along with subsequent placement of a transvenous implantable cardioverter-defibrillator (ICD).

D. **Preoperative considerations**

1. A biplane left ventriculogram is helpful in identifying regions of akinesia and dyskinesia and assessing the function of noninfarcted segments. Echocardiography

is best for assessing ventricular size and dimensions, wall motion of the noninfarcted segments, the presence of thrombus, and mitral valve function, which is often abnormal with dilated cardiomyopathies.

2. The patient should be maintained on heparin up to the time of surgery if left ventricular thrombus is present.

E. **Surgical procedures**

1. Standard aneurysmectomy entails a ventriculotomy through the aneurysm, resection of the aneurysm wall, including part of the septum if involved, and linear closure over felt strips (Figure 1.5).[77]

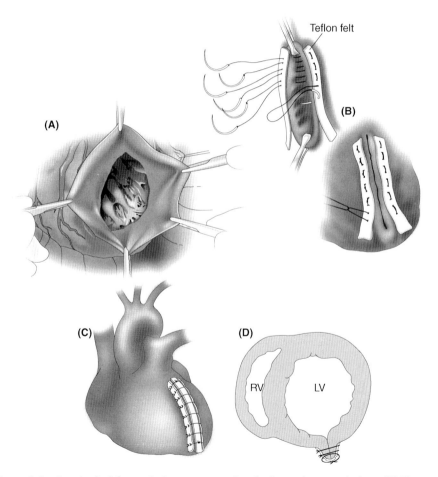

Figure 1.5 • Repair of a left ventricular aneurysm using the linear closure technique. (A) The thinned-out scar tissue is opened and partially resected. Any left ventricular thrombus is removed. (B) The aneurysm is then closed with mattress sutures over felt strips. (C) An additional over-and-over suture is placed over a third felt strip. (D) Cross-section of the final repair.

2. Endoventricular reconstruction techniques are applicable to large aneurysms or akinetic segments with the intent of reducing ventricular volume and restoring an elliptical shape.

    a. The "endoaneurysmorrhaphy" technique is used for large aneurysms. A pericardial or Dacron patch is sewn to the edges of viable myocardium at the base of the aneurysm and the aneurysm wall is reapproximated over the patch (Figure 1.6). This preserves left ventricular geometry and improves ventricular function to a greater degree than the linear closure method.

    b. A slightly more elaborate endoventricular reconstruction involves the endoventricular circular patch plasty technique of Dor, which is termed "surgical ventricular restoration" (SVR). This can be applied to left ventricular aneurysms as well as cases of ischemic cardiomyopathy with anterior akinesis (Figure 1.6D).[78,79] The procedure involves placement of an encircling suture at the junction of the contracting and noncontracting segments, and then

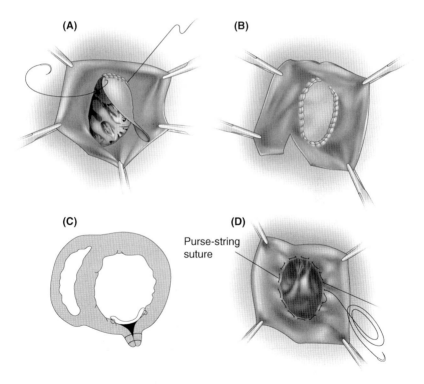

Figure 1.6 • Repair of a left ventricular aneurysm using the endoaneurysmorrhaphy technique. (A,B) A pericardial patch is sewn at the base of the defect at the junction of scar and normal myocardium to better preserve ventricular geometry. The resected edges of the left ventricle are closed in a similar fashion to the linear technique. (C) Cross-section of the final repair. (D) The Dor procedure is a modification of this technique in which a circumferential pursestring suture is placed at the base of the defect to restore a normal orientation to the ventricle. A patch is then sewn over the defect.

exclusion of the noncontracting segment with a patch. This produces an elliptical contour of the heart and results in significant improvement in ventricular size and function. This procedure is generally done on a beating heart to allow for better differentiation of akinetic and normal segments of the heart.

    c. Although SVR is associated with a reduction in LV volume, clinical improvement is not uniform. Several studies have suggested that the addition of SVR to a CABG improves clinical status and long-term survival.[80,81] However, the STICH trial of patients with CAD-related anterior akinesia or dyskinesia with EF <35% was unable to demonstrate that reduction in LV size was associated with an improvement in symptoms or a reduction in mortality after 4 years (see also page 62).[82]

3. Coronary bypass grafting of critically diseased vessels should be performed. Bypass of the LAD and diagonal arteries should be considered if septal reperfusion can be accomplished.

4. Mitral valve repair with a complete annuloplasty ring is indicated when the severity of mitral regurgitation (MR) is 2+ or greater. MR is usually related to apical tethering of the leaflets due to ventricular dilatation or may result from annular dilatation.

III. Ventricular Septal Rupture

A. Pathophysiology. Extensive myocardial damage subsequent to occlusion of a major coronary vessel may result in septal necrosis and rupture. This usually occurs within the first week of an infarction, more commonly in the anteroapical region (from occlusion of the left anterior descending artery), and less commonly in the inferior wall (usually from occlusion of the right coronary artery). It is noted in fewer than 1% of acute MIs, and the incidence has been reduced by use of early reperfusion therapy for STEMIs. The presence of a ventricular septal defect (VSD) is suggested by the presence of a loud holosystolic murmur that reflects the left-to-right shunting across the ruptured septum. The patient usually develops acute pulmonary edema and cardiogenic shock from the left-to-right shunt.[83]

B. Indications for surgery. Surgery is indicated on an emergency basis for nearly all postinfarction VSDs to prevent the development of progressive multisystem organ failure. The overall surgical mortality rate is about 30%, but once the patient develops cardiogenic shock (which is often present), the surgical mortality rate is even higher.[84,85] Occasionally, a small VSD with a shunt of <2:1 can be managed medically, but it usually should be repaired after 6 weeks to prevent future hemodynamic problems.

C. Preoperative considerations

    1. Prompt diagnosis can be made using a Swan-Ganz catheter, which detects a step-up of oxygen saturation in the right ventricle. Two-dimensional echocardiography can confirm the diagnosis of a VSD and differentiate it from acute MR, which can produce a similar clinical scenario.

    2. Inotropic support and reduction of afterload, usually with an IABP, are indicated in all patients with VSDs in anticipation of emergent cardiac catheterization and surgery.

    3. Cardiac catheterization with coronary angiography should be performed to confirm the severity of the shunt and to identify associated coronary artery disease.

D. Surgical procedures

1. The traditional surgical treatment for postinfarct VSDs had been the performance of a ventriculotomy through the infarcted zone, resection of the area of septal necrosis, and Teflon felt or pericardial patching of the septum and free wall. This technique requires transmural suturing and is prone to recurrence.

2. The preferred approach is to perform circumferential pericardial patching around the border of the infarcted ventricular muscle. This technique excludes the infarcted septum to eliminate the shunt and reduces recurrence rates, because suturing is performed to viable myocardium away from the area of necrosis (Figure 1.7).[86]

3. Coronary bypass grafting of critically diseased vessels should be performed, since it has been shown to improve short- and long-term survival after surgery.[85,87]

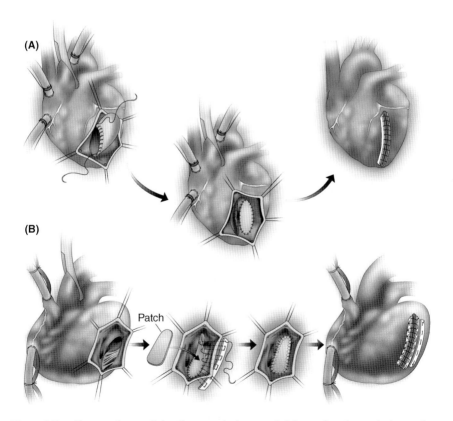

Figure 1.7 • Closure of a postinfarction ventricular septal defect using the exclusion technique. (A) Anterior VSD. (B) Inferior VSD. The pericardial patch is anchored to viable myocardium away from the site of the defect, thus eliminating shunt flow across the septal defect.

IV. Aortic Stenosis

A. **Pathophysiology.**[88] Aortic stenosis (AS) results from thickening, calcification, and/or fusion of the aortic valve leaflets, which produce an obstruction to left ventricular outflow. In younger patients, AS usually develops on congenitally bicuspid valves, whereas in older patients, degenerative change in trileaflet valves is more common. Aortic sclerosis is a very common finding in elderly patients, and may be a manifestation of atherosclerosis, but usually does not progress to aortic stenosis. Progression of AS may be related to endothelial cell activation and atherogenesis, but it has not been shown conclusively that statins will slow the progression of degenerative AS.[89,90] In contrast, there is some evidence that statins may retard the progression of rheumatic AS.[91]

   1. The impairment to cusp opening leads to pressure overload, compensatory left ventricular hypertrophy (LVH), and reduced ventricular compliance. The development of LVH maintains normal wall stress and a normal EF.

   2. If the increase in wall thickness does not increase in proportion to the rise in intraventricular pressure, wall stress will increase and EF will fall. It is important to assess whether a reduced EF in patients with severe AS is the result of excessive afterload (i.e., inadequate hypertrophy to overcome the obstruction) or depressed contractility. If the latter is present, surgical risk is higher.

   3. In patients with excessive and inappropriate degrees of LVH, wall stress is low and the heart will become hyperdynamic with a very high EF. This finding portends a worse prognosis after surgical correction.[92]

B. **Symptoms**. Angina may result from the increased myocardial oxygen demand caused by increased wall stress, from reduction in blood supply per gram of hypertrophied tissue, and/or from limited coronary vasodilator reserve. Hypertrophied hearts are more sensitive to ischemic injury, and exercise may induce subendocardial ischemia, inducing systolic or diastolic dysfunction. Thus, angina may occur with or without concomitant epicardial CAD. Congestive heart failure results from elevation of filling pressures (LV end-diastolic pressure) with diastolic dysfunction and eventually by progressive decline in LV systolic function. Cardiac output is relatively fixed across the valve orifice and can lead to syncope in the face of peripheral vasodilation. The development of atrial fibrillation leads to clinical deterioration because the hypertrophied ventricle relies on atrial contraction to maintain a satisfactory stroke volume.

C. **Diagnosis**. The severity of AS can be readily diagnosed by either echocardiography or cardiac catheterization. In some patients with a critically narrowed valve, it may not be possible to cross the valve with a catheter to measure the gradient. In most cases, echocardiography should be sufficient in assessing the degree of AS, and because of the increased risk of embolic stroke during catheterization, hemodynamic assessment of AS during catheterization is not recommended (a class III recommendation) unless echo results are equivocal.[93] Coronary angiography is indicated before surgery to identify whether CAD is present.

   1. Doppler echocardiography assesses the severity of aortic stenosis by measuring the maximum jet velocity and the mean transvalvular gradient, and allows for calculation of the aortic valve area using the continuity equation. Echo imaging can also measure the valve area directly by planimetry in the short-axis view (Table 1.1).

Table 1.1 • Correlation of Echocardiographic Measurements with the Severity of Aortic Stenosis

Indicator	Mild	Moderate	Severe
Jet velocity (m/s)	< 3.0	3.0–4.0	> 4.0
Mean gradient (mm Hg)	< 25	25–40	> 40
Aortic valve area (cm^2)	> 1.5	1.0–1.5	< 1.0
Aortic valve area index (cm^2/m^2)			< 0.6
Dimensionless index			≤ 0.25

2. At catheterization, the degree of valve stenosis (effective valve area) is assessed by a measurement of transvalvular flow (essentially the cardiac output or stroke volume) with a calculation of the peak or mean pressure gradient across the valve calculated from pressures obtained on a catheter pull-back from the left ventricle into the aorta (Figure 2.4, page 97). A valve area is calculated using the Gorlin formula:

$$AVA = \frac{CO/(SEP \times HR)}{44.3 \times \sqrt{\text{mean gradient}}}$$

where:

AVA = aortic valve area in cm^2 (normal = 2.5–3.5 cm^2)

CO = cardiac output in mL/min

SEP = systolic ejection period/beat

HR = heart rate

Since the pressure gradient is related to both the orifice area and the transvalvular flow, low gradients may be noted in low cardiac output states despite severe AS; conversely, high gradients may be noted in high output states in the absence of severe AS. This concept may account for apparent inconsistencies in the degree of AS using different measurements and in different clinical states.

3. Assessing the severity of aortic stenosis in a patient with a low gradient and poor ventricular function can be problematic. A patient may have a calculated valve area consistent with severe AS, although the degree of AS may not be significant. Dobutamine stress echocardiography (DSE) can be used in this circumstance to determine whether poor ventricular function with a low stroke volume is primarily related to afterload mismatch from true severe AS or is due to contractile dysfunction.

   a. If dobutamine produces an increase in stroke volume and cardiac output with little increase in gradient, the valve area will increase, indicating that the severity of valve stenosis was overestimated and surgery is not indicated.

   b. In contrast, if dobutamine increases both the stroke volume and the gradient, the valve area will remain the same, confirming that true aortic stenosis is present that will benefit from surgery.

    c. If dobutamine fails to produce an increase in stroke volume, the patient has poor contractile reserve and is a poor candidate for surgery.[88,94,95] However, despite a high operative mortality, patients with poor contractile reserve (<20% increase in stroke volume with DSE) still have a better long-term prognosis with surgery than with medical management. In these patients, an alternative approach to aortic valve replacement (AVR), such as a transcatheter valve replacement, may be preferable.[95]

    d. Interestingly, studies have suggested that an elevated B-type natriuretic peptide (BNP) level (>550) is a very strong predictor of operative mortality, even more important than contractile reserve documented by DSE.[96]

D. Indications for surgery. The grading of indications for surgery and the levels of evidence for all types of valve surgery listed in the next few sections (see Appendix 1) are based on 2008 ACC guidelines[88] and are available at www.acc.org.

  1. The presence of symptoms (angina, CHF, syncope or resuscitation from sudden death) with severe AS is a class I indication for surgery, because once symptoms are present, the average survival is only about 2 years with a less than 20% chance of surviving 5 years.[88,97] Generally, mean survival is 1 year for patients with CHF, 2 years with syncope, and 4 years with angina.[97] Surgery will improve survival even in patients with LV dysfunction not caused by excessive afterload, although LV dysfunction and symptoms may not completely resolve.

  2. In contrast, surgery has traditionally not been considered for the asymptomatic patient, no matter how severe the degree of stenosis, because the risk of sudden death is considered to be low (estimated at <1%/year), and the risk of the AVR may exceed the potential benefit of surgery.[98] However, patients with severe AS need to be followed carefully for the development of symptoms or rapidly progressive valve stenosis. Failure to perform surgery once patients become symptomatic is the most important risk factor for late mortality.[99]

    a. It is estimated that up to 40% of patients with severe AS will become symptomatic within 2 years and about 67% will be symptomatic by 5 years.[100,101] However, in patients with high jet velocities, LV hypertrophy, or severe valve calcification, the rate of progression of valve stenosis is faster and the symptom-free interval is shorter.[101]

    b. On the average, the annual increase in jet velocity is 0.3 m/sec, the increase in mean gradient is 7 mm, and the decrease in valve area is 0.1 cm^2. However, the rate of progression of AS can be quite variable, and serial Doppler echos should be used to assess the rate of hemodynamic progression of the AS, which is predictive of clinical outcome.

  3. Indications for surgery in the asymptomatic patient are:

    a. Class I: LV systolic dysfunction (EF <50%)

    b. Class IIb

      i. Abnormal response to exercise (hypotension, symptoms) – note that stress testing is contraindicated in the symptomatic patient with severe AS

      ii. Severe AS with high likelihood of progression (elderly patients, calcified valve, presence of CAD) or if there will be a potential delay from symptom onset to surgery

      iii. Extremely severe AS (AVA <0.6 cm^2, mean gradient >60 mm Hg, jet velocity >5.0 m/s)

4. AVR is generally indicated for patients undergoing other cardiac surgery if the AVA is <1.2 cm², and possibly as high as 1.4 cm². Invariably, a native valve with at least moderate stenosis will require surgery within a few years for progressive obstruction, thus mandating a reoperative procedure at higher risk. Clearly, it is essential that the prosthetic valve being placed have hemodynamics as good as and hopefully better than the valve being replaced. Nonetheless, one must remember that placing a prosthetic valve introduces at least a 1–2% annual risk for each of the prosthetic-related complications, including endocarditis, thromboembolism, and bleeding.

5. When indications for aortic valve surgery are met and an enlarged aorta ≥ 4.5 cm is present, the ascending aorta should also be replaced. Although this is a standard criterion for bicuspid valves, it is not inappropriate for patients with trileaflet valves.

E. **Preoperative considerations**

1. Coronary angiography should be performed in any patient over the age of 40 or in a younger patient with coronary risk factors, angina, or a positive stress test.

2. Ischemic syndromes in patients with AS require judicious management. Medications that must be used very cautiously are those that can reduce preload (nitroglycerin), afterload (calcium channel blockers), or heart rate (β-blockers), because they may lower cardiac output and precipitate cardiac arrest in a patient with critical AS. The ventricular response to atrial fibrillation must be controlled, and cardioversion should be performed if this rhythm is poorly tolerated.

3. Dental work should be performed before surgery to minimize the risk of prosthetic valve endocarditis unless it is felt to be a prohibitive risk.

4. Selection of the appropriate procedure and valve type depends on a number of factors, including the patient's age, contraindications to long-term anticoagulation, and the patient's desire to avoid anticoagulation.

F. **Surgical procedures**

1. Aortic valve procedures may be performed through a full median sternotomy incision or through a minimally invasive incision. These include an upper or lower sternotomy with a "J" or "T" incision into the third or fourth intercostal space, or an anterior right second or third interspace incision.[102,103] Cannulation for CPB for minimally invasive approaches can be performed either through the incision or using the femoral vessels.

2. Aortic valve replacement with either a tissue or mechanical valve is the standard treatment for AS (Figure 1.8).

   a. In general, tissue valves are selected for patients >age 65 to avoid use of warfarin. Current-generation tissue valves have anticalcification treatment to reduce the risk of structural valve deterioration, and thus these valves are being used more commonly in younger patients.

   b. A stentless valve may be selected to provide a larger effective orifice area and may be placed in the subcoronary position or as a root replacement.[104] Significant clinical benefits of this valve are controversial, and the operation is more complex (Figure 1.9).

   c. The Ross procedure, in which the patient's own pulmonary valve is used to replace the aortic root, with the pulmonary valve replaced with a homograft

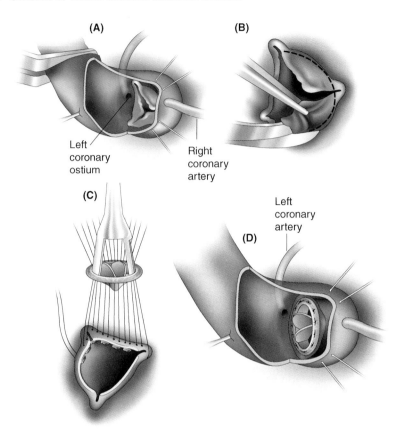

Figure 1.8 • Aortic valve replacement. (A) A transverse aortotomy incision is made and holding sutures are placed. (B) The valve is excised, and the annulus is debrided and sized. (C,D) Pledgeted mattress sutures are placed through the annulus and through the sewing ring of the valve, which is tied into position. The aortotomy is then closed.

(basically a double valve operation for single valve disease), is an even more complicated procedure generally reserved for patients younger than age 50 who wish to avoid anticoagulation (Figure 1.10).[105]

   d. Homografts are usually reserved for patients with aortic valve endocarditis, although other types of prostheses arguably provide comparable results.[106–109]

   e. An aortic root replacement, usually as a valved conduit, is indicated when the ascending aorta must also be replaced (Figure 1.11).[110] If the sinuses of Valsalva are not dilated, replacing the aortic valve and using a supracoronary graft simplifies the procedure.

3. Reparative procedures, such as commissurotomy or debridement, have little role in the management of critical aortic stenosis. However, debridement may be

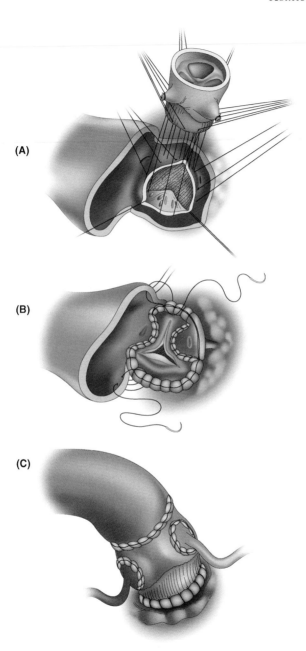

Figure 1.9 • Stentless valves have a larger effective orifice than stented valves, allowing for more regression of LV hypertrophy. (A) The proximal suture line sews the lower Dacron skirt of the prosthesis to the aortic annulus. (B) Subcoronary implantation of a Medtronic Freestyle valve. This requires scalloping of two sinuses with the distal suture line carried out below the coronary ostia. (C) A stentless valve can be used as a root replacement, requiring reimplantation of buttons of the coronary ostia. The distal suture line is an end-to-end anastomosis to the aortic wall.

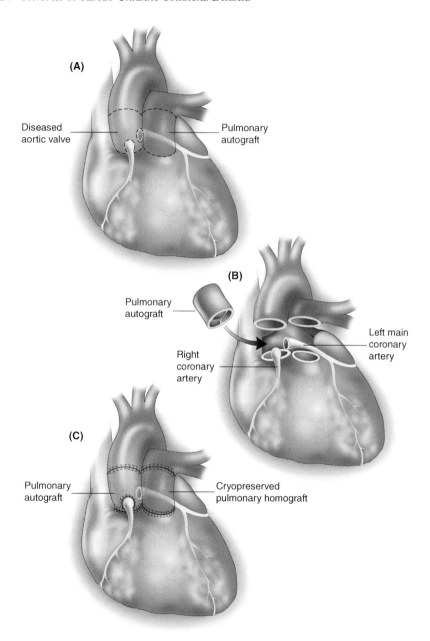

Figure 1.10 • Ross procedure. (A) The aorta is opened and the diseased aortic valve is removed. The pulmonic valve and main pulmonary artery are carefully excised and the coronary arteries are mobilized. (B) The pulmonary autograft is then transposed to the aortic root. (C) The coronary arteries are reimplanted and the RV outflow tract is reconstructed with a cryopreserved pulmonary valved homograft.

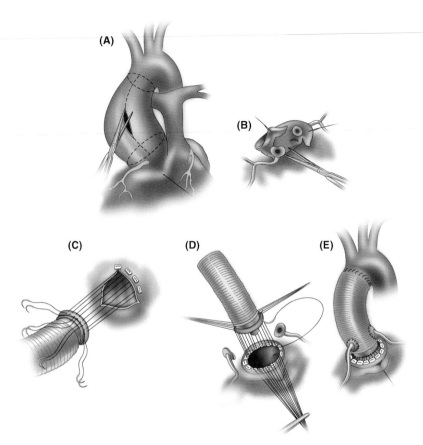

Figure 1.11 • Bentall procedure. (A) The aorta is opened longitudinally and then divided proximally and distally. (B) Coronary ostial buttons are mobilized. (C,D) A valve incorporated into the proximal end of the conduit is then sewn to the aortic annulus. (E) The coronary ostial buttons are reimplanted and the distal suture line is completed.

considered in the patient with moderate AS in whom the valve disease is not severe enough to warrant valve replacement, but in whom decalcification may delay surgery for a number of years.

4. Transcatheter aortic valve implantation (TAVI) involves placement in the aortic root of a tissue valve mounted on a catheter that is advanced either antegrade through the LV apex (via a left thoracotomy) or retrograde through the femoral vessels (Figure 1.12). Using rapid ventricular pacing, the device is positioned fluoroscopically at the level of the aortic annulus amidst the diseased valve and then inflated manually. Potential serious complications include migration, coronary obstruction, and stroke. Technical complications noted during apical implantation include acute aortic and mitral regurgitation, septal hematomas, and apical rupture. Early trials have limited inclusion criteria primarily to patients considered too high

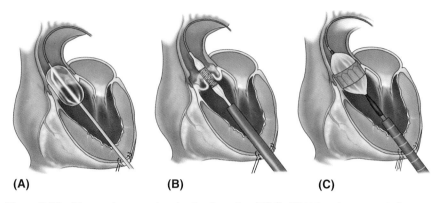

(A) **(B)** **(C)**

Figure 1.12 • Transcatheter aortic valve implantation (TAVI). (A) Using the transapical approach, a wire is placed through the aortic valve over which a balloon is used to dilate the valve. (B) Using fluoroscopic imaging, the catheter is positioned across the valve, and (C) the valve is inflated.

risk for surgery, with a resultant mortality rate consistently exceeding 10%. The role for transcatheter AVR in patients who are surgical candidates has yet to be defined.[111–115] Matched for annular size, percutaneous valves have been shown to be superior in hemodynamic performance to both stented and stentless bioprosthetic valves.[116]

V. Aortic Regurgitation

A. **Pathophysiology.**[88] Aortic regurgitation (AR) results from abnormalities in the aortic valve leaflets (calcific degeneration, bicuspid valves, destruction from endocarditis) or from aortic root dilatation that prevents leaflet coaptation (idiopathic root dilatation causing annuloaortic ectasia, aortic dissection with cusp prolapse).

1. Acute AR usually results from endocarditis or a type A dissection. The ventricle is unable to dilate acutely to handle the sudden increase in regurgitant volume which increases the LV end-diastolic volume (LVEDV) and pressure (LVEDP), resulting in acute LV failure, cardiogenic shock, and pulmonary edema. Dramatic elevations in filling pressures may occur if acute AR is superimposed on a hypertrophic ventricle. Acute myocardial ischemia may result from increased afterload (LV dilatation), compensatory tachycardia, and a reduction in perfusion pressure as the LVEDP approaches the aortic diastolic pressure. As a result, sudden death may occur.

2. Chronic AR produces pressure and volume overload of the left ventricle, resulting in progressive LV dilatation (increase in LVEDV) with an increase in wall stress, an increase in ventricular compliance, and progressive hypertrophy. Most patients remain asymptomatic for decades, even with severe AR, because recruitment of preload reserve and compensatory hypertrophy maintain a normal EF despite the increased afterload. The increased stroke volume maintains forward output and is manifest by an increase in pulse pressure with bounding peripheral pulses. Eventually, increased afterload and impaired contractility lead to LV systolic dysfunction and a fall in EF. Usually at this point, the patient becomes symptomatic with

dyspnea, and impairment of coronary flow reserve may cause angina. The normalization of a depressed EF may occur after surgery when afterload excess is the cause of LV systolic dysfunction, but is less likely when it is caused by depressed myocardial contractility.

B. Diagnosis. Echocardiography and aortic root aortography at the time of catheterization can delineate the degree of AR (Figure 2.8, page 99). Echo is valuable in assessing the valve morphology, aortic root size, LV cavity dimensions, wall thickness, and systolic function. Color and pulsed wave Doppler findings can be used to assess the degree of AR.

C. Indications for surgery

1. **Symptomatic patients** with severe AR, irrespective of LV systolic function or LV size, should undergo surgery (class I). Without surgery, the estimated mortality rate is >10%/year for patients with angina and >20%/year for patients with CHF. Symptomatic patients with LV dysfunction and severely dilated hearts are considered high risk, because they often have irreversible myocardial damage.

2. Endocarditis with hemodynamic compromise, persistent bacteremia or sepsis, conduction abnormalities, recurrent systemic embolization from vegetations, large mobile vegetations, or annular abscess formation should prompt urgent surgery (see section IX, pages 39−41).

3. **Asymptomatic patients** must be followed closely for the development of symptoms or evidence of ventricular decompensation. Although the rate of progression to symptoms or LV dysfunction in asymptomatic patients with normal LV systolic function is only about 4%/year, about 25% of patients may develop LV dysfunction or die before they become symptomatic. Both medical survival and surgical operative and long-term survival are influenced significantly by impaired LV function. Thus, in asymptomatic patients, surgery is indicated at the earliest signs of LV decompensation:

   a. Class I: EF <50% at rest. Symptoms develop in these patients at a rate of 25%/year.[88]

   b. Class IIa: EF >50% but severe LV dilatation (end-diastolic dimension >75 mm or end-systolic dimension >55 mm). These patients are at high risk for sudden death.

   c. Class IIb: EF >50% with less severe LV dilatation (end-diastolic dimension >70 mm or end-systolic dimension >50 mm when there is evidence of progressive dilatation, declining exercise tolerance, or abnormal hemodynamic response to exercise.

4. In patients with severe AR from annuloaortic ectasia with an enlarged aortic root, it is recommended that the aorta be replaced if it exceeds 4.5 cm in diameter (and perhaps 4.0 cm in patients with Marfan syndrome).

D. Preoperative considerations

1. Systemic hypertension should be controlled with vasodilators to increase forward flow and reduce the degree of regurgitation. However, excessive afterload reduction may reduce diastolic coronary perfusion pressure and exacerbate ischemia. β-blockers for control of ischemia must be used cautiously because a slow heart rate increases the amount of regurgitation. They are contraindicated in acute AR because they will block the compensatory tachycardia.

2. Placement of an IABP for control of anginal symptoms is contraindicated.

3. As for all valve patients, dental work should be completed before surgery.

4. Contraindications to warfarin should be identified so that the appropriate valve can be selected.

E. **Surgical procedures**

1. Aortic valve replacement has traditionally been the procedure of choice for adults with AR. This may involve use of a tissue or mechanical valve, the Ross procedure, or a cryopreserved homograft.

2. Aortic valve repair, involving resection of portions of the valve leaflets and reapproximation to improve leaflet coaptation (especially for bicuspid valves), often with a suture annuloplasty, has been performed successfully. This is valuable in the younger patient in whom a valve-sparing procedure is preferable to valve replacement.[117]

3. A valved conduit (Bentall procedure) is placed if an ascending aortic aneurysm ("annuloaortic ectasia") is also present (Figure 1.11). In younger patients, manufactured mechanical valved conduits are preferable, but if there is a strong indication for avoiding anticoagulation, sewing a tissue valve into a graft can easily be accomplished.[118,119] Alternatively, a Medtronic Freestyle stentless valve can be placed with distal graft extension to replace an aortic aneurysm.[120]

4. Aortic valve-sparing root replacement is feasible in some patients with significant AR if adequate remodeling of the root can be accomplished, and it can be used successfully even in patients with bicuspid valves or Marfan syndrome (Figure 1.13).

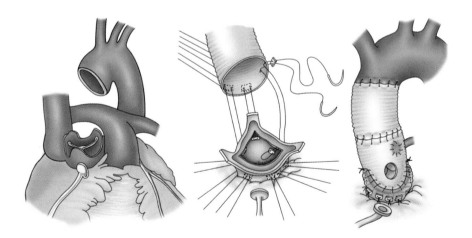

Figure 1.13 • Aortic valve-sparing root replacement. (A) The aortic root is resected, sparing the pillars that support the commissures and excising the coronary arteries as buttons. (B) Sutures are placed at the subannular level in a horizontal plane and passed through a tubular graft. (C) The graft is tied down and the aortic valve is reimplanted within the graft by elevating the commissural posts, suspending them from the graft, and sewing the aortic remnants to the graft. Finally, the coronary buttons are reimplanted.

The aorta is resected, sparing commissural pillars. A graft is then sewn at the subannular level, the aortic valve is resuspended within the graft, and the aortic remnants are sewn to the graft. Coronary ostial buttons are then sewn to the graft.[121–123]

5. Transcatheter AVR is generally not applicable to cases of AR because the absence of calcification prevents adequate seating of the valve.

VI. Mitral Stenosis

A. **Pathophysiology.**[88] Mitral stenosis (MS) occurs nearly exclusively as a consequence of rheumatic fever. Thickening of the valve leaflets with commissural fusion, and thickening and shortening of the chordae tendineae gradually reduce the size of the mitral valve orifice and the efficiency of LV filling. The increase in the diastolic transmitral gradient increases the left atrial and pulmonary venous pressures, leading to CHF. An adaptive measure that can minimize symptoms is a decrease in pulmonary microvascular permeability and the development of pulmonary arteriolar vasoconstriction and thickening, which leads to pulmonary hypertension (PH). This may then lead to right-sided heart failure and functional tricuspid regurgitation (TR). As the severity of MS and PH worsen, the cardiac output is compromised at rest and fails to increase with exercise. The development of atrial fibrillation further increases LA pressures, decreases ventricular filling, and compromises cardiac output.

B. **Natural history.** MS is a slowly progressive process which may not produce symptoms for several decades. The minimally symptomatic patient has an 80% 10-year survival, but once the patient becomes significantly symptomatic, survival is very poor, with less than a 15% 10-year survival. Severe pulmonary hypertension (pulmonary artery [PA] pressure >60 mm Hg) is associated with an average survival of less than 3 years. Therefore, intervention should be considered when the patient develops class II–III symptoms.

C. **Diagnosis.** The severity of MS can be determined by echocardiography or cardiac catheterization (Table 1.2). Echo is valuable in assessing the severity of MS by the continuity equation, estimating the PA pressure from the tricuspid velocity jet, and evaluating valve morphology using an echo score.[124] This assesses leaflet mobility, thickening, calcification, and subvalvular thickening and can be used to determine whether the valve is amenable to balloon valvuloplasty.

Table 1.2 • Measurement of the Severity of Mitral Stenosis

Indicator	Mild	Moderate	Severe
Mean gradient (mm Hg)	<5	5–10	>10
PA systolic pressure (mm Hg)	<30	30–50	>50
Mitral valve area (cm²)	>1.5	1.0–1.5	<1.0

At catheterization, the mitral valve area is calculated from measurements of the cardiac output and the transvalvular mean gradient (pulmonary capillary wedge pressure [PCWP] minus the LV mean diastolic pressure). The PA pressure should be measured by right-heart catheterization.

$$MVA = \frac{CO/(DFP \times HR)}{37.7 \times \sqrt{\text{mean gradient}}}$$

where:

MVA = mitral valve area in cm^2 (normal = 4–6 cm^2)

DFP = diastolic filling period/beat

mean gradient = PCWP − left ventricular mean diastolic pressure

D. Indications for intervention

1. An interventional procedure is indicated for a patient in NYHA class III–IV with moderate or severe mitral stenosis (MVA <1.5 cm^2). It may also be considered for patients with class II symptoms when critical MS (MVA <1 cm^2) is present and for other patients with lesser degrees of MS when exercise testing precipitates significant hemodynamic changes.

2. **Percutaneous balloon mitral valvuloplasty** (PBMV) is the procedure of choice for patients with moderate-to-severe MS if valve morphology is favorable by echo score. This generally results in a doubling of the valve area and a 50% reduction in the mean gradient, with excellent long-term results. The presence of left atrial thrombus or more than 2+ MR usually contraindicates this procedure.

   a. Class I: symptomatic class II–IV patients

   b. Class IIa: symptomatic class III–IV patients with moderate or severe MS with nonpliable calcified valves who are not good surgical candidates

   c. Class IIb
      • Symptomatic class II–IV patients with MVA >1.5 cm^2 but hemodynamically significant MS (PA >60 mm Hg, PCWP >25 mm Hg, or mean gradient >15 mm Hg with exercise or dobutamine stress echo)
      • Asymptomatic patients with pulmonary hypertension (PA >50 mm Hg at rest or >60 mm Hg with exercise) or new-onset atrial fibrillation

3. **Surgery** is indicated when PBMV is contraindicated or not feasible due to unfavorable valve morphology, left atrial thrombus, or 3−4 + MR.

   a. Class I
      • Symptomatic class III–IV patients with MVA <1.5 cm^2
      • Symptomatic patients with moderate-to-severe MS and moderate-to-severe MR

   b. Class IIa: symptomatic class I–II patients with severe MS and PA >60 mm Hg − surgery is generally indicated with these hemodynamics even if the patient is asymptomatic

   c. Class IIb: asymptomatic patients with MVA <1.5 cm^2 with recurrent embolism on anticoagulation if valve repair can be performed

E. Preoperative considerations

1. Hemodynamic performance is frequently compromised by a low cardiac output state, which can be worsened by the presence of atrial fibrillation. A rapid

ventricular response will shorten the diastolic filling period, reduce LV preload, and elevate LA pressures. Thus, the ventricular response to AF is best controlled in the perioperative period by β-blockers or calcium channel blockers, although many patients are on digoxin for chronic rate control, which can be continued up to the time of surgery. There is usually a delicate balance between fluid overload, which can precipitate pulmonary edema, and hypovolemia from aggressive diuresis, which can compromise renal function when the cardiac output is marginal. Thus, preload must be adjusted judiciously to ensure adequate LV filling across the stenotic valve.

2. Many patients with long-standing MS are cachectic and at increased risk for developing respiratory failure. Aggressive preoperative diuresis and nutritional supplementation may reduce morbidity in the early postoperative period.

3. Warfarin used for AF, left atrial thrombus, or a history of systemic embolism should be stopped 4 days before surgery. If the patient is considered at high risk for embolization, outpatient low-molecular-weight heparin may be prescribed, but must be stopped at least 18–24 hours before surgery. Admission for unfractionated heparin the day before surgery may be considered once the international normalized ratio (INR) falls below the therapeutic range.

F. Surgical procedures

1. Closed mitral commissurotomy has been supplanted by PBMV, which produces superior results. Either should be considered in the pregnant patient with critical MS in whom CPB should be avoided.

2. Open mitral commissurotomy is performed if PBMV is not considered to be feasible or there is evidence of left atrial thrombus. It produces better hemodynamics than either a PBMV or a closed commissurotomy and is associated with improved long-term event-free survival, especially in patients with high echo scores or atrial fibrillation.[125] Although recurrent symptoms are noted in 60% of patients after 9 years, most symptoms are related to the development of MR or CAD, not to recurrent MS.[88]

3. Mitral valve replacement (MVR) is indicated if the valve leaflets are calcified and fibrotic or there is significant subvalvular fusion (Figure 1.14).

4. A Maze procedure should be considered in a patient with either paroxysmal or persistent AF. The "cut and sew" Cox-Maze procedure has been replaced by use of energy sources (usually radiofrequency, cryoablation, or high-frequency ultrasound) that can be applied to create transmural ablation lines in well-described patterns to ablate this arrhythmia with fairly good success rates (see section XIII, pages 54–57).[126–128]

5. Although functional TR usually improves after left-sided surgery, tricuspid valve repair is recommended for patients with significant TR. It has also been recommended for patients with significant RV dilatation with lesser degrees of TR, especially when the pulmonary vascular resistance (PVR) is elevated, AF is present, or the left atrium is significantly enlarged.[129–131] However, although tricuspid valve repair may improve the functional outcome in patients with significant TR and may prevent the progression of TR in those with lesser degrees of TR, neither strategy may improve long-term survival.[132]

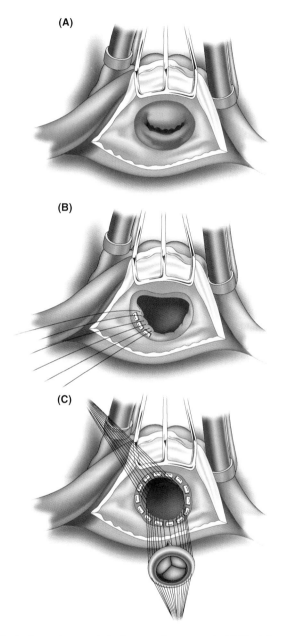

Figure 1.14 • Mitral valve replacement via the posterior approach. (A) The left atrium is opened behind the intraatrial groove and the retractor is positioned. Although both leaflets may be retained, the anterior leaflet is usually resected. (B) The posterior leaflet is retained and imbricated into the suture line. (C) Pledgeted mattress sutures are placed through the annulus, through or around the valve tissue, and into the sewing ring. The valve is then tied into position. The left atrial appendage may be oversewn from inside the left atrium.

VII. Mitral Regurgitation

A. **Pathophysiology.**[88,133] Mitral regurgitation (MR) may result from abnormalities of the annulus (dilatation), valve leaflets (myxomatous change with redundancy and prolapse, leaflet defect or damage from endocarditis, leaflet shrinkage from rheumatic disease), chordae tendineae (rupture, elongation), or papillary muscles (rupture, ischemic dysfunction).

1. Acute MR usually results from myocardial ischemia or infarction with papillary muscle rupture, from endocarditis, or from idiopathic chordal rupture. Acute left ventricular volume overload develops with a reduction in forward output and regurgitant flow into a small noncompliant left atrium. This may result in both cardiogenic shock and acute pulmonary edema.

2. Chronic MR is a condition of volume overload that is characterized by a progressive increase in compliance of the left atrium and ventricle, followed by progressive increase in LVEDV as the LV dilates. The increase in preload increases overall stroke volume and maintains forward cardiac output. At the same time, there is a decrease in afterload due to ventricular unloading into the left atrium, so that a normal EF may be maintained despite contractile dysfunction. Patients are usually asymptomatic during this compensatory phase and may remain so even as ventricular decompensation occurs. Eventually, prolonged volume overload causes significant contractile dysfunction, more LV dilatation, an increase in end-systolic volume and elevated filling pressures. This reduces forward output and worsens symptoms of CHF. The progression of MR and assessment of LV dimensions and function should be followed by serial echocardiograms.

3. "Ischemic MR" may be acute or chronic. Acute MR may be the result of a mechanical complication, such as papillary muscle rupture, or it may be functional, due to ongoing ischemia. Chronic "ischemic MR" may develop following a myocardial infarction either from annular dilatation that prevents leaflet coaptation or from papillary muscle displacement from LV remodeling that produces apical tethering of the leaflets. The prognosis of ischemic MR is worse because the MR results from LV dysfunction, not from primary disease of the mitral valve or chordae tendineae.

B. **Diagnostic evaluation**

1. Left ventriculography may be used to assess LV function and the degree of MR, but it is frequently insensitive in assessing its severity, which may depend on catheter position, the amount and force of contrast injection, the size of the left atrium or ventricle, and the presence of arrhythmias or ischemia.

2. Transesophageal echocardiography (TEE) is the best technique to determine the degree and nature of the MR, and it also assesses the status of LV function and provides an estimate of PA pressures. It can define whether MR is functional on the basis of a dilated annulus or enlarged LV with apical tethering of the leaflets, or whether it is primarily from leaflet prolapse with chordal elongation or rupture. Generally, single-leaflet prolapse produces eccentric jets (Figure 2.16, page 109) whereas annular dilatation causes central MR. Apical tethering will also produce eccentric jets. TEE assessment is invaluable to the surgeon in helping to determine whether a valve can be repaired, what type of repair may be necessary, or whether replacement is indicated from the outset.

3. A discrepancy is often noted between the degree of MR identified preoperatively in the awake patient and that assessed under general anesthesia, which alters systemic resistance and loading conditions. Thus, a preoperative TEE is important to quantitate the degree of MR and define the precise anatomic mechanism for the MR.

C. **Indications for surgery**

1. Class I
   - Symptomatic acute MR (usually CHF or cardiogenic shock)
   - Symptomatic class II−IV patients with chronic severe MR as long as EF >30% and/or end-systolic dimension >55 mm
   - Acute endocarditis with hemodynamic compromise, persistent bacteremia or sepsis, annular abscess, recurrent systemic embolization from vegetations, or threatened embolization from large vegetations (Figure 2.17, page 110)
   - Asymptomatic patients with chronic severe MR and EF 30−60% and/or end-systolic dimension ≥ 40 mm

2. Class IIa: patients with very advanced MR with class III−IV symptoms, EF <30%, and/or end-systolic dimension >55 mm if repair is highly likely.

3. Class IIb: asymptomatic patients with chronic severe MR and EF >60% with end-systolic dimension <40 mm (if repair likely), new onset of atrial fibrillation, or PA >50 mm Hg at rest or >60 mm Hg with exercise. In many experienced centers, repair is recommended in asymptomatic patients with severe MR and normal LV function to prevent the long-term sequelae of chronic MR.

4. Persistence of AF after mitral valve surgery alone is more likely when LA size exceeds 50 mm or AF has been present over 6 months. Because of the adverse influence of postoperative AF on outcome in patients with nonischemic MR (reduced survival, late cardiac function, and freedom from late stroke), a Maze procedure with obliteration of the left atrial appendage is recommended.[134,135] It should also be considered in patients with AF and ischemic MR, primarily to reduce the risk of stroke. Reducing the size of a dilated left atrium may improve atrial mechanical function and improve the results of a Maze procedure.[136]

5. In patients with CAD requiring CABG who also have concomitant MR, degenerative MR of grade 3−4 + should generally be repaired. Although ischemic MR may improve after myocardial revacularization, this is often unpredictable, and moderate-to-severe ischemic MR should be addressed by mitral repair or replacement. The effect of residual moderate MR on long-term survival is unclear, being comparable in some studies and worse in others.[137,138]

6. In patients with concomitant severe AS and moderate MR, the severity of MR improves in about two-thirds of patients after AVR, with comparable survival to those in whom mitral valve repair is performed.[139] However, the likelihood of improvement is greater in patients with functional MR, a small left atrium, preoperative CHF, and AR as the indication for surgery.[140] If degenerative MR is present with single-leaflet prolapse and eccentric jets, it is unlikely that the MR will improve after relief of the outflow tract obstruction, and consideration should be given to repairing 2−3+ MR.

D. **Preoperative considerations**

1. Patients with acute MR are susceptible to pulmonary edema and multisystem organ failure from a reduced forward cardiac output. Use of inotropes, vasodilators, and an

IABP can transiently improve myocardial function and forward flow in anticipation of urgent cardiac catheterization and surgery. Intubation and mechanical ventilation are frequently required for progressive hypoxia or hypercarbia. Diuretics must be used judiciously to improve pulmonary edema while not creating prerenal azotemia. Some patients with chordal rupture who present with acute pulmonary edema may stabilize and develop chronic MR that can be treated electively.

2. Patients with chronic MR are managed with diuretics to reduce preload and with vasodilators, such as the ACE inhibitors, to improve forward flow. However, ACE inhibitors are only indicated if the patient is symptomatic and has hypertension or systolic dysfunction. ACE inhibitors should not be given the morning of surgery because of concerns about perioperative hypotension associated with their use.

3. Adequate preload must be maintained to ensure forward output while carefully monitoring the patient for evidence of CHF. Systemic hypertension should be avoided because it will increase the amount of regurgitant flow. If the patient has ischemic MR or a borderline cardiac output, use of systemic vasodilators or an IABP generally improves forward flow.

E. **Surgical procedures**

1. Mitral valve reconstruction is applicable to more than 90% of patients with degenerative MR, although success rates are greater for posterior than anterior leaflet repairs. Techniques include annuloplasty rings, leaflet repairs, and chordal transfers and replacement (Figure 1.15).[141,142] These reparative techniques can also be applied to patients with mitral valve endocarditis.[143–145] Mitral valve repair gives a survival advantage over mitral valve replacement in patients with degenerative MR and coexisting CAD,[146] but advantages of repair over replacement for ischemic MR are not as well defined.[147,148] Thus, the decision to repair or replace a valve for ischemic MR can be difficult and depends on an understanding of the pathophysiology of the MR and patient-related factors.

2. Mitral valve replacement (MVR) is indicated when satisfactory repair cannot be accomplished. Acute MR from papillary muscle rupture usually requires MVR. Chordal preservation of at least the posterior leaflet should be considered for all MVRs performed for MR. This improves ventricular function and will minimize the risk of LV rupture.

3. Traditional mitral valve operations have been performed through a median sternotomy incision. Other "minimal access" approaches, such as an upper sternotomy incision (using the "superior" approach to the valve between the aorta and superior vena cava), a right parasternal incision (using the biatrial transseptal approach), or a right anterolateral thoracotomy or lower sternotomy incision (using the posterior approach behind the interatrial septum) can also be considered. CPB can be established either directly through the chest or through the femoral vessels. Minimally invasive video-assisted surgery has seen increasing applicability in patients undergoing mitral valve repairs and replacements, whereas a robotic approach has been limited primarily to patients undergoing mitral valve repairs.[149–152]

4. A concomitant Maze procedure should be performed in patients with either paroxysmal or persistent AF.

5. Functional TR should be managed as noted on page 31 above.

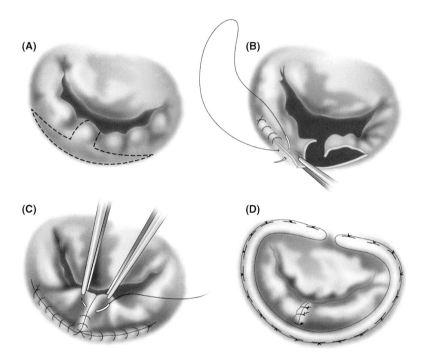

Figure 1.15 • Mitral valve repair. The most common pathology involves a flail posterior mitral leaflet. (A) A quadrangular excision is made as indicated by the dotted lines and the flail segment is resected. The remaining leaflet tissue may be incised along the annulus. (B) It is then advanced and reattached to the annulus ("sliding plasty"). (C) The leaflet tissue is then approximated, and (D) an annuloplasty ring is placed.

VIII. Tricuspid Valve Disease

A. **Pathophysiology.**[153] Tricuspid stenosis (TS) is very rare, usually developing as a result of rheumatic heart disease in association with mitral stenosis. Tricuspid regurgitation (TR) most commonly is "functional" in nature, occurring as a consequence of advanced mitral valve disease which leads to pulmonary hypertension, RV dilatation, and tricuspid annular dilatation. RV systolic dysfunction contributes to elevated right atrial and systemic venous pressures, producing signs of right-sided heart failure. Atrial fibrillation is common. Forward output may also be reduced, resulting in fatigue and a low output state. Other common causes of TR include endocarditis (usually with intravenous drug abuse, an indwelling pacemaker wire, or hemodialysis catheter) and pulmonary hypertension, independent of etiology.

B. **Diagnosis**. Clinical examination in TR will reveal a systolic murmur that increases with inspiration, prominent jugular venous pulsations, and occasionally a pulsatile liver. The diagnosis is confirmed by echocardiography, which can assess the tricuspid valve anatomy, the severity of TR, RV size and function, provide estimates of PA and RV pressures, and identify associated contributing pathology.

C. Indications for surgery

1. Tricuspid stenosis. Surgery is indicated for class III–IV symptoms, including hepatic congestion, ascites, and peripheral edema that are refractory to salt restriction and diuretics.

2. Tricuspid regurgitation

   a. Class I: TV repair is indicated when severe TR is present with mitral valve disease requiring mitral valve surgery.

   b. Class IIa: TV repair (annuloplasty) or replacement (if leaflets not amenable to repair) is reasonable for symptomatic, severe primary TR. Note that the surgical risk is high in the presence of severe pulmonary hypertension (PA systolic > 60 mm Hg) in the absence of left-sided valve disease, especially if RV dysfunction is present.

   c. Class IIb: TV annuloplasty is reasonable if less than severe TR is noted at the time of mitral valve surgery, but pulmonary hypertension or a dilated tricuspid annulus is present. These patients may subsequently develop RV dysfunction and worsening TR, although the impact on long-term clinical outcome is not clear.[129–132]

   d. Persistent sepsis or recurrent pulmonary embolization from tricuspid valve vegetations is an indication for surgery.

   e. Class III: surgery should not be considered in asymptomatic patients with a PA pressure < 60 mm Hg and no mitral valve disease.

D. Preoperative considerations

1. Passive congestion of the liver resulting from elevated right-heart pressures frequently leads to coagulation abnormalities, which should be treated aggressively before and during surgery. Frequently, these patients have uncorrectable INRs before surgery.

2. Salt restriction and diuretics may improve hepatic function, but significant improvement in liver function tests may not be possible until after surgery.

3. Maintenance of an elevated central venous pressure is essential to achieve satisfactory forward flow. A normal sinus mechanism provides better hemodynamics than atrial fibrillation, although the latter is frequently present. Slower heart rates are preferable for TS, and faster heart rates for TR.

E. Surgical procedures

1. Tricuspid commissurotomy can be performed for rheumatic TS.

2. Tricuspid annuloplasty with a ring (Carpentier) or suture technique (DeVega or bicuspidization) is feasible and preferred for the majority of patients with annular dilatation and functional TR (Figure 1.16).[154]

3. Tricuspid valve replacement (TVR) is necessary when leaflet shrinkage and poor coaptation prevent an annuloplasty technique from eliminating the TR. There is no particular preference for valve selection. Tissue valves have a lower risk of thromboembolism than mechanical valves when placed in the right heart, and valve survival may be better due to lower stress on the valve leaflets. Tissue valves may also be preferable because long-term survival after TVR is somewhat limited, most likely because it reflects more advanced multivalvular disease. The overall mortality rate for TVR is consistently about 20%, because most patients are in a higher functional class and have pulmonary hypertension.[155–158]

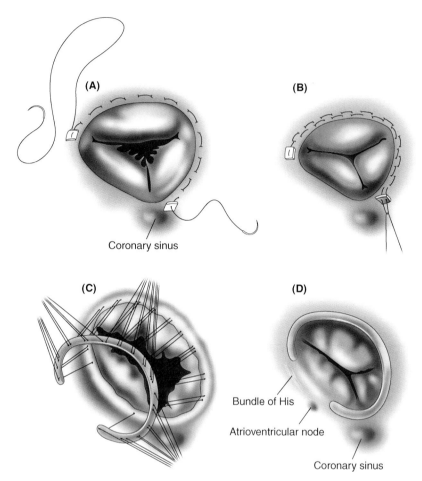

Coronary sinus

Figure 1.16 • Tricuspid valve repair involves reduction of annular dilatation to correct functional tricuspid regurgitation. (A,B) The circumferential suturing technique (DeVega repair). (C,D) Placement of an annuloplasty ring. Note the location of the coronary sinus and the proximity of the conduction system to the repair.

4. Due to the necessity of placing sutures near the conduction system, patients are more prone to developing heart block after tricuspid valve surgery. If there are concerns that permanent pacing may be required, epicardial pacing leads should be placed on the right ventricle, pacing and sensing thresholds are determined, and the pacing leads are buried in a subcutaneous pocket for later attachment to a permanent pacemaker. In one report, more than 20% of patients required postoperative permanent pacemakers.[159]

5. The management of tricuspid valve endocarditis is noted in the next section.

IX. Endocarditis

A. **Pathophysiology.** Endocarditis can result in the destruction of valve leaflets, invasion of surrounding myocardial tissue, systemic embolization of valve vegetations, or persistent systemic sepsis. Embolization is more likely with mitral than aortic valve involvement, staphylococcal organisms, and large or mobile vegetations. Native valve endocarditis is most commonly caused by *Streptococcus viridans, Staphylococcus aureus*, or coagulase-negative staph. Tricuspid valve endocarditis is usually caused by intravenous drug abuse, although the left-sided valves are actually more commonly involved with IV drug abusers.[160] The incidence of prosthetic valve endocarditis (PVE) is approximately 0.5–1% per patient-year for most mechanical and tissue valves. It is most commonly caused by staph organisms.

B. **Indications for surgery in native valve endocarditis**[88]

  1. Class I indications include:

    a. Presence of moderate-to-severe CHF from regurgitant lesions. Surgery should not be delayed if cardiogenic shock is present unless the likelihood of recovery from complications (severe stroke) is remote.

    b. Hemodynamically significant regurgitant lesions (elevated LVEDP or LA pressures or moderate-to-severe pulmonary hypertension)

    c. Evidence of local extension resulting in aortic or annular abscesses (usually manifest by heart block) or destructive lesions (intracardiac fistulas, mitral leaflet perforation from aortic valve endocarditis)

    d. Organisms unlikely to be adequately treated with antibiotics alone, especially fungal endocarditis

    e. Persistent sepsis or bacteremia despite antibiotics for more than 1 week, especially with staph infections. This is commonly noted with the above two indications and should be considered an indication for proceeding with urgent surgery, although not listed as an indication in the ACC guidelines. Surgery during septic shock portends a very poor prognosis with an operative mortality rate exceeding 50%.[161]

  2. Class IIa: recurrent embolization and persistent vegetations despite antibiotic treatment. Note that the incidence of embolization decreases significantly once antibiotic therapy has been initiated, but evidence of increasing vegetation size on antibiotics may predict later embolization.[162,163]

  3. Class IIb: mobile vegetations >10 mm in diameter even in the absence of documented embolization. These vegetations, especially on the mitral valve, have an increased risk of embolization.

C. **Indications for surgery in prosthetic valve endocarditis (PVE)**[164]

  1. Class I

    a. Heart failure

    b. Valve dehiscence (unstable prosthesis or perivalvular leak)

    c. Evidence of increasing valvular obstruction or worsening regurgitation

    d. Complications, such as abscess formation or heart block

    e. Fungal etiology

  2. Class IIa

    a. Persistent bacteremia or recurrent emboli despite antibiotics

    b. Relapsing infection

D. Preoperative considerations

1. TEE is the gold standard for the identification of endocarditis and is more sensitive and specific than transthoracic echocardiography in identifying and quantifying the size and mobility of vegetations, detecting annular destruction, and identifying valvular abnormalities (Figure 2.17, page 110).

2. Ideally, the patient should receive a 6-week course of antibiotics prior to surgery to reduce the risk of PVE, because the risk of prosthetic valve endocarditis is lowered from about 10% to 2% once a successful course of antibiotics has been completed. However, hemodynamic deterioration and intracardiac invasion are compelling indications that mandate earlier surgery. Attempts should be made to optimize hemodynamic and renal status before operation, but surgery should not be delayed if there is evidence of progressive organ system deterioration.

3. Appropriate timing of surgery in patients suffering cerebral embolization is controversial. Some reports suggest that the risk of exacerbating a cerebral insult is greatest if surgery is performed within 2−3 weeks of the embolic event, primarily from cerebral edema rather than from hemorrhage.[165,166] However, others suggest that earlier surgery can be performed safely and should be considered within several days to prevent recurrent embolization from persistent vegetations, as long as an immediate preoperative CT scan shows no hemorrhage.[167−169] In these situations, the benefit of surgery usually exceeds the risk. However, in patients with a hemorrhagic stroke, the risk of early surgery is high and it should be delayed at least 3−4 weeks, if possible.

4. The appropriate antibiotics should be given for a total perioperative course of 6 weeks. However, if intraoperative cultures are positive, 6 weeks of postoperative antibiotics are generally recommended.

5. Patients with aortic valve endocarditis may have evidence of heart block from involvement of the conduction system by periannular infection. This may require preoperative placement of a transvenous pacing wire.

6. Coronary angiography should be avoided, if possible, if mobile aortic valve vegetations are identified.

E. Surgical procedures

1. Surgery entails excision of all infected valve tissue, drainage and debridement of abscess cavities, and repair or replacement of the damaged valves. An aortic valve homograft is arguably the valve of choice because of its increased resistance to infection and adaptability to disrupted tissue in the aortic root.[106] However, homograft replacement is technically quite complex and the operative mortality may be greater when performed by surgeons without extensive experience with these conduits. Aortic valve replacement with either mechanical or tissue valves is a satisfactory alternative.[108,109] The risk of prosthetic valve endocarditis on tissue or mechanical valves is fairly comparable.[164]

2. Mitral endocarditis can frequently be repaired, especially if leaflet perforation is the primary pathology, and there are proponents of earlier surgery in mitral valve endocarditis to preserve the patient's native valve.[143−145] More advanced stages of endocarditis usually require valve replacement.

3. Tricuspid valve repair is recommended for tricuspid endocarditis and should be attempted aggressively in intravenous drug abusers, who are more prone to reinfection if a valve replacement is performed.[160,170,171] If repair cannot be accomplished, tricuspid valvulectomy can be performed in patients without

pulmonary hypertension with few adverse hemodynamic sequelae.[172] Otherwise, a tricuspid valve should be placed, accepting the higher risk of recurrence in IV drug abusers.

X. Hypertrophic Obstructive Cardiomyopathy

A. **Pathophysiology.** Hypertrophic obstructive cardiomyopathy (HOCM) is character-ized by diastolic dysfunction and varying degrees of dynamic left ventricular outflow tract obstruction. The latter most commonly results from hypertrophy of the basal septum with mitral–septal apposition from systolic anterior motion of the mitral valve (SAM). This also contributes to mitral regurgitation from incomplete leaflet apposi-tion. An anomalous papillary muscle insertion into the leaflets can also cause mitral regurgitation and may contribute to midcavity obstruction, especially with excessive midventricular hypertrophy. Four different clinical patterns may be noted and they dictate how HOCM should be managed.[173–175]

1. Patients generally become symptomatic with congestive heart failure, which is related to both **diastolic dysfunction** and **outflow tract obstruction**. The latter is most predictive of a worse prognosis. Angina may develop because of abnormal coronary microvasculature and inadequate capillary density for the degree of hypertrophy. Syncope may also occur.

2. The risk of **sudden death** is estimated at 1%/year, but is increased in patients with any of the following major risk factors: a history of cardiac arrest, sustained ventricular tachycardia (VT) or repetitive prolonged bursts of nonsustained VT, a family history of premature HOCM-related death, unexplained syncope, a hypotensive blood pressure response to exercise, or extreme LVH with wall thickness over 30 mm.

3. Advanced heart failure may develop with remodeling and **systolic dysfunction** that may require heart transplantation.

4. **Atrial fibrillation** may develop due to left atrial enlargement in 20–25% of patients and may contribute to an embolic stroke.

B. **Indications and options for intervention**[174]

1. No pharmacologic regimen has been shown conclusively to reduce the risk of sudden death. Therefore, medications are used to alleviate symptoms, which are usually related to diastolic heart failure. β-blockers or verapamil can be recommended to patients with or without obstruction. Disopyramide can be added when there is significant outflow tract obstruction as it will decrease SAM and the outflow gradient.

2. ICD placement should be considered in patients at high risk for sudden death (as noted above).[176]

3. Dual-chamber pacing with a short atrioventricular delay to ensure complete ventricular-paced activation is effective in reducing the gradient by approximately 35% and in improving symptoms.[177] Biventricular pacing has been found beneficial in a few reports of patients with either intraventricular conduction delay or normal conduction.[178,179]

4. Further intervention is indicated in patients with a peak gradient >50 mm Hg and persistent symptoms despite medications. It may also be considered in asymptom-atic patients considered at high risk for sudden death, including younger patients and those with a peak gradient >80 mm Hg.

5. Alcohol septal ablation of the upper septal perforator branch of the LAD produces an infarct of the upper septum. This should reduce basal septal thickness, enlarging the LV outflow tract and reducing SAM in appropriately selected patients. It has been shown to produce a substantial reduction in gradient with improvement in symptoms and exercise tolerance. Potential complications include need for a permanent pacemaker in about 10% of patients (up to 40% at 3 years) and the potential creation of an arrhythmogenic focus.[180,181] Comparative studies of alcohol ablation and myectomy have shown comparable clinical improvement, but a lower gradient and less requirement for pacing with a myectomy.[181]

C. **Preoperative considerations**

1. Measures that produce hypovolemia or vasodilation must be avoided because they increase the outflow tract gradient. Volume infusions should be used to maintain preload with the use of α-agonists to maintain systemic resistance.

2. Use of β-blockers and calcium channel blockers to reduce heart rate and contractility are the mainstay of medical management of HOCM and should be continued up to the time of surgery.

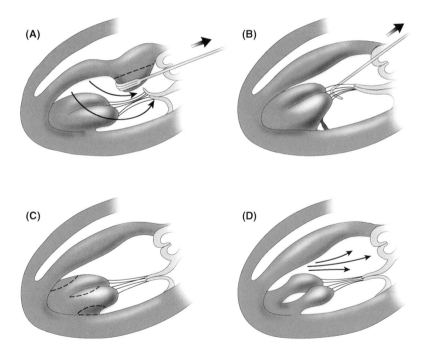

Figure 1.17 • (A) Hypertrophic obstructive cardiomyopathy is characterized by septal hypertrophy which orients the outflow jet into the anterior leaflet of the mitral valve, producing systolic anterior motion (SAM). An extensive septal myectomy is performed, often requiring a midventricular resection. (B,C) Using a nerve hook to provide traction, the atypical attachments of hypertrophied anomalous papillary muscles are partially detached from the ventricular wall and trimmed. (D) After this procedure, the outflow jet is directed more anteriorly.

D. Surgical procedures

1. The traditional surgical approach of a left ventricular septal myectomy entailed resection of a 1.5 × 4 cm wedge of septum below the right coronary aortic leaflet through an aortotomy incision.

2. With further understanding of the mechanism of SAM, the current operation is more elaborate and involves performing an extended septal myectomy to the base of the papillary muscles, mobilization and partial excision of the papillary muscles off the ventricular wall to allow the papillary muscles to assume a more posterior position in the left ventricle, and anterior mitral leaflet plication if there is any redundancy. This reduces chordal and leaflet slack that can produce SAM (Figure 1.17). Resection of midventricular obstruction or anomalous chords and relief of papillary muscle fusion may be necessary. A successful operation dramatically reduces the gradient, eliminates mitral regurgitation, improves functional status, and may reduce the risk of sudden death.[182–186]

3. Mitral valve replacement is indicated if the septal thickness is less than 18 mm, or if there is atypical septal morphology, significant MR, or failure of the other procedures to relieve the outflow tract gradient.

XI. Aortic Dissections

A. **Pathophysiology.** An aortic dissection results from an intimal tear that allows passage of blood into the media, creating a false channel. This channel is contained externally by the outer medial and adventitial layers of the aorta. With each cardiac contraction, the dissected channel can extend proximally or distally, potentially causing branch artery compromise or rupture as the outer wall weakens. Dissections involving the ascending aorta are classified as Stanford type A (DeBakey type I–II, or proximal), whereas those not involving the ascending aorta are called Stanford type B (DeBakey type III, or distal) dissections (Figure 1.18). The dissection is termed acute when it is diagnosed within 2 weeks of its onset; otherwise, it is termed chronic.[187,188]

B. **Presentation**

1. **Type A dissection.** This is a life-threatening condition that must be considered in any patient presenting to the emergency room with the acute onset of chest pain. Failure to be aware of the various presentations of type A dissections has led to a misdiagnosis in up to 40% of patients.[189]

   a. The traditional notion is that patients develop tearing, ripping chest pain that radiates to the back, but this has been found to be less common than non-radiating sharp chest pain according to contemporary analyses published by the International Registry of Acute Aortic Dissections (IRAD).[190,191] Two key elements to the pain are that it is invariably acute in onset and severe in nature – usually the worst pain the patient has ever experienced. The pain is associated with the tearing of the aortic wall and its extension; it often abates and may wax and wane – this may be deceptive to the clinician if this fact is not appreciated.

   b. Depending on the location of the intimal tear and the extent of the dissection, potential complications include cardiac tamponade from hemopericardium (the most common cause of death), aortic regurgitation, myocardial infarction,

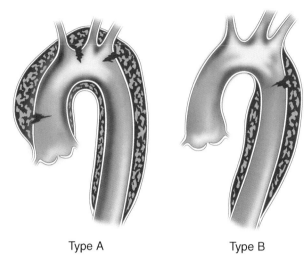

Type A   Type B

Figure 1.18 • Classification of aortic dissection. Type A dissections involve the ascending aorta. Type B dissections usually originate distal to the left subclavian artery and do not involve the ascending aorta. If they do extend retrograde, they are then considered type A dissections.

stroke, and branch artery compromise causing malperfusion. The latter may involve the brachiocephalic vessels, causing syncope, a stroke, or a discrepancy in upper-extremity blood pressures; the intercostal vessels, causing paraplegia; the mesenteric or renal vessels, compromising blood flow to the bowel or the kidneys; or the iliofemoral vessels, reducing distal blood flow to the legs.

   c. An elevation in D-dimer levels is usually, but not always, noted in acute dissections and may be useful in supporting suspicion of the diagnosis.[192,193] Another biomarker that is being studied is smooth muscle myosin heavy chain protein that is released from damaged aortic medial smooth muscle.

  2. Type B dissection. This usually presents with back pain that may radiate into the abdomen. It generally does not cause anterior chest wall pain since the ascending aorta is not involved. Potential rupture into the mediastinum, pleural spaces or abdomen may occur. Malperfusion from branch artery compromise from the descending thoracic and abdominal aorta may occur as noted above.

C. Indications for surgery

  1. Type A dissection. Surgery is indicated for all patients unless it is considered to carry a prohibitive risk because of patient age, overall medical condition and comorbidities, or the development of extensive renal, myocardial, or bowel infarction or massive stroke. In selected cases of mesenteric malperfusion, fenestration and stenting may be indicated prior to surgical repair of the site of the dissection.[194,195] Surgery is also indicated for virtually all patients with chronic type A dissections.

  2. Type B dissections. Patients with uncomplicated type B dissections are usually treated medically. Interventional (endovascular) or surgical procedures are reserved for patients with complicated dissections, i.e., persistent pain, uncontrollable hypertension, evidence of aneurysmal expansion or rupture, or visceral, renal, or lower-extremity vascular compromise.[196,197] The long-term prognosis of medically treated dissections is not ideal and is influenced by the potential for subsequent aneurysmal expansion.[198] This is more likely if the patient's heart rate and blood pressure are not well controlled, the false lumen remains patent, or the initial false lumen diameter is >40–45 mm.[199–202] Because of this concern, studies are being done to assess whether low-risk patients with uncomplicated type B dissections might benefit from surgery or endovascular stenting to prevent subsequent expansion and improve long-term survival. Chronic type B dissections should be operated upon when they reach 6–6.5 cm in diameter.

D. Preoperative considerations and diagnostic testing

1. Upon suspicion of the diagnosis, all patients must be treated pharmacologically to reduce the blood pressure (to about 110 mm Hg systolic), the heart rate (to 60–70 bpm), and the force of cardiac ejection (dp/dt). The patient should be carefully monitored and must undergo diagnostic testing as soon as possible to establish or exclude the diagnosis.

2. Recommended antihypertensive regimens include a β-blocker (esmolol, metoprolol, or labetalol) with or without addition of sodium nitroprusside (see Table 11.8, page 497, for doses). Aggressive management up to the time of surgery is essential to prevent rupture.

3. A careful pulse examination may indicate the extent of the dissection. Particular attention should be paid to the carotid, radial, and femoral pulses. Differential upper-extremity blood pressures in a young patient with chest pain is a strong clue to the presence of a dissection. Cardiac evaluation may reveal the presence of an aortic regurgitation murmur.

4. A detailed preoperative neurologic examination is essential because a deficit recognized postoperatively may have been present at the time of presentation. A change in neurologic status may indicate progressive compromise of cerebral perfusion that can resolve with emergency surgery. However, cerebral malperfusion during CPB may also cause a significant cerebral insult. Evidence of renal dysfunction (rising BUN or creatinine, oliguria) or bowel ischemia (abdominal pain, acidosis) may necessitate modification of the surgical approach. Recurrent chest or back pain usually indicates extension, expansion, or rupture of the dissection.

5. The chest x-ray will usually demonstrate either a widened mediastinum or irregularity of the aortic contour, but may be normal in 10–15% of patients with type A dissections.[190]

6. In a patient with severe chest pain, one might suspect that an abnormal ECG would be more consistent with an acute coronary syndrome, and a normal ECG would suggest the diagnosis of dissection. However, IRAD data showed that only 33% of patients with type A dissections had a normal ECG.[190] Nonspecific ST changes were noted in about 40% of patients and about 20% had ischemic changes, possibly related to coronary ostial involvement with the dissection.

7. Dissections can be diagnosed by a variety of techniques.

    a. In most hospitals, a CT scan **with contrast** is performed first. It has about 90% sensitivity and specificity in identifying intimal flaps and differential flow into true and false lumens (Figure 2.23, page 117). 64-slice CT scanning, especially with three-dimensional reconstruction, can provide beautiful images of aortic dissections (Figure 2.24, page 118) and can demonstrate branch artery compromise as well.

    b. TEE is the best procedure for identifying intimal flaps, evidence of tamponade, and aortic regurgitation (Figure 2.18, page 111). If the diagnosis of a type A dissection is unequivocal on CT scanning, TEE is best deferred until the patient is anesthetized. If the diagnosis is in doubt, TEE should be performed **very cautiously** because sedation may lead to hypotension in a patient with a pericardial effusion, and acute hypertension in an inadequately sedated patient could precipitate rupture. A transthoracic echo may be valuable in ruling out a significant pericardial effusion before proceeding with a TEE.

    c. Magnetic resonance imaging (MRI) may be the most sensitive and specific diagnostic technique to identify a dissection, but only rarely can it be obtained on an emergency basis (Figure 2.27, page 121). Furthermore, there are usually limitations to its performance in a patient requiring careful monitoring and intravenous drug infusions.

    d. There is little role for aortography in the evaluation of an acute dissection; branch vessel perfusion in the abdomen can be identified by CT angiography.

    e. Coronary angiography is usually not indicated in cases of acute aortic dissection because of the necessity of urgent surgical repair. Evidence of significant ECG changes may lead to coronary angiography as the initial diagnostic test, only to find that coronary ostial compromise is caused by an aortic dissection. In contrast, coronary angiography is helpful in planning surgical strategy in patients with chronic dissections.

E. **Surgical procedures**

1. **Type A dissections**

    a. Repair involves resuspension or replacement of the aortic valve (if AR is present), resection of the intimal tear, and placement of an interposition graft to reapproximate the aortic wall (Figure 1.19). Biologic glue (preferably BioGlue) can be used to improve tissue integrity for grafting. If the root is destroyed and cannot be reconstructed, a Bentall procedure (valved conduit) is performed. If the tear extends across the arch, consideration should be given to replacing the entire arch, often with an elephant trunk, using standard techniques of cerebral perfusion to protect the brain.[203] Patients with visceral malperfusion have a high mortality rate and may benefit from a fenestration procedure prior to repair of the ascending aorta.[204] Iliofemoral malperfusion may require additional revascularization procedures after the ascending aorta is replaced.

    b. Repair of any type A dissection should be performed during a period of deep hypothermic circulatory arrest (DHCA) (see page 52).

    c. The complex situation of the type A dissection with a tear in the descending aorta can be managed by an initial repair via a median sternotomy, leaving an

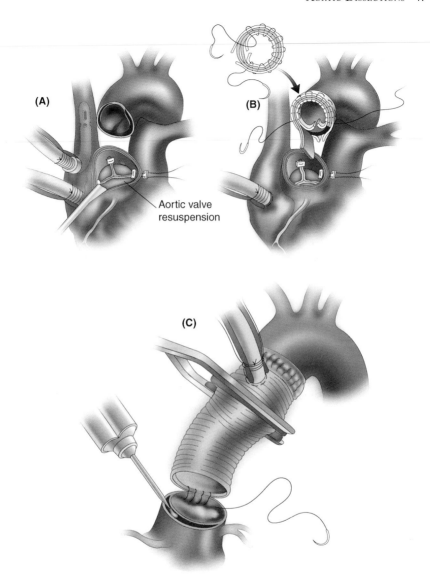

Figure 1.19 • Repair of a type A aortic dissection. (A) During circulatory arrest without aortic cross-clamping, the aorta is opened and the entry site is resected. The aortic valve is resuspended. (B) The proximal and distal suture lines are fragile and are reinforced. Two felt strips are shown for the distal suture line, being placed inside the true lumen and outside the adventitia. (C) After the distal suture line is completed, the graft is cannulated to reestablish antegrade cardiopulmonary bypass flow with proximal application of a cross-clamp. BioGlue may be injected to stabilize the distal and proximal (shown here) suture lines, and the proximal graft anastomosis is performed, again using felt reinforcement.

elephant trunk for repair of the descending aorta. Alternatively, an endovascular stent can be placed through the arch into the descending aorta.[205,206] A retrograde dissection occurring after placement of an endovascular stent for a type B dissection is a difficult problem that usually requires open surgery through a sternotomy.[207]

2. **Type B dissections**

   a. The traditional surgical approach to complicated type B dissections involves resection of the intimal tear and interposition graft replacement to reapproximate the aortic wall. The risk of paraplegia is greater than in patients with atherosclerotic aneurysms because less collateral flow is present. Thus, measures to reduce spinal cord ischemia by maintaining distal perfusion should be taken (see page 53). Visceral malperfusion may improve with restoration of flow into the true lumen. Otherwise a percutaneous fenestration procedure to produce a communication between the true and false lumens or additional grafting may be necessary to improve organ system or distal limb perfusion.[208]

   b. Due to the substantial morbidity and mortality associated with surgical repair, endovascular stenting is becoming increasingly popular.[209–211] This procedure should seal the entry site to allow for thrombosis of the false lumen. It has been used primarily in complicated type B dissections, as it is not yet clear whether endografting for uncomplicated type B dissections will provide superior results to medical management. Additional fenestration and stenting may be required if reconstitution of true channel flow does not correct malperfusion.

XII. Thoracic Aortic Aneurysms

A. **Pathophysiology**. Ascending aortic (AAo) aneurysms usually result from medial degeneration or atherosclerosis, whereas those in the distal arch, descending thoracic, and thoracoabdominal aorta are generally atherosclerotic in nature. Aneurysms in any location may result from expansion of chronic dissections. Although progressive enlargement may result in compression of adjacent structures, most deaths result from aneurysm rupture or dissection. Natural history studies have been used to correlate aneurysm size with the risk of rupture or dissection in an attempt to provide objective data on when surgery should be performed.[212]

B. **Indications for surgery**

   1. **Ascending aortic aneurysms**

      a. Symptomatic, expanding, or $\geq$ 5.5 cm without Marfan syndrome.[212] These recommendations are based on natural history studies that suggest that the risk of rupture or dissection is <5%/year for an aortic diameter <6 cm and 16–34% once the aorta reaches 6 cm.[212] Although the Society of Thoracic Surgeons (STS) consensus document noted that 15% of aortas that dissect in patients with bicuspid valves or Marfan syndrome are <5 cm in size, other reports (including one IRAD study) indicate that 60% of aortic dissections occur in aortas that measure <5.5 cm and 40% occur when the aorta is <5 cm.[213–215] Although studies have correlated initial aortic size with the risk of rupture or dissection (Figure 1.20), it has been proposed that indexing the aortic size to the patient's size rather than using aortic size alone may provide better guidelines for resection (Figure 1.21).[215] The risk is low for an aortic size

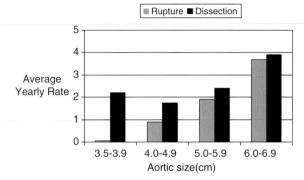

Figure 1.20 • Risk of aortic dissection or rupture based on the initial aortic size. (Adapted with permission from Davies et al., *Ann Thorac Surg* 2002;73:17–27.)

index (ASI) $<2.75\ cm/m^2$, moderate for an ASI of $2.75–4.25\ cm/m^2$, and significant once the ASI exceeds $4.25\ cm/m^2$.

b. Aneurysms ≥ 5 cm in patients with bicuspid aortic valves

c. Aneurysms ≥ 4.5 cm if an operation is indicated for aortic stenosis or regurgitation. One study showed that the risk of developing an aortic dissection following AVR was more than 25% if the aortic size exceeds 5 cm at the time of AVR, but current recommendations are to replace an aorta ≥ 4.5 cm, probably for both bicuspid and trileaflet valves.[216]

d. Aneurysms ≥ 4.5 cm in Marfan syndrome

e. Virtually all acute type A dissections (as noted above)

f. Mycotic aneurysms

2. **Transverse arch aneurysms**

   a. Ascending aortic aneurysms that require replacement that also extend into the arch. It should be noted that the "aortopathy" associated with bicuspid valves tends to involve the arch in 75% of patients in whom hemiarch or arch replacement should be performed.[217]

   b. Acute arch dissections with intimal tear in the arch or evidence of arch expansion or rupture

   c. Aneurysms $\geq 5–6$ cm in diameter

3. **Descending thoracic (DAo) and thoracoabdominal aneurysms** (see Figure 1.22 for classification)

   a. Symptomatic aneurysms

   b. Aneurysms ≥ 6.5 cm in diameter (atherosclerotic or chronic dissections)

   c. Complicated acute type B dissections (uncomplicated if low risk patient)

C. **Preoperative considerations**

1. Coronary angiography is required before surgery for ascending aortic and proximal arch aneurysms (not acute dissections). If significant coronary disease is present, it is bypassed at the time of the aneurysm resection.

2. Myocardial perfusion stress imaging (dipyridamole–thallium or sestamibi) is indicated in patients with descending thoracic aneurysms because of the

Aortic Size (cm)

BSA	3.5	4.0	4.5	5.0	5.5	6.0	6.5	7.0	7.5	8.0
1.30	2.69	3.08	3.46	3.86	4.23	4.62	5.00	5.38	5.77	6.15
1.40	2.50	2.86	3.21	3.57	3.93	4.29	4.64	5.00	5.36	5.71
1.50	2.33	2.67	3.00	3.33	3.67	4.00	4.33	4.67	5.00	5.33
1.60	2.19	2.50	2.80	3.13	3.44	3.75	4.06	4.38	4.69	5.00
1.70	2.05	2.35	2.65	2.94	3.24	3.53	3.82	4.12	4.41	4.71
1.80	1.94	2.22	2.50	2.78	3.06	3.33	3.61	3.89	4.17	4.44
1.90	1.84	2.11	2.37	2.63	2.89	3.16	3.42	3.68	3.95	4.22
2.00	1.75	2.00	2.25	2.50	2.75	3.00	3.25	3.50	3.75	4.00
2.10	1.67	1.90	2.14	2.38	2.62	2.86	3.10	3.33	3.57	3.80
2.20	1.59	1.82	2.05	2.27	2.50	2.72	2.95	3.18	3.41	3.64
2.30	1.52	1.74	1.96	2.17	2.39	2.61	2.83	3.04	3.26	3.48
2.40	1.46	1.67	1.88	2.08	2.29	2.50	2.71	2.92	3.13	3.33
2.50	1.40	1.60	1.80	2.00	2.20	2.40	2.60	2.80	3.00	3.20

☐ = low risk (~1% per yr);   ▨ = moderate risk (~8% per yr);   ■ = severe risk (~20% per yr);

Figure 1.21 • Risk of aortic complications (dissection, rupture, and death) correlating the patient's body surface area and the aortic size in cm measured by CT scan. The values within the chart reflect the aortic size index (ASI). The risk is moderate with an ASI > 2.75 cm/m^2 and significant once the ASI exceeds 4.25 cm/m^2. BSA, body surface area. (Reproduced with permission from Davies et al., *Ann Thorac Surg* 2006;81:169–77.)

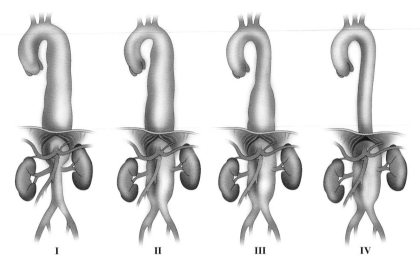

Figure 1.22 • Crawford classification of thoracoabdominal aneurysms.

likelihood of coexistent CAD. If the scan is positive, coronary angiography should be performed. The presence of significant coronary disease usually warrants some form of intervention (PCI or CABG) to reduce the risk of cardiac complications associated with repair of the aneurysm.

3. A careful preoperative baseline neurologic evaluation is important because of the risks associated with circulatory arrest (stroke, seizures) and aortic cross-clamping (paraplegia). A detailed informed-consent discussion with the patient about these devastating complications is essential and must be documented.

4. An assessment of aortoiliac disease is essential prior to any endovascular stenting procedure. Severe stenosis, tortuosity, or extensive atherosclerotic disease may necessitate an alternative site for arterial access or may lead to abandonment of the proposed procedure.

5. Pulmonary status must be optimized prior to surgery. Many patients with aneurysmal disease have concomitant chronic obstructive pulmonary disease, and the use of a thoracotomy incision, lung manipulation during surgery, anticoagulation, and multiple blood transfusions may have a detrimental effect on pulmonary function.

6. Renal function must be monitored carefully after angiography, especially in diabetic patients. The creatinine should be allowed to return to baseline before surgery to reduce the risk of renal dysfunction associated with aortic cross-clamping.

D. Surgical procedures

1. Ascending aortic aneurysms

   a. Supracoronary interposition graft placement is performed if the aneurysm develops above the sinotubular junction, thus sparing the segment from which the coronary arteries arise.

b. If the sinuses are aneurysmal, they should be resected and replaced. Most commonly a valved conduit (Bentall procedure) is placed (Figure 1.11).[110,218] However, an aortic valve-sparing operation can be performed even if aortic regurgitation is present, and is applicable to patients with Marfan syndrome or bicuspid valves (Figure 1.13).[121–123,219–221] The design of this procedure depends on the extent of the aneurysm and the pathophysiology of aortic regurgitation.

c. CPB is required for repair of AAo aneurysms. Depending on the site of the distal anastomosis, simple aortic cross-clamping or a period of DHCA may be necessary. Arterial access for CPB can be achieved through the femoral artery or the axillary artery if significant descending aortic atherosclerosis is present.[222]

d. For DHCA, the central core temperature should be lowered to 18 °C, at which time there is presumed to be electroencephalographic silence. This should provide 45–60 minutes of safe arrest with minimal risk of neurologic insult. Adjuncts to improve cerebral protection during a period of DHCA include methylprednisolone 30 mg/kg, packing the head in ice, and either continuous retrograde cerebral perfusion (RCP) through the superior vena cava (SVC) or preferably antegrade cerebral perfusion (ACP) directly or through the axillary artery.[223,224] With the latter approach, the operation can be done at moderate systemic hypothermia.[225]

2. **Transverse arch aneurysms**[226]

   a. Hemiarch repair using DHCA with RCP or ACP is performed if the ascending aorta and proximal arch are involved. A graft is sewn to the undersurface of the arch leaving the brachiocephalic vessels attached to the native aorta.

   b. Extended arch repair involves placement of an interposition graft sewn to the proximal descending aorta and reimplantation of a brachiocephalic island during a period of circulatory arrest. Alternatively, a debranching operation with use of individual trifurcation grafts to the arch vessels may be performed. This should reduce the duration of DHCA and improve cerebral protection, potentially reducing neurologic morbidity (Figure 1.23).[226,227]

   c. Distal arch repair can be performed via a left thoracotomy without cardiopulmonary bypass. Use of CPB and a period of DHCA through either a sternotomy or thoracotomy incision may be useful when clamping is not feasible for the proximal anastomosis or for more complex operations. Several creative operations for distal arch aneurysms have been described, such as open transaortic stent endografting of distal arch aneurysms with carotid artery bypass.[228]

   d. If it is anticipated that a descending aortic repair may be necessary in the future, a piece of graft material is left dangling from the distal anastomosis and can be retrieved at a subsequent operation through the left chest (the "elephant trunk" procedure).[229]

3. **Descending thoracic aorta**

   a. Graft replacement of the diseased aorta is performed with reimplantation of intercostal vessels at the level of T8–T12 for more extensive aneurysms. This is performed through a left thoracotomy or thoracoabdominal incision with use of one-lung anesthesia.

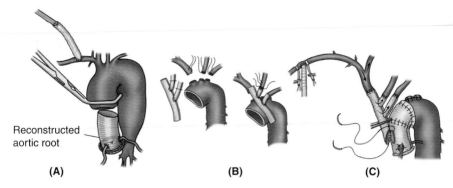

(A)　　　**(B)**　　　**(C)**

Reconstructed aortic root

Figure 1.23 • Aortic arch replacement using a trifurcation graft (TG). (A) Using axillary cannulation for CPB, the aorta is clamped and the proximal root reconstruction is performed. (B) During DHCA, the arch vessels are divided 1 cm from their origins, and individual anastomoses are sequentially performed to the arch vessels with side limbs off the trifurcation graft. (C) Flow is then restored to the brain with a clamp on the proximal segment of the trifurcation graft. The distal arch anastomosis is constructed and the two aortic grafts are reapproximated. Finally, the trifurcation graft is sewn to the proximal portion of the aortic graft.

    b. Consideration should be given to the use of adjuncts (medications, cerebrospinal fluid [CSF] drainage, shunting) to prevent spinal cord ischemia during the period of aortic cross-clamping, which may reduce the risk of paraplegia to less than 5%.[230,231] Shunting can be accomplished by draining blood from a site proximal to the aortic cross-clamp (inferior pulmonary vein/left atrium/proximal aorta) and returning it distally (distal aorta/femoral artery) to perfuse the spinal cord and kidneys. A BioMedicus centrifugal pump, which actively returns blood to the patient at a designated rate, can be used with or without oxygenation. Left-heart bypass alone has been shown to reduce the incidence of paraplegia during surgery for thoracoabdominal aneurysms, but not necessarily more limited descending thoracic aneurysms.[232,233]

    c. Femoro-femoral bypass can be used to provide distal protection. It can also be used along with DHCA when clamping is not possible due to extensive disease or calcification. This technique also provides visceral and spinal cord protection.[234–236]

    d. Arterial monitoring lines are inserted in the right radial and femoral arteries to monitor proximal and distal pressures during the period of aortic cross-clamping, especially if left-heart bypass is used.

    e. Because of the inherent risk of descending aortic clamping, thoracic endovascular aortic repair (TEVAR) has become popularized for the treatment of descending thoracic and thoracoabdominal aneurysms. This may reduce the risk of early death and postoperative complications, including paraplegia, acute kidney injury, bleeding, pneumonia, and cardiac morbidity.[212,237–239]

XIII. Atrial Fibrillation

A. Pathophysiology

1. Atrial fibrillation (AF) results from the presence of multiple reentrant circuits that prevent the synchronous activation of adequate atrial tissue to generate mechanical contraction. It is perpetuated by the variable refractoriness of atrial tissue to the generation of these circuits. Atrial distention may predispose to this arrhythmia, which then promotes progressive atrial dilatation and remodeling, leading to permanent AF. Atrial fibrillation can lead to:

   a. Loss of atrioventricular (AV) synchrony, which reduces ventricular filling and stroke volume. This can produce dizziness, fatigue, and shortness of breath, especially in hypertrophied hearts and when the ventricular rate is high.

   b. Thrombus formation in the left atrium with a predisposition to thromboembolism and stroke

   c. Symptoms of an irregular heartbeat (palpitations)

   d. A cardiomyopathy if the rate is not controlled

2. Atrial fibrillation may occur as an isolated entity ("lone AF") in patients with no structural heart disease or in patients with underlying heart disease. It is more common in patients with hypertension and valvular heart disease. It is categorized as paroxysmal (recurrent AF that terminates spontaneously within 7 days), persistent (lasts >7 days and responds to cardioversion), or long-standing persistent or permanent (fails to respond to medications or cardioversion and lasts over 1 year). In paroxysmal AF, the atrial foci that serve as the trigger are usually located in the tissue surrounding the pulmonary veins as they enter the left atrium. The reentrant circuits in patients with persistent AF usually originate in the left atrium.

B. Management considerations and indications for surgery

1. AF is managed with medications to control the ventricular rate (β-blockers, calcium channel blockers, digoxin) and prevent thromboembolism (warfarin). When the rate cannot be controlled, symptoms are disabling, thromboembolism occurs on anticoagulation, or anticoagulation cannot be tolerated or is not desirable, an ablative procedure should be considered.

2. In the absence of the above indications, surgery for AF is generally not indicated. However, with the use of thoracoscopic approaches and advances in catheter ablation technology, the indications have been liberalized to include patients with lone AF. Transcatheter ablations are very successful in ablating paroxysmal AF arising from pulmonary veins, and with adequate mapping, reasonable success (about 60%) can be achieved in patients with persistent AF.

3. The ability to restore sinus rhythm with an ablative procedure during concomitant cardiac surgery improves long-term survival and may also improve cardiac function and reduce the incidence of stroke.[134,135,240] Therefore, it is strongly recommended during mitral valve surgery, and can be considered in patients undergoing other types of cardiac surgery.

4. Medications used for rate control or for AF prophylaxis should be continued up to the time of surgery. Because reversion to sinus rhythm may not occur immediately after surgery, these medications are generally continued afterwards.

C. Surgical procedures[241]

1. In 1986, Cox designed a technically complex "cut-and-sew" operation called the "Maze" procedure that was designed to ablate AF, restore AV synchrony, and preserve atrial transport function. This was subsequently redesigned as the Cox-Maze III operation, in which the incisions not only interrupted the microreentrant circuits, but also allowed the sinus node to function, and directed propagation of the sinus impulse through both atria. Atrial fibrillation was eliminated in about 90% of patients, but about 10% of patients still required pacemakers.

2. Various ablation technologies have now been developed to mimic the suture lines of the Cox-Maze III operation, the best of which appear to be cryoablation, radiofrequency, and high-frequency ultrasound (HIFU). To achieve success, the lesions created must achieve transmurality. Since the left atrium is usually the primary focus of reentry, a left-sided Maze is most commonly performed.

3. The basic operation involves bilateral pulmonary vein isolation with obliteration of the left atrial appendage. This can be performed epicardially and thus is amenable to bilateral thoracosopic approaches. It is only applicable with good success to patients with paroxysmal AF.[242] However, an additional ablation line that mimics the mitral isthmus lesion of a left atrial Maze procedure can be performed epicardially across the left atrial dome from the left fibrous trigone at the mitral valve annulus to the base of the noncoronary cusp of the aortic valve (Figure 1.24). This should improve the success rate in patients with persistent AF.[243,244]

4. A left-sided Maze operation is usually performed in conjunction with mitral valve surgery (Figure 1.25). This procedure produces ablation lines that encircle and connect the right and left pulmonary veins ("box lesion"), and one that

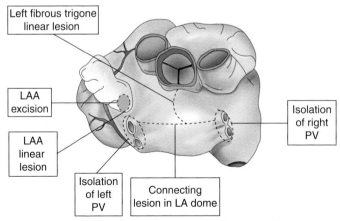

Left fibrous trigone linear lesion

LAA excision

LAA linear lesion

Isolation of left PV

Connecting lesion in LA dome

Isolation of right PV

LAA = left atrial appendage; PV = pulmonary veins

Figure 1.24 • Epicardial lesion set for thoracoscopic approaches to atrial fibrillation. Bilateral pulmonary vein isolation and a connecting lesion between the right- and left-sided pulmonary veins are performed. In addition, a linear lesion over the dome of the left atrium is created extending from the left fibrous trigone at the anterior mitral valve annulus to the base of the junction of the left and noncoronary cusps to mimic the mitral isthmus lesion performed endocardially.

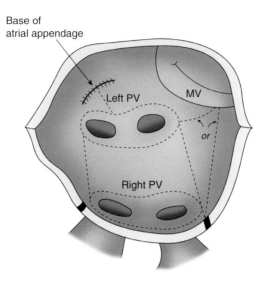

Figure 1.25 • The left-sided Maze involves ablation lines that encircle and connect the right and left pulmonary veins and one that extends from the inferior box lesion near the right or left inferior pulmonary vein to the mitral valve annulus. The left atrial appendage is amputated and an additional ablation line is placed from the base of the appendage to the left pulmonary veins. The base of the left atrial appendage is then oversewn.

extends from the inferior pulmonary vein ablation line to the mitral valve annulus.[245,246] The left atrial appendage is amputated and an ablation line carried from the base of the appendage to the left pulmonary vein encircling line. Left atrial volume reduction may be helpful when the LA dimension exceeds 6 cm.[136,247] Use of ganglionic plexi mapping and ablation with confirmation of conduction block by pacing may improve results.[248]

5. The right-sided Maze includes amputation of the right atrial appendage (or an ablation line across its base) and an incision into the right atrium from the septum towards the AV groove. Through this incision, ablation lines are extended laterally up the SVC and down to the inferior vena cava (IVC), across the fossa ovalis down to the coronary sinus, from the IVC to the coronary sinus and from the sinus to the tricuspid annulus (isthmus lesions). Additional ablation lines extend from the anterior tricuspid leaflet to the base of the excised RA appendage and from the posterior tricuspid leaflet to the AV groove (Figure 1.26).

XIV. Ventricular Tachycardia and Sudden Death

A. Pathophysiology

1. Nonidiopathic ventricular tachycardia (VT) occurs in association with structural heart disease, and may be subdivided into ischemic and nonischemic etiologies.

    a. Ischemic VT is caused either by active ischemia (usually from a ruptured plaque or induced during hemodynamic stress) or from a previous myocardial infarction (MI) that produces scar tissue and impaired LV function. The latter results from heterogeneous myocardial damage that produces the electrophysiologic substrate for the development of a reentrant rhythm. This

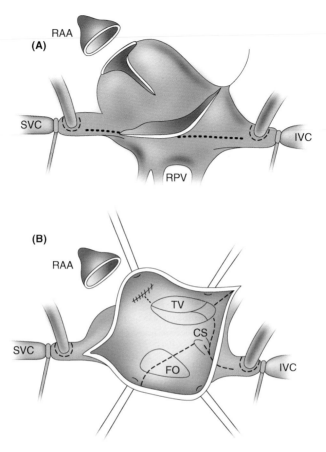

Figure 1.26 • (A) The right-sided Maze includes ablation of the base of the right atrial appendage and an incision in the right atrial wall through which multiple bipolar and unipolar ablation lines can be carried out. (B) Sites for endocardial ablation are shown by the dotted lines (see text).

commonly occurs at the border zone of an LV aneurysm between dense subendocardial scar tissue and normal myocardium. Premature stimuli delivered during electrophysiologic testing may initiate an impulse that triggers the reentrant circuit of monomorphic VT ("inducible VT").

b. Nonischemic VT may result from reentrant circuits or triggered automaticity. It is most commonly noted in patients with dilated cardiomyopathies and markedly depressed ventricular function, as well as less common entities such as arrhythmogenic RV dysplasia. In these conditions, the arrhythmogenic focus frequently cannot be adequately mapped and it is difficult to ablate with catheter intervention.

2. Idiopathic VT occurs in the absence of structural heart disease and may arise along the RV outflow tract or in the left posterior fascicle of the left ventricle. It is usually caused by triggered activity related to a high adrenergic state. As such, it can be treated by medical therapy, or, if that fails, by radiofrequency catheter ablation.

3. Out-of-hospital cardiac arrest (so-called sudden cardiac death [SCD]) is estimated to be the first manifestation of coronary disease in 40% of patients, usually as a result of rupture of an unstable plaque. Other patients have no identifiable cause for such an event and may or may not have inducible arrhythmias.

B. **Interventional procedures and their indications**

1. The presence of malignant ventricular arrhythmias mandates an assessment for potentially correctable causes. Surgery, such as a CABG or LVA resection, can be considered based on standard indications with the understanding that no antiarrhythmic benefit may be achieved. In these situations, and in patients in whom no cardiac surgical procedure is indicated, ICD implantation can be considered to improve survival. The recommendations for ICD implantation are based upon the 2008 guidelines, which evaluated numerous primary and secondary prevention trials.[249,250]

2. Class I indications (ICD implantation is indicated)

   a. Survivors of cardiac arrest due to VF/VT not due to a reversible cause

   b. Spontaneous sustained VT with structural heart disease (usually a dilated cardiomyopathy)

   c. Unexplained syncope if hemodynamically significant sustained VT or VF is inducible during an electrophysiology (EP) study

   d. In patients with prior MI:

      i. LVEF < 40% if nonsustained VT (NSVT) or inducible VF or sustained VT at EP study

      ii. LVEF < 35% at least 40 days post-MI in NYHA class II–III

      iii. LVEF < 30% at least 40 days post-MI in NYHA class I

      iv. LVEF ≤ 35% with nonischemic dilated cardiomyopathy in NYHA class II–III

3. Class IIa indications (ICD implantation is reasonable)

   a. Unexplained syncope, significant LV dysfunction, and nonischemic dilated cardiomyopathy

   b. Sustained VT and normal or near-normal LV function

   c. HOCM with one or more major risk factors for SCD (see page 41)

   d. Other conditions of nonschemic VT, including outpatients awaiting transplantation

4. Class IIb indications (ICD implantation should be considered)

   a. Nonischemic heart disease with LVEF ≤ 35% in NYHA class I

   b. Unexplained syncope with advanced structural heart disease

5. The 2008 guidelines do not provide specific recommendations on how to manage postoperative cardiac surgical patients who develop sustained or nonsustained VT or have a preoperative EF <30%, but inferences can be drawn.

   a. Since patients undergoing cardiac surgery generally have structural heart disease, the occurrence of postoperative sustained VT is both a class I and IIa indication for an ICD, independent of LVEF.

    b. In patients with NSVT, the decision can be based on LVEF and EP studies.

      i. For LVEF >40%, an ICD is not recommended and β-blockers are generally prescribed.

      ii. For LVEF of 30–40%, an EP study is indicated. A noninducible patient is considered at low risk for sudden death and β-blockers are prescribed. If inducible, an ICD is placed.

      iii. For LVEF <30%, an ICD is indicated if the patient is at least 40 days post-MI, even in the absence of VT. However, this ACC/AHA/HRS recommendation does not specifically address patients who have NSVT, recent revascularization (in the MADIT-II trial, patients with LVEF <30% had to be more than 3 months post-CABG), or depressed LVEF from symptomatic yet repaired valvular heart disease. If the patient has NSVT and depressed LV function, the options are to (1) place an ICD, (2) rely on an EP study to assess for inducibility, or (3) simply use β-blockers until the patient is 40 days after an MI and then place an ICD. Most centers would probably place an ICD prior to patient discharge. If the patient has an EF <30% but no VT, elective evaluation and placement of an ICD are indicated.

C. Preoperative considerations

    1. A thorough preoperative evaluation should be undertaken to determine whether structural heart disease is present. Preliminary cardiac catheterization should be performed to ascertain whether myocardial revascularization is indicated. This may lower the risk of ICD implantation, and may also reduce the risk of recurrent VT if it was occurring on an ischemic basis.

    2. Many patients with cardiomyopathies are maintained on warfarin, which must be held for several days to prevent bleeding into the ICD pocket. Infection developing in the pocket implies infection of the entire lead system and mandates its removal.[251]

    3. Careful monitoring and provisions for cardiac resuscitation (trained personnel and equipment) are essential during ICD implantation.

D. Surgical procedures

    1. Myocardial revascularization should be performed in the patient with reversible ischemia and bypassable anatomy. It provides excellent results in patients with ischemic VT/VF.[252] The role of PCI in such patients is undefined. Standard indications for ICD implantation, including EP testing for inducibility, should then be followed.

    2. Blind endocardial resection should be performed when ischemic ventricular tachycardia is present in a patient undergoing resection of an LV aneurysm. Aggressive resection of scar tissue, including that on the septum, with cryoablation at the periphery of the scar tissue and reconstruction of the ventricle by geometric modeling (SVR noted on page 62) should be performed. These procedures have supplanted the map-guided surgery performed in the mid-1990s that achieved success rates greater than 75% and reached 90% with the addition of medications. In high-risk patients with depressed ventricular function, one study showed that long-term survival was fairly similar with direct VT surgery or placement of an ICD, often with associated CABG.[253]

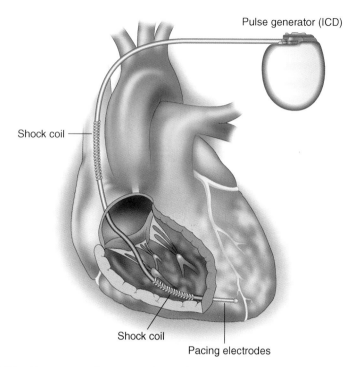

Figure 1.27 • Transvenous ICD system. The single-chamber system consists of one right ventricular lead that contains shocking coils that lie within the SVC and the right ventricle, and bipolar sensing and pacing electrodes that lie within the ventricle.

3. ICD implantation is performed in the EP lab. Most patients receive biventricular ICD systems that can perform AV sequential pacing and antitachycardia pacing. The device is implanted in a prepectoral pocket. Testing of the leads for sensing and defibrillation thresholds (DFTs) is performed. The generator is then connected to the leads and the system is retested (Figure 1.27).

4. Prior to the development of transvenous systems, ICD implantation was performed through left thoracotomy, median sternotomy, subcostal, or sub-xiphoid approaches. Device replacement and removal of infected lead systems mandate an understanding of their implantation methods. These systems usually involved two rate-sensing electrodes placed into the right or left ventricular epicardium and two titanium mesh patches for defibrillation placed over the ventricles, either inside or outside the pericardium.

XV. End-Stage Heart Failure

A. **Pathophysiology**. End-stage heart failure is a clinical syndrome that develops due to progressive deterioration in LV function associated with LV remodeling. It is most commonly the result of multiple infarctions from coronary artery disease (ischemic cardiomyopathy), but may result from a dilated cardiomyopathy or end-stage valvular heart disease. As ventricular function deteriorates, the left ventricle dilates and changes from an elliptical to a spherical shape. This increases wall stress, which then increases oxygen requirements, causes pathologic cardiomyocyte hypertrophy that further compromises contractile function, and induces functional MR. These changes lead to intractable heart failure. In addition, ventricular remodeling increases the tendency to develop ventricular arrhythmias.

1. Neurohormonal activation, with elevated levels of angiotensin II, aldosterone, norepinephrine, endothelin, vasopressin, and cytokines, may contribute to remodeling. These increase sodium retention and produce peripheral vasoconstriction, increasing hemodynamic stress. They also have direct toxic effects on myocardial cells, stimulating the development of fibrosis. This relationship between neurohormonal activation and worsening of CHF forms the basis of the medical approach to CHF.

2. Patients with long-standing hypertension tend to develop diastolic heart failure, although both systolic and diastolic components coexist in most patients.

3. The ACC/AHA guidelines have defined four stages in the progression of CHF: stage A (high risk for development of CHF), stage B (structural heart disease with LVH and reduced EF without CHF), stage C (structural heart disease with CHF), and stage D (refractory CHF requiring specialized intervention). Stage A patients should have their risk factors aggressively addressed. Stage B and C patients should receive more aggressive medical therapy with consideration of the surgical procedures listed below. Stage D patients may require destination assist devices or cardiac transplantation.[254,255]

B. **Medical therapy.** The prognosis for patients with end-stage heart failure with NYHA class III–IV CHF is very poor, with a markedly impaired quality of life and a limited life span. Clinical improvement and improved survival have been noted with use of ACE inhibitors or angiotensin receptor blockers (ARBs), β-blockers such as carvedilol, bisoprolol and metoprolol, and diuretics, such as the aldosterone blockers (spironolactone or eplerenone). However, even with optimal medical therapy, annual mortality rates exceed 12%/year. Thus, alternative strategies are essential to treat this growing segment of the population.

C. **Indications for surgery and surgical procedures.** A variety of surgical procedures can be utilized to treat the patient with end-stage heart failure, depending on the pathophysiology of the disease.[256]

1. Coronary bypass surgery should be performed in patients with an ischemic cardiomyopathy if they have angina or documentation of ischemic, viable, hibernating myocardium. This can reduce anginal symptoms, in many cases will improve ventricular function and symptoms of CHF, may lower the risk of sudden cardiac death, and may improve survival.[257] Patients with fewer viable segments of LV dyssynchrony do poorly.[258] Clearly, revascularization earlier in a patient's course will produce a better clinical outcome.

2. Mitral valve repair with a small restrictive annuloplasty ring can be offered to patients with chronic severe MR and ischemic cardiomyopathies. This can promote reverse remodeling (usually a reduction in end-systolic volume index >15%), restore normal geometric relationships, alleviate symptoms of CHF, and prevent recurrent MR.[259] Although a restrictive annuloplasty is usually successful

in improving symptoms, an improvement in long-term survival is less evident.[260-262] Poor results are noted when mitral valve repair if performed in patients with severely dilated ventricles (LV end-diastolic dimension >65 mm) and in many patients with nonischemic cardiomyopathy.[263,264] The 2009 ACCF/AHA guidelines consider mitral valve repair a class IIb indication in stage D patients since its effectiveness is not well-established.[255] Percutaneous approaches to annular remodeling via the coronary sinus and edge-to-edge apposition techniques (MitraClip [Abbott]) are being investigated.

3. Cardiac resynchronization therapy (CRT) (atrial-synchronized biventricular pacing) has been demonstrated to improve heart failure symptoms and exercise tolerance and promote reverse remodeling. It is applicable to patients with an EF ≤ 35%, NYHA class II–III symptoms, and a QRS duration ≥ 120 msec. In these patients, ventricular dyssynchrony produces suboptimal ventricular filling, a reduction in contractility, paradoxical septal wall motion, and worsening MR. By activating both ventricles in a synchronized manner, CRT is able to increase LV filling time, decrease septal dyskinesis, and reduce MR.[255,265] An ICD can also be considered in these patients. In patients in NYHA class III–IV who are dependent on ventricular pacing, CRT is considered a reasonable approach.

4. An ICD is indicated in many patients with stage B–D heart failure because of the frequent association of a dilated dysfunctional ventricle with ventricular tachyarrhythmias.

   a. Ischemic cardiomyopathy with EF ≤ 30%, at least 40 days post-MI in Stage B (NYHA class I)

   b. Nonischemic cardiomyopathy with EF ≤ 35% in Stage B (NYHA class I)

   c. Stage C with current or past symptoms of CHF, reduced EF, and a history of cardiac arrest, VF, or unstable VT (class I recommendation for secondary prevention)

   d. Stage C (NYHA II–III) with EF <35% of any etiology

5. Surgical ventricular restoration (SVR) can be used for patients who develop akinesia or dyskinesia subsequent to a single-territory MI.

   a. It has been shown that LV end-systolic volume index (ESVI) is a major determinant of survival in patients with ischemic cardiomyopathy.[266] Thus, combining CABG with resection of nonfunctioning tissue to decrease ventricular size and restore geometry should improve ventricular function, produce symptomatic improvement, and improve survival. These benefits have been documented in some studies comparing CABG + SVR with CABG alone, although an improvement in survival may not be evident.[80,267,268] However, the STICH trial of patients with CAD-related anterior akinesia or dyskinesia with an ejection fraction <35% was unable to demonstrate that reduction in LV size was associated with an improvement in symptoms or reduction in mortality after 4 years.[82] The methodology of this report has been criticized, because the literature suggests a benefit to adjunctive SVR with proper patient selection (ESVI >60 mL/m^2, more than 35% akinesia from anterior wall necrosis), and appropriately performed surgery (ensuring a 30% reduction in ESVI at follow-up).[269] Some patients in the STICH trial did not satisfy these criteria.

b. In patients with mild-to-moderate MR, CABG + SVR may reduce MR by reducing sphericity of the LV, thus reducing the longitudinal and transverse dimensions of the LV that increase the interpapillary muscle distance and cause apical tethering of the leaflets.[270] However, in patients with 3−4+ MR, mitral repair should be considered. Resecting viable myocardium simply to reduce the size of the ventricle (Batista procedure) is not recommended.

6. Techniques and devices that prevent ventricular dilatation, such as a cardiomyoplasty, the CorCap restraint device (Acorn International), and the Myocor myosplint and Coapsys devices, have been investigated as means of improving symptoms of CHF. These have been shown to reduce end-diastolic dimensions, reduce wall stress, improve EF, and reduce MR.[271,272]

7. When the patient has advanced heart failure and is not a candidate for any of the above procedures, more advanced interventional therapy may be required.

   a. Cardiac transplantation should be considered in patients with end-stage heart failure who have an EF <15% and a peak VO_2 <10−15 mL/min/m^2 with maximal exercise testing. In potential transplanat recipients, insertion of a left ventricular or even biventricular assist device (VAD) may be necessary if the patient develops progressive hemodynamic deterioration despite maximal pharmacologic therapy and an IABP. This can serve as a bridge to transplantation.[273]

   b. VADs can be considered for destination therapy in patients who are not considered transplant candidates (usually because of age). Several devices, including the Thoratec HeartMate II, the Jarvik 2000, and the Micromed Heart Assist 5 (DeBakey) axial flow pumps have been used for destination therapy, with numerous other devices undergoing evaluation.[274−276]

8. Muscle and stem cell transplantation into areas of infarcted myocardium are being investigated as a means of improving ventricular function.[277,278]

XVI. Pericardial Disease

A. **Pathophysiology and diagnostic techniques.** The pericardium may become involved in a variety of systemic disease processes that produce either pericardial effusions or constriction. The most common causes of effusions are idiopathic (probably viral), malignant, uremic, pyogenic, and tuberculous. The most common causes of constriction are idiopathic, radiation, and tuberculous. Early and late postoperative cardiac tamponade due to hemopericardium are discussed on pages 372 and 660.

1. Large effusions result in tamponade physiology with progressive low output states. They are best documented by two-dimensional echocardiography, which delineates their size and provides hemodynamic evidence of tamponade. Findings include right atrial and ventricular diastolic collapse, increased reversal of flow in the hepatic veins during atrial systole, a dilated IVC with lack of inspiratory collapse, and decreased SVC flow during diastole.[279] Equilibration of intracardiac pressures (RVEDP = PCWP = LVEDP) will be detected by cardiac catheterization.

2. Constriction can also produce a low output state despite preserved systolic function. Cardiac catheterization will demonstrate a "square-root sign" in the

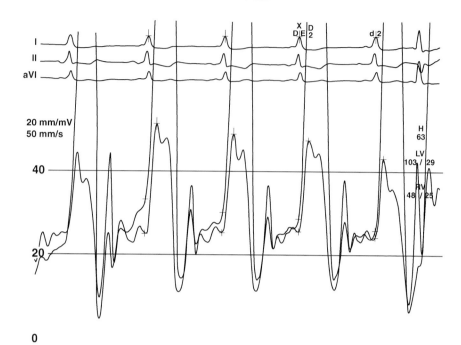

Figure 1.28 • Simultaneous right and left ventricular pressure tracings in constrictive pericarditis. Note the "dip-and-plateau" pattern as diastolic filling of the ventricular chambersis abruptly truncated by the constriction. Note also the equilibration of diastolic ventricular pressures. (Reproduced with permission from Myers and Spodick, *Am Heart J* 1999;138:219–32.)[281]

right ventricular tracing, indicating rapid early filling and a diastolic plateau caused by severe impairment to RV filling (Figure 1.28).[280,281] Cardiovascular CT and MRI scanning can be done to assess the thickness of the pericardium.[282] The differentiation of constriction, which is surgically correctable, from restriction, which is not, can be difficult because they have many findings in common. Although restrictive pathology is associated with diastolic dysfunction, it may or may not be associated with systolic dysfunction. However, the presence of significant pulmonary hypertension suggests a restrictive process, since it is rarely seen with constriction. A number of echocardiographic methods are helpful in differentiating constriction from restriction.[283,284]

B. Indications for surgery

　　1. Large effusions that fail to respond to noninvasive measures (dialysis for uremia, antibiotics for infection, radiation or chemotherapy for malignancy, thyroid replacement for myxedema) may be treated initially by a percutaneous drainage procedure (either pericardiocentesis with catheter drainage or balloon pericardiostomy).[285,286] Echocardiography is helpful in localizing the effusion and determining whether it is easily accessible to a percutaneous needle or not. If these procedures cannot be performed or the effusion recurs, surgical drainage should be performed.

2. Constriction that produces a refractory low output state, hepatomegaly, or peripheral edema should be treated by a pericardiectomy. Lesser degrees of constriction may resolve spontaneously or respond to a course of nonsteroidal antiinflammatory medications or steroids. Factors that compromise the long-term results of pericardiectomy include radiation-induced constriction, higher PA pressures, worse LV systolic function, and the presence of hyponatremia or renal dysfunction.[287]

C. Preoperative considerations

1. The subacute development of cardiac tamponade increases systemic venous pressures with eventual compromise in organ system perfusion from a low cardiac output syndrome. Patients frequently develop oliguric renal dysfunction, worsening respiratory status, and hepatic congestion. None of these will improve until drainage is accomplished. Fresh frozen plasma should be available if there is a preexisting coagulopathy.

2. Both tamponade and constriction are associated with low cardiac output states. Intrinsic compensatory mechanisms to maintain blood pressure and cardiac output include a tachycardia and increased sympathetic tone. Maintenance of adequate preload is essential to increase cardiac output. β-blockers and vasodilators must be avoided. Patients with low output states from severe constriction may benefit from a few days of inotropic support prior to surgery. Patients with abnormal LV contractility and relaxation properties before surgery have a higher inotropic requirement after surgery with a higher mortality rate and worse long-term outcome. They might benefit the most from preoperative support.[288]

3. Preliminary pericardiocentesis for a very large effusion improves the safety of anesthetic induction, which can produce vasodilation, a fall in filling pressures, and profound hypotension.

4. Prepping and draping the patient prior to the induction of anesthesia may be a prudent maneuver in patients with extremely tenuous hemodynamic status.

D. Surgical procedures

1. **Pericardial effusions.** If percutaneous drainage is inadequate or contraindicated, surgery should be performed.

   a. A subxiphoid pericardiostomy opens the pericardium, drains the pericardial space, allows for obtaining a small biopsy specimen, and obliterates the pericardial space by promoting the formation of adhesions with several days of chest tube drainage (Figure 1.29). It is the safest approach in the unstable patient and the best for patients with malignancies and a limited life span. Recurrence rate is lower with this procedure than with percutaneous catheter drainage.[285]

   b. A pericardial window, created with a balloon technique, a videothoracoscopic approach (VATS), or a limited thoracotomy, can be used to drain the effusion into the pleural space and obtain a biopsy specimen. The latter two procedures require general anesthesia and are best utilized when there is suspicion of underlying pleuropulmonary pathology. One study suggested that a VATS approach produced a lower recurrence rate than a subxiphoid drainage procedure.[289]

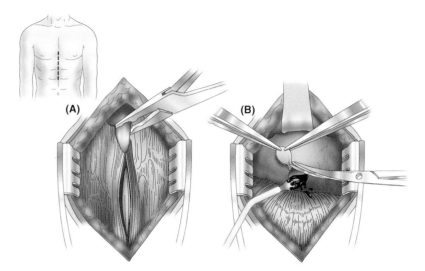

Figure 1.29 • The subxiphoid approach to pericardial disease. (A) An incision is made over the xiphisternal junction, extending inferiorly for 5 cm. The rectus fascia is incised and the xiphoid process is removed. (B) With upward traction on the distal sternum, the preperitoneal fat is swept away. The pericardium is grasped and incised and a small specimen may be removed. A finger is insinuated to break up any loculations, and pericardial fluid is aspirated with a suction catheter. One or two chest tubes are then placed within the pericardium.

2. **Constrictive pericarditis**[290]

   a. Pericardiectomy is best performed through a median sternotomy approach with pump standby. The pericardium is removed to within 2 cm of the phrenic nerves on either side, or at least as far as exposure allows. Dissection of the aorta and pulmonary arteries should be performed first, followed by the left and then the right ventricle to avoid pulmonary edema. One comparative study of sternotomy vs. thoracotomy approaches found both approaches to be effective, but generally the thoracotomy approach is associated with more pulmonary complications and should be reserved for cases of infectious pericarditis (usually tuberculosis) to avoid a sternal infection.[291–293]

   b. When there is no dissection plane between the thickened pericardium and the epicardium, the operation can be quite difficult. When dense calcific adhesions are present without a cleavage plane, use of CPB may allow for a safer dissection, although bleeding may be increased by heparinization. It is frequently prudent to leave heavily calcified areas adherent to the heart to minimize bleeding and pericardial damage.

   c. Rarely, patients will develop epicardial constriction with a severe inflammatory response postoperatively, anecdotally noted in some patients with prior mediastinal radiation. This problem is approached using a "waffle" procedure, which entails multiple crisscrossing incisions in the scar tissue to optimize ventricular expansion and filling.[294]

XVII. Congenital Heart Disease: Atrial Septal Abnormalities

A. Pathophysiology

1. The atrial septum is comprised embryologically of two separate septa which form a flap-like orifice that permits right-to-left blood flow as part of the fetal circulation. After birth, the septum seals, producing an intact atrial septum. In 25% of patients, it remains patent and is called a "patent foramen ovale" or PFO. The risk of a PFO is that of paraxodical embolism associated with right-to-left shunting when the RA pressure exceeds the LA pressure. This may be noted during straining, heavy lifting, and coughing, but can be present in more than half of patients at rest.

2. An atrial septal aneurysm (ASA) reflects redundant tissue in the area of the fossa ovalis that produces excessive mobility of the septum. This promotes adherence of platelet–fibrin debris to the left atrial side which can embolize into the systemic circulation, most commonly when there is a right-to-left shunt, which is present in 50–80% of patients with these aneurysms. This may result from a PFO or perforations developing within the aneurysm. Aneurysms are present in only 2% of patients with PFOs, but when present, the likelihood of sustaining a stroke is four times greater than with PFOs alone. Overall, PFOs are noted in 40% of patients with cryptogenic stroke, with 10% having both an ASA and a PFO.[295,296]

3. A small percentage of patients born with congenital atrial septal defects (ASDs) will reach adult life with a persistent left-to-right communication that may remain asymptomatic for decades. The increased shunt flow results in right atrial and right ventricular enlargement, eventually leading to pulmonary hypertension, atrial fibrillation, and tricuspid regurgitation. An untreated large ASD will eventually cause reversal of shunt flow, which is an inoperable situation.

B. Clinical presentation

1. **PFO.** Most patients with a PFO are asymptomatic. Clinical presentation is usually a transient ischemic attack (TIA) or stroke, or migraine-like headaches. In one study, a PFO and/or ASA could be identified in about 30% of patients <age 55 and 40% >age 55 who were diagnosed with a cryptogenic stroke.[297] Shunting through a PFO is believed to be the mechanism in platypnea–orthodeoxia syndrome (dyspnea and deoxygenation when sitting or standing up from a recumbent position).

2. **ASDs.** Depending on the size of the ASD, the degree of shunt flow, and the presence of partial anomalous pulmonary venous drainage (noted with sinus venosus defects), a patient may develop shortness of breath, fatigue, exercise intolerance, frequent pulmonary infections, and palpitations from atrial arrhythmias. Although the flow is predominantly left-to-right, paradoxical embolism is noted in about 15% of patients.[298]

C. Evaluation

1. **PFO.** Transesophageal echocardiography with agitated saline injection should be performed in patients with cryptogenic stroke to detect right-to-left shunting through a PFO. Transcranial Doppler studies with agitated saline are also helpful. Noninvasive lower-extremity venous studies tend to be negative

because the embolus usually arises from the heart or consists of platelet–fibrin particles that are too small to detect.

2. **ASDs.** An echocardiogram can define the location and size of the septal defect, which can determine whether percutaneous closure is feasible. It should also quantitate the degree of left-to-right shunting, and assess RA and RV dilatation, RV dysfunction, and the degree of pulmonary hypertension.

D. Indications for intervention

1. There is no indication for a prophylactic intervention in an asymptomatic patient with a PFO, because alone it is not an independent risk factor for stroke.[296]

2. There is increasing interest in PFO closures in patients with migraine headaches and documented ischemic cerebral events.[299]

3. The optimal treatment for patients with prior TIA or cryptogenic stroke associated with a PFO is controversial.[300] Medical therapy with aspirin and/or warfarin can be recommended, because the risk of recurrent stroke is fairly low (about 2.5% at 4 years).[301] However, excellent results have been obtained with percutaneous closure, which is safe and effective, and thus might be justifiable.[302] Closure can be recommended for patients with coexistent PFO and ASA, in whom the risk of recurrent stroke is significantly greater (15% at 4 years).[301]

4. An ASD associated with symptoms, RA and RV enlargement (even if asymptomatic), or shunt flow exceeding 1.5 : 1 should be closed.[303] Surgery can improve clinical status and prevent RV dilatation independent of the patient's age, although patients undergoing closure after age 30 tend to have higher PA pressures and a greater incidence of atrial fibrillation, which are predictive of an increase in late death from arrhythmias or heart failure. An intervention can be offered as long as the PA pressure is less than 2/3 systemic or responds to vasodilators; irreversible pulmonary hypertension contraindicates closure.[304–306]

E. Interventions

1. Percutaneous closure can be performed for PFOs and secundum ASDs that are less than 38 mm in size and have a satisfactory tissue rim. Anticoagulation with antiplatelet therapy (aspirin +/– clopidogrel) is indicated for 6 months after placement of the device (Amplatzer).

2. Surgical closure, usually with a patch, is indicated in large secundum ASDs not amenable to percutaneous closure and for all non-secundum ASDs, including sinus venosus defects close to the SVC with associated anomalous pulmonary venous drainage, and ostium primum defects. This can frequently be done through a minithoracotomy incision.[307]

XVIII. Adults with Other Congenital Heart Disease

For the management of adults with all other forms of congenital heart disease, the reader is referred to the ACC/AHA guidelines available at www.acc.org.[303]

References

1. Kim H, Yang DH, Park Y, et al. Incremental prognostic value of C-reactive protein and N-terminal proB-type natriuretic peptide in acute coronary syndrome. *Circ J* 2006;70:1379–84.

2. Jneid H, Bhatt DL, Corti R, Badimon JJ, Fuster V, Francis GS. Aspirin and clopidogrel in acute coronary syndromes: therapeutic insights from the CURE study. *Arch Intern Med* 2003;163:1145–53.

3. Fox KA, Mehta SR, Peters R, et al. Benefits and risks of the combination of clopidogrel and aspirin in patients undergoing surgical revascularization for non-ST elevation acute coronary syndrome: the Clopidogrel in Unstable Angina to prevent Recurrent Ischemic Events (CURE) trial. *Circulation* 2004;110:1202–8.

4. Keller TT, Squizzato A, Middeldorp S. Clopidogrel plus aspirin versus aspirin alone for preventing cardiovascular disease. *Cochrane Database Syst Rev* 2007;3:CD005158.

5. Berger JS, Frye CB, Harshaw Q, Edwards FH, Steinhubl SR, Becker RC. Impact of clopidogrel in patients with acute coronary syndromes requiring coronary artery bypass surgery: a multicenter analysis. *J Am Coll Cardiol* 2008;52:1693–701.

6. Bhatt DL, Flather MD, Hacke W, et al. Patients with prior myocardial infarction, stroke, or symptomatic peripheral vascular disease in the CHARISMA trial. *J Am Coll Cardiol* 2007;49:1982–8.

7. Antman EM, Hand M, Armstrong PW, et al. 2007 focused update of the ACC/AHA 2004 guidelines for the management of patients with ST-elevation myocardial infarction. A report of the American College of Cardiology/American Heart Association Task Force on Practice Guidelines (2007 writing group to review new evidence and update the ACC/AHA 2004 guidelines for the management of patients with ST-elevation myocardial infarction). *J Am Coll Cardiol* 2008;51:210–47.

8. Armstrong PW. Contemporary therapy of acute ST-elevation myocardial infarction. *Tex Heart Inst J* 2009;36:273–81.

9. Anderson JL, Adams CD, Antman EM, et al. ACC/AHA 2007 guidelines for the management of patients with unstable angina/non ST-elevation myocardial infarction: a report of the American College of Cardiology/American Heart Association task force on practice guidelines (writing committee to review the 2002 guidelines for the management of patients with unstable angina/non-ST elevation myocardial infarction) developed in collaboration with the American College of Emergency Physicians, the Society for Cardiovascular Angiography and Intervention, and the Society of Thoracic Surgeons endorsed by the American Association of Cardiovascular and Pulmonary Rehabilitation and the Society for Academic Emergency Medicine. *J Am Coll Cardiol* 2007;50:1965–72 or *Circulation* 2007;116:e148–304 (available online at acc.org).

10. Giugliano RP, Braunwald E. The year in non-ST-segment elevation acute coronary syndrome. *J Am Coll Cardiol* 2008;52:1095–1103.

11. Ebrahimi R, Dyke C, Mehran R, et al. Outcomes following pre-operative clopidogrel administration in patients with acute coronary syndromes undergoing coronary artery bypass surgery. The ACUITY (Acute Catheterization and Urgent Intervention Triage strategY) Trial. *J Am Coll Cardiol* 2009;53:1965–72.

12. Patel MR, Dehmer GJ, Hirshfeld JW, Smith PK, Spertus JA. ACCF/SCAI/AATS/AHA/ASNC 2009 appropriateness criteria for coronary revascularization. *J Am Coll Cardiol* 2009;53:530–53.

13. Katritsis DM, Meier B. Percutaneous coronary intervention for stable coronary artery disease. *J Am Coll Cardiol* 2008;52:889–93.

14. Holmes DR Jr, Gersh BJ, Whitlow P, King SB III, Dove JT. Percutaneous coronary intervention for chronic stable angina. A reassessment. *JACC Cardiovasc Interv* 2008;1:34–43.

15. Hannan EL, Wu C, Walford G, et al. Drug-eluting stents vs. coronary-artery bypass grafting in multivessel coronary disease. *N Engl J Med* 2008;358:331–41.

16. Booth J, Clayton T, Pepper J, et al. Randomized, controlled trial of coronary artery bypass surgery versus percutaneous coronary intervention in patients with multivessel coronary artery disease: six-year follow-up from the Stent or Surgery trial (SoS). *Circulation* 2008;118:381–8.

17. Serruys PW, Morice MC, Kappetein AP, et al. Percutaneous coronary intervention versus coronary-artery bypass grafting for severe coronary artery disease. *N Engl J Med* 2009;360:961–72.

18. Mack MJ, Prince SL, Herbert M, et al. Current clinical outcomes of percutaneous coronary intervention and coronary artery bypass grafting. *Ann Thorac Surg* 2008;86:496–503.

19. Smith PK. Treatment selection for coronary artery disease: the collision of a belief system with evidence. *Ann Thorac Surg* 2009;87:1328–31.

20. May SA, Wilson JM. The comparative efficacy of percutaneous and surgical coronary revascularization in 2009. *Tex Heart Inst J* 2009;36:375–86.

21. Seung KB, Park DW, Kim YH, et al. Stents versus coronary-artery bypass grafting for left main coronary artery disease. *N Engl J Med* 2008;358:1781–92.

22. Ellis SG. Percutaneous left main intervention. An evolving perspective. *JACC Cardiovasc Interv* 2010;3:642–7.

23. Garg S, Stone GW, Kappetein AP, Sabik JF, Simonton C, Serruys PW. Clinical and angiographic risk assessment in patients with left main stem lesions. *JACC Cardiovasc Interv* 2010;3:891–901.

24. Sianos G, Morel MA, Kappetein AP, et al. The SYNTAX score: an angiographic tool grading the complexity of coronary artery disease. *Eurointervention* 2005;1:219–27.

25. Capodanno D, Capranzano P, Di Salvo ME, et al. Usefulness of SYNTAX score to select patients with left main coronary artery disease to be treated with coronary artery bypass graft. *JACC Cardiovasc Interv* 2009;2:731–8.

26. Roukoz H, Bavry AA, Sarkees ML, et al. Comprehensive meta-analysis on drug-eluting stents versus bare-metal stents during extended follow-up. *Am J Med* 2009; 122;581.e1–10.

27. Garg P, Cohen DJ, Gaziano T, Mauri L. Balancing the risks of restenosis and stent thrombosis in bare-metal versus drug-eluting stents. *J Am Coll Cardiol* 2008;51:1844–53.

28. Grines CL, Bonow RO, Casey DE Jr, et al. Prevention of premature discontinuation of dual antiplatelet therapy in patients with coronary artery stents: a science advisory from the American Heart Association, American College of Cardiology, Society for Cardiovascular Angiography and Interventions, American College of Surgeons, and American Dental Association, with representation from the American College of Physicians. *Circulation* 2007;115:813–8 and *J Am Coll Cardiol* 2007;49:734–9.

29. Byrne JG, Leacche M, Vaughan DE, Zhao DX. Hybrid cardiovascular procedures. *JACC Cardiovasc Interv* 2008;1:459–68.

30. Hholzey DM, Jacobs S, Mochalski M, et al, Minimally invasive hybrid coronary artery revascularization. *Ann Thorac Surg* 2008;86:1856–60.

31. Society of Thoracic Surgeons Blood Conservation Task Force, Ferraris VA, Ferraris SP, Saha SP, et al. Perioperative blood transfusion and blood conservation in cardiac surgery: the Society of Thoracic Surgeons and the Society of Cardiovascular Anesthesiologists clinical practice guideline. *Ann Thorac Surg* 2007;83(5 suppl):S27–86.

32. Bell ML, Grunwald GK, Baltz JH, et al. Does preoperative hemoglobin independently predict short-term outcomes after coronary artery bypass surgery? *Ann Thorac Surg* 2008;86:1415–23.

33. Kuduvalli M, Oo AY, Newall N, et al. Effect of peri-operative red blood cell transfusion on 30-day and 1-year mortality following coronary artery bypass surgery. *Eur J Cardiothorac Surg* 2005;27:592–8.

34. Scott BH, Seifert FC, Grimson R. Blood transfusion is associated with increased resource utilisation, morbidity and mortality in cardiac surgery. *Ann Card Anaesth* 2008;11:15–9.

35. Spiess BD. Choose one: damned if you do/damned if you don't! *Crit Care Med* 2005;33:1871–3.

36. Ereth MH, Nuttall GA, Orszulak TA, Santrach PJ, Cooney WP IV, Oliver WC Jr. Blood loss from coronary angiography increases transfusion requirements for coronary artery bypass graft surgery. *J Cardiothorac Vasc Anesth* 2000;14:177–81.

37. Karkouti K, Beattie WS, Wijeysundera DN, et al. Hemodilution during cardiopulmonary bypass is an independent risk factor for acute renal failure in adult cardiac surgery. *J Thorac Cardiovasc Surg* 2005;129:391–400.

38. Karkouti K. Djaiani G, Borger MA, et al. Low hematocrit during cardiopulmonary bypass is associated with increased risk of perioperative stroke in cardiac surgery. *Ann Thorac Surg* 2005;80:1381–7.

39. DeFoe GR, Ross CS, Olmstead EM, et al. Lowest hematocrit on bypass and adverse outcomes associated with coronary artery bypass grafting. Northern New England Cardiovascular Disease Study Group. *Ann Thorac Surg* 2001;71:769–76.

40. Kalyani SD, Miller NR, Dong LM, Baumgartner WA, Alejo DE, Gilbert TB. Incidence of and risk factors for perioperative optic neuropathy after cardiac surgery. *Ann Thorac Surg* 2004;78:34–7.

41. Ferguson TB, Coombs LP, Peterson ED. Preoperative beta-blocker use and mortality and morbidity following CABG surgery in North America. *JAMA* 2002;287:2221–7.

42. Warkentin TE, Greinacher A, Koster A, Lincoff AM. Treatment and prevention of heparin-induced thrombocytopenia. American College of Chest Physicians evidence-based clinical practice guidelines (8th edition). *Chest* 2009;133:340S–80S.

43. Gibbs NM, Weightman WM, Thackray NM, Michalopoulos N, Weidmann C. The effects of recent aspirin ingestion on platelet function in cardiac surgical patients. *J Cardiothorac Vasc Anesth* 2001;15:55–9.

44. Ferraris VA, Ferraris SP, Moliterno DJ, et al. The Society of Thoracic Surgeons practice guidelines series: aspirin and other antiplatelet agents during operative coronary revascularization (executive summary). *Ann Thorac Surg* 2005;79:1454–61.

45. Bybee KA, Powell BD, Valeti U, et al. Preoperative aspirin therapy is associated with improved postoperative outcomes in patients undergoing coronary artery bypass grafting. *Circulation* 2005; 112(9 Suppl):I-286–92.

46. Sun JC, Whitlock R, Cheng J, et al. The effect of pre-operative aspirin on bleeding, transfusion, myocardial infarction, and mortality in coronary artery bypass surgery: a systematic review of randomized and observational studies. *Eur Heart J* 2008;29:1057–71.

47. Mahla E, Metzler H, Tantry US, Gurbel PA. Controversies in oral antiplatelet therapy in patients undergoing aortocoronary bypass surgery. *Ann Thorac Surg* 2010; 90:1040–51.

48. Aranki SF, Body SC. Antiplatelet agents used for early intervention in acute coronary syndrome: myocardial salvage versus bleeding complications. *J Thorac Cardiovasc Surg* 2009;138:807–10.

49. Maltais S, Perrault LP, Do QB. Effect of clopidogrel on bleeding and transfusions after off-pump coronary artery bypass graft surgery: impact of discontinuation prior to surgery. *Eur J Cardiothorac Surg* 2008;34:127–31.

50. Mitchell LB, Exner DV, Wyse DG, et al. Prophylactic oral amiodarone for the prevention of arrhythmias that begin early after revascularization, valve replacement or repair: PAPABEAR: a randomized controlled trial. *JAMA* 2005;294:3093–100.

51. Kourliouros A, De Souza A, Roberts N, et al. Dose-related effect of statins on atrial fibrillation after cardiac surgery. *Ann Thorac Surg* 2008;85:1515–20.

52. Liakopoulos OJ, Choi YH, Kuhn EW, et al. Statins for prevention of atrial fibrillation after cardiac surgery: a systematic literature review. *J Thorac Cardiovasc Surg* 2009;138:678–86.

53. Liakopoulos OJ, Choi YH, Haldenwang PL, et al. Impact of preoperative statin therapy on adverse postoperative outcomes in patients undergoing cardiac surgery: a meta-analysis of over 30,000 patients. *Eur Heart J* 2008;29:1548–59.

54. Whitlock RP, Chan S, Devereaux PJ, et al. Clinical benefit of steroid use in patients undergoing cardiopulmonary bypass: a meta-analysis of randomized trials. *Eur Heart J* 2008;29:2592–600.

55. Liakopoulos OJ, Schmitto JD, Kazmaier S, et al. Cardiopulmonary and systemic effects of methylprednisolone in patients undergoing cardiac surgery. *Ann Thorac Surg* 2007;84:110–9.

56. Halonen J, Halonon P, Jarvinen O, et al. Corticosteroids for the prevention of atrial fibrillation after cardiac surgery. A randomized controlled trial. *JAMA* 2007;297:1562–7.

57. Morariu AM, Loef BG, Aarts LP, et al. Dexamethasone benefit and prejudice for patients undergoing on-pump coronary artery bypass grafting: a study on myocardial, pulmonary, renal, intestinal, and hepatic injury. *Chest* 2005;128:2677–87.

58. Ouzounian M, Hassan A, Buth KJ, et al. Impact of endoscopic versus open saphenous vein harvest techniques on outcomes after coronary artery bypass grafting. *Ann Thorac Surg* 2010;89:403–9.

59. Lopes RD, Hafley GE, Allen KB, et al. Endoscopic versus open vein-graft harvesting in coronary-artery bypass surgery. *N Engl J Med* 2009;361:235–44.

60. Rousou LJ, Taylor KB, Lu XG, et al. Saphenous vein conduits harvested by endoscopic technique exhibit structural and functional damage. *Ann Thorac Surg* 2009;87:62–70.

61. Zacharias A, Schwann TA, Riordan CJ, Durham SJ, Shah AS, Habib RH. Late results of conventional versus all-arterial revascularization based on internal thoracic and radial artery grafting. *Ann Thorac Surg* 2009;87:19–26.

62. Tatoulis J, Buxton BF, Fuller JA, et al. Long-term patency of 1108 radial arterial-coronary angiograms over 10 years. *Ann Thorac Surg* 2009;88:23–30.

63. Nasso G, Coppola R, Bonifazi R, Piancone F, Bozzetti G, Speziale G. Arterial revascularization in primary coronary artery bypass grafting: direct comparison of 4 strategies – results of the Stand-in-Y mammary study. *J Thorac Cardiovasc Surg* 2009;137:1093–100.

64. Carrier M, Cossette M, Pellerin M, et al. Statin treatment equalizes long-term survival between patients with single and bilateral internal thoracic artery grafts. *Ann Thorac Surg* 2009;88:789–95.

65. Vuković PM, Radak SS, Perić MS, Nežić DG, Knezević AM. Radial artery harvesting for coronary artery bypass grafting: a stepwise-made decision. *Ann Thorac Surg* 2008;86:828–31.

66. Reyes AT, Frame R, Brodman RF. Technique for harvesting the radial artery as a coronary artery bypass graft. *Ann Thorac Surg* 1995;59:118–26.

67. Connolly MW, Torrillo LD, Stauder MJ, et al. Endoscopic radial artery harvesting: results of the first 300 patients. *Ann Thorac Surg* 2002;74:502–5.

68. Attaran S, John L, El-Gamel A. Clinical and potential use of pharmacological agents to reduce radial artery spasm in coronary artery surgery. *Ann Thorac Surg* 2008;85:1483–9.

69. Bergsland J, Lingaas PS, Skulstad H, et al. Intracoronary shunt prevents ischemia in off-pump coronary artery bypass surgery. *Ann Thorac Surg* 2009;87:54–61.

70. Sellke FW, DiMaio JM, Caplan LR, et al. Comparing on-pump and off-pump coronary artery bypass grafting: numerous studies but few conclusions: a scientific statement from the American Heart Association council on cardiovascular surgery and anesthesia in collaboration with the interdisciplinary working group on quality of care and outcomes research. *Circulation* 2005;111:2858–64.

71. Puskas JD, Kilgo PD, Lattouf OM, et al. Off-pump coronary bypass provides reduced mortality and morbidity and equivalent 10-year survival. *Ann Thorac Surg* 2008;86:1139–46.

72. Møller CH, Penninga L, Wetterslev J, Steinbrüchel DA, Gluud C. Clinical outcomes in randomized trials of off- vs. on-pump coronary artery bypass surgery: systematic review with meta-analyses and trial sequential analyses. *Eur Heart J* 2008;29:2601–16.

73. Chu D, Bakaeen FG, Dao TK, LeMaire SA, Coselli JS, Huh J. On-pump versus off-pump coronary artery bypass grafting in a cohort of 63,000 patients. *Ann Thorac Surg* 2009;87:1820–7.

74. Holzhey DM, Jacobs S, Mochalski M, et al. Seven-year follow-up after minimally invasive direct coronary artery bypass: experience with more than 1300 patients. *Ann Thorac Surg* 2007;83:108–14.

75. Bonatti J, Schachner T, Bonaros N, et al. How to improve performance of robotic totally endoscopic coronary artery bypass grafting. *Am J Surg* 2008;195:711–6.

76. Bridges CR, Horvath KA, Nugent WC, et al. The Society of Thoracic Surgeons practice guideline series: transmyocardial laser revascularization. *Ann Thorac Surg* 2004;77:1494–502.

77. Shapira OM, Davidoff R, Hilkert RJ, Aldea GS, Fitzgerald CA, Shemin RJ. Repair of left ventricular aneurysm: long-term results of linear repair versus endoaneurysmorrhaphy. *Ann Thorac Surg* 1997;63:701–5.

78. Dor V, Di Donato M, Sabatier M, Montiglio F, Civaia F; RESTORE group. Left ventricular reconstruction by endoventricular circular patch plasty repair: a 17-year experience. *Semin Thorac Cardiovasc Surg* 2001;13:435–7.

79. Athanasuleas C, Buckberg GD, Stanley AW, et al. Surgical ventricular restoration in the treatment of congestive heart failure due to post-infarction ventricular dilatation. *J Am Coll Cardiol* 2004;44:1439–45.

80. Di Donato M, Castelvecchio S, Kukulski T, et al. Surgical ventricular restoration: left ventricular shape influence on cardiac function, clinical status, and survival. *Ann Thorac Surg* 2009;87:455–62.

81. Dzemali O, Risteski P, Bakhtiary F, et al. Surgical ventricular remodeling leads to better long-term survival and exercise tolerance than coronary artery bypass grafting alone in patients with moderate ischemic cardiomyopathy. *J Thorac Cardiovasc Surg* 2009;138:663–8.

82. Jones RH, Velazquez EJ, Michler RE, et al. Coronary bypass surgery with or without surgical ventricular reconstruction. *N Engl J Med* 2009;360:1705–17.

83. Birnbaum Y, Fishbein MC, Blanche C, Siegel RJ. Ventricular septal rupture after acute myocardial infarction. *N Engl J Med* 2002;347:1426–32.

84. Poulsen SH, Praestholm M, Munk K, Wierup P, Egeblad H, Nielsen-Kudsk JE. Ventricular septal rupture complicating acute myocardial infarction: clinical characteristics and contemporary outcome. *Ann Thorac Surg* 2008;85:1591–6.

85. Lundblad R, Abdelnoor M, Geiran OR, Svennevig JL. Surgical repair of postinfarction ventricular septal rupture: risk factors of early and late death. *J Thorac Cardiovasc Surg* 2009;137:862–8.

86. David TE, Armstrong S. Surgical repair of postinfarction ventricular septal defect by infarct exclusion. *Semin Thorac Cardiovasc Surg* 1998;10:105–10.

87. Muehrcke DD, Daggett WM Jr, Buckley MJ, Akins CW, Hilgenberg AD, Austen WG. Postinfarct ventricular septal defect repair: effect of coronary artery bypass grafting. *Ann Thorac Surg* 1992;54:876–83.

88. Bonow RO, Carabello BA, Chatterjee K, et al. 2008 focused update incorporated into the ACC/ AHA 2006 guidelines for the management of patients with valvular heart disease. A report of the American College of Cardiology/American Heart Association task force on practice guidelines (Writing committee to revise the 1998 guidelines for the management of patients with valvular heart disease). Endorsed by the Society of Cardiovascular Anesthesiologists, Society for Cardiovascular Angiography and Interventions, and Society of Thoracic Surgeons. *J Am Coll Cardiol* 2008;52:1–142 (available at www.acc.org).

89. Cowell SJ, Newby DE, Prescott RJ, et al. A randomized trial of intensive lipid-lowering in calcific aortic stenosis. *N Engl J Med* 2005;352:2389–97.

90. Rossebø AB, Pedersen TR, Boman K, et al. Intensive lipid lowering with simvastatin and ezetimibe in aortic stenosis. *N Engl J Med* 2008;359:1343–56.

91. Antonini-Canterin F, Leiballi E, Enache R, et al. Hydroxymethylglutaryl coenzyme-A reductase inhibitors delay the progression of rheumatic aortic valve stenosis. A long-term echocardiographic study. *J Am Coll Cardiol* 2009;53:1874–9.

92. Bartunek J, Sys SU, Rodrigues AC, Scheurbeeck EV, Mortier L, de Bruyne B. Abnormal systolic intracavity flow velocities after valve replacement for aortic stenosis. Mechanisms, predictive factors, and prognostic significance. *Circulation* 1996;93:712–9.

93. Omran H, Schmidt H, Hackenbroch M, et al. Silent and apparent cerebral embolism after retrograde catheterisation of the aortic valve in valvular stenosis: a prospective, randomised study. *Lancet* 2003;361:1241–6.

94. Levy F, Laurent M, Monin JL. et al. Aortic valve replacement for low-flow/low-gradient aortic stenosis. Operative risk stratification and long-term outcome: a European Multicenter study. *J Am Coll Cardiol* 2008;51:1466–72.

95. Tribouilloy C, Lévy F, Rusinaru D, et al. Outcome after aortic valve replacement for low-flow/low-gradient aortic stenosis without contractile reserve on dobutamine stress echocardiography. *J Am Coll Cardiol* 2009;53:1865–73.

96. Bergler-Klein J, Mundigler G, Pibarot P, et al. B-type natriuretic peptide in low-flow, low-gradient aortic stenosis: relationship to hemodynamics and clinical outcome: results from the Multicenter Truly or Pseudo-Severe Aortic Stenosis (TOPAS) study. *Circulation* 2007;115:2848–55.

97. Horstkotte D, Loogen F. The natural history of aortic valve stenosis. *Eur Heart J* 1988;9Suppl E:57–64.

98. Dal-Bianco JP, Khandheria BK, Mookadam R, Gentile F, Sengupta P.P. Management of asymptomatic severe aortic stenosis. *J Am Coll Cardiol* 2008;52:1279–92.

99. Brown ML, Pellikka PA, Schaff HV, et al. The benefits of early valve replacement in asymptomatic patients with severe aortic stenosis. *J Thorac Cardiovasc Surg* 2008;135:308–15.

100. Pellikka PA, Nishimura RA, Bailey KR, Tajik AJ. The natural history of adults with asymptomatic, hemodynamically significant aortic stenosis. *J Am Coll Cardiol* 1990;15:1012–7.

101. Pellikka PA, Sarano ME, Nishimura RA, et al. Outcome of 622 adults with asymptomatic, hemodynamically significant aortic stenosis during prolonged follow-up. *Circulation* 2005;111:3290–5.

102. Brown ML, McKellar SH, Sundt TM, Schaff HV. Ministernotomy versus conventional sternotomy for aortic valve replacement: systematic review and meta-analysis. *J Thorac Cardiovasc Surg* 2009;137:670–9.

103. Plass A, Scheffel H, Alkadhi H, et al. Aortic valve replacement through a minimally invasive approach: preoperative planning, surgical technique, and outcome. *Ann Thorac Surg* 2009;88:1851–6.

104. Ennker JAC, Albert AA, Rosendahl UP, Ennker IC, Dalladaku F, Florath I. Ten-year experience with stentless aortic valves: full-root versus subcoronary implantation. *Ann Thorac Surg* 2008;85:445–53.

105. de Kerchove L, Rubay J, Pasquet A, et al. Ross operation in the adult: long-term outcomes after root replacement and inclusion techniques. *Ann Thorac Surg* 2009;87:95–102.

106. Grinda JM, Mainardi JL, D'Attellis N, et al. Cryopreserved aortic viable homograft for active aortic endocarditis. *Ann Thorac Surg* 2005;79:767–71.

107. Gulbins H, Kilian E, Roth S, Uhlig A, Kreuzer E, Reichart B. Is there an advantage in using homografts in patients with acute infective endocarditis of the aortic valve? *J Heart Valve Dis* 2002;11:492–7.

108. Avierinos JF, Thuny F, Chalvignac V, et al. Surgical treatment of active aortic endocarditis: homografts are not the cornerstone of outcome. *Ann Thorac Surg* 2007;84:1935–42.

109. Gaudino M, De Filippo C, Pennestri F, Possati G. The use of mechanical prostheses in native aortic valve endocarditis. *J Heart Valve Dis* 1997;6:79–83.

110. Mataraci I, Polat A, Kiran B, et al. Long-term results of aortic root replacement: 15 years' experience. *Ann Thorac Surg* 2009;87:1783–8.

111. Walther T, Dewey T, Borger MA, et al. Transapical aortic valve implantation: step by step. *Ann Thorac Surg* 2009;87:276–83.

112. Wong DR, Ye J, Cheung A, Webb JG, Carere RG, Lichtenstein SV. Technical considerations to avoid pitfalls during transapical aortic valve implantation. *J Thorac Cardiovasc Surg* 2010;140:196–202.

113. Masson JB, Kovac J, Schuler G, et al. Transcatheter aortic valve implantation. Review of the nature, management, and avoidance of procedural complications. *JACC Cardiovasc Interv* 2009;2:811–20.

114. Al-Attar N, Ghodbane W, Himbert D, et al. Unexpected complications of transapical aortic valve implantation. *Ann Thorac Surg* 2009;88:90–4.

115. Zajarias A, Cribier AG. Outcomes and safety of percutaneous aortic valve replacement. *J Am Coll Cardiol* 2009;53:1829–36.

116. Clavel MA, Webb JG, Pibarot P, et al. Comparison of the hemodynamic performance of percutaneous and surgical bioprostheses for the treatment of severe aortic stenosis. *J Am Coll Cardiol* 2009;53:1883–91.

117. Pettersson GB, Crucean AC, Savage R, et al. Toward predictable repair of regurgitant aortic valves. A systematic morphology-directed approach to bicommissural repair. *J Am Coll Cardiol* 2008;52:40–9.

118. Tabata M, Takayama H, Bowdish ME, Smith CR, Stewart AS. Modified Bentall operation with bioprosthetic valved conduit: Columbia University experience. *Ann Thorac Surg* 2009;87:1969–70.

119. Etz CD, Homann TM, Rane N, et al. Aortic root reconstruction with a bioprosthetic valved conduit: a consecutive series of 275 procedures. *J Thorac Cardiovasc Surg* 2007;133:1455–63.

120. Zannis K, Deux JF, Tzvetkov B, et al. Composite Freestyle stentless xenograft with Dacron graft extension for ascending aortic replacement. *Ann Thorac Surg* 2009;87:1789–94.

121. Boodhwani M, de Kerchove L, El Khoury G. Aortic root replacement using the reimplantation technique: tips and tricks. *Interact Cardiovasc Thorac Surg* 2009;8:584–6.

122. Sareyyupoglu B, Suri RM, Schaff HV, et al. Survival and reoperation risk following bicuspid aortic-valve sparing root replacement. *J Heart Valve Dis* 2009;18:1–8.

123. David TE, Armstrong S, Maganti M, Colman J, Bradley TJ. Long-term results of aortic valve-sparing operations in patients with Marfan syndrome. *J Thorac Cardiovasc Surg* 2009;138:859–64.

124. Wilkins GT, Weyman AE, Abascal VM, Block PC, Palacios IF. Percutaneous balloon dilatation of the mitral valve: an analysis of echocardiographic variables related to outcome and the mechanism of dilatation. *Br Heart J* 1988;60:299–308.

125. Song JK, Kim MJ, Yun SC, et al. Long-term outcome of percutaneous mitral balloon valvuloplasty versus open cardiac surgery. *J Thorac Cardiovasc Surg* 2010;139:103–10.

126. Kim JB, Yun TJ, Chung CH, Choo SJ, Hong H, Lee JW. Long-term outcome of modified maze procedure combined with mitral valve surgery: analysis of outcomes according to type of mitral valve surgery. *J Thorac Cardiovasc Surg* 2010;139:111–7.

127. Halkos ME, Craver JM, Thourani VH, et al. Intraoperative radiofrequency ablation for the treatment of atrial fibrillation during concomitant cardiac surgery. *Ann Thorac Surg* 2005;80:210–6.

128. Jahangiri M, Weir G, Mandal K, Savelieva I, Camm J. Current strategies in the management of atrial fibrillation. *Ann Thorac Surg* 2006;82:35–64.

129. Raja SG, Dreyfus GD. Surgery for functional tricuspid regurgitation: current techniques, outcomes, and emerging concepts. *Expert Rev Cardiovasc Ther* 2009;7:73–84.

130. Matsumaya K, Matsumoto M, Sugita T, Nishizawa J, Tokuda Y, Matsuo T. Predictors of residual tricuspid regurgitation after mitral valve surgery. *Ann Thorac Surg* 2003;75:1826–8.

131. Anyanwu AC, Chikwe J. Adams DH. Tricuspid valve repair for treatment and prevention of secondary tricuspid regurgitation in patients undergoing mitral valve surgery. *Curr Cardiol Rep* 2008;10:110–7.

132. Chan V, Burwash IG, Lam BK, et al. Clinical and echocardiographic impact of functional tricuspid regurgitation repair at the time of mitral valve replacement. *Ann Thorac Surg* 2009;88:1209–15.

133. Carabello BA. The current therapy for mitral regurgitation. *J Am Coll Cardiol* 2008;52:319–26.

134. Chua YL, Schaff HV, Orszulak TA, Morris JJ. Outcome of mitral valve repair in patients with preoperative atrial fibrillation: should the maze procedure be combined with mitral valvuloplasty? *J Thorac Cardiovasc Surg* 1994;107:408–15.

135. Bando K, Kasegawa H, Okada Y, et al, Impact of preoperative and postoperative atrial fibrillation on outcome after mitral valvuloplasty for nonischemic mitral regurgitation. *J Thorac Cardiovasc Surg* 2005;129:1032–40.

136. Marui A, Saji Y, Nishina T, et al. Impact of left atrial reduction concomitant with atrial fibrillation surgery on left atrial geometry and mechanical function. *J Thorac Cardiovasc Surg* 2008;135:1297–305.

137. Di Donato M, Frigiola A, Menicanti L, et al. Moderate ischemic mitral regurgitation and coronary artery bypass surgery: effect of mitral repair on clinical outcome. *J Heart Valve Dis* 2003;12:272–9.

138. Paparella D, Mickleborough LL, Carson S, Ivanov J. Mild to moderate mitral regurgitation in patients undergoing coronary bypass grafting: effects on operative mortality and long-term significance. *Ann Thorac Surg* 2003;76:1094–100.

139. Wan CKN, Suri RM, Li Z, et al. Management of moderate functional mitral regurgitation at the time of aortic valve replacement: is concomitant mitral valve repair necessary? *J Thorac Cardiovasc Surg* 2009;137:635–40.

140. Waisbren EC, Stevens LM, Avery EG, Picard MH, Vlahakes GJ, Agnihotri AK. Changes in mitral regurgitation after replacement of the stenotic aortic valve. *Ann Thorac Surg* 2008;86:56–63.

141. Gillinov AM, Blackstone EH, Nowicki ER, et al. Valve repair versus valve replacement for degenerative mitral valve disease. *J Thorac Cardiovasc Surg* 2008;135:885–93.

142. Gillinov AM, Blackstone EH, Alaulaqi A, et al. Outcomes after repair of the anterior mitral leaflet for degenerative disease. *Ann Thorac Surg* 2008;86:708–17.

143. Shimokawa T, Kasegawa H, Matsuyama S, et al. Long-term outcome of mitral valve repair for infective endocarditis. *Ann Thorac Surg* 2009;88:733–9.

144. de Kerchove L, Vanoverschiede JL, Poncelet A, et al. Reconstructive surgery in active mitral valve endocarditis: feasibility, safety and durability. *Eur J Cardiothorac Surg* 2007;31:592–9.

145. Shang E, Forrest GN, Chizmar T, et al. Mitral valve infective endocarditis: benefit of early operation and aggressive use of repair. *Ann Thorac Surg* 2009;87:1728–34.

146. Gillinov AM, Faber C, Houghtaling PL, et al. Repair versus replacement for degenerative mitral valve disease with coexisting ischemic heart disease. *J Thorac Cardiovasc Surg* 2003;125:1350–62.

147. Borger MA, Alam A, Murphy PM, Doenst T, David TE. Chronic ischemic mitral regurgitation: repair, replace or rethink? *Ann Thorac Surg* 2006;81:1153–61.

148. Gillinov AM, Wierup PN, Blackstone EH, et al. Is repair preferable to replacement for ischemic mitral regurgitation? *J Thorac Cardiovasc Surg* 2001;122:1125–41.

149. Suri RM, Schaff HV, Meyer SR, Hargrove WC III. Thoracoscopic versus open mitral valve repair: a propensity score analysis of early outcomes. *Ann Thorac Surg* 2009;88:1185–90.

150. Modi P, Rodriguez E, Hargrove WC III, Hassan A, Szeto WY, Chitwood WR Jr. Minimally invasive video-assisted mitral valve surgery: a 12-year 2-center experience in 1178 patients. *J Thorac Cardiovasc Surg* 2009;137:1481–7.

151. Modi P, Hassan A, Chitwood WR Jr. Minimally invasive mitral valve surgery: a systematic review and meta-analysis. *Eur J Cardiothorac Surg* 2008;34:943–52.

152. Chitwood WR Jr, Rodriguez E, Chu MW, et al. Robotic mitral valve repair in 300 patients: a single-center experience. *J Thorac Cardiovasc Surg* 2008;136:436–41.

153. Shah PM, Raney A. Tricuspid valve disease. *Cur Probl Cardiol* 2008;33:47–84.

154. Rivera R, Duran E, Ajuria M. Carpentier's flexible ring versus De Vega's annuloplasty.a prospective randomized study. *J Thorac Cardiovasc Surg* 1985;89:196–203.

155. Filsoufi F, Anyanwu AC, Salzberg SP, Frankel T, Cohn LH, Adams DH. Long-term outcome of tricuspid valve replacement in the current era. *Ann Thorac Surg* 2005;80:845–50.

156. Iscan ZH, Vural KM, Bahar I, Mavioglu L, Saritas A. What to expect after tricuspid valve replacement? Long-term results. *Eur J Cardiothorac Surg* 2007;32:296–300.

157. Civelek A, Ak K, Akgün S, Isbir SC, Arsan S. Tricuspid valve replacement: an analysis of risk factors and outcomes. *Thorac Cardiovasc Surg* 2008;56:456–60.

158. Moraca RJ, Moon MR, Lawton JS, et al. Outcomes of tricuspid valve repair and replacement: a propensity analysis. *Ann Thorac Surg* 2009;87:83–9.

159. Jokinen JJ, Turpeinen AK, Pitkänen O, Hippeläinen MJ, Hartikainen JEK. Pacemaker therapy after tricuspid valve operations: implications on mortality, morbidity, and quality of life. *Ann Thorac Surg* 2009;87:1806–15.

160. Carozza A, De Santo LS, Romano G, et al. Infective endocarditis in intravenous drug abusers: patterns of presentation and long-term outcomes of surgical treatment. *J Heart Valve Dis* 2006;15:125–31.

161. Hill EE, Herrogods MC, Vanderschueren S, Claus P, Peetermans WE, Herijgers P. Outcome of patients requiring valve surgery during active infective endocarditis. *Ann Thorac Surg* 2008;85:1564–9.

162. Vilacosta I, Grampner C, San Roman A, et al. Risk of embolization after institution of antibiotic therapy for infective endocarditis. *J Am Coll Cardiol* 2002;39:1489–95.

163. Dickerman SA, Abrutyn E, Barsic B, et al. The relationship between the initiation of antimicrobial therapy and the incidence of stroke in infective endocarditis: analysis from the ICE prospective cohort study (ICS-PCS). *Am Heart J* 2007;154:1086–94.

164. Vlessis AA, Khaki A, Grunkemeier GL, Li HH, Starr A. Risk, diagnosis, and management of prosthetic valve endocarditis: a review. *J Heart Valve Disease* 1997;6:443–65.

165. Eishi K, Kawazoe K, Kuriyama Y, Kitoh Y, Kawashima Y, Omae T. Surgical management of infective endocarditis associated with cerebral complications: multi-center retrospective study in Japan. *J Thorac Cardiovasc Surg* 1995;110:1745–55.

166. Gillinov AM, Shah RV, Curtis WE, et al. Valve replacement in patients with endocarditis and acute neurologic deficit. *Ann Thorac Surg* 1996;61:1125–9.

167. Parrino PE, Kron IL, Ross SD, et al. Does a focal neurologic deficit contraindicate operation in a patient with endocarditis? *Ann Thorac Surg* 1999;67:59–64.

168. Piper C, Wiemer M, Schulte HD, Hortskotte D. Stroke is not a contraindication for urgent valve replacement in acute infective endocarditis. *J Heart Valve Dis* 2001;10:703–11.

169. Ruttmann E, Willeit J, Ulmer H, et al. Neurological outcome of septic cardioembolic stroke after infective endocarditis. *Stroke* 2006;37:2094–9.

170. Miró JM, Moreno A, Mestres CA. Infective endocarditis in intravenous drug abusers. *Curr Infect Dis Rep* 2003;5:307–16.

171. Carozza A, Renzulli A, De Feo M, et al. Tricuspid repair for infective endocarditis. Clinical and echocardiographic results. *Tex Heart Inst J* 2001;28:96–101.

172. Arbulu A, Holmes RJ, Asfaw I. Tricuspid valvulectomy without replacement. Twenty years' clinical experience. *J Thorac Cardiovasc Surg* 1991;102:917–22.

173. Maron BJ, McKenna WJ, Danielson GK, et al. American College of Cardiology/European Society of Cardiology Clinical Expert Consensus Document on Hypertrophic Cardiomyopathy. A report of the American College of Cardiology Foundation Task Force on Clinical Expert Consensus Documents and the European Society of Cardiology Committee for Practice Guidelines. *J Am Coll Cardiol* 2003;42:1687–713.

174. Marian AJ. Contemporary treatment of hypertrophic cardiomyopathy. *Tex Heart Inst J* 2009;36:194–204.

175. Sherrid MV, Chaudhry FA, Swistel DG. Obstructive hypertrophic cardiomyopathy: echocardiography, pathophysiology, and the continuing evolution of surgery for obstruction. *Ann Thorac Surg* 2003;75:620–32.

176. Maron BJ, Spirito P, Shen WK, et al. Implantable cardioverter-defibrillator and prevention of sudden cardiac death in hypertrophic cardiomoyopathy. *JAMA* 2007;298:405–12.

177. Galve E, Sambola A, Saldaña G, et al. Late benefits of dual-chamber pacing in obstructive hypertrophic cardiomyopathy. A 10-year follow-up study. *Heart* 2010;96:352–6.

178. Rinaldi CA, Bucknall CA, Gill JS. Beneficial effects of biventricular pacing in a patient with hypertrophic cardiomyopathy and intraventricular conduction delay, *Heart* 2002;87:e6.

179. Komsuoglu B, Vural A, Agacdiken A, Ural D. Effect of biventricular pacing on left ventricular outflow tract pressure gradient with hypertrophic cardiomyopathy and normal interventricular conduction. *J Cardiovasc Electrophysiol* 2006;17:207–9.

180. Agarwal S, Tuzcu EM, Desai MY, et al. Updated meta-analysis of septal alcohol ablation versus myectomy for hypertrophic cardiomyopathy. *J Am Coll Cardiol* 2010;55:823–34.

181. Ralph-Edwards A, Woo A, McCrindle BW, et al. Hypertropic cardiomyopathy: comparison of outcomes after myectomy or alcohol ablation adjusted by propensity score. *J Thorac Cardiovasc Surg* 2005;129:351–8.

182. Dearani JA, Ommen SR, Gersh BJ, Schaff HV, Danielson GK. Surgical insight: septal myectomy for obstructive hypertrophic cardiomyopathy – the Mayo Clinic experience. *Nat Clin Pract Cardiovasc Med* 2007;4:503–12.

183. Smedira NG, Lytle BW, Lever HM, et al. Current effectiveness and risks of isolated septal myectomy for hypertrophic obstructive cardiomyopathy. *Ann Thorac Surg* 2008;85:127–33.

184. Minakata K, Dearani JA, Schaff HV, O'Leary PW, Ommen SR, Danielson GK. Mechanisms for recurrent left ventricular outflow tract obstruction after septal myectomy for obstructive hypertrophic cardiomyopathy. *Ann Thorac Surg* 2005;80:851–6.

185. Minakata K, Dearani JA, Nishimura RA, Maron BJ, Danielson GK. Extended septal myectomy for hypertrophic obstructive cardiomyopathy with anomalous papillary muscles or chordae. *J Thorac Cardiovasc Surg* 2004;127:481–9.

186. Kaple RK, Murphy RT, DiPaola L.M. et al. Mitral valve abnormalities in hypertrophic cardiomyopathy: echocardiographic features and surgical outcomes. *Ann Thorac Surg* 2008; 85:1527–36.

187. Khan IA, Nair CK. Clinical, diagnostic, and management perspectives of aortic dissection. *Chest* 2002;122:311–28.

188. Golledge J, Eagle KA. Acute aortic dissection. *Lancet* 2008;372:55–66.

189. Hansen MS, Nogareda GJ, Hutchison FJ. Frequency of and inappropriate treatment of misdiagnosis of acute aortic dissection. *Am J Cardiol* 2007;99:852–6.

190. Hagan PG, Nienaber CA, Isselbacher EM, et al. The international registry of acute aortic dissection (IRAD). New insights into an old disease. *JAMA* 2000;283:897–903.

191. Trimarchi S, Nienaber C, Rampoldi V, et al. Contemporary results of surgery in acute type A dissection: the International Registry of Acute Aortic Dissection experience. *J Thorac Cardiovasc Surg* 2005;129:112–22.

192. Suzuki T, Distante A, Zizza A, et al. Diagnosis of acute aortic dissection by D-Dimer: the International Registry of Acute Aortic Dissection Substudy on Biomarkers (IRAD-Bio) experience. *Circulation* 2009;119:2702–7.

193. Paparella D, Malvindi PG, Scrascia G, et al. D-dimers are not always elevated in patients with acute dissection. *J Cardiovasc Med (Hagerstown)* 2009;10:212–4.

194. Patel HJ, Williams DM, Dasika NL, Suzuki Y, Deeb GM. Operative delay for peripheral malperfusion syndrome in acute type A aortic dissection: a long-term analysis. *J Thorac Cardiovasc Surg* 2008;135:1288–96.

195. Yagdi T, Atay Y, Engin C, et al. Impact of organ malperfusion on mortality and morbidity in acute type A aortic dissections. *J Card Surg* 2006;21:363–9.

196. Estera AL, Miller CC, Goodrick J, et al. Update on outcomes of acute type B aortic dissection. *Ann Thorac Surg* 2007;83:S842–5.

197. Trimarchi S, Nienaber CA, Rampoldi V, et al. Role and results of surgery in acute type B dissection. Insights from the International Registry of Acute Aortic Dissection (IRAD). *Circulation* 2006;114 (1 Suppl):I-357–64.

198. Umana JP, Lai DT, Mitchell RS, et al. Is medical therapy still the optimal treatment strategy for patients with acute type B aortic dissections? *J Thorc Cardiovasc Surg* 2002;124:896–910.

199. Kodama K, Nishigami K, Sakamoto T, et al. Tight heart rate control reduces secondary adverse events in patients with type B acute aortic dissection. *Circulation* 2008;118(14 Suppl): S167–70.

200. Kunishige H, Myojin K, Ishibashi Y, Ishii K, Kawasaki M, Oka J. Predictors of surgical indications for acute type B dissection based on enlargement of aortic diameter during the chronic phase. *Jpn J Thorac Cardiovasc Surg* 2006;54:477–82.

201. Song JM, Kim SD, Kim JH, et al. Long-term predictors of descending aorta aneurysmal change in patients with aortic dissection. *J Am Coll Cardiol* 2007;50:799–804.

202. Onitsuka S, Akashi H, Tayama K, et al. Long-term outcome and prognostic indicators of medically treated acute type B aortic dissections. *Ann Thorac Surg* 2004;78:1268–73.

203. Watanuki H, Ogino H, Minatoya K, et al. Is emergency total arch replacement with a modified elephant trunk technique justified for acute type A aortic dissection? *Ann Thorac Surg* 2007;84:1585–91.

204. Geirsson A, Szeto WY, Pochettino A, et al. Significance of malperfusion syndromes prior to contemporary surgical repair for acute type A dissection: outcomes and need for additional revascularization. *Eur J Cardiothorac Surg* 2007;32:255–62.

205. Hanafusa Y, Ogino H, Sasaki H, et al. Total arch replacement with elephant trunk procedure for retrograde dissection. *Ann Thorac Surg* 2002;74:S1836–9.

206. Sun L, Qi R, Chang Q, et al. Surgery for acute type A dissection with the tear in the descending aorta using a stented elephant trunk procedure. *Ann Thorac Surg* 2009;87:1177–81.

207. Dong ZH, Fu WG, Wang YQ, et al. Retrograde type A aortic dissection after endovascular stent graft placement for treatment of type B dissection. *Circulation* 2009;119:735–41.

208. Patel HJ, Williams DM, Meekov M, et al. Long-term results of percutaneous management of malperfusion in acute type B aortic dissection: implications for thoracic aortic endovascular repair. *J Thorac Cardiovasc Surg* 2009;138:300–8.

209. Feezor RJ, Martin TD, Hess PJ Jr, Beaver TM, Klodell CT, Lee WA. Early outcomes after endovascular management of acute complicated type B aortic dissection. *J Vasc Surg* 2009;49:561–6.

210. Parker JD, Golledge J. Outcome of endovascular treatement of acute type B aortic dissection. *Ann Thorac Surg* 2008;86:1707–12.

211. Szeto WY, McGarvey M, Pochettino A, et al. Results of a new surgical paradigm: endovascular repair for acute complicated type B aortic dissection. *Ann Thorac Surg* 2008;86:87–93.

212. Svensson LG, Kouchoukos NT, Miller DC. Expert consensus document on the treatment of descending thoracic aortic disease using endovascular stent-grafts. *Ann Thorac Surg* 2008;85:S1–41.

213. Parish LM, Gorman JH 3rd, Kahn S, et al. Aortic size in acute type A dissection: implications for preventive ascending aortic replacement. *Eur J Cardiothorac Surg* 2009;35:941–5.

214. Pape LA, Tsai TT, Isselbacher EM, et al. Aortic diameter >or = 5.5 cm is not a good predictor of type A aortic dissection: observations from the International Registry of Acute Aortic Dissection (IRAD). *Circulation* 2007;116:1120–7.

215. Elefteriades JA, Farkas EA. Thoracic aortic aneurysm. Clinically pertinent controversies and uncertainties. *J Am Coll Cardiol* 2010;55:841–57.

216. Prenger K, Pieters F, Cheriex E. Aortic dissection after valve replacement: incidence and consequences for strategy. *J Card Surg* 1994;9:495–8.

217. Fazel SS, Mallidi HR, Lee RS, et al. The aortopathy of bicuspid aortic valve disease has distinctive patterns and usually involves the transverse aortic arch. *J Thorac Cardiovasc Surg* 2008;135:901–7.

218. Etz CD, Homann TM, Silovitz D, et al,. Long-term survival after the Bentall procedure in 206 patients with bicuspid aortic valves. *Ann Thorac Surg* 2007;84:1186–93.

219. David TE, Ivanov J, Armstrong S, Feindel CM, Webb GD. Aortic valve-sparing operations in patients with aneurysms of the aortic root or ascending aorta. *Ann Thorac Surg* 2002;74:S1758–61.

220. Cameron DE, Alejo DE, Patel ND, et al. Aortic root replacement in 372 Marfan patients: evolution of operative repair over 30 years. *Ann Thorac Surg* 2009;87:1344–9.

221. Volguina IV, Miller DC, LeMaire SA, et al. Valve-sparing and valve-replacing techniques for aortic root replacement in patients with Marfan syndrome: analysis of early outcome. *J Thorac Cardiovasc Surg* 2009;137:1124–32.

222. Etz CD, Plestis KA, Kari FA, et al. Axillary cannulation significantly improves survival and neurologic outcome after atherosclerotic aneuruysm repair of the aortic root and ascending aorta. *Ann Thorac Surg* 2008;86:441–6.

223. Apostolakis E, Akinosoglou K. The methodologies of hypothermic circulatory arrest and of antegrade and retrograde cerebral perfusion for aortic arch surgery. *Ann Thorac Cardiovasc Surg* 2008;14:138–48.

224. Halkos ME, Kerendi F, Myung R, Kilgo P, Puskas JD, Chen EP. Selective antegrade cerebral perfusion via right axillary artery cannulation reduces morbidity and mortality after proximal aortic surgery. *J Thorac Cardiovasc Surg* 2009;138:1081–9.

225. Minatoya K, Ogino H, Matsuda H, et al. Evolving selective cerebral perfusion for aortic arch replacement: high flow rate with moderate hypothermic circulatory arrest. *Ann Thorac Surg* 2008;86:1827–31.

226. Strauch JT, Spielvogel D, Lauten A, et al. Technical advances in total aortic arch replacement. *Ann Thorac Surg* 2004;77:581–9.

227. Spielvogel D, Etz CD, Silovitz D, Lansman SL, Griepp RB. Aortic arch replacement with a trifurcated graft. *Ann Thorac Surg* 2007;83:S791–5.

228. Uchida N, Ishihara H, Sakashita M, Kanou M, Sumiyoshi T. Repair of the thoracic aorta by transaortic stent grafting (open stenting). *Ann Thorac Surg* 2002;73:444–9.

229. Etz CD, Plestis KA, Kari FA, et al. Staged repair of thoracic and thoracoabdominal aortic aneurysms using the elephant trunk technique: a consecutive series of 215 first stage and 120 complete repairs. *Eur J Cardiothorac Surg* 2008;34:605–14.

230. Estrera AL, Miller CC III, Chen EP, et al. Descending thoracic aortic aneurysm repair: a 12-year experience using distal aortic perfusion and cerebrospinal fluid drainage. *Ann Thorac Surg* 2005;80:1290–6.

231. Estrera AL, Sheinbaum R, Miller CC, et al. Cerebrospinal fluid drainage during thoracic aortic repair: safety and current management. *Ann Thorac Surg* 2009;88:9–15.

232. Coselli JS, LeMaire SA, Conklin LD, Adams GJ. Left heart bypass during descending thoracic aortic aneurysm repair does not reduce the incidence of paraplegia. *Ann Thorac Surg* 2004;77:1298–303.

233. Coselli JS, Lemaire SA, Koksoy C, Schmittling ZC, Curling PE. Cerebrospinal fluid drainage reduces paraplegia after thoracoabdominal aortic aneurysm repair: results of a randomized clinical trial. *J Vasc Surg* 2002;3:631–9.

234. Patel HJ, Sillingford MS, Mihalik S, Proctor MC, Deeb GM. Resection of the descending thoracic aorta: outcomes after use of hypothermic circulatory arrest. *Ann Thorac Surg* 2006;82:90–6.

235. Fehrenbacher JW, Hart DW, Huddleston E, Siderys H, Rice C. Optimal end-organ protection for thoracic and thoracoabdominal aneurysm repair using deep hypothermic circulatory arrest. *Ann Thorac Surg* 2007;83:1041–6.

236. Misfeld M, Sievers HH, Hadlak M, Gorski A, Hanke T. Rate of paraplegia and mortality in elective descending and thoracoabdominal aortic repair in the modern surgical era. *Thorac Cardiovasc Surg* 2008;56:342–7.

237. Bavaria JE, Appoo JJ, Makaroun MS, et al. Endovascular stent grafting versus open surgical repair of descending thoracic aortic aneurysms in low-risk patients: a multicenter comparative trial. *J Thorac Cardiovasc Surg* 2007;133:369–77.

238. Cheng D, Martin J, Shennib H, et al. Endovascular aortic repair versus open surgical repair for descending thoracic aortic disease. A systematic review and meta-analysis of comparative studies. *J Am Coll Cardiol* 2010;55:986–1001.

239. Hnath JC, Mehta M, Taggert JB, et al. Strategies to improve spinal cord ischemia in endovascular thoracic aortic repair: outcomes of a prospective cerebrospinal fluid drainage protocol. *J Vasc Surg* 2008;48:836–40.

240. Louagie Y, Buche M, Eucher P, et al. Improved patient survival with concomitant Cox Maze III procedure compared with heart surgery alone. *Ann Thorac Surg* 2009;87:440–7.

241. Saltman AE, Gillinov AM. Surgical approaches for atrial fibrillation. *Cardiol Clin* 2009;27:179–88.

242. Li H, Li Y, Sun L, et al. Minimally invasive surgical pulmonary vein isolation alone for persistent atrial fibrillation: preliminary results of epicardial atrial electrogram analysis. *Ann Thorac Surg* 2008;86:1219–26.

243. Edgerton JR, McClelland JH, Duke D, et al. Minimally invasive surgical ablation of atrial fibrillation: six-month results. *J Thorac Cardiovasc Surg* 2009;138:109–14.

244. Edgerton JR, Jackman WM, Mack MJ. A new epicardial lesion set for minimal access left atrial Maze: the Dallas lesion set. *Ann Thorac Surg* 2009;88:1655–7.

245. Gillinov AM. Choice of surgical lesion set: answers from the data. *Ann Thorac Surg* 2007;84:1786–92.

246. Voeller RK, Bailey MS, Zierer A, et al. Isolating the entire posterior left atrium improves surgical outcomes after the Cox maze procedure. *J Thorac Cardiovasc Surg* 2008;135:870–7.

247. Scherer M, Dzemali O, Aybek T, Wimer-Greinecker G, Moritz A. Impact of left atrial size reduction on chronic atrial fibrillation in mitral valve surgery. *J Heart Valve Dis* 2003;12:469–74.

248. Doll N, Pritzwald-Stegmann P, Czesla M, et al. Ablation of ganglionic plexi during combined surgery for atrial fibrillation. *Ann Thorac Surg* 2008;86:1659–63.

249. Tung R, Zimetbaum P, Josephson ME. A critical appraisal of implantable cardioverter-defibrillator therapy for the prevention of sudden cardiac death. *J Am Coll Cardiol* 2008;52:1111–21.

250. Epstein AE, DiMarco JP, Ellenbogen KA, et al. ACC/AHA/HRS 2008 guidelines for device-based therapy of cardiac rhythm abnormalities: executive summary. A report of the American College of Cardiology/American Heart Association task force on practice guidelines (Writing committee to revise the ACC/AHA/NASPE 2002 guideline update for implantation of cardiac pacemakers and antiarrhythmia devices). *J Am Coll Cardiol* 2008;51:2085–2105 (available at www.acc.org).

251. del Rio A Anguera I, Miro JM, et al. Surgical treatment of pacemaker and defibrillator lead endocarditis: the impact of electrode lead extraction on outcome. *Chest* 2003;124:1451–9.

252. Ngaage DL, Cale ARJ, Cowen ME, Griffin S, Guvendik L. Early and late survival after surgical revascularization for ischemic ventricular fibrillation/tachycardia. *Ann Thorac Surg* 2008;85:1278–82.

253. Ferguson TB Jr, Smith JM, Cox JL, Cain ME, Lindsay BD. Direct operation versus ICD therapy for ischemic ventricular tachycardia. *Ann Thorac Surg* 1994;58:1291–6.

254. Hunt SA, Abraham WT, Chin MH, et al. ACC/AHA 2005 guideline update for the diagnosis and management of chronic heart failure in the adult: summary article. A report of the American College of Cardiology/American Heart Association task force on practice guidelines (Writing committee to update the 2001 guidelines for the evaluation and management of heart failure). *J Am Coll Cardiol* 2005;46:1116–43.

255. Jessup M, Abraham WT, Casey DE, et al. 2009 Focused update: ACCF/AHA guidelines for the diagnosis and management of heart failure in adults. A report of the American College of Cardiology Foundation/American Heart Association task force on the practice guidelines in collaboration with the International Society for Heart and Lung Transplantation. *J Am Coll Cardiol* 2009;53:1343–82 (available at www.acc.org).

256. Nicolini F, Gherli T. Alternatives to transplantation in the surgical therapy for heart failure. *Eur J Cardiothorac Surg* 2009;35:214–28.

257. Pocar M, Moneta A, Grossi A, Donatelli F. Coronary artery bypass for heart failure in ischemic cardiomyopathy: a 17-year follow-up. *Ann Thorac Surg* 2007;83:468–74.

258. Maruskova M, Gregor P, Bartunek J, Tintera J, Penicka M. Myocardial viability and cardiac dyssynchrony as strong predictors of perioperative mortality in high-risk patients with ischemic cardiomyopathy having coronary artery bypass surgery. *J Thorac Cardiovasc Surg* 2009;138:62–8.

259. Di Salvo TG, Acker MA, Dec GW, Byrne JG. Mitral valve surgery in advanced heart failure. *J Am Coll Cardiol* 2010;55:271–82.

260. Gorman JH 3rd, Gorman RC. Mitral valve surgery for heart failure: a failed innovation? *Semin Thorac Cardiovasc Surg* 2008;18:135–8.

261. Fattouch K, Guccione F, Sampognaro R, et al. POINT: Efficacy of adding mitral valve restrictive annuloplasty to coronary artery bypass grafting in patients with moderate ischemic mitral valve regurgitation: a randomized trial. *J Thorac Cardiovasc Surg* 2009;138:278–85.

262. Trento A, Goland S, De Robertis MA, Czer LSC. COUNTERPOINT: Efficacy of adding mitral valve restrictive annuloplasty to coronary artery bypass grafting in patients with moderate ischemic mitral valve regurgitation. *J Thorac Cardiovasc Surg* 2009;138:286–8.

263. Braun J, van de Veire NR, Klautz RJ, et al. Restrictive mitral annuloplasty cures ischemic mitral regurgitation and heart failure. *Ann Thorac Surg* 2008;85:430–6.

264. Onarati G, Rubino AS, Marturano D, et al. Mid-term clinical and echocardiographic results and predictors of mitral regurgitation recurrence following restrictive annuloplasty for ischemic cardiomyopathy. *J Thorac Cardiovasc Surg* 2009;138:654–62.

265. Hansky B, Vogt J, Zittermann A, et al. Cardiac resynchronization therapy: long-term alternative to cardiac transplantation? *Ann Thorac Surg* 2009;87:432–9.

266. Yamaguchi A, Ino T, Adachi H, et al. Left ventricular volume predicts postoperative course in patients with ischemic cardiomyopathy. *Ann Thorac Surg* 1998;65:434–8.

267. Prucz RB, Weiss ES, Patel ND, Nwakanma LU, Baumgartner WA, Conte JV. Coronary artery bypass grafting with or without surgical ventricular restoration: a comparison. *Ann Thorac Surg* 2008;86:806–14.

268. Maxey TS, Reece TB, Ellman PI, et al. Coronary artery bypass with ventricular restoration is superior to coronary artery bypass alone in patients with ischemic cardiomyopathy. *J Thorac Cardiovasc Surg* 2004;127:428–34.

269. Buckberg GD, Athanasuleas CL. The STICH trial: misguided conclusions. *J Thorac Cardiovasc Surg* 2009;138:1060–4.

270. Prucz RB, Weiss ES, Patel ND, Nwakanma LU, Shah AS, Conte JV. The impact of surgical ventricular restoration on mitral valve regurgitation. *Ann Thorac Surg* 2008;86:726–34.

271. Starling RC, Jessup M, Oh JK, et al. Sustained benefits of the CorCap cardiac support device on left ventricular remodeling: three year follow-up results from the Acorn clinical trial. *Ann Thorac Surg* 2007;84:1236–42.

272. Mishra YK, Mittai S, Jaguri P, Trehan N. Coapsys mitral annuloplasty for chronic functional ischemic mitral regurgitation: 1-year results. *Ann Thorac Surg* 2006;81:42–6.

273. John R, Kamdar F, Liao K, Colvin-Adams M, Boyle A, Joyce L. Improved survival and decreasing incidence of adverse events with the HeartMate II left ventricular assist device as bridge-to-transplant therapy. *Ann Thorac Surg* 2008;86:1227–34.

274. Lietz K, Miller LW. Destination therapy: current results and future promise. *Semin Thorac Cardiovasc Surg* 2008;20:225–33.

275. Slaughter MS, Rogers JG, Milano CA, et al. Advanced heart failure treated with continuous-flow left ventricular assist device. *N Engl J Med* 2009;361:2241–51.

276. John R. Current axial-flow devices – the HeartMate II and Jarvik 2000 left ventricular assist devices. *Semin Thorac Cardiovasc Surg* 2008;20:264–72.

277. Guo C, Haider HK, Wang C, et al. Myoblast transplantation for cardiac repair: from automyoblast to allomyoblast transplantation. *Ann Thorac Surg* 2008;86:1841–8.

278. Atoui R, Shum-Tim D, Chiu RCJ. Myocardial regenerative therapy: immunologic basis for potential "universal donor cells". *Ann Thorac Surg* 2008;86:327–34.

279. Tsang TSM, Oh JK, Seward JB. Diagnosis and management of cardiac tamponade in the era of echocardiography. *Clin Cardiol* 1999;22:446–52.

280. Schwefer M, Aschenbach R, Heidemann J, Mey C, Lapp H. Constrictive pericarditis: still a diagnostic challenge: comprehensive review of clinical management. *Eur J Cardiothorac Surg* 2009;36:502–10.

281. Myers RB, Spodick DH. Constrictive pericarditis: clinical and pathophysiologic characteristics. *Am Heart J* 1999;138:219–32.

282. Yared K, Baggish AL, Picard MH, Hoffmann U, Hung J. Multimodality imaging of pericardial diseases. *JACC Cardiovasc Imaging* 2010;3:650-60.

283. Garcia MJ. Constriction vs. restriction: how to evaluate? *ACC Current Journal Review* Jul/Aug 2003.

284. Rajagopalan N, Garcia MJ, Rodriguez L, et al. Comparison of new Doppler echocardiographic methods to differentiate constrictive pericardial disease and restrictive cardiomyopathy. *Am J Cardiol* 2001;87:86-94.

285. McDonald JM, Meyers BF, Guthrie TJ, Battafarano RJ, Cooper JD, Patterson GA. Comparison of open subxiphoid pericardial drainage with percutaneous catheter drainage for symptomatic pericardial effusion. *Ann Thorac Surg* 2003;76:811-6.

286. Ziskind AA, Pearce AC, Lemmon CC, et al. Percutaneous balloon pericardiotomy for the treatment of cardiac tamponade and large pericardial effusions: description of technique and report of the first 50 cases. *J Am Coll Cardiol* 1993;21:1-5.

287. Bertog SC, Thambidorai SK, Parakh K, et al. Constrictive pericarditis: etiology and cause-specific survival after pericardiectomy. *J Am Coll Cardiol* 2004;43:1445-52.

288. Ha HW, Oh JK, Schaff HV, et al. Impact of left ventricular function on immediate and long-term outcomes after pericardiectomy in constrictive pericarditis. *J Thorac Cardiovasc Surg* 2008;136: 1136-41.

289. O'Brien PK, Kucharczuk JC, Marshall MB, et al. Comparative study of subxiphoid versus video-thoracoscopic pericardial "window". *Ann Thorac Surg* 2005;80:2013-9.

290. Sengupta PP, Eleid MF, Khandheria BK. Constrictive pericarditis. *Circ J* 2008;72:1555-62.

291. Tiruvoipati R, Naik RD, Loubani M, Billa GN. Surgical approach for pericardiectomy: a comparative study between median sternotomy and left anterolateral thoracotomy. *Interact Cardiovasc Thorac Surg* 2003;2:322-6.

292. Clare GC, Troughton RW. Management of constrictive pericarditis in the 21st century. *Curr Treat Options Cardiovasc Med* 2007;9:436-42.

293. Choudhury UK, Subramaniam GK, Kumar AS, et al. Pericardiectomy for constrictive pericarditis: a clinical, echocardiographic, and hemodynamic evaluation of two surgical techniques. *Ann Thorac Surg* 2006;81:522-30.

294. Anderson CA, Rodriguez E, Shammas RL, Kypson AP. Early constrictive epicarditis after coronary artery bypass surgery. *Ann Thorac Surg* 2009;87:642-3.

295. Meissner I, Khandheria BK, Heit JA, et al. Patent foramen ovale: innocent or guilty? Evidence from a prospective population-based study. *J Am Coll Cardiol* 2006;47:440-5.

296. Lamy C, Giannesini C, Zuber M, et al. Clinical and imaging findings in cryotogenic stroke patients with and without patent foramen ovale: The PFO-ASA study. Atrial Septal Aneurysm. *Stroke* 2002;33:706-11.

297. Handke M, Harloff A, Olschewski M, Hetzel A, Geibel A. Patent foramen ovale and crytogenic stroke in older patients. *N Engl J Med* 2007;357:2262-8.

298. Bannan A, Shen R, Silverstry FE, Herrmann HC. Characteristics of adult patients with atrial septal defects presenting with paradoxical embolism. *Catheter Cardiovasc Interv* 2009;74:1066-9.

299. Papa M, Gaspardone A, Fracasso G, et al. Usefulness of transcatheter patent foramen ovale closure in migraineurs with moderate to large right-to-left shunt and instrumental evidence of cerebrovascular damage. *Am J Cardiol* 2009;104:434-9.

300. Kedia G, Tobis J, Lee MS. Patent foramen ovale: clinical manifestations and treatment. *Rev Cardiovasc Med* 2008;9:168-73.

301. Mas JL, Arquizan C, Lamy C, et al. Recurrent cerebrovascular events associated with patent foramen ovale, atrial septal aneurysm, or both. *N Engl J Med* 2001;345:1740-6.

302. Ford MA, Reeder GS, Lennon RJ, et al. Percutaneous device closure of patent foramen ovale in patients with presumed cryptogenic stroke or transient ischemic attack. The Mayo Clinic experience. *JACC Cardiovasc Interv* 2009;2:404-11.

303. Warnes CA, Williams RG, Bashore TM, et al. ACC/AHA 2008 guidelines for the management of adults with congenital heart disease: executive summary. A report of the American College of Cardiology American Heart Association Task Force on Practice Guidelines (Writing committee to develop guidelines for the management of adults with congenital heart disease). *J Am Coll Cardiol* 2008;52:1890-947.

304. Hörer J, Müller S, Schreiber C, et al. Surgical closure of atrial septal defect in patients older than 30 years: risk factors for late death from arrhythmia or heart failure. *Thorac Cardiovasc Surg* 2007;55:79–83.

305. Gatzoulis MA, Freeman MA, Siu SC, Webb GD, Harris L. Atrial arrhythmia after surgical closure of atrial septal defects in adults. *N Engl J Med* 1999;340:839–46.

306. Ghosh S, Chatterjee S, Black E, Firmin RK. Surgical closure of atrial septal defects in adults: effect of age at operation on outcome. *Heart* 2002;88:485–7.

307. Doll N, Walther T, Falk V, et al. Secundum ASD closure using a right lateral minithoracotomy: five-year experience in 122 patients. *Ann Thorac Surg* 2003;75:1527–31.

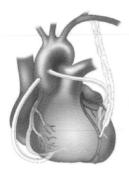

CHAPTER 2

Diagnostic Techniques in Cardiac Surgery

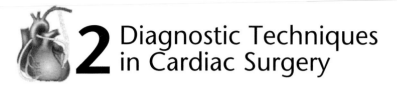

2 Diagnostic Techniques in Cardiac Surgery

Although the general nature of a patient's cardiac disease can usually be ascertained from a thorough history and physical examination, diagnostic tests are essential to define the pathology and extent of cardiac disease more precisely. A variety of noninvasive and invasive modalities can be used to identify the presence and severity of cardiovascular abnormalities that may require surgery. This chapter will briefly review the basic types of diagnostic tests available to the clinician and define their role in preoperative evaluation. Updated detailed discussions of the indications, uses, and interpretation of several diagnostic tests can be found in the ACC/AHA www.cardiosource.com/guidelines website. Summaries with extensive references can be found at online medical websites such as www.uptodate.com or www.emedicine.medscape.com.

I. Chest Radiography

A. A PA and lateral chest x-ray should be obtained on all patients before surgery. It should be consistent with the patient's cardiac diagnosis and can provide a wealth of potential information to the surgeon (Figure 2.1).

1. Compatibility with the clinical diagnosis:

   a. Left ventricular (LV) enlargement in patients with volume overload (aortic regurgitation/mitral regurgitation) or a dilated cardiomyopathy

   b. LV hypertrophy (LVH) (aortic stenosis, hypertension)

   c. Enlarged cardiac silhouette (pericardial effusion)

   d. Large left atrium or calcified mitral valve or annulus (mitral valve disease)

   e. Wide superior mediastinum (aortic dissection or aortic aneurysm)

   f. Pulmonary vascular redistribution (congestive heart failure)

2. Identify other potentially relevant abnormalities:

   a. Pulmonary: emphysema, pneumonia, parenchymal nodules, interstitial disease, previous pulmonary resection

   b. Pleural space: effusions, pneumothorax

   c. Mediastinum: tumors or widened mediastinum consistent with aortic disease

   d. Bone: pectus excavatum, rib resection from a previous thoracotomy

   e. Foreign bodies: sternal wires from a previous sternotomy, type of prosthetic heart valve, pacemaker wires, central venous catheters, position of an intra-aortic balloon pump (IABP)

Manual of Perioperative Care in Adult Cardiac Surgery, 5th Edition. By Robert M. Bojar.
Published 2011 by Blackwell Publishing Ltd.

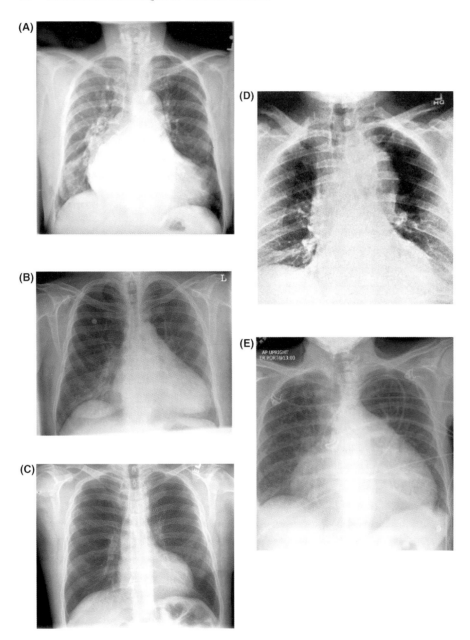

Figure 2.1 • Chest x-rays obtained preoperatively. (A) Patient with advanced mitral stenosis demonstrating marked enlargement of the left atrium projecting to the right of the cardiac silhouette. (B) Left ventricular enlargement from volume overload in a patient with chronic mitral regurgitation. (C) Aortic stenosis with left ventricular hypertrophy. (D) A wide mediastinum in a patient with an aortic dissection. (E) A markedly enlarged cardiac silhouette in a patient with a large pericardial effusion.

B. The chest x-ray can also provide important information that may influence operability or operative technique.

   1. Calcification of the ascending aorta or arch is an important finding that may increase the risk of stroke. This may require an alternative cannulation site (femoral or axillary artery), avoidance of aortic cross-clamping (beating or fibrillating heart surgery), or avoidance of both cannulation and aortic cross-clamping (off-pump surgery). It may necessitate use of deep hypothermic circulatory arrest to perform an aortic valve replacement. This approach may not be tolerated in some patients, especially the elderly, in whom percutaneous valve placement may be preferable. Epiaortic echocardiography may be indicated during surgery to evaluate for ascending aortic atherosclerosis. Suspicion of ascending aortic calcification by chest x-ray (usually on the lateral film) or cardiac catheterization may be further defined by noncontrast CT scanning (see Figure 2.9, page 100). Calcification of the aortic knob alone is a common finding on chest x-ray but is usually of little significance.

   2. An elevated hemidiaphragm on one side might deter the surgeon from using the contralateral internal thoracic artery (ITA), especially in diabetic patients, who arguably are more prone to phrenic nerve paresis.[1,2]

   3. Mitral annular calcification in patients with mitral regurgitation makes mitral valve repair or replacement more difficult and may necessitate creative surgical techniques.

   4. For patients undergoing reoperation, PA and lateral films are essential. The PA film may identify the proximity of the ITA pedicle (identified by metallic clips) to the midline, although this usually requires a selective ITA angiogram to detect its true course. However, the lateral film will demonstrate the proximity of an aortic aneurysm, the right ventricle, and occasionally the ITA to the posterior sternal table. If there is a concern about potential damage to any of these structures with a sternotomy, groin cannulation and even initiation of cardiopulmonary bypass prior to sternotomy may be indicated. Alternatively, a thoracotomy incision should be considered, especially for redo mitral valve surgery (right chest) or redo coronary surgery to the left-sided vessels (left chest).

   5. The location and orientation of the heart should be considered when selecting the appropriate incision for minimally invasive surgery. For example, in thin patients and those with emphysema, the heart has a vertical orientation and lies quite caudad in the chest. Thus, for aortic valve surgery, a more distal intercostal space incision may be necessary with either a partial upper sternotomy incision or anterior thoracotomy approach to obtain appropriate exposure.

   6. The patient in profound congestive heart failure may benefit from aggressive diuresis or hemofiltration during bypass.

II. Electrocardiography

   A. A 12-lead ECG must be reviewed prior to surgery because it can yield valuable information about the nature of the patient's disease, the urgency of surgery, the appropriate management of arrhythmias, and other considerations in perioperative management.

   B. Disorders of rate and rhythm

      1. The presence of sinus tachycardia in a patient with coronary disease suggests that the patient is inadequately β-blocked. This may predispose the patient to the development of ischemia preoperatively and to atrial fibrillation (AF) after surgery.

2. Patients with sinus bradycardia usually require temporary postoperative pacing and may not tolerate β-blockers or amiodarone that might otherwise be used prophylactically to prevent postoperative AF. Patients with sick sinus or tachycardia/bradycardia syndrome are more likely to require a permanent pacemaker postoperatively.

3. A rapid ventricular response to AF must be controlled pharmacologically. It can precipitate myocardial ischemia in the patient with coronary artery disease (CAD) and can compromise the cardiac output, especially in patients with LVH. If longstanding persistent AF has been present, the use of prophylactic medications to prevent postoperative AF is usually of little benefit, but postoperative anticoagulation is indicated to prevent a thromboembolic stroke. A Maze procedure may be considered as an adjunct to other cardiac operations in patients with either paroxysmal or persistent AF.

4. Ventricular tachyarrhythmias may result from active ischemia or remote myocardial infarction. If revascularization is indicated, a postoperative electrophysiology study should be considered in patients with sustained VT. An implantable cardioverter-defibrillator (ICD) should be inserted if VT is inducible or the ejection fraction remains <35% a few months after surgery (see pages 58–59 for the indications for ICD placement).

C. Conduction problems

1. The presence of a left bundle branch block increases the risk of asystole during insertion of a Swan-Ganz pulmonary artery catheter. This should be deferred until after the sternotomy has been performed so that immediate epicardial pacing can be achieved.

2. Ischemic ECG changes are difficult to assess in the patient with a bundle branch block. Early catheterization may be indicated in patients with acute coronary syndromes considered at high risk based on clinical criteria.

3. The development of conduction abnormalities in a patient with aortic valve endocarditis suggests annular extension of the infection, which is an indication for urgent surgery.

4. Patients sustaining an inferior infarction may develop heart block and require temporary pacing preoperatively.

D. Evidence of ischemia and infarction

1. ST and T wave changes consistent with ischemia require aggressive management. This may entail use of intravenous nitrates, antiplatelet agents (aspirin, clopidogrel, glycoprotein IIb/IIIa inhibitors), heparin, and/or placement of an IABP. An early invasive strategy with urgent percutaneous coronary intervention (PCI) or surgery is usually indicated. Evidence of recent infarction may influence the timing and risk of surgery. Waiting several days may lower the surgical risk in stable patients, but is inadvisable if the patient develops recurrent chest pain or ischemia or has threatening coronary anatomy.

2. In patients with depressed LV function, an ECG with Q waves is more consistent with transmural infarction, but the absence of Q waves suggests that the myocardium may be chronically ischemic and hibernating, rather than infarcted. Further evaluation with viability studies may be indicated to determine whether surgery will prove beneficial in improving LV function and survival.

E. Transvenous pacemaker and ICD issues

   1. The function of a permanent transvenous pacing system can be disrupted by use of electrocautery at the time of surgery. A magnet must be available to convert the pacemaker into a fixed pacing mode.

   2. ICD units should be inactivated prior to surgery.

   3. Because the right atrial lead of a dual-chamber pacemaker may be displaced during surgery or the pulse generator may be damaged by electrocautery, all permanent pacemaker systems must be interrogated immediately after surgery to ensure appropriate sensing and pacing.

III. Stress Testing and Myocardial Perfusion Imaging

A. Stress testing plays a major role in detecting the potential presence and functional significance of coronary artery disease. In addition to basic exercise stress testing, rest and stress myocardial perfusion imaging (MPI) have greater sensitivity and specificity in identifying viable and ischemic myocardium that will benefit from an interventional procedure. The technology has become very sophisticated, and only the salient features are presented.[3–5]

B. Types of stress testing

   1. In patients who can exercise, stress testing to maximal exercise is performed on a treadmill with a graded protocol (Figure 2.2).[6] ECG changes of ischemia can be difficult to detect in patients with a left bundle branch block or ST changes on baseline ECG. The following findings are consistent with multivessel coronary disease and an adverse prognosis, especially when they occur at a low workload (<6 mets):

      a. Development of anginal symptoms

      b. More than 2 mm ST depression in multiple leads and persisting more than 5 minutes into recovery

      c. ST segment elevation

      d. Failure to increase blood pressure to higher than 120 mm Hg or a sustained decrease in blood pressure greater than 10 mm Hg or below rest levels

      e. Sustained ventricular tachycardia

   2. Radionuclide myocardial perfusion imaging (rMPI) may be performed as part of an exercise protocol or with pharmacologic stress using a vasodilator (either dipyridamole or adenosine). The accuracy is fairly comparable whether exercise- or pharmacologic-based, with sensitivities and specificities of 80–90%.[5,7–9] In patients with contraindications to these medications, such as hypotension, sick sinus syndrome, high-degree AV block, bronchospastic lung disease, or use of theophylline, dobutamine can be used for MPI.[10]

      a. Planar images or single proton emission computed tomographic scanning (SPECT) can be performed using thallium-201, technetium-99m sestamibi (Cardiolite), or technetium-99m tetrofosmin (Myoview). A common protocol is a 4-minute infusion of dipyridamole followed 8 minutes later by injection of the tracer, and then scintigraphy is performed. Planar or SPECT thallium-201 scanning has a high false-positive rate for image attenuation artifacts.

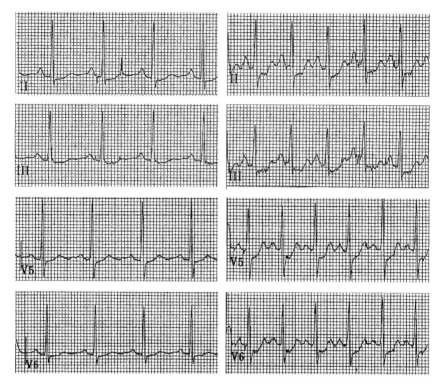

Figure 2.2 • Positive exercise stress test. (Left) Baseline ECG before exercise (leads II, III, V5, V6. (Right) Exercise ECG after 4 minutes of stage 2. At a heart rate of 157 bpm, note the presence of 3 mm of ST depression in these leads, reflecting inferolateral ischemia.

b. The basic principle of MPI is that vasodilators produce coronary vasodilation, and in the absence of CAD, blood flow will increase accordingly (coronary flow reserve). Thus, nonischemic viable tissue will exhibit tracer uptake and "light up".[11] However, with flow-limiting stenosis, there is less flow reserve and thus less tracer uptake by the myocardium. At peak stress, lack of tracer update ("cold spot") may be consistent with either irreversible infarction or ischemia. Muscle that "lights up" on a delayed basis due to redistribution (Figure 2.3) reflects reversibility and ischemia. In some patients, stress-redistribution imaging may underestimate the degree of ischemic and viable myocardium, but reinjection will improve sensitivity.[12]

c. Left ventricular dilatation resulting from an impairment in subendocardial flow is a strong indicator of significant ischemia and is a high risk marker for adverse cardiac events.

d. Positron-emission tomography (PET) scanning using rubidium-82 or ^{13}N-ammonia or dobutamine may provide superior diagnostic accuracy to SPECT scanning.[13]

3. Exercise radionuclide angiography using a bicycle can be used to identify myocardial ischemia. The development of a regional wall motion abnormality or

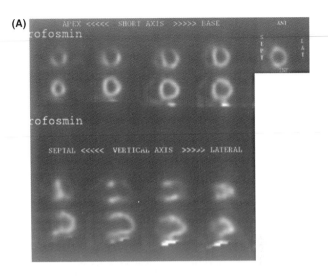

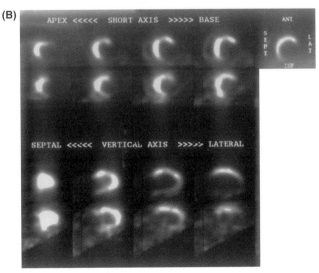

Figure 2.3 • Stress imaging studies with Tc-99m tetrofosmin. (A) Short-axis (upper two rows) and vertical long-axis views (lower two rows) at stress (top image of each pair) and redistribution (lower image of each pair). The stress images demonstrate reduced tracer uptake in the anteroapical region that improves during the redistribution phase, consistent with anteroapical ischemia. (B) Similar views demonstrating a defect in the inferolateral region in the stress images that does not improve with redistribution. This is consistent with infarction. (Courtesy of Dr. David Bader, Department of Radiology, Saint Vincent Hospital, Worcester, MA.)

fall in ejection fraction with exercise is indicative of ischemia. Technetium-labeled tracers can be used to assess both myocardial perfusion and ventricular function.[8]

4. **Exercise echocardiography** is based on the principle that stress-induced ischemia caused by coronary artery stenosis will produce regional wall motion abnormalities. These tests may be performed using bicycle or treadmill exercise. An alternative to exercise is the use of **dobutamine** to increase myocardial oxygen demand (dobutamine stress echocardiogram or DSE). If this cannot be met by an increase in blood flow, ischemia will produce regional wall motion abnormalities in the distribution of the stenotic coronary artery. These tests have provided comparable results to those of exercise nuclear imaging.[9,14,15]

C. **Viability studies**. Myocardial viability studies are useful in patients with severe left ventricular dysfunction to distinguish areas of myocardial necrosis from "hibernating myocardium" that may recover function after revascularization. Usually improvement in LV function is associated with symptomatic improvement and increased survival, and this may be noted in patients with congestive heart failure with or without angina.[16–22] In some patients, reperfusion of zones with stress-induced ischemia will improve symptoms but will not be associated with any improvement in global or regional function. Extensive remodeling and high end-systolic volumes are associated with less improvement in LV function.[21] Among the modalities available to detect viability are the following:

1. **Thallium-201 rMPI with SPECT** is the most common means of assessing viability. Thallium uptake reflects cell membrane integrity, so that viable zones, whether ischemic or not, will perfuse and retain thallium at rest. With rest-redistribution imaging, nonischemic viable tissue will retain thallium at rest. However, if there is rest ischemia, a defect may be evident initially, but may show redistribution 4 hours later, indicating viability. With stress-redistribution imaging, an area of ischemia that produces a defect at stress may demonstrate redistribution either with reinjection of thallium or on delayed imaging up to 18–24 hours later.[12]

2. **SPECT imaging with Tc-99m tracers** (sestamibi or tetrofosmin) is based on intact mitochondrial function reflecting viability. Its accuracy in assessing viability is comparable to thallium. Gated SPECT scanning allows for assessment of ventricular function as well as viability.

3. ^{18}**F-deoxyglucose (FDG) uptake** using PET or SPECT imaging is a very sensitive test of viability. FDG is a marker of glucose uptake by the myocardium, thus assessing metabolism and cell viability. An assessment is made of perfusion with ^{13}N-ammonia or rubidium-82, and then ^{18}FDG is injected to assess metabolism. Zones with matching perfusion and metabolism are either not ischemic or are infarcted. Evidence of preserved metabolic activity in zones of reduced perfusion indicates viable, hibernating myocardium. These studies may detect viability in zones considered nonviable by thallium imaging.[20]

4. **Dobutamine stress echo (DSE)** can be used to identify contractile reserve, which suggests viability.[10,15] Low doses of dobutamine are administered during echocardiography to assess any change in global and regional wall motion. A biphasic response during dobutamine echocardiography (improvement in function at low dose and worsening of function at peak stress from high doses of dobutamine) is highly predictive of recovery of regional contractile function in patients with LV

dysfunction.[23] Another use for this test is in patients with low-flow, low-gradient aortic stenosis (AS), in whom an improvement in LV function and an increase in the gradient with dobutamine suggests that the patient will benefit from an aortic valve replacement.[24]

5. **Contrast-enhanced magnetic resonance imaging (MRI)** holds promise as a means of assessing viability. Hyperenhancement by gadolinium is noted in regions of transmural nonviability. MRI-defined diastolic wall thickness >5.5 mm and dobutamine-induced systolic wall thickening >2 mm are predictive of contractile recovery after CABG. MRI provides excellent image quality with precise identification of epicardial and endocardial borders to allow for assessment of wall motion and thickening.[16,25,26]

6. In a meta-analysis of PET, SPECT, and DSE in patients with LV dysfunction, all three tests showed relatively comparable efficacy in demonstrating the association between viability and improved survival after myocardial revascularization. PET and SPECT scanning were more sensitive, but DSE was more specific in predicting functional improvement.[17]

IV. Cardiac Catheterization

A. The gold standard for the diagnosis of most forms of cardiac disease remains cardiac catheterization.[27,28] It is indicated in most patients whose clinical presentation and diagnostic testing suggest that an interventional procedure (PCI or open-heart surgery) may be indicated. The exceptions are acute type A aortic dissections, which are surgical emergencies, and aortic valve endocarditis with vegetations, with which catheter manipulation in the root may cause embolization.

B. **Techniques** (Tables 2.1 and 2.2; Figures 2.4 and 2.5)

1. **Right-heart catheterization** is performed in patients with valve disease and those with coronary disease and left ventricular dysfunction. It involves placement of a Swan-Ganz catheter to obtain intracardiac pressures and measure oxygen saturations from each chamber to detect intracardiac shunts (atrial or ventricular septal defects). The mixed venous oxygen saturation from the pulmonary artery (PA) port indirectly reflects the cardiac output. A thermodilution cardiac output is obtained and can be used along with pressure gradients obtained from right- and left-heart catheterization to calculate valve areas using the Gorlin formula (see pages 19 and 30).

2. **Left-heart catheterization** involves advancing a catheter from the aorta through the aortic valve into the left ventricle. This allows for the measurement of the left ventricular end-diastolic pressure (LVEDP), obtaining a left ventriculogram to assess the ejection fraction (end-diastolic volume minus end-systolic volume divided by the end-diastolic volume) (Figure 2.6), and identification of mitral regurgitation (Figure 2.7). A Fick cardiac output can be calculated. The aortic valve gradient can be measured during pullback of the catheter, but in patients with aortic stenosis, this has been reported to increase the risk of stroke.[29] Therefore, this should not be performed if severe aortic stenosis is confirmed by echocardiography.

3. Evaluation of both left- and right-heart pressures is invaluable in making the diagnosis of constrictive pericarditis (Figure 1.28, page 64).[30]

Table 2.1 • Information Obtained From Right and Left Heart Catheterization

Elevated RA pressure	Tricuspid stenosis (large "a" wave) Tricuspid regurgitation (large "v" wave) RV dysfunction (pulmonary hypertension, RV infarction) Constrictive pericarditis/tamponade/restrictive disease
Elevated RV pressure	RV dysfunction (pulmonary hypertension, RV infarction) Constrictive pericarditis (square root sign; rapid "x" and "y" descent) Restrictive disease Cardiac tamponade (absent "y" descent)
Elevated PA pressure	Mitral stenosis/regurgitation LV systolic or diastolic dysfunction (ischemic, dilated cardiomyopathy, aortic stenosis/regurgitation) Pulmonary hypertension of other etiologies Constrictive pericarditis/tamponade/restrictive disease
Elevated PCW pressure	Mitral stenosis (large "a" wave if sinus rhythm) Mitral regurgitation (large "v" wave) LV systolic or diastolic dysfunction (ischemic, dilated cardiomyopathy, aortic stenosis/regurgitation) Constrictive pericarditis/tamponade
Elevated LVEDP	LV systolic or diastolic dysfunction (ischemic, dilated cardiomyopathy, aortic stenosis/regurgitation) Constrictive pericarditis/tamponade

RA, right atrial; RV, right ventricular; PA, pulmonary artery; LV, left ventricular; PCW, pulmonary capillary wedge; LVEDP, left ventricular end-diastolic pressure.

4. An **aortogram** ("root shot") should be performed in patients with aortic valve disease to assess the degree of aortic regurgitation (Figure 2.8). Both an aortogram and a left ventriculogram will give an estimate of aortic size that might necessitate replacement of the ascending aorta. Excessive whip of an angiographic catheter may also suggest the presence of a dilated aortic root. A CT scan or echocardiogram can assess the size of the aorta more precisely, since magnification of the aorta is very common during aortography.

5. **Fluoroscopy** can yield valuable information, including:

   a. Calcification of the ascending aorta that may require further evaluation by noncontrast CT scanning (Figure 2.9)

   b. Severe coronary calcification or extensive coronary stenting that may make bypass grafting virtually impossible

   c. The location of intravascular catheters or position of an IABP

   d. "Rocking" of a prosthetic valve suggestive of endocarditis with annular invasion and possible dehiscence

   e. Limitation of movement of prosthetic valve discs, consistent with valve thrombosis or restriction by pannus ingrowth (Figure 2.10)

Table 2.2 • Hemodynamic Norms During Cardiac Catheterization

Location	Pressures (mm Hg)
Right atrium	Mean 3–8
Right ventricle	Systolic 15–30 Diastolic 3–8
Pulmonary artery	Systolic 15–30 Diastolic 5–12 Mean 9–16
PCW position	5–12
Left atrium	5–12
Left ventricle	Systolic 90–140 End–diastolic 5–12
Aorta	Systolic 90–140 Diastolic 60–90 Mean 70–105

PCW, pulmonary capillary wedge.

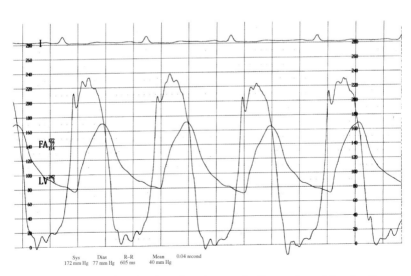

Sys 172 mm Hg   Dias 77 mm Hg   R–R 605 ms   Mean 40 mm Hg   0.04 second

Figure 2.4 • Left heart catheterization of aortic stenosis. Comparison of the simultaneous peak left ventricular and femoral artery pressures demonstrates a peak gradient of 60 mm Hg. If there is a discrepancy between the central aortic and femoral artery pressures, the pullback gradient is calculated as the catheter is withdrawn from the left ventricle into the aorta.

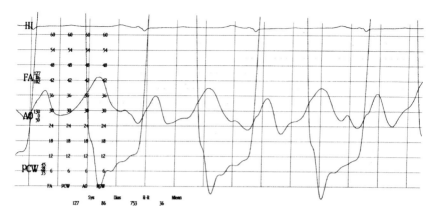

Figure 2.5 • Left heart catheterization of mitral stenosis. There is a pressure difference (gradient) of approximately 20 mm Hg between the pulmonary capillary wedge pressure and the mean left ventricular end-diastolic pressure.

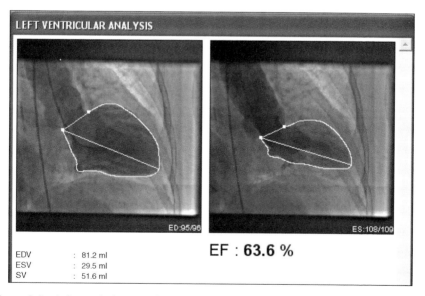

Figure 2.6 • Left ventriculogram. The ejection fraction (EF) is calculated by dividing the end-distolic volume (left) minus the end-systolic volume (right) by the end-diastolic volume.

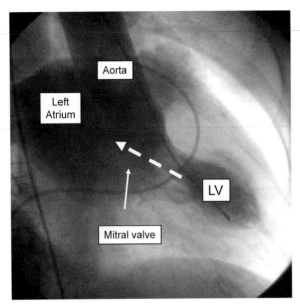

Figure 2.7 • Left ventriculogram obtained at end-systole demonstrating severe mitral regurgitation into a dilated left atrium.

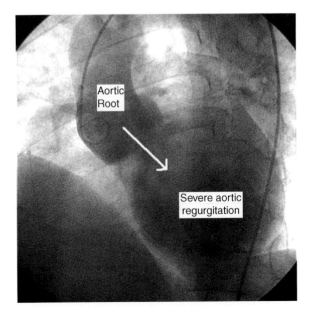

Figure 2.8 • A "root shot" with a pigtail catheter in the proximal aorta will demonstrate the size of the aorta and the degree of aortic regurgitation, which in this patient was severe.

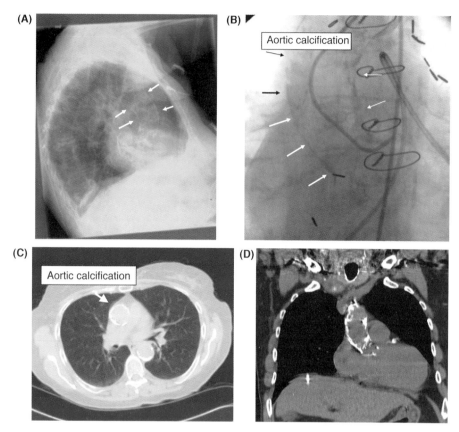

Figure 2.9 • (A) Lateral chest x-ray demonstrating severe ascending aortic calcification. (B) Using fluoroscopy prior to injection of contrast, significant calcification can be seen in the wall of the ascending aorta. A noncontrast CT scan in the transverse (C) and coronal (D) cuts further defines the degree of calcification, which produced essentially a "porcelain" aorta.

V. Coronary Angiography

A. Coronary angiography is performed as part of the cardiac catheterization procedure by placing special preformed catheters directly into the coronary ostia and injecting contrast into the coronary arteries (Figures 2.11 and 2.12).[27,28] Angiography will assess whether the circulation is right- or left-dominant (i.e., whether the posterior descending artery arises from the right or left system), and it will define the location, extent, and degree of coronary stenoses (Figure 2.13). This information is then used to determine if an interventional procedure is indicated and whether PCI or CABG is preferable. Among the factors to be considered when contemplating surgery are the quality and bypassability of the target vessels based on their size and the extent of distal disease.

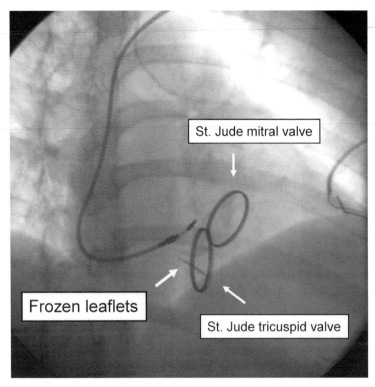

Figure 2.10 • Fluoroscopy of a patient with St. Jude Medical valves in the mitral and tricuspid positions. The leaflets of the prosthetic tricuspid valve were completely immobile during the cardiac cycle, producing both stenosis and regurgitation of the valve. Note how important the projection is in identifying the leaflets – the mitral valve leaflets are not seen.

    B. Anteroposterior, right anterior oblique, and left anterior oblique views are obtained at varying degrees of cranial and caudal angulation to optimally visualize each of the coronary arteries. For reoperative procedures, imaging of the ITA pedicle in a true AP projection is indicated to identify whether the ITA pedicle is very close to the midline (Figure 2.14). A lateral projection can identify its relationship to the posterior sternal table.

    C. Coronary angiography is still considered the gold standard for the identification of coronary artery disease, but it has limitations which need to be understood when interpreting the significance of blockage and making a decision to proceed with an interventional approach.

        1. Lesions can be concentric or eccentric. For purely concentric stenosis, the correlation of diameter and cross-sectional area (CSA) loss is estimated as follows:

- 50% diameter = 75% loss of CSA
- 67% diameter = 90% loss of CSA

        Thus, >50% diameter stenosis is considered significant.

        2. The calculation of % diameter stenosis with contrast injection is based upon a comparison of the luminal diameter of a narrowed segment to that of the largest

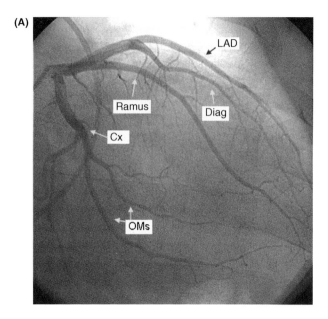

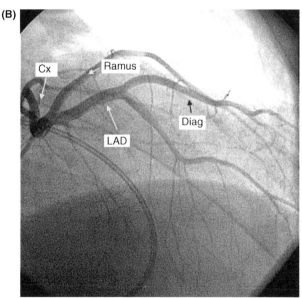

Figure 2.11 • Left coronary angiograms in four projections. (A) Right anterior oblique (RAO) nicely demonstrates the circumflex (Cx) marginal system. (B) RAO with cranial angulation best demonstrates the left anterior descending (LAD) and the origin of its diagonal branches.

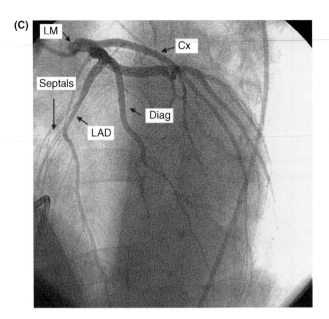

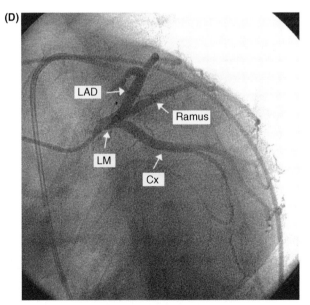

Figure 2.11 • *(Continued)* (C) Left anterior oblique (LAO) provides a good view of the LAD system and the origin of the circumflex. (D) LAO caudal "spider view" shows the left main giving rise to three vessels, including a large ramus intermedius. LM, left main; OM, obtuse marginal artery.

(A)

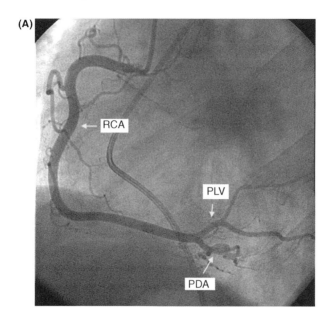

(B)

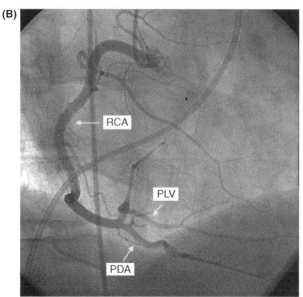

Figure 2.12 • Right coronary angiograms in the (A) LAO and (B) RAO projections. The right coronary artery (RCA) divides at the crux into the posterior left ventricular branch (PLV), best seen in the LAO view, and the posterior descending artery (PDA), best seen in the RAO projection.

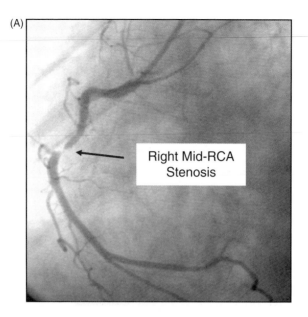

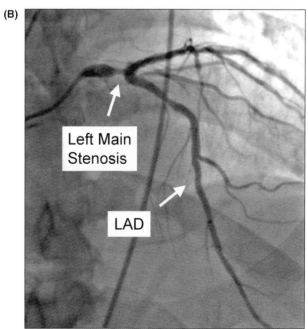

Figure 2.13 • Significant coronary stenoses. (A) A 99% stenosis of the mid-right coronary artery, best managed by PCI. (B) A 75% left main stenosis.

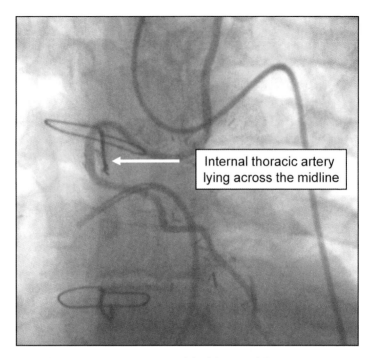

Figure 2.14 • Selective coronary angiogram of the left internal thoracic artery (ITA) in the anteroposterior (AP) projection. The pedicle has been pushed medially by the lung and extends to the midline, risking damage during a midline redo sternotomy.

segment of an artery, unless the artery is ectatic. In patients with diffuse CAD, the large segment may not reflect normal vessel diameter, and thus angiography will underestimate the extent of disease. **Intravascular ultrasound** (IVUS) can visualize the entire vessel wall and give a more precise calculation of the true extent of narrowing, measured as a "minimal luminal area" (MLA) in mm^2 (Figure 2.15). IVUS can be used to identify a stenosis that may benefit from stenting and it is particularly helpful in indeterminate left main stenoses. A left main MLA $<7\,mm^2$ in a symptomatic patient or $<5.5{-}6\,mm^2$ in an asymptomatic patient is considered significant.[31,32] An MLA $<4\,mm^2$ in the other proximal arteries is considered significant.

3. The correlation of the degree of stenosis and its functional significance is imprecise. **Fractional flow reserve** (FFR) measurements using a pressure wire can help to determine whether an intervention is indicated.[33–37] A catheter is placed through the stenosis in the coronary artery, and proximal and distal pressure measurements are obtained after inducing a hyperemic response with either intracoronary or intravenous adenosine. If the distal/proximal pressure ratio (FFR) is ≤ 0.8, the lesion is considered to be functionally significant, and revascularization will provide a clinical benefit; otherwise, intervention is generally not indicated.[34] This is also beneficial in sorting out the significance of left main lesions.[33,36]

4. Occluded vessels that are underfilled via collateral flow may represent large vessels that are good surgical targets (but not always). Symptomatic patients with viable

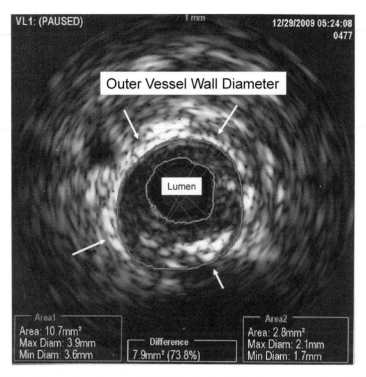

Figure 2.15 • Intravascular ultrasound (IVUS) study of the left main coronary artery. A 2 Fr echo probe is introduced into the vessel, producing images of the lumen and the surrounding vessel wall. This allows for calculation of a minimal luminal area (MLA). In this case, the MLA was < 4 mm², consistent with severe left main stenosis.

myocardium subtended by occluded vessels may benefit from PCI of the chronically occluded vessel or from CABG.

D. Important indications for coronary angiography include:

1. Any patient with suspected CAD in whom an interventional procedure might be indicated on a clinical basis. This includes patients presenting with ST-elevation myocardial infarctions (STEMIs), acute coronary syndromes (NSTEMI or unstable angina), chronic stable angina with positive stress tests, or ischemic pulmonary edema.

2. Patients > age 40 who require open-heart surgery for other reasons. Angiography should also be considered in younger patients with multiple risk factors for premature coronary artery disease.

3. Annual follow-up of the cardiac transplant patient to detect the development of silent allograft coronary artery disease.

E. The risk of complications resulting from cardiac catheterization is very low, with development of a groin hematoma being most common. This is more likely to occur in patients undergoing PCI who have received aspirin, clopidogrel, prasugrel, either heparin or bivalirudin, and often a glycoprotein IIb/IIIa inhibitor in the cath lab. Patients with critical left main disease may not tolerate catheter manipulation, and are more prone to develop a myocardial infarction, arrhythmias, hemodynamic compromise, or death. To a great degree, morbidity and mortality following catheterization or PCI are dependent on the patient's clinical status and on preexisting comorbidities, especially renal dysfunction. Patients taking metformin for diabetes should withhold this medication starting the day before their catheterization. Hydration and use of a sodium bicarbonate infusion or N-acetylcysteine are common strategies in patients with renal dysfunction. **Sodium bicarbonate** 150 mEq (1 mEq/mL) is added to 850 mL of D5W with an initial infusion of 3 mL/kg over 1 hour starting just prior to catheterization followed by a 1 mL/kg/h infusion for up to 12 hours. **N-acetylcysteine** (NAC) may be given orally 600 mg bid prior to and for four doses after catheterization.[38–41] There is some evidence that the combination of both may provide the best renal protection.[42]

VI. Echocardiography

A. Echocardiography provides real-time two- or three-dimensional (3-D) imaging of the thoracic aorta and cardiac structures. It is an invaluable noninvasive means of evaluating ventricular and valvular function before, during, and after surgery.[43,44] Although a transthoracic study is usually the initial study performed in the preoperative patient, transesophageal echocardiography (TEE) provides superior imaging because of the proximity of the probe to the heart. Routine evaluation includes multiplane two-dimensional imaging, pulsed wave Doppler, and color flow Doppler analysis. TEE is very important in the preoperative evaluation of the patient with mitral regurgitation (MR) because it provides an assessment of the nature and degree of MR, which may be different during intraoperative evaluation due to altered loading conditions (Figure 2.16). It also provides excellent images of vegetations in patients

(A)

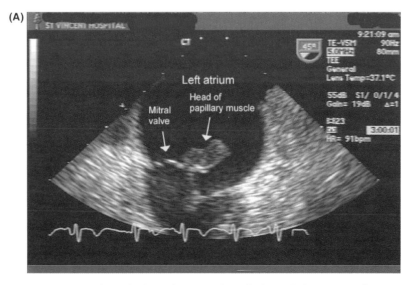

Figure 2.16 • Transesophageal echocardiograms of mitral valve pathology. (A) Papillary muscle rupture and acute mitral regurgitation. Note the flail anterior leaflet with the attached papillary muscle head.

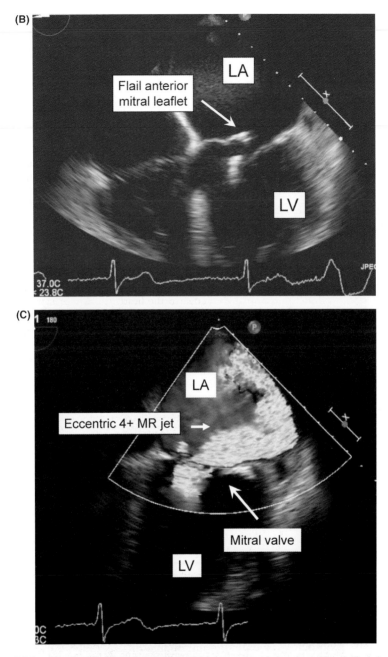

Figure 2.16 • *(Continued)* (B) Flail anterior leaflet from ruptured chordae with calcified chords. (C) Color flow Doppler showing a posteriorly directed jet with 4 + mitral regurgitation (a bright mosaic yellow/green jet on the color image).

with endocarditis (Figure 2.17), has become the gold standard for the diagnosis of aortic dissections (Figure 2.18), and is the best technique to identify the location and sites of attachment of cardiac tumors (Figure 2.19). Three-dimensional imaging is especially beneficial in evaluating mitral valve pathology and its amenability to repair (Figure 2.20).[44]

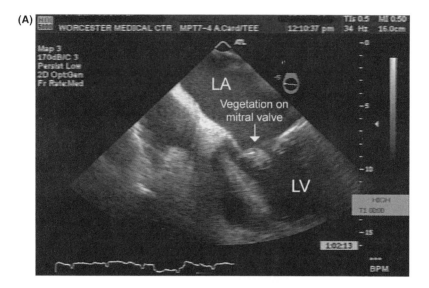

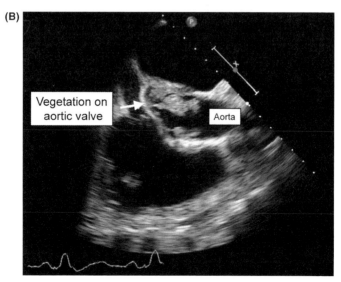

Figure 2.17 • Transesophageal echocardiograms of two patients with endocarditis. (A) Vegetation on the anterior mitral valve leaflet. (B) Vegetation on the aortic valve seen in the long-axis view.

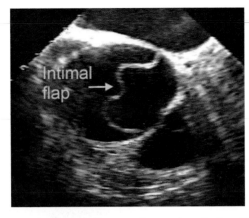

Figure 2.18 • Transesophageal echocardiogram of a type A aortic dissection. Note the intimal flap separating the true and false lumens.

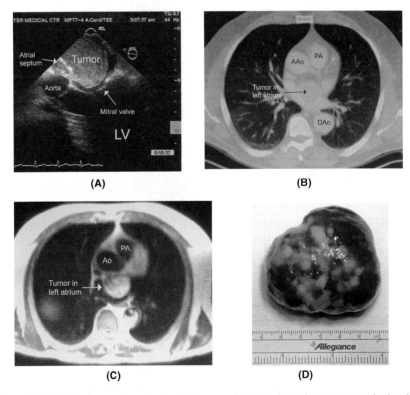

Figure 2.19 • (A) Transesophageal echocardiogram of a large left atrial myxoma attached to the superior aspect of the atrial septum. This mass was initially detected on a CT scan (B), and an MRI (C) was also obtained before the TEE was performed. (D) Intraoperative photograph of the resected myxoma. Ao, aorta; AAo, ascending aorta; DAo, descending aorta; LV, left ventricle; PA, pulmonary artery.

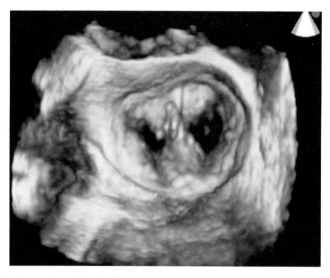

Figure 2.20 • Three-dimensional echo images of mitral regurgitation related to flail of the P2 scallop of the posterior leaflet. (Image courtesy of Dr. Feroze Mahmood, Beth Israel Deaconess Medical Center, Boston, MA)

B. Dobutamine stress echocardiography can be used to identify ischemia and myocardial viability (see pages 94–95) and to determine the severity of aortic stenosis in patients with low-flow, low-gradient AS (see pages 19–20).[15,23,24]

C. Examples of information that can be derived from preoperative and postoperative echocardiography are noted in Tables 2.3 and 2.4. The utility of TEE in the operating room is noted in Table 4.1 (page 181). Diagrams of common views obtained by TEE are shown in Figures 4.6–4.8, pages 183–185.

VII. Noninvasive Coronary Angiography

A. Tremendous technological advances in noninvasive imaging have led to the use of CT and MRI scanning for the evaluation of coronary anatomy. The temporal or spatial resolution is approaching that of invasive coronary angiography and is quite sensitive in ruling out obstructive disease, but it is not yet clear whether it will imminently replace routine angiography.[45–49] Most guidelines as of 2010 recommended noninvasive imaging only in patients with equivocal stress tests, intermediate coronary risk, or atypical symptoms. These studies are not yet recommended as a screening tool in asymptomatic patients, nor in patients with typical symptoms that may warrant PCI or CABG.

B. **Multidetector row or multislice CT scanning** (MDCT or MSCT) that can acquire at least 64 slices per gantry rotation provides adequate imaging of a beating heart with little motion artifact when the heart rate is slowed to less than 70 bpm with beta-blockers.[46–51]

Table 2.3 • *Information Obtained From Preoperative Echocardiography*

All patients	Global and regional wall motion abnormalities Signs of diastolic dysfunction Valve function Aortic atherosclerosis Pericardial fluid and thickening Presence of an intracardiac shunt
Coronary artery disease	Global and regional wall motion abnormalities Signs of diastolic dysfunction Left ventricular mural thrombus Presence of mitral regurgitation Stress imaging for ischemic zones
Aortic stenosis	Gradient calculation from flow velocity Planimetry of valve area Annular diameter (root enlargement, selection of homo- graft size) Stress imaging if low-flow/low-gradient stenosis Presence of mitral regurgitation
Aortic regurgitation	Degree of regurgitation Annular diameter (selection of homograft size)
Ascending aortic aneurysm	Size of sinuses, ascending aorta and proximal arch
Aortic dissection	Location of intimal flap Detection of aortic regurgitation Presence of pericardial effusion
Mitral stenosis	Size of left atrium Mean diastolic gradient Planimetry of valve area Presence of left atrial thrombus

Mitral regurgitation	Size of left atrium
	Degree of regurgitation
	Nature of pathology (annular dilatation, anterior or
	    posterior leaflet prolapse, elongated or torn chords,
	    papillary muscle rupture)

Tricuspid valve disease	Calculation of pulmonary artery pressure from tricuspid regurgitation jet velocity ($4V^2$) Gradient (stenosis) or degree of regurgitation
Endocarditis	Vegetations Annular abscesses Valvular regurgitation
Cardiac masses	Location and relationship to cardiac structures of tumors, thrombus, vegetations
Pericardial tamponade	Diastolic collapse of atrial or ventricular chambers Location of fluid around heart

Table 2.4 • Indications for Postoperative Echocardiography

Low output states	LV or RV systolic dysfunction LV diastolic dysfunction Cardiac tamponade Hypovolemia
New/persistent murmur (recurrent congestive heart failure)	Paravalvular leak Inadequate valve repair Outflow tract gradient from small valve or systolic anterior motion (SAM) of anterior mitral valve leaflet Recurrent ventricular septal defect
Evaluation of ventricular recovery after assist device insertion	LV or RV systolic function

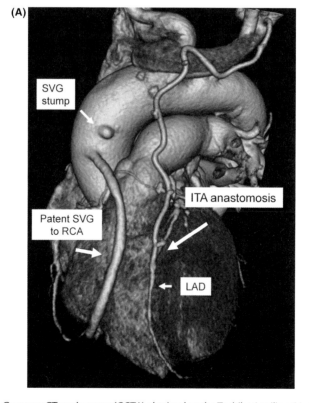

(A)

SVG stump

ITA anastomosis

Patent SVG to RCA

LAD

Figure 2.21 • Coronary CT angiograms (CCTA) obtained on the Toshiba Aquilion 64-slice scanner. (A) This patient with prior surgery has a patent LITA to the LAD and a patent saphenous vein graft (SVG) to the right coronary artery (RCA); a nubbin of an occluded SVG is noted on the aorta.

Coventry University
Lanchester Library
Tel 02476 887575

Item Title	Due Date
38001004295741	
Physiotherapy in respiratory c	13/06/2011
38001003666470	
Cardiopulmonary physiothera	13/06/2011
38001005739192	
Searching skills toolkit	13/06/2011
38001005113091	
Randomised controlled trials	13/06/2011
38001005397181	
How to read a paper	13/06/2011
38001005119148	
Rehabilitation research	13/06/2011
38001005716489	
Respiratory physiotherapy	18/06/2011
38001005024082	
Clinical management notes a	18/06/2011
38001005920867	
Manual of perioperative care	29/06/2011

Indicates items borrowed today
Thankyou
www.coventry.ac.uk

(B)

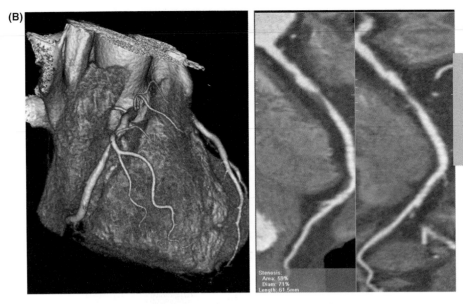

Stenosis:
Area: 59%
Diam: 71%
Length: 61.5mm

Figure 2.21 • *(Continued)* (B) Evaluation of the native circulation identifies a tight stenosis in the proximal to mid-right coronary artery. (Images courtesy of Toshiba-America).

1. Coronary CT angiography (CCTA) provides excellent imaging of native coronary arteries and bypass grafts (Figure 2.21). It does require contrast and radiation and produces suboptimal imaging with an irregular heart rhythm, severe coronary calcification, or very small vessels. Although stents do interfere with imaging, CCTA is quite accurate in assessing in-stent stenosis.[50] It is contraindicated in patients with renal dysfunction or an allergy to contrast. The sensitivity and specificity of CCTA in identifying coronary stenoses is about 80–90% and will improve with faster 256- and 320-slice scanners which can provide extraordinary images with less radiation.

2. The ability to assess physiologic significance simultaneously with anatomic findings can be achieved using combined CCTA with SPECT MPI. This combination has improved the accuracy of CCTA.[51]

3. CCTA is very sensitive and specific in evaluating stenosis in bypass grafts.[52–54] It is also beneficial in identifying the proximal course of the coronary arteries near the great vessels in patients with coronary anomalies.

C. **Cardiovascular magnetic resonance imaging (CMRI)** is able to visualize the proximal portions of coronary arteries, but it is not quite as sensitive and specific as CCTA and therefore is not recommended for the routine identification of coronary disease (Figure 2.22).[55–57]

1. The advantages of CMRI are the lack of irradiation or contrast, less interference from coronary calcification, and less motion artifact at higher heart rates. However, suboptimal images will be obtained in patients with stents, arrhythmias, or irregular breathing patterns. CMRI is contraindicated in patients with pacemakers or ICDs.

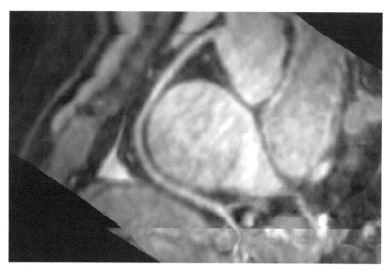

Figure 2.22 • A cardiovascular MR image (CMRI) of the right coronary artery. (Image courtesy of Timothy Albert, MD, FACC, Salinas Valley Memorial Cardiovascular Diagnostic Center)

    2. The primary indications for CMRI in the assessment of coronary artery disease are:

        a. Coronary anomalies, by identifying their proximal course (especially in young patients)

        b. Coronary aneurysms

        c. Saphenous vein graft and internal thoracic artery stenosis. CMRI has a sensitivity and specificity >90% in identifying significant lesions.[58,59] However, if the patient is symptomatic and may require an intervention, CMRI is usually not indicated unless the graft cannot be selectively cannulated by routine angiography. CMRI and CCTA have similar accuracy in assessing bypass grafts.

VIII. Evaluation of Aortic and Cardiac Disease by CT and MR Scanning

  A. **Computerized tomography (CT) scanning** is used primarily for the evaluation of aortic disease, but has several other potential uses in identifying chest pathology in addition to CCTA. 64-slice CT angiography with color volume-rendered multiplanar reformation provides excellent angiographic images.

    1. Identification of an aortic dissection in a patient with a typical or atypical presentation (Figures 2.23 and 2.24). This requires a CT scan with contrast and can also simultaneously rule out a pulmonary embolism. CT scans can also be used for postoperative follow-up to identify distal aneurysmal disease.

(A)

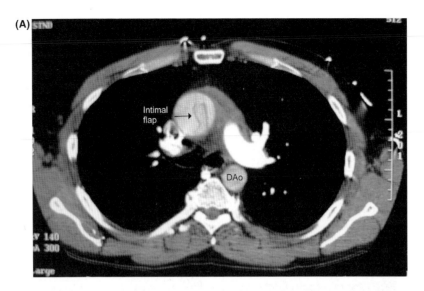

(B)

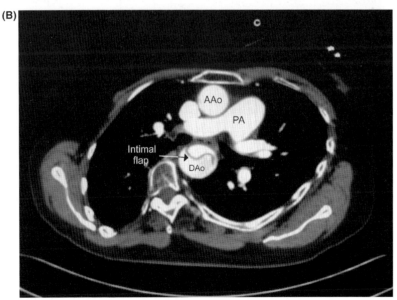

Figure 2.23 • CT scan with contrast of aortic dissections. (A) Type A involving only the ascending aorta. (B) Type B starting just distal to the left subclavian artery without any involvement of the ascending aorta. Note the intimal flap separating the true and false lumens. AAo, ascending aorta; DAo, descending aorta; PA, pulmonary artery.

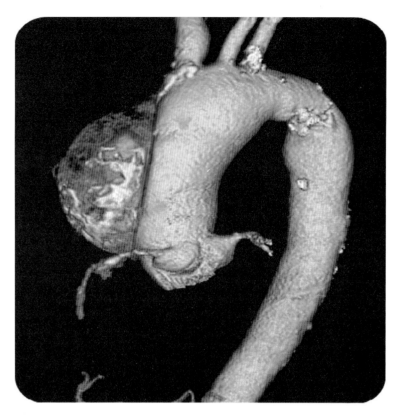

Figure 2.24 • 64-slice 3-D reconstruction of a chronic type A aortic dissection (Image courtesy of Grayson Wheatley III, MD, Arizona Heart Institute)

2. Assessment of aortic size

   a. When the standard angiogram (left ventriculogram or root shot) suggests ascending aortic enlargement, a contrast CT scan with three-dimensional reconstruction can provide transverse, sagittal, and coronal cuts as well as a rotational three-dimensional image (Figure 2.25). This can provide an exact measurement of aortic diameter, since an obliquely coursing structure (such as a tortuous or ectatic segment of aorta) will give a spuriously increased measurement on transverse cuts which will not reflect the true diameter of the aorta. Three-dimensional imaging also gives a better appreciation of the distal extent of disease. If the aneurysm tapers proximal to the arch, it may be possible to sew a distal anastomosis with a clamp in place. If it extends into the proximal arch, this will require circulatory arrest.

   b. Descending thoracic aneurysms (Figure 2.26)

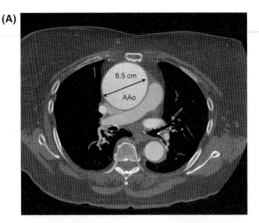

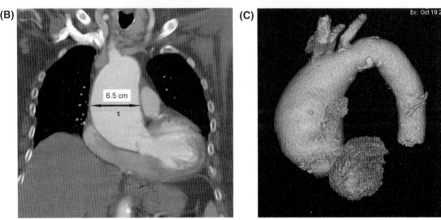

Figure 2.25 • (A) CT scan demonstrating a 6.5 cm ascending aorta (AAo) that will need to be replaced at the time of aortic valve surgery by a valved conduit. (B) The coronal slice is somewhat helpful in defining the aortic anatomy, but (C) a three-dimensional reconstruction using a 64-slice scanner provides an image which can be rotated and provides an even better delineation of the extent of the aneurysm, especially at the level of the arch. (Images courtesy of Robert Hagberg, MD, Beth Israel Deaconess Medical Center, Boston, MA.)

3. Evaluation of ascending aortic calcification suggested by chest x-ray or fluoroscopy (Figure 2.9). This should be done without contrast.

4. Location of right ventricle, aorta, saphenous vein grafts, or ITA graft in planning of reoperative surgery.[60]

5. Identification of pericardial (and pleural) effusions or the thickness of the pericardium in cases of constrictive pericarditis.

6. Identification of intracardiac masses (Figure 2.19B).

7. Identification of pulmonary or mediastinal abnormalities on preoperative chest x-ray. Obtaining a baseline CT scan prior to cardiac surgery

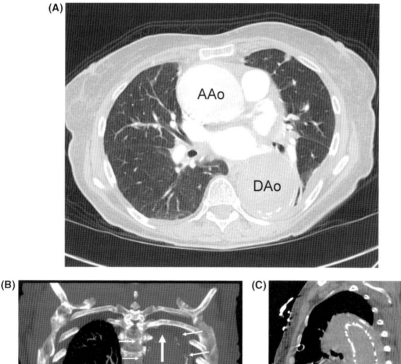

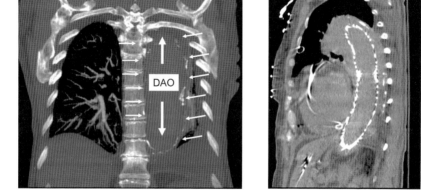

Figure 2.26 • (A) CT scan of ascending and descending thoracic aneurysms. (B) The coronal cut demonstrates the large descending thoracic aneurysm (no contrast present). (C) An endovascular stent has been placed to repair the aneurysm. AAo, ascending aorta; DAo, descending aorta.

eliminates the potential distortion of pulmonary pathology by postoperative changes.

   B. **Cardiovascular magnetic resonance imaging (CMRI)** is useful in the identification of cardiac disease and imaging of the aorta and its branches, in addition to its ability to provide adequate images of coronary arteries and bypass grafts.[61]

      1. CMRI cannot be performed in patients with pacemakers or ICDs, but it can be performed in patients with coronary stents, current-generation

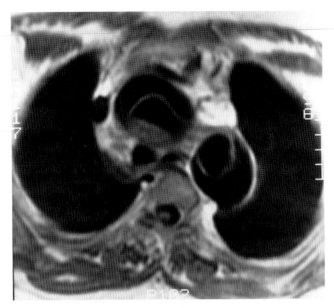

Figure 2.27 • MRI scan demonstrating the intimal flap separating the true and false lumens in a patient with an extensive aortic dissection involving both the ascending and descending thoracic aorta.

mechanical prosthetic heart valves (note that most bileaflet valves are composed of carbon and silicone and not metal), and retained epicardial pacing wires. Manufacturers of coronary stents have indicated that MRI scanning with magnetic fields less than 3-tesla are safe for newly implanted stents, and several studies indicate that there are no adverse long-term effects of performing an MRI soon after stent implantation.[62,63] The major advantage of MRI is the avoidance of radiation, and therefore it is preferable in the young patient. Contraindications to MRI are noted on multiple websites under a search for this topic.

2. CMRI is the most sensitive and specific test for detection of an aortic dissection (Figure 2.27). It can demonstrate differential flow velocities in the true and false channels and can identify branch artery compromise. However, it generally cannot be performed in the unstable patient requiring careful monitoring and often intravenous infusions. However, it should be considered when the clinical suspicion of a dissection is very high, yet other tests have been inconclusive. Most commonly, it is used in the follow-up of patients who have had repair of an aortic dissection to assess the status of the false channel or distal aneurysmal expansion.

3. Aortic and cerebrovascular diseases can be defined by magnetic resonance angiography (MRA) using time-of-flight (TOF) MRA and gadolinium-enhanced MRA (Figure 2.28). Spin-echo and cine CMRI can also be used

(A)

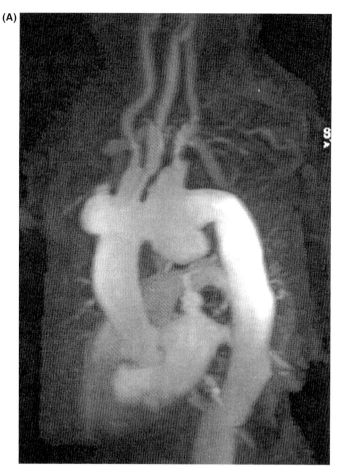

Figure 2.28 • (A) MRA with gadolinium demonstrating aneurysms of the aortic arch on a rotational image that were poorly delineated in transverse images.

to provide excellent three-dimensional images of aortic disease, including true and false aneurysms and periaortic abscesses or perigraft fluid collections.

4. Cine CMRI allows for differentiation of blood (bright images) from cardiac tissue (dark images). It is useful in the assessment of ventricular function, valvular pathology, and intracardiac masses (Figure 2.19C).

5. CMRI is useful in the assessment of pericarditis or tumor invasion into the pericardium.

6. Pharmacologic stress CMRI using dobutamine, dipyridamole, or adenosine is used when assessing for ischemia. Myocardial viability may be evaluated using

(B)

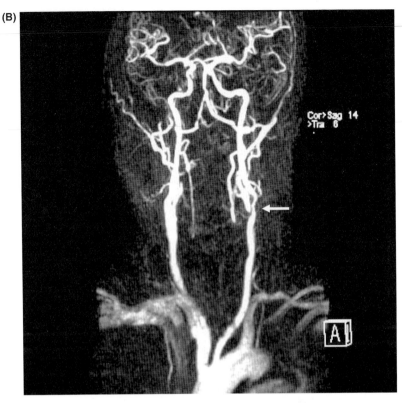

Figure 2.28 • *(Continued)* (B) MRA nicely demonstrating extracranial carotid stenosis (arrow) as well as the intracranial vessels to the circle of Willis.

gadolinium (to distinguish hibernating from infarcted myocardium) or dobutamine (systolic wall thickening being predictive of functional recovery). CMRI is comparable or superior to dobutamine stress echocardiography in predicting functional recovery after revascularization.[64,65]

References

1. Merino-Ramirez MA, Juan G, Ramón M, et al. Electrophysiologic evaluation of phrenic nerve and diaphragm function after coronary bypass surgery: prospective study of diabetes and other risk factors. *J Thorac Cardiovasc Surg* 2006;132:530–6.

2. Yamazaki K, Kato H, Tsujimoto S, Kitamura R. Diabetes mellitus, internal thoracic artery grafting, and the risk of an elevated hemidiaphragm after coronary artery bypass surgery. *J Cardiothorac Vasc Anesth* 1994;8:437–40.

3. San Román SA, Vilacosta I, Castillo JA, et al. Selection of the optimal stress test for the diagnosis of coronary artery disease. *Heart* 1998;80:370–6.

4. Gibbons RJ, Balady GJ, Bricker JT, et al. ACC/AHA 2002 guidelines for exercise testing: summary article. A report of the American College of Cardiology/American Heart Association Task Force on Practice Guidelines (Committee to Update the 1997 Exercise Testing Guidelines). *J Am Coll Cardiol* 2002;40:1531–40.

5. Kim C, Kwok YS, Heagerty P, Redberg R. Pharmacologic stress testing for coronary disease diagnosis: a meta-analysis. *Am Heart J* 2001;142:934–44.

6. Tavel ME. Stress testing in cardiac evaluation. Current concepts with emphasis on the ECG. *Chest* 2001;119:907–25.

7. Klocke FJ, Baird MG, Lorell BH, et al. ACC/AHA/ASNC guidelines for the clinical use of cardiac radionuclide imaging – executive summary: a report of the American College of Cardiology/American Heart Association Task Force on Practice Guidelines (ACC/AHA/ASNC Committee to Revise the 1995 Guidelines for the Clinical Use of Cardiac Radionuclide Imaging). *J Am Coll Cardiol* 2003;42:1318–33.

8. Hendel RC, Berman DS, Di Carli MF, et al. ACCF/ASNC/ACR/AHA/SCCT/SCMR/SNM 2009 appropriate use criteria for cardiac radionuclide imaging A report of the American College of Cardiology Foundation Appropriate Use Criteria Task Force, the American Society of Nuclear Cardiology, the American College of Radiology, the American Heart Association, the American Society of Echocardiography, the Society of Cardiovascular Computed Tomography, the Society for Cardiovascular Magnetic Resonance, and the Society of Nuclear Medicine. *J Am Coll Cardiol* 2009;53:2201–29 (available at www.cardiosource.com/guidelines).

9. Heller GV, Kapetanopoulos A. Pharmacologic stress radionuclide myocardial perfusion imaging: testing methodologies and safety. www.utdol.com, 2009.

10. Elhendy A, Bax JJ, Poldermans D. Dobutamine stress myocardial perfusion imaging in coronary artery disease. *J Nucl Med* 2002;43:1634–46.

11. Gould KL. Coronary flow reserve and pharmacologic stress perfusion imaging: beginnings and evolution. *JACC Cardiovasc Imaging* 2009;2:664–9.

12. Dilsizian V, Rocco TP, Freedman NM, Leon MB, Bonow RO. Enhanced detection of ischemic but viable myocardium by the reinjection of thallium after stress-redistribution imaging. *N Engl J Med* 1990;323:141–6.

13. Bateman TM, Heller GV, McGhie AI, et al. Diagnostic accuracy of rest/stress ECG-gated Rb-82 myocardial perfusion PET: comparison with ECG-gated Tc-99m sestamibi SPECT. *J Nucl Cardiol* 2006;13:24–33.

14. Douglas PS, Khandheria B, Stainback RF, et al. ACCF/ASE/ACEP/AHA/ASNC/SCAI/SCCT/SCMR 2008 appropriateness criteria for stress echocardiography. A report of the American College of Cardiology Foundation Appropriateness Criteria Task Force, American Society of Echocardiography, American College of Emergency Physicians, American Heart Association, American Society of Nuclear Cardiology, Society for Cardiovascular Angiography and Interventions, Society of Cardiovascular Computed Tomography, and Society for Cardiovascular Magnetic Resonance. Endorsed by the Heart Rhythm Society and the Society of Critical Care Medicine. *J Am Coll Cardiol* 2008;51:1127–47 (available at content.onlinejacc.org).

15. Pellikka PA. Stress echocardiography for the diagnosis of coronary artery disease: progress towards quantification. *Curr Opin Cardiol* 2005;20:395–8.

16. Soman P, Udelson JE. Assessment of myocardial viability by nuclear imaging in coronary heart disease. www.utdol.com, 2009.

17. Allman KC, Shaw LJ, Hachamovitch R, Udelson JE. Myocardial viability testing and impact of revascularization on prognosis in patients with coronary artery disease and left ventricular dysfunction: a meta-analysis. *J Am Coll Cardiol* 2002;39:1151–8.

18. Di Carli MF, Hachamovitch R, Berman DS. The art and science of predicting postrevascularization improvement in left ventricular (LV) function in patients with severely depressed LV function. *J Am Coll Cardiol* 2002;40:1744–7.

19. Bax JJ, Poldermans D, Elhendy A, Boersma E, Rahimtoola SH. Sensitivity, specificity, and predictive accuracies of various noninvasive techniques for detecting hibernating myocardium. *Curr Probl Cardiol* 2001;26:147–86.

20. Schinkel AF, Bax JJ, Biagini E, et al. Myocardial technetium-99m-tetrofosmin single-photon emission computed tomography compared with 18F-fluorodeoxyglucose imaging to assess myocardial viability. *Am J Cardiol* 2005;95:1223–5.

21. Schinkel AF, Poldermans D, Rizzello V, et al. Why do patients with ischemic cardiomyopathy and a substantial amount of viable myocardium not always recover in function after revascularization? *J Thorac Cardiovasc Surg* 2004;127:385–90.

22. Marzullo P, Parodi O, Reisenhofer B, et al. Value of rest thallium-201/technetium-99m sestamibi scans and dobutamine echocardiography for detecting myocardial viability. *Am J Cardiol* 1993;71:166–72.

23. Cornel JH, Bax JJ, Elhendy A, et al. Biphasic response to dobutamine predicts improvement of global left ventricular function after surgical revascularization in patients with stable coronary artery disease: implications of time course of recovery on diagnostic accuracy. *J Am Coll Cardiol* 1998;31:1002–10.

24. Picano E, Pibarot P, lLancellotti P, Monin JL, Bonow RO. The emerging role of exercise testing and stress echocardiography in valvular heart disease. *J Am Coll Cardiol* 2009;54:2251–60.

25. Kim RJ, Wu E, Rafael A, et al. The use of contrast-enhanced magnetic resonance imaging to identify reversible myocardial dysfunction. *N Engl J Med* 2000;343:1445–53.

26. Shan K, Constantine G, Sivananthan M, Flamm SD. Role of cardiac magnetic resonance imaging in the assessment of myocardial viability. *Circulation* 2004;109:1328–34.

27. Baim DS. *Grossman's Cardiac Catheterization, Angiography, and Intervention*, 7th edition. Philadelphia: Lippincott, Williams & Wilkins, 2005.

28. Ragosta M. Cardiac Catheterization: an Atlas and DVD, 4th edition. Philadelphia: WB Saunders, 2009.

29. Meine TJ, Harrison JK. Should we cross the valve: the risk of retrograde catheterization of the left ventricle in patients with aortic stenosis. *Am Heart J* 2004;148:41–2.

30. Talreja DR, Nishimura RA, Oh JK, Holmes DR. Constrictive pericarditis in the modern era: novel criteria for diagnosis in the cardiac catheterization laboratory. *J Am Coll Cardiol* 2008;51:315–9.

31. Tobis J, Azarbal B, Slavin L. Assessment of intermediate severity coronary lesions in the catheterization laboratory. *J Am Coll Cardiol* 2007;49:839–48.

32. Fassa AA, Wagatsuma K, Higano ST, et al. Intravascular ultrasound-guided treatment for angiographically indeterminate left main coronary artery disease: a long-term follow-up study. *J Am Coll Cardiol* 2005;45:204–11.

33. Arora H, Posligua W, Mesa A. Use of fractional flow reserve and intravascular ultrasonography to evaluate ambiguous left main coronary artery stenosis. *Tex Heart Inst J* 2008;35:329–33.

34. Blows LJ, Redwood SR. The pressure wire in practice. *Heart* 2007;93:419–22.

35. Bishop AH, Samady H. Fractional flow reserve: critical review of an important physiologic adjunct to angiography. *Am Heart J* 2004;147:792–802.

36. Courtis J, Rodés-Cabau J, Larose E, et al. Usefulness of coronary fractional flow reserve measurements in guiding clinical decisions in intermediate or equivocal left main coronary stenoses. *Am J Cardiol* 2009;103:943–9.

37. Tonino PA, Fearon WF, De Bruyne B, et al. Angiographic versus functional severity of coronary artery stenoses in the FAME study: fractional flow reserve versus angiography in multivessel evaluation. *J Am Coll Cardiol* 2010;55:2816–21.

38. Kelly AM, Dwamena B, Cronin P, Bernstein SJ, Carlos RC. Meta-analysis: effectiveness of drugs for preventing contrast-induced nephropathy. *Ann Intern Med* 2008;148:284–94.

39. Ozcan EE, Guneri S, Akdeniz B, et al. Sodium bicarbonate, N-acetylcysteine, and saline for prevention of radiocontrast-induced nephropathy. A comparison of 3 regimens for protecting contrast-induced nephropathy in patients undergoing coronary procedures. A single-center prospective controlled trial. *Am Heart J* 2007;154:539–44.

40. Hogan SE, L'Allier P, Chetcuti S, et al. Current role of sodium bicarbonate-based preprocedural hydration for the prevention of contrast-induced acute kidney injury: a meta-analysis. *Am Heart J* 2008;156:414–21.

41. Maioli M, Toso A, Leoncini M, et al. Sodium bicarbonate versus saline for the prevention of contrast-induced nephropathy in patients with renal dysfunction undergoing coronary angiography or intervention. *J Am Coll Cardiol* 2008;52:599–604.

42. Brown JR, Block CA, Malenka DJ, O'Connor GT, Schoolwerth AC, Thompson CA. Sodium bicarbonate plus N-acetylcysteine prophylaxis: a meta-analysis. *JACC Cardiovasc Interv* 2009;2:1116–24.

43. Oh JK, Seward JB, Tajik AJ. *The Echo Manual*, 3rd edition. Philadelphia: Lippincott Williams & Wilkins, 2007.

44. Grewal J, Mankad S, Freeman WK, et al. Real-time three-dimensional transesophageal echocardiography in the intraoperative assessment of mitral valve disease. *J Am Soc Echocardiogr* 2009;22:34–41.

45. Gerber TC, Manning WJ. Noninvasive coronary angiography with cardiac computed tomography and cardiovascular magnetic resonance. www.utdol.com, 2009.

46. Budoff MJ, Cohen MC, Garcia MJ, et al. ACCF/AHA clinical competence statement on cardiac imaging with computed tomography and magnetic resonance: a report of the American College of Cardiology Foundation/American Heart Association/American College of Physicians Task Force on Clinical Competence and Training. *J Am Coll Cardiol* 2005;46:383–402 and online at content.onlinejacc.org.

47. Budoff MJ, Dowe D, Jollis JG, et al. Diagnostic performance of 64-multidetector row coronary computed tomographic angiography for evaluation of coronary artery stenosis in individuals without known coronary artery disease: results from the prospective multicenter ACCURACY (Assessment by Coronary Computed Tomographic Angiography of Individuals Undergoing Invasive Coronary Angiography) Trial. *J Am Coll Cardiol* 2008;52:1724–32.

48. Miller JM, Rochitte CE, Dewey M, et al. Diagnostic performance of coronary angiography by 64-row CT. *N Engl J Med* 2008;359:2324–36.

49. Min JK, Shaw LJ, Berman DS. The present state of coronary computed tomography angiography. A process in evolution. *J Am Coll Cardiol* 2010;55:957–65.

50. Ehara M, Kawai M, Surmely JF, et al. Diagnostic accuracy of coronary in-stent stenosis using 64-slice computed tomography: comparison with invasive coronary angiography. *J Am Coll Cardiol* 2007;49:951–9.

51. Rispler S, Keidar Z, Ghersin E, et al. Integrated single-photon emission computed tomography and computed tomography coronary angiography for the assessment of hemodynamically significant coronary artery lesions. *J Am Coll Cardiol* 2007;49:1059–67.

52. Meyer TS, Martinoff S, Hadamitzky M, et al. Improved noninvasive assessment of coronary artery bypass grafts with 64-slice computed tomographic angiography in an unselected patient population. *J Am Coll Cardiol* 2007;49:946–50.

53. Ropers D, Pohle RK, Kuettner A, et al. Diagnostic accuracy of noninvasive coronary angiography in patients after bypass surgery using 64-slice spiral computed tomography with 330-ms gantry rotation. *Circulation* 2006;114:2334–41.

54. Jones CM, Athanasiou T, Dunne N, et al. Multi-detector computed tomography in coronary artery bypass graft assessment: a meta-analysis. *Ann Thorac Surg* 2007;83:341–8.

55. Schuijf JD, Bax JJ, Shaw LJ, et al. Meta-analysis of comparative diagnostic performance of magnetic resonance imaging and multislice computed tomography for noninvasive coronary angiography. *Am Heart J* 2006;151:404–11.

56. Dewey M, Teige F, Schnapauff D, et al. Noninvasive detection of coronary artery stenoses with multislice computed tomography or magnetic resonance imaging. *Ann Intern Med* 2006;145:407–15.

57. Nandalur KR, Dwamena BA, Choudhri AF, Nandalur MR, Carlos RC. Diagnostic performance of stress cardiac magnetic resonance imaging in the detection of coronary artery disease. A meta-analysis. *J Am Coll Cardiol* 2007;50:1343–53.

58. Langerak SE, Vliegen HW, Jukema JW, et al. Value of magnetic resonance imaging for the noninvasive detection of stenosis in coronary artery bypass grafts and recipient coronary arteries. *Circulation* 2003;107:1502–8.

59. Salm LP, Bax JJ, Vliegen HW, et al. Functional significance of stenoses in coronary artery bypass grafts. Evaluation by single-photon emission computed tomography perfusion imaging, cardiovascular magnetic resonance, and angiography. *J Am Coll Cardiol* 2004;44:1877–82.

60. Kamdar AR, Meadows TA, Roselli EE, et al. Multidetector computed tomographic angiography in planning of reoperative cardiothoracic surgery. *Ann Thorac Surg* 2008;85:1239–46.

61. Fuisz AR, Pohost GM. Clinical utility of cardiovascular magnetic resonance imaging. www.utdol.com, 2009.

62. Kaya MG, Okyay K, Yazici H, et al. Long-term clinical effects of magnetic resonance imaging in patients with coronary artery stent implantation. *Coron Artery Dis* 2009;20:138–42.

63. Syed MA, Carlson K, Murphy M, Ingkanisorn WP, Rhoads KL, Arai AE. Long-term safety of cardiac magnetic resonance imaging performed in the first few days after bare-metal stent implantation. *J Magn Reson Imaging* 2006;24:1056–61.

64. Baer FM, Theissen P, Crnac J, et al. Head to head comparison of dobutamine-transesophageal echocardiography and dobutamine-magnetic resonance imaging for the prediction of left ventricular functional recovery in patients with chronic coronary disease. *Eur Heart J* 2000; 21:981–91.

65. Wellnehofer E, Olariu A, Klein C, et al. Magnetic resonance low-dose dobutamine test is superior to SCAR quantification for the prediction of functional recovery. *Circulation* 2004;109:2172–4.

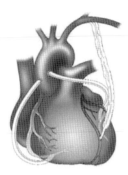

CHAPTER 3

General Preoperative Considerations and Preparation of the Patient for Surgery

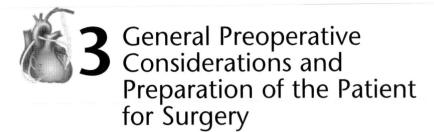

3 General Preoperative Considerations and Preparation of the Patient for Surgery

I. General Considerations

A. Once a patient is considered a candidate for cardiac surgery, a comprehensive evaluation of the patient's overall medical condition and comorbidities is essential. This includes a detailed history and physical examination, which may identify cardiac and noncardiac problems that might need to be addressed perioperatively to minimize postoperative morbidity (Table 3.1). On occasion, the severity of comorbidities and an assessment of the patient's quality of life may contraindicate a surgical procedure that might otherwise seem to be indicated. Attention should also be paid to identifying new cardiac abnormalities that may have arisen since the initial cardiac evaluation that may warrant further work-up. Baseline laboratory tests, if not recently performed, are also obtained, and further evaluation and consultation are performed, if indicated.

B. Evaluation of demographic factors, cardiac disease, and noncardiac comorbidities can afford both the surgeon and the patient an insight into the risk of surgery. A variety of bedside and computerized risk models are available that can provide risk assessment for individual patients, not just for operative mortality, but also for the occurrence of significant postoperative morbidities (see section VIII, pages 155–163). Data entry into software programs compatible with the Society of Thoracic Surgeons (STS) database allows surgeons to obtain an extensive analysis of their hospital's unadjusted and risk-adjusted results and a comparison with national norms (Table 3.2).

C. A cardiac anesthesiologist should interview and examine the patient and discuss issues related to sedation, anesthetic medications, monitoring lines, awakening from anesthesia, and mechanical ventilation. The anesthesiologist should also carefully review the patient's medications and make recommendations (in conjunction with the surgeon's policies) about whether certain medications should be modified or discontinued preoperatively.

D. Providing patients with information booklets related to their cardiac disease and proposed procedure is invaluable in alleviating some of the stress and anxiety of having to undergo open-heart surgery. If possible, nurses or physician assistants with experience

Manual of Perioperative Care in Adult Cardiac Surgery, 5th Edition. By Robert M. Bojar.
Published 2011 by Blackwell Publishing Ltd.

Table 3.1 • Preoperative Evaluation for Open-Heart Surgery

History

1. Bleeding issues: antiplatelet or anticoagulant medications, bleeding history
2. Smoking (COPD, bronchospasm)
3. Alcohol (cirrhosis, DTs)
4. Diabetes (wound infections, risk of protamine reaction)
5. Neurologic symptoms (transient ischemic attacks, remote stroke, previous carotid endarterectomy)
6. Vein stripping (alternative conduits)
7. Distal vascular reconstruction (alternative conduits)
8. Urologic symptoms (antibiotics, catheter placement problems)
9. Ulcer disease/GI bleeding (stress prophylaxis)
10. Active infections (urinary tract)
11. Current medications
12. Drug allergies

Physical Examination

1. Skin infections/rash
2. Dental caries (valve surgery)
3. Vascular examination: carotid bruits (stroke), abdominal aneurysm and peripheral pulses (IABP placement, groin cannulation for minimally invasive procedures or aortic surgery)
4. Differential arm blood pressures (pedicled ITA grafts)
5. Heart/lungs (congestive heart failure, new murmur)
6. Varicose veins (alternative conduits)

Laboratory Data

1. Hematology: CBC, PT, PTT, platelet count
2. Chemistry: electrolytes, BUN, creatinine, blood glucose, liver function tests (baseline for use of statins)
3. Arterial blood gases if room air O_2 saturation $< 90\%$
4. TSH (if amiodarone to be used)
5. Hemoglobin A1c level (assessment of diabetic control)
6. BNP level
7. Urinalysis
8. Chest x-ray PA and lateral
9. Electrocardiogram

in postoperative care should discuss a simplified critical pathway so that the patient has a realistic expectation of what will transpire during the hospital stay. Informing the patient of what procedures will take place and when, what is expected of him/her on each day, when discharge should be anticipated, and what the options are for post-hospital discharge care (home health care, rehabilitation facility, or skilled nursing facility) are extremely beneficial in enhancing the patient's involvement in his/her own care and promoting a prompt recovery from surgery and early hospital discharge.

Table 3.2 • Risk Factors for Operative Mortality in the Society of Thoracic Surgeons (STS) Database

Demographics	Cardiac Disease
Age	History of MI <24 h
Gender	Left main disease
BSA	Ejection fraction
Race	Number of diseased vessels
	Associated valve disease

Comorbidities	Preoperative Status
Renal failure/dialysis	Salvage status
Cerebrovascular disease	Cardiogenic shock
COPD	Preoperative IABP
Diabetes	Reoperation
Peripheral vascular disease	NYHA class
Hypertension	Failed PCI <6 h
Hypercholesterolemia	
Immunosuppressive therapy	

Factors are listed in order of their relative risk ratio for operative mortality within each category (i.e., the factor associated with the highest mortality is noted first and achieves greater weighting in the risk assessment models).

A partial list of definitions from the 2011 STS specification publication is noted in Appendix 13.

II. History

    A. The nature, duration, and pattern of the patient's cardiac symptoms should be briefly summarized to allow for symptomatic classification using either the Canadian Classification System (for angina) or the New York Heart Association (NYHA) system (for both angina and heart failure symptoms). The results of diagnostic tests previously performed should be noted.

    B. Review of the patient's prior and current medications is important. Particular attention should be paid to antiischemic and antiplatelet/anticoagulant medications which should be either continued or stopped prior to surgery, depending on the clinical situation (Tables 3.3 and 3.4).

        1. Aspirin (ASA) is beneficial for the primary and secondary prevention of cardiovascular disease and is given routinely to patients presenting with acute coronary syndromes (ACS). Furthermore, its preoperative use has been shown to improve outcomes in patients undergoing coronary artery bypass grafting (CABG).[1,2] Aspirin irreversibly acetylates platelet cyclooxygenase, impairing thromboxane A_2 formation and inhibiting platelet aggregation for the life span of the platelet (7–10 days). Thus, aspirin will be superimposing impaired platelet dysfunction on the clotting derangements induced by cardiopulmonary bypass (CPB).

Table 3.3 • Platelet Inhibitors To Be Stopped Prior to Surgery

	Mechanism of Action	Duration of Effect	Discontinue Preoperatively
Aspirin	Inhibits cyclooxygenase	7 days (life span of platelets)	3–7 days
Clopidogrel	Inhibits ADP receptor P2Y12 (irreversible)	7 days (life span of platelets)	5–7 days
Prasugrel	Inhibits ADP receptor P2Y12 (irreversible)	7 days (life span of platelets)	7 days
Ticagrelor	Inhibits ADP receptor P2Y12 (reversible)	1–2 days ($t_{1/2} = 7$–8 h)	24–36 hours
Tirofiban	Inhibits IIb/IIIa receptor	4–6 hours	4 hours
Eptifibatide	Inhibits IIb/IIIa receptor	4–6 hours	4 hours
Abciximab	Inhibits IIb/IIIa receptor	>24 hours	24 hours

Table 3.4 • Other Anticoagulants to Be Stopped Prior to Surgery

	Mechanism of Action	Duration of Effect	Discontinue Preoperatively
Warfarin	Inhibits clotting factor synthesis	4–5 days	4–5 days
Unfractionated heparin	Binds to antithrombin III, primarily inhibiting thrombin and factor Xa	4 hours	4 hours
LMWH	Inhibits factors Xa and II	12–18 h ($t_{1/2} = 4.5$ h)	18–24 hours
Fondaparinux	Inhibits factor Xa	48 h ($t_{1/2} = 17$–21 h)	48 hours
Bivalirudin	Direct thrombin inhibitor	2 h ($t_{1/2} = 25$ min)	1–2 hours

a. Most studies have shown that preoperative use of aspirin increases perioperative blood loss, but this is generally noted in patients taking 325 mg daily, not with lower doses. Thus, it is advisable to continue aspirin 81 mg daily up to the day of surgery in ACS patients.[3–10]

b. In elective patients, aspirin may be stopped 3–5 days preoperatively.[5] Significant improvement of platelet function occurs within 3 days of the last dose, at which time there is regeneration of half of the platelet pool, resulting in normalization of bleeding times and thromboxane B_2 levels.[11,12] Because of the potential benefits of preoperative aspirin in reducing the risk of perioperative myocardial infarction (MI) and mortality, it is not unreasonable to continue aspirin in all patients up to the time of surgery.

c. Studies have shown that there is enhanced platelet aggregation and thromboxane formation in the early postoperative period, even in patients receiving preoperative aspirin.[13] This is more common following off-pump (OPCAB) than on-pump cases.[14] Use of preoperative aspirin and initiation of aspirin within 6–8 hours after surgery to mitigate the extent of platelet activation and aggregation might improve graft patency, reduce the occurrence of perioperative MI, and improve operative survival.

d. A variety of platelet aggregometry tests are available to assess the antiplatelet effect of aspirin, but they may not necessarily correlate with the degree of platelet inhibition, and are rarely indicated before surgery.[15,16] It is likely that the 20% of patients who have "aspirin resistance" with inadequate inhibition of platelet function will exhibit minimal intraoperative bleeding, while those who are aspirin responders may bleed more. Patients taking higher doses of aspirin and those with conditions associated with platelet dysfunction, such as uremia and von Willebrand's disease, may also exhibit more bleeding. In addition, there are a few patients considered to be "hyperresponders" to aspirin who exhibit very prolonged bleeding times and thus may be more predisposed to perioperative bleeding.[5] If these patients are recognized, it may be advisable to stop aspirin a few days before surgery.

2. **Clopidogrel** (Plavix) is a thienopyridine that is biotransformed into an active metabolite which inhibits platelet function by irreversibly modifying the platelet adenosine diphosphate (ADP) receptor $P2Y_{12}$, inhibiting ADP-mediated activation of the glycoprotein IIb/IIIa receptor. Genetic polymorphisms in the CYP2C19 allele reduce conversion to the active metabolite, resulting in clopidogrel resistance. The drug is commonly administered to patients with an ACS and to those in whom percutaneous coronary intervention (PCI) is contemplated. It is usually given as a loading dose of 300–600 mg, which achieves about 40% platelet inhibition within a few hours. This effect lasts for the life span of the platelet. Platelet transfusions given within 6 hours of a loading dose or 4 hours after a maintenance dose may be less effective because some of the active metabolite may bind exogenous platelets. Virtually all patients receiving clopidogrel also receive aspirin, producing dual antiplatelet activity.

a. Most studies have shown that clopidogrel taken within 5 days of surgery (perhaps 3 days for off-pump surgery) is associated with an increased risk of bleeding and increased rates of transfusion and reexploration for bleeding.[3–6,17–23] For patients undergoing elective surgery, clopidogrel should be discontinued 5–7 days preoperatively. The role of platelet function testing to assess the degree of platelet inhibition by clopidogrel prior to surgery is undefined. However, it is feasible that if some degree of clopidogrel resistance is present, surgery could be performed early than the recommended 5–7-day waiting period without incurring an increased risk of bleeding.

b. For patients receiving clopidogrel who require urgent surgery, the surgery should not be delayed if clinically indicated. The surgeon should be aware of the potential for increased bleeding and the necessity for platelet transfusions.

c. Patients on aspirin/clopidogrel following placement of coronary stents who present for urgent or elective surgery (of any kind) pose a potential dilemma. The risk of stent thrombosis is increased within the first month with bare-metal stents (BMS) and within 1 year for patients with drug-eluting stents (DES) if clopidogrel is stopped, and this is associated with a significant mortality risk of 40–50%.[3–6,24–26] In these patients, it is not unreasonable to stop the clopidogrel 3 days before surgery, which may provide some residual antiplatelet benefits for the stent, yet minimize the increased risk of bleeding. However, it is also reasonable to continue the clopidogrel up to the time of surgery and use platelets if necessary for excessive bleeding.

3. **Prasugrel** is a third-generation thienopyridine that produces irreversible antagonism of the ADP $P2Y_{12}$ receptor. It is approximately 10 times more potent than clopidogrel (60 mg prasugrel >600 mg clopidogrel), producing 80% platelet inhibition with a more rapid onset of action. There is less interpatient variability in the antiplatelet effects achieved than with clopidogrel, since its activity is not influenced by genetic variations in CYP2C19. Although clinically superior in ACS patients undergoing PCI, it may be associated with a higher risk of bleeding. Despite a short half-life of 7 hours (comparable to clopidogrel), the irreversible effect on platelet function mandates that it be stopped at least 7 days before surgery.[27] Similar to clopidogrel, platelet transfusions may be less effective when given within 4–6 hours of a dose of prasugrel.

4. **Ticagrelor** is a reversible inhibitor of the $P2Y_{12}$ receptor that has a more rapid onset of action and more pronounced inhibition of platelet function than clopidogrel. It has been found to be more effective in reducing death in patients with an ACS with a comparable rate (12%) of major bleeding. It is given as a 180 mg oral load followed by 90 mg twice a day. Its reversible effect on platelet function with a half-life of 7–8 hours should translate into a lower risk of operative bleeding if held for 1–2 days prior to surgery.[28]

5. **Cangrelor** is an intravenous reversible inhibitor of $P2Y_{12}$ which produces nearly 100% platelet inhibition with rapid onset of action since it does not require conversion to an active metabolite. It has a half-life of 3–6 minutes with reversal of effect in 30–60 minutes. Its availability may be limited by an increased risk of bleeding during PCI without significantly greater clinical efficacy.[29]

6. **Heparin** is given to patients with an ACS before and after cardiac catheterization if urgent surgery is recommended. It is also used in patients in whom an intra-aortic balloon pump (IABP) is placed preoperatively. It may also be used as a bridge to surgery in patients taking preoperative warfarin.

a. **Unfractionated heparin (UFH)** is given using a weight-based protocol (see Appendix 7) and requires monitoring by a partial thromboplastin time (PTT) to ensure a therapeutic range of approximately 50–60 seconds. In patients being bridged, heparin is usually stopped about 4 hours before surgery. However, in patients with critical coronary artery disease, it is best to continue heparin into the operating room. This should not pose a significant risk during insertion of central lines. When heparin is given for several days, the platelet count should be checked on a daily basis to assess for the development of heparin-induced thrombocytopenia (HIT) (see page 201).

b. **Low-molecular-weight heparin (LMWH)** (enoxaparin) is commonly used in patients with an ACS (1 mg/kg SC twice a day) due to its simplicity of use, with no requirement for blood monitoring. It may be used for venous thromboembolism (VTE) prophylaxis in a dose of 40 mg SC once daily. LMWH is also an alternative to UFH during cardiac catheterization procedures. LMWH has demonstrated comparable if not superior efficacy to UFH in ACS patients, because it not only inhibits the conversion of prothrombin to thrombin, but also inhibits activated factor X (factor Xa). Enoxaparin has an elimination half-life of 4.5 hours, but still exhibits 30% of anti-factor Xa activity at 12 hours. Furthermore, only 60% of LMWH can neutralized by protamine. Therefore it is recommended that the last dose should be given 18–24 hours prior to surgery to minimize perioperative bleeding.[5,30–32]

7. **Fondaparinux** (Arixtra) is an indirect factor Xa inhibitor that acts by catalyzing factor Xa inhibition by antithrombin. It is given in a daily dose of 2.5 mg SC for VTE prophylaxis and in a higher weight-based protocol for established thrombosis (5 mg if <50 kg, 7.5 mg if 50–100 kg, 10 mg if >100 kg). Its use in patients with ACS is being evaluated. Its effects cannot be reversed by protamine and, because of its long elimination half-life of 17–21 hours, the dose should be withheld for at least 48 hours prior to surgery.[33]

8. **Bivalirudin** (Angiomax) is a direct thrombin inhibitor that is approved as an alternative to UFH during PCI. Its benefits are a short half-life (25 minutes) and avoidance of exposure to heparin. The usual dose is a 0.7 mg/kg IV bolus followed by an infusion of 1.75 mg/kg/h during the procedure. Due to its short half-life, the potential risk for significant surgical bleeding (other than from the femoral artery puncture) would be increased only if an emergency procedure were required within 1–2 hours of its administration.

9. **Warfarin** is given primarily to patients with mechanical prosthetic valves, atrial fibrillation (AF), a history of VTE or pulmonary embolism, or hypercoagulable disorders. Warfarin should be stopped 4–5 days prior to surgery. Although the risk of thromboembolism is low during a brief period of underanticoagulation, this risk is difficult to quantitate and could be clinically significant if complications occur.[34,35]

a. If there are concerns about an increased risk of thromboembolism, short-acting anticoagulants should be considered. LMWH may be given as an outpatient for a few days (enoxaparin 1 mg/kg SC bid) but should be avoided in the 24 hours prior to surgery. The patient may then be admitted to the hospital the day before surgery for UFH.

b. If the patient requires urgent surgery and has an elevated international normalized ratio (INR), administration of 5 mg of vitamin K (given intravenously over 30 minutes) should significantly reduce the INR within 12–24 hours. This always runs the risk of an anaphylactic reaction, but the incidence is extremely low. Fresh frozen plasma may be necessary if more emergent surgery is indicated. Oral vitamin K (5 mg) is safer than parenteral administration, but it takes longer to reverse the INR and is best used in less urgent situations. Subcutaneous vitamin K has unpredictable and delayed absorption and is not recommended.[35]

10. **Glycoprotein IIb/IIIa inhibitors** are commonly used in patients with an ACS and non-ST-elevation myocardial infarctions (NSTEMI) in whom an early invasive strategy is planned. They are usually continued after catheterization along with heparin if CABG is considered the best option for revascularization.

  a. **Eptifibatide** (Integrilin) and **tirofiban** (Aggrastat) are short-acting reversible antagonists of fibrinogen binding to the IIb/IIIa receptor.

   i. Eptifibatide is given as a 180 µg bolus followed by an infusion of 2.0 µg/kg/min for 72–96 hours. Tirofiban is given in a dose of 0.4 µg/kg/min for 30 minutes followed by an infusion of 0.1 µg/kg/min for 48–96 hours.

   ii. The time course of platelet inhibition parallels their plasma level. It is estimated that platelet aggregation returns to 90% of normal within 4–8 hours after stopping tirofiban and to 50–80% of normal within 4 hours of stopping eptifibatide. It is recommended that these medications be stopped approximately 4 hours prior to surgery (see Table 3.4).[36,37] It is noteworthy, however, that some studies have not identified an increased risk of postbypass bleeding even if these medications are stopped 2 hours preoperatively or even as late as the time of skin incision. This may be attributable to their transient "platelet anesthesia" effects, which may offset the adverse influence of CPB on platelet number and function.[38]

  b. **Abciximab** (ReoPro) is the Fab fragment of a monoclonal antibody that binds to the IIb/IIIa receptor on the surface of platelets. Platelet aggregation is significantly inhibited by preventing the binding of fibrinogen and von Willebrand's factor to this receptor site on activated platelets. This drug has a half-life of 12 hours and platelet function may take up to 48 hours to recover. If possible, surgery should be delayed for at least 24 hours after a patient has received abciximab. If emergency surgery is indicated, significant bleeding can be anticipated. Platelet transfusions are effective in producing hemostasis by reducing the overall number of platelet receptors bound to abciximab.[39] A hemoconcentrator can remove some of the residual free abciximab, allowing platelets to function more for hemostasis than for binding free antibody.[40] Fortunately, this medication has been supplanted in most centers by the shorter-acting reversible IIb/IIIa antagonists.

11. Surgery should be delayed at least 24 hours, if possible, in patients receiving **thrombolytic therapy** for an acute evolving ST-elevation infarction (STEMI). Increased perioperative bleeding may result from the persistent systemic hemostatic defects of thrombolytic agents that outlive their short half-lives (less than 30 minutes for most recombinant tissue plasminogen activator preparations). These effects include depletion of fibrinogen, reduction in factor II, V, and VIII levels, impairment of platelet aggregation, and the appearance of fibrin split products. When surgery must be performed on an emergency basis, the antifibrinolytic agents noted in Chapter 4 (page 199) and a variety of clotting factors are usually necessary to control mediastinal hemorrhage.

12. **Nonsteroidal anti-inflammatory drugs** have a reversible effect on platelet cyclooxygenase, and their antiplatelet effects are primarily determined by their

dosing and half-life. Generally, they only need to be stopped a few days before surgery.[41]

13. **Omega-3 fatty acids (fish oils)** have been shown to enhance platelet inhibition,[42] although one study suggested this only occurred when given with aspirin.[43] Flaxseed oil, garlic, vitamin E, and ginkgo preparations all have antiplatelet activity and should be stopped as soon as possible before surgery.[43–47] Even flavonoids in purple grape juice have been shown to inhibit platelet function.[48] All of these vitamins and herbal remedies may be of benefit to patients with coronary artery disease, but can contribute to significant perioperative bleeding if not recognized and stopped prior to surgery. It is imperative to specifically ask the patient if these products are being taken, since they are usually not volunteered when a list of medications is reviewed.

C. Inquiry should be made about any known clinical bleeding disorder or hypercoagulable state. This may direct perioperative anticoagulant management or provide direction in the treatment of bleeding problems.

1. **Antiphospholipid syndrome** is an autoimmune disorder in which antiphospholipid (APL) antibodies (anticardiolipin antibodies) and/or lupus anticoagulant are present. It is a rare phenomenon, but has been associated with valvular pathology. These antibodies produce a hypercoagulable state that may cause arterial and venous thrombosis even though the coagulation profile shows an elevated PTT and commonly thrombocytopenia. The APL antibodies affect the kaolin-activated activated clotting time (ACT), so celite ACTs have been recommended for intraoperative monitoring. However, a target ACT is difficult to define because the ACT is considered unreliable in assessing the degree of heparinization during surgery. Most reports recommend maintaining a high target ACT to minimize clotting risks or, preferably, use of a heparin–protamine titration test, aiming for a heparin level of 3.4 units/mL.[49–51] Alternatively, bivalirudin might be considered as a substitute anticoagulant during bypass (see Chapter 4).

2. Other hypercoagulable states, such as **factor V Leiden mutation** or **protein C or S deficiency,** are usually not recognized until the patient sustains a postoperative thrombotic event. However, if these syndromes are known to be present and the patient was taking preoperative warfarin, aggressive anticoagulant measures should be taken to reduce the risk of postoperative thrombosis. Admission for preoperative heparinization should be considered when the INR is subtherapeutic. If the patient has an **antithrombin III deficiency,** which is also a hypercoagulable condition, either fresh frozen plasma or antithrombin III concentrate (Thrombate) may be required to achieve adequate heparinization during cardiopulmonary bypass.[52]

D. **Chronic obstructive pulmonary disease** (COPD) is a term often applied to patients with a significant smoking history independent of the degree of respiratory impairment. However, the degree of COPD is best defined by pulmonary function testing (PFTs). Although this is not essential in patients without functional limitations, failure to perform spirometry testing may lead to underreporting of COPD and thus an underestimation of the risk of adverse outcomes in the STS database.[53]

1. The definitions of chronic lung disease in the 2011 STS database specifications are as follows:

    a. Mild: forced expiratory volume in the first second (FEV_1) 60–75% of predicted and/or on chronic inhaled or oral bronchodilator therapy

    b. Moderate: FEV_1 50–59% of predicted and/or on chronic steroid therapy

    c. Severe: FEV_1 <50% predicted and/or room air PO_2 <60 torr or PCO_2 >50 torr

2. Significant COPD, especially in elderly patients and those on steroids, is associated with an increased incidence of prolonged ventilation, sternal wound complications, longer ICU stays, and increased operative mortality.[54]

3. Baseline pulse oximetry on room air should be obtained on every patient, and if the oxygen saturation is less than 90%, arterial blood gases (ABGs) on room air should be obtained. If the patient has significant COPD, these can be valuable for comparison with postoperative values when weaning the patient from the ventilator. An elevated PCO_2 is a significant marker for postoperative pulmonary morbidity and mortality. Additionally, patients on home oxygen or with a baseline PO_2 <60 torr are extremely borderline operative candidates.

4. The patient's physiologic reserve and functional status, including the ability to walk up a flight of stairs or several hundred feet on a level surface, are sometimes as important, if not more important, than spirometric values in determining whether the patient can tolerate a surgical procedure.[55] Nonetheless, PFTs might identify patients at such high pulmonary risk that surgery may be contraindicated (generally an FEV_1 <0.6). Occasionally, especially in patients with valve disease and congestive heart failure (CHF), it may be difficult to determine the cardiac contribution to abnormal PFTs or diffusion capacity (<20% of predicted is an ominous sign of impaired ability to oxygenate). In this situation, careful clinical judgment must be used in deciding whether surgery will improve the patient's pulmonary status or will leave the patient a pulmonary cripple.

5. In addition to significant COPD, pulmonary complications are more common in patients who actively smoke and in those with advanced age, obesity, diabetes, preoperative cardiac instability, pulmonary hypertension, history of cerebrovascular disease, a productive cough, or lower respiratory tract colonization.[56,57] A logistic risk model to predict respiratory failure after valve surgery found the following to be independent predictors of respiratory failure: more complex surgery (multiple valves > valve-CABG > CABG), age >70, diabetes, reoperations or emergency operations, surgery for endocarditis, prior MI, CHF, and bypass times over 3 hours (Figure 10.2, page 397).[58]

6. Actively smoking patients should be advised to terminate smoking at least 4 weeks (and preferably 2 months) before surgery to decrease the volume of airway secretions and improve mucociliary transport.[59,60] Use of medications to assist smokers to quit, such as varenicline (Chantix) or bupropion HCL (Zyban), should be recommended as soon as possible once the patient understands the adverse influence of smoking on the perioperative course and long-term results of surgery. However, some patients have extreme difficulty stopping smoking due to their nicotine addiction and simply cannot stop prior to surgery. Unfortunately, not smoking for just a few days before surgery is probably of little benefit and may increase airway secretions. If a patient indicates that he/she has stopped smoking, further inquiry as to when this occurred is important, because being off of cigarettes for a few days ("Yes, I quit") while hospitalized still places the patient at increased risk of pulmonary complications.

7. An active pulmonary or bronchitic process (evidenced by a productive cough) should be resolved before surgery using antibiotics. Bronchospastic disease should be treated with bronchodilators and, if severe, with steroids. Pulmonary consultation may be indicated in this situation. Short-term pulmonary rehabilitation is effective in improving perioperative pulmonary function in patients with significant COPD and can reduce the risk of pulmonary complications.[61]

8. B-type natriuretic peptide (BNP) is secreted by the atria and ventricles in patients with systolic and diastolic dysfunction, with levels generally correlating with the patient's ejection fraction.[62] BNP levels are helpful in differentiating whether dyspnea is primarily of cardiac or pulmonary origin. A BNP level <100 pg/mL indicates that a patient's dyspnea is most likely related to a primary pulmonary process, such as exacerbation of COPD. In contrast, dyspnea in a patient with a BNP level >500 pg/mL is usually caused by decompensated heart failure. Intermediate values may be associated with LV dysfunction without decompensation, but a pulmonary process must also be considered in the differential diagnosis.[63]

9. Some patients on chronic high-dose amiodarone therapy are prone to the development of pulmonary toxicity and adult respiratory distress syndrome (ARDS) after surgery. This is manifested by dyspnea, hypoxia, radiographic infiltrates, and a decrease in diffusion capacity, and carries a very high mortality rate.[64] Evidence of preoperative pulmonary toxicity with a decrease in diffusion capacity may contraindicate a cardiac surgical procedure. Avoidance of potential contributing causes, such as a high inspired oxygen fraction, long duration of bypass, and fluid overload, is critical. On rare occasions, this syndrome may occur after a very short course of amiodarone, and it appears to be an idiosyncratic or hypersensitivity reaction.[65] Although baseline PFTs are not necessary in patients on a short-term course of amiodarone for atrial fibrillation prophylaxis, they should be considered when it is anticipated that the amiodarone may be given for more than 1 month (e.g. after a Maze procedure).

E. A history of heavy **alcohol** abuse identifies potential problems with intraoperative bleeding and postoperative hepatic dysfunction, agitation, and alcohol withdrawal. Prevention of postoperative delirium tremens (DTs) with thiamine, folate, and benzodiazepines should be considered. Bioprosthetic valves should be selected to avoid postoperative anticoagulation.

1. Mildly elevated liver function tests (LFTs) are often of unclear significance and usually do not require further evaluation. However, in a patient with a drinking history, they do not exclude the possibility of alcoholic hepatitis or cirrhosis, and a gastrointestinal (GI) consultation may be indicated. A common cause of mildly elevated LFTs is use of a statin medication for hypercholesterolemia.

2. A history of GI bleeding, an elevated prothrombin time (reported as the INR), a low serum albumin indicating impaired synthetic function or malnutrition, or a low platelet count, may suggest the presence of severe cirrhosis with portal hypertension and/or hypersplenism. A liver biopsy may be indicated to evaluate the risk of surgery and the potential for postoperative hepatic failure.

3. Two risk models have been used in cirrhotic patients to predict outcomes – the Child-Turcotte-Pugh (CTP) and the Mayo End-Stage Liver Disease (MELD) scores. Patients with CTP class A cirrhosis (Table 3.5) will usually tolerate CPB, but

Table 3.5 • Child-Turcotte-Pugh Classification of Cirrhosis

Total bilirubin (mg/dL)	Albumin (g/dl)	INR
<2: 1 point	>3.5: 1 point	<1.7: 1 point
2–3: 2 points	2.8–3.5: 2 points	1.71–2.2: 2 points
>3: 3 points	<2.8: 3 points	>2.2: 3 points
Ascites	**Encephalopathy**	**CTP Class**
None: 1 point	None: 1 point	Class A: 5–6 points
Controlled: 2 points	Controlled medically: 2 points	Class B: 7–9 points
Poorly controlled: 3 points	Poorly controlled: 3 points	Class C: 10–15 points

may have a higher risk of postoperative complications, including infections, bleeding, GI complications, respiratory and renal failure. Patients with advanced alcoholic cirrhosis (class B or C) or CTP score ≥ 8 are generally not candidates for cardiac surgery. The mortality rate for these patients is very high, with several studies showing mortality rates of 50–67% for class B and 100% for class C patients.[66-69]

4. The MELD score includes both hepatic and renal variables and may therefore be a more sensitive indicator of surgical risk. It is calculated from a summation of multiples of natural logarithms of the INR, serum creatinine, and total bilirubin (see calculator at www.mayoclinic.org/meld). Surgical risk is very high with a MELD score exceeding 13, especially if associated with a platelet count less than 96,000/µL (reflecting advanced liver fibrosis).[70]

5. With recognition that CPB is a major contributing factor to adverse outcomes, off-pump surgery should be considered in patients with advanced liver disease if their lifestyle and life span are compromised primarily by their heart disease.

F. **Diabetes mellitus** is a condition associated with more extensive and diffuse atherosclerotic disease due to metabolic derangements and a proinflammatory and prothrombotic state.[71] It may range in severity from mild hyperglycemia controlled with diet or oral medications to patients requiring insulin. The more severe and uncontrolled the diabetes, the greater the risk of obesity, congestive heart failure, peripheral vascular disease, extensive coronary artery disease, and chronic kidney disease.[72]

1. Generally, diabetes is associated with an increased postoperative risk of stroke, infection, and renal dysfunction, an increased operative mortality, a decrease in saphenous vein graft patency, and worse long-term survival.[71-74] Non-insulin dependent diabetics tend to fare somewhat better, with a lower immediate risk of postoperative complications, including respiratory and renal failure and mediastinitis. Their long-term prognosis is favorable in the absence of significant comorbidities.[71,75]

2. An elevated hemoglobin A1c (>7%) is a marker for poorly controlled diabetes in the previous 3–4 months and has been associated with more adverse outcomes, including infection, stroke, renal failure, and myocardial infarction, as well as reduced long-term survival after CABG.[76-78] One study showed that the CABG mortality risk increased fourfold when the hemoglobin A1c level was >8.6%.[77]

3. To optimize perioperative care, careful attention to potential diabetic-related complications is essential.

   a. Any preexisting infections must be treated (urinary infections are particularly common in diabetic women).

   b. Oral hypoglycemics and insulin are held the morning of surgery. Monitoring of intraoperative glucose levels and aggressive treatment to maintain blood glucose <180 mg/dL is essential to reduce neurologic morbidity and the risk of infection.

   c. In patients with any element of chronic kidney disease, steps must be taken during cardiac catheterization and surgery to optimize renal function (see Chapter 12).

   d. Although saphenous vein graft patency is compromised in diabetics, use of bilateral internal thoracic artery (ITA) bypass grafting is relatively contraindicated. Multiple studies have shown an increased risk of deep sternal wound infection, especially in insulin-dependent, obese women.[79,80] Notably, diabetics may be more prone to phrenic nerve dysfunction after ITA harvesting, so cautery near the phrenic nerve must be avoided.[81]

   e. Patients taking NPH insulin are at increased risk of experiencing an allergic reaction to protamine.[82]

   f. Management of postoperative hyperglycemia with a defined protocol (see Appendix 6) is an essential element of perioperative care and has been documented to reduce operative morbidity and mortality.[83,84] An endocrine consultation may be helpful in patients with refractory hyperglycemia.

G. **Neurologic symptoms** whether active (transient ischemic attack [TIA]) or remote (history of a stroke), increase the risk of perioperative stroke and warrant evaluation.[85,86] Generally, a carotid noninvasive study with ultrasound imaging and measurement of flow velocities should be performed in the patient with neurologic symptoms, a history of a carotid endarterectomy, or asymptomatic carotid bruits to assess for significant stenoses or flow-limiting lesions. A peak systolic velocity (PSV) >230 cm/sec in the internal carotid artery (ICA), an ICA/common carotid artery PSV >4.0, or an end-diastolic velocity >100 cm/sec associated with significant plaque burden by ultrasonic imaging are consistent with significant stenosis. Approximately 10–15% of patients requiring CABG have significant carotid disease. Selective screening limited to patients > age 65, or those with carotid bruits, TIA, or stroke can identify most patients at high risk.[87] Patients with hypertension, peripheral vascular disease, and particularly women with left main disease or calcified aortas are also at higher risk and should be screened. Further evaluation by carotid arteriography (usually magnetic resonance angiography) may be considered if noninvasive studies are inconclusive or more precise visualization of the carotid vessels is desired.

1. Actively symptomatic carotid disease always warrants carotid endarterectomy (CEA) either prior to or at the time of cardiac surgery. A combined CABG-CEA should be performed in the patient with unstable angina or significant myocardium at risk if neurologic symptoms are present.

2. The management of asymptomatic carotid lesions in patients requiring cardiac surgery is controversial and is noted below in the discussion of carotid bruits (see page 145).

H. A history of **saphenous vein strippings and/or ligation** or **distal vascular reconstructive procedures** using saphenous vein alerts the surgeon to potential problems obtaining satisfactory conduit for bypass grafting. Noninvasive venous mapping of the lower extremities may identify satisfactory greater or lesser saphenous veins for use, but is not always reliable. Doppler assessment of the palmar arch or digital plethysmography with radial compression can be performed to assess the feasibility of using the radial artery as a bypass conduit (i.e., confirming that the arm is ulnar-dominant). Informing the patient of potential complications of radial artery harvesting, specifically numbness of the dorsum of the thumb and part of the thenar eminence or thumb weakness from trauma to the superficial radial nerve, is essential.[88–90] An increased incidence of forearm neurologic deficits has been noted in smokers, older patients, and those with diabetes, obesity, and peripheral vascular disease.[91] Venipunctures and IV catheters should be avoided in the arm from which the radial artery will be harvested. The anesthesiologist should also be alerted to avoid placing a radial artery line or intravenous catheter in that arm in the operating room!

I. **Urologic symptoms** suggest the presence of an active urinary tract infection that must be treated before surgery. In men, a history of prostatic cancer treated by irradiation, a prior transurethral resection, or other urinary symptoms consistent with prostatic hypertrophy identify potential problems with Foley catheter placement in the operating room. Use of a coudé catheter may be necessary. Urologic consultation should be obtained if a catheter cannot be passed. Either a catheter may be placed after dilating the urethra or a suprapubic tube may be inserted. Prolonged postoperative urinary drainage should be anticipated until the patient is fully ambulatory or until further urologic evaluation is performed.

J. A history of significant **ulcer disease** or **gastrointestinal bleeding** may necessitate further evaluation by endoscopy, especially if the patient will require postoperative anticoagulation. However, invasive diagnostic tests may need to be deferred in patients with significant coronary disease. Use of postoperative proton pump inhibitors, H_2 blockers, or sucralfate should be considered in these patients.[92]

K. The risk of **infection** is increased if another infectious source is present in the body (commonly a urinary tract or skin infection). Concurrent infections must be identified and treated before surgery. An upper respiratory infection may increase the risk of pulmonary complications, and bacterial infections may increase the risk of a hematogenous sternal wound infection and can seed a prosthetic heart valve. Patients at risk for methicillin-resistant *Staphylococcus aureus* (MRSA) infections or with positive nasal swabs should receive additional prophylaxis with nasal mupirocin with use of vancomycin for perioperative prophylaxis (see page 155).

L. The patient's **medications and allergies** should be reviewed. Most cardiac medications should be continued up to the time of surgery. Some must be stopped in advance (warfarin, antiplatelet drugs depending on the clinical circumstance, metformin, angiotensin-converting enzymes [ACE] inhibitors), and others may require specific attention during anesthesia and the early postoperative course (steroids, insulin, alternative antibiotics for antibiotic allergies). See section VI (page 150).

M. Other significant past medical history, such as chronic use of steroids, prior chest irradiation for cancer (usually for mediastinal lymphoma, breast, or lung cancer), or psychiatric history, should be detailed in the medical record. A thorough review of systems should be able to identify other comorbid conditions likely to affect the outcome of surgery.

III. Physical Examination

A. The patient's general appearance, mental status, and affect should be evaluated and noted in the medical record as a baseline for comparison with the postoperative period.

B. An active **skin infection or rash** that might be secondarily infected must be treated before surgery to minimize the risk of sternal wound infection.

C. **Dental caries** must be treated before operations during which prosthetic material (valves, grafts) will be placed.[93,94] Dental extractions, however, should be recommended cautiously in patients with severe ischemic heart disease or critical aortic stenosis. Cardiac complications may occur even if dental procedures are performed under local anesthesia.

D. **Carotid bruits** are a marker, although an insensitive one, of carotid disease, which is present in about 10–15% of patients with significant coronary disease. Carotid noninvasive studies are warranted in virtually all patients with bruits to assess for high-grade unilateral or bilateral disease because of the association of severe carotid disease with postoperative stroke.[95,96]

1. The management of an asymptomatic carotid lesion in a patient requiring open-heart surgery is controversial. Some studies have shown a similar risk of stroke comparing combined CABG-CEA procedures with isolated CABGs, although mortality and other adverse events may be greater with combined procedures.[97] Other studies have reported an increased risk of stroke, but this may be neutralized by risk-factor matching, indicating that the procedure itself may not be an independent risk factor for stroke.[98,99] Long-term follow-up studies do indicate that patients have a reduced short- and long-term risk of stroke following combined operations, although postoperative carotid surgery when indicated might offset this perceived benefit.[100] Because carotid disease is a marker for aortic atherosclerosis, it is not surprising that stroke risk is greater in patients with aortic calcification or atherosclerosis, likely explaining why half of perioperative strokes following combined operations occur contralateral to the operated side.[100,101]

2. If the patient presents with an acute coronary syndrome or has a large degree of myocardium at risk, most surgeons would consider performing a combined CABG-CEA for a unilateral carotid stenosis > 90%. The risk of stroke in a combined operation for unilateral asymptomatic disease is very low (most studies combine symptomatic and asymptomatic patients) and this approach reduces the subsequent risk of stroke. In contrast, preliminary CEA is the preferred approach in patients with stable angina, and may result in a lower overall risk of stroke, myocardial infarction, and death. Studies comparing preoperative carotid artery stenting with combined operations have demonstrated a reduced risk of stroke with

the former approach, perhaps indicating that a "hybrid" approach with stenting immediately followed by CABG is preferable.[102,103]

3. The risk of stroke with bilateral disease (>75% bilaterally) is significant during isolated CABG (as high as 10–15%), especially in patients with unilateral stenosis with contralateral occlusion.[95] However, it remains quite significant even with a combined operation. Thus, the operations should be staged with the carotid endarterectomy performed first if cardiac disease permits. If this is not possible because of unstable angina, left main or severe three-vessel disease with a large amount of "myocardium in jeopardy", preliminary carotid stenting or a combined operation should be performed, with the understanding that the risk of stroke is somewhat increased.

E. **Bilateral arm blood pressures** should be measured. Differential pressures may identify possible subclavian artery stenosis, a contraindication to use of a pedicled ITA graft. This finding is also noted in some patients presenting with a type A aortic dissection.

F. The presence of a **heart murmur** may warrant a preoperative echocardiogram if no valvular abnormality had been identified at the time of catheterization. Occasionally, new-onset ischemic mitral regurgitation or unsuspected aortic valve disease will be detected. In terms of valve selection, risk assessment, and informed consent, it is certainly preferable if this is recognized before surgery, rather than being identified for the first time in the operating room.

G. An **abdominal aortic aneurysm** detected upon palpation should be evaluated by ultrasound. IABP placement through the femoral artery should be avoided to prevent distal atheroembolism.

H. Severe **peripheral vascular disease** (PVD) must be assessed by a careful pulse examination. It is often associated with cerebrovascular disease and may prompt a preoperative carotid noninvasive study. PVD is a risk factor for operative mortality and is also an independent predictor of impaired long-term survival.[104] Weak femoral pulses may be indicative of "inflow" aortoiliac disease. This may dictate the unsuitability of the femoral arteries for cannulation, especially for minimally invasive valve surgery, or for placement of an IABP. If the ascending aorta is also significantly diseased and an alternative cannulation site must be utilized, the axillary artery should be considered.[105]

1. Aortoiliac disease must be identified in patients in whom endovascular stenting is contemplated. This may require exposure of the iliac artery with grafting to allow for stent-graft placement.

2. PVD may contribute to poor leg wound healing, although this is generally not a significant problem with endoscopic vein harvesting. If there are plans for future peripheral vascular reconstruction, the vein should be harvested from the opposite leg.

I. The presence of **varicose veins** identifies potential problems with conduits for CABG. The distribution of varicosities may indicate whether or not the greater saphenous vein is involved. Noninvasive venous mapping may identify a normal greater saphenous vein despite significant varicosities. The lesser saphenous vein distribution should be inspected to determine whether it might serve as a potential conduit. Assessment of the radial artery, as noted above, should be considered.

IV. Laboratory Assessment

A. Complete blood count (CBC), PT, PTT, and platelet count

1. Patients with moderate anemia (hemoglobin <10 g/dL) have a significantly higher risk of postoperative adverse events (renal and neurologic) as well as a higher operative mortality. This is probably more related to conditions associated with anemia, such as CHF or renal dysfunction.[106,107] Patients with unstable ischemic syndromes should be transfused to a hematocrit of at least 28% in anticipation of surgery. This is beneficial in reducing potential preoperative cardiac ischemia as well as reducing the extent of hemodilution during surgery. Profound anemia increases the need for intraoperative transfusions of blood and blood components, which are risk factors for morbidity and mortality. It is noteworthy that many patients experience a significant fall in hematocrit following cardiac catheterization, approximating 5.4% on the average, either from hydration, external blood loss, groin hematomas, or retroperitoneal bleeding.[108]

2. An elevated WBC may be associated with an infectious process that should be identified before surgery. However, it may also be a generalized marker of inflammation. Studies indicate that preoperative leukocytosis is associated with increased perioperative myonecrosis (CK elevation), stroke, and operative mortality, and decreased 1-year survival.[109-111]

3. It is important to check a daily platelet count in patients maintained on heparin to allow for prompt recognition of potential HIT. If this is suspected based on a falling platelet count, further workup is indicated with testing for heparin-induced platelet aggregation (usually by the serotonin release assay) or serologic testing for heparin antibodies.[112] If these tests are positive, an alternative means of anticoagulation during bypass may be necessary (see page pages 202–204). The mere presence of heparin antibodies in the absence of thrombocytopenia should not contraindicate use of heparin during surgery. Routine assessment for heparin antibodies in the absence of thrombocytopenia is not recommended.[113]

4. Preoperative platelet aggregation testing may be beneficial in assessing the residual antiplatelet effects of aspirin and, in particular, clopidogrel, and may influence the appropriate timing of surgery. If not utilized, it should be anticipated that some patients receiving these medications will bleed more than desired, and standard guidelines for their cessation should be followed, as noted on page 134. Postbypass point-of-care testing may provide objective evidence of qualitative platelet dysfunction that justifies platelet transfusions in the bleeding patient.

B. Electrolytes, BUN, creatinine, blood glucose.

Patients with a serum creatinine (Scr) >1.4 mg/dL or a glomerular filtration rate (GFR) < 60 mL/min, especially if diabetic, are more prone to acute kidney injury after surgery and have a higher operative mortality and lower long-term survival.[114,115] Measures should be taken during cardiac catheterization to minimize renal toxicity (see pages 595–597). The Scr should be rechecked afterwards in patients at increased risk of developing renal dysfunction. If the Scr has increased, surgery should be deferred, if clinically feasible, until it has returned to baseline. However, surgery should not be delayed in critically ill patients with hemodynamic compromise and worsening renal function, since delay will often lead to less reversible renal failure and multisystem organ failure. Specific intraoperative measures and postoperative hemodynamic support are critical to minimize the renal insult (see Chapter 12).

C. **Liver function tests (LFTs)** including bilirubin, alkaline phosphatase, alanine aminotransferase, aspartate aminotransferase, albumin, and serum amylase should be obtained. Abnormalities suggestive of hepatitis or cirrhosis may warrant further evaluation. Those associated with chronic passive congestion (tricuspid valve pathology, right heart failure or constriction) may not improve until after surgery has been performed. Occasionally, emergency surgery is indicated in patients with cardiogenic shock and an acute hepatic insult with markedly increased liver enzymes. In this situation, there is a higher risk of severe hepatic dysfunction after surgery. Baseline LFTs are also valuable because all patients should be placed on pre- and postoperative statins, the most common side effect of which is elevation in LFTs.

D. **Other laboratory tests to be considered**

1. **Thyroid-stimulating hormone (TSH)** levels should be measured preoperatively in the event that amiodarone will be used either prophylactically or therapeutically after surgery for atrial fibrillation. Amiodarone is an iodine-rich compound that can have a variety of effects on thyroid function, producing either thyrotoxicosis or hypothyroidism in about 15% of patients receiving chronic amiodarone therapy.[116,117]

2. **BNP levels** may be drawn to differentiate among the causes of dyspnea. In patients with systolic or diastolic dysfunction, BNP levels are invariably elevated. Elevated BNP levels are associated with postoperative ventricular dysfunction and a higher mortality rate after CABG and also correlate with a worse short- and long-term outcome in patients undergoing aortic valve replacement for symptomatic aortic stenosis.[118,119]

3. **C-reactive protein** levels are elevated in patients with infections or inflammatory processes. An elevated preoperative level (>10 mg/L) is associated with increased operative mortality, and a level >5 mg/L is associated with reduced long-term survival following CABG.[120] Elevated levels are also associated with an increased incidence of graft occlusion.

E. **Urinalysis.** If an initial urinalysis suggests contamination, a "clean-catch" specimen with proper cleansing should be obtained. If there is a suggestion of a urinary tract infection, a culture should be obtained. An appropriate antibiotic should be given for several days prior to elective surgery. If the patient requires urgent bypass surgery, one or two doses of an antibiotic providing gram-negative coverage should suffice, although a few days of treatment might be considered before performing valve surgery.

F. **Chest x-ray (PA and lateral).** The x-ray is essential to rule out any active pulmonary disease that should be treated prior to surgery. Identification of pulmonary nodules should be further evaluated by a preoperative chest CT scan, since radiographic interpretation can be difficult postoperatively. Evidence of severe aortic calcification should prompt a careful review of the aortic root from the catheterization films and often a noncontrast CT scan to identify ascending aortic calcification. If present, this may necessitate modification of the operative approach, and in some elderly patients a determination of inoperability. A lateral film should always be obtained before reoperation through a median sternotomy incision. This gives an assessment of the proximity of the cardiac structures and the ITA pedicle clips to the posterior sternal table. It also allows for optimal planning of minimally invasive incisions. Additional significant information that can be derived from a chest x-ray is noted on page 87.

G. Electrocardiogram (ECG). A baseline study should be obtained for comparison with postoperative ECGs. Evidence of an interval infarction or new ischemia since the time of catheterization may warrant reevaluation of ventricular function and, on occasion, a repeat coronary angiogram. Patients being evaluated for elective surgery with active ischemia on ECG should be hospitalized and undergo prompt surgery.

1. If atrial fibrillation (AF) is present, it should be rate-controlled and its duration should be ascertained. The likelihood of conversion to sinus rhythm after surgery is nearly 80% for patients in atrial fibrillation less than 6 months, but it is unlikely if the AF has been of longer duration. Thus, the duration of AF would influence the aggressiveness of postoperative treatment and possibly influence the decision to perform a Maze procedure in addition to the planned operation.

2. The presence of a left bundle branch block raises the risk of complete heart block occurring during the insertion of a Swan-Ganz catheter. Advancement of the catheter into the pulmonary artery may be delayed until after the chest is open unless other provisions for urgent pacing (external pads, transvenous pacing wires) are available. The presence of a bundle branch block also makes it more difficult to detect ischemia.

3. Patients with significant preoperative bradycardia, especially if not taking β-blockers, will often require pacing after surgery. Both atrial and ventricular pacing wires should be placed during surgery. Care must be taken to avoid β-blockers and amiodarone after surgery as prophylactic measures to prevent atrial fibrillation, since profound bradycardia might occur.

H. Most test results are acceptable when performed within 1 month of surgery. However, it is beneficial to have a CBC, electrolytes, BUN, and creatinine checked within a few days of surgery.

V. Preoperative Blood Donation

A. Preoperative autologous blood donation is a feasible objective in patients with stable angina or valvular heart disease.[121] However, its limited use can be ascribed to several factors: (1) the urgency of surgery in most cases; (2) concerns about precipitating angina in patients with severe coronary disease; (3) lessened concern about the transmission of hepatitis C and human immunodeficiency virus; (4) questions about its cost-effectiveness with the availability of other measures to reduce blood loss, such as antifibrinolytic drugs, cell-saving devices, and off-pump surgery; and (5) logistic blood bank considerations. Thus, it is commonly neither necessary nor encouraged.

1. One unit of blood may be donated every week as long as the hematocrit exceeds 33%, allowing an additional 2−3 weeks before surgery for the hematocrit to return to normal.

2. The use of recombinant erythropoietin with iron supplementation can induce erythropoiesis very rapidly. This is particularly helpful in anemic patients, patients who donate their own blood, and Jehovah's Witness patients.[122] A common dose is 100 units/kg three times a week SC starting at least 1 week before surgery because the onset of action is considered to be 4−6 days. However, it has been shown that a single dose given IV only 4 days prior to surgery can rapidly produce erythropoiesis and reduce transfusion requirements.[123]

B. The percentage of patients requiring blood transfusions after coronary surgery has gradually been decreasing, and fewer than 50% of patients receive any blood products. In addition to the measures mentioned above, a lower transfusion trigger has evolved with the recognition that postoperative hematocrits as low as 22−24% are safe.[124,125]

C. Refinement in testing for hepatitis C (1/250,000−1/1,500,000 units) and human immunodeficiency virus (1/750,000 units) has lowered their risks to extremely low levels. This has allayed the morbid fear of many patients of receiving transfusions. Nonetheless, blood transfusions may still cause febrile, allergic, or transfusion reactions and may adversely affect respiratory and hemodynamic function when given in massive amounts. It has been well documented that perioperative transfusions raise the risk of infection, renal dysfunction, respiratory complications, and overall mortality. A conscientious blood conservation program is beneficial in reducing the need for transfusions (see Chapter 9).[126]

VI. Preoperative Medications

A. All antianginal medications should be continued up to and including the morning of surgery to prevent recurrence of ischemia. The substitution of a shorter-acting β-blocker or calcium channel blocker for a longer-acting one (metoprolol for nadolol, diltiazem for Cardizem CD) should be considered. The use of preoperative β-blockers has been shown to lower the mortality rate of coronary bypass surgery.[127]

B. Diuretics, β-blockers, or calcium channel blockers used for hypertension can be given preoperatively to prevent rebound hypertension and provide for a more stable anesthetic course. However, angiotensin-converting enzyme (ACE) inhibitors or angiotensin receptor blockers (ARBs) should be withheld the morning of surgery because they are associated with reduced systemic resistance and a vasoplegic state during and after cardiopulmonary bypass.[128,129] In fact, preoperative use of ACE inhibitors may be associated with higher mortality rates, an increasing need for inotropic support, more atrial fibrillation, and arguably more postoperative acute kidney injury.[130−132]

C. Digoxin should be given the morning of surgery if used for rate control.

D. Diuretics are continued up to the morning of surgery. Hypokalemia from diuretics is usually not a problem intraoperatively because of the high doses of potassium present in the cardioplegia solutions used for myocardial protection.

E. Anticoagulants and antiplatelet agents (see pages 133−139)

  1. Aspirin 81 mg should be continued up to the time of surgery in patients with critical coronary disease or advanced symptoms; it may be stopped 3−5 days prior to noncoronary surgery or in patients undergoing truly elective CABG.

  2. Clopidogrel or prasugrel should be stopped 5−7 days prior to surgery. If the patient has received a bare-metal stent within the past month or a drug-eluting stent within the past year, clopidogrel should be either continued up to the time of surgery or possibly stopped for only 3 days before surgery. Patients requiring surgery after use of ticagrelor should wait 24−36 hours after the last dose before surgery, if possible.

3. Warfarin should be stopped 4–5 days before surgery to allow for normalization of the INR. If the INR remains elevated, 5 mg of oral vitamin K is effective in reducing the INR within 1–2 days. If more urgent reversal is necessary, 5 mg of IV vitamin K and occasionally fresh frozen plasma may be used.

4. Intravenous heparin is generally continued up to the time of surgery in patients with critical coronary disease, but when used as a bridge, it can be stopped about 4 hours before surgery.

5. LMWH should be stopped 18–24 hours preoperatively.

6. Fondaparinux has a long half-life and surgery should be delayed at least 48 hours after the last dose.

7. Short-acting IIb/IIIa inhibitors should be stopped 4 hours preoperatively.

8. Surgery should be delayed 12–24 hours in patients receiving abciximab or thrombolytic therapy.

9. If the patient requires truly urgent or emergency surgery, platelets and clotting factors must be available to combat the lingering antihemostatic effects of any of the above drugs.

F. Diabetic patients should refrain from taking insulin or oral hypoglycemic medications the morning of surgery. Blood glucose should be routinely checked in the operating room and treated with intravenous insulin to maintain the blood glucose <180 mg/dL.

G. Antiarrhythmic therapy should be continued until the time of surgery. Long-term use of **amiodarone** may be associated with postoperative respiratory failure, and it should be stopped as soon as surgery is being contemplated if there is evidence of any pulmonary complications.[64] Otherwise, there is little benefit in stopping it for a short period of time to reduce perioperative risks because it has a very long half-life. Amiodarone may be used for atrial fibrillation prophylaxis, either starting with a preoperative oral load over several days (10 mg/kg/day) or initiating it intravenously in the operating room.[133]

H. **Statins** should be given to all patients undergoing cardiac surgery, as they have been shown to reduce the risk of atrial fibrillation and operative mortality.[134–137] One study showed that statins also reduce the risk of postoperative delirium.[138]

I. Perioperative use of **steroids** (methylprednisolone, dexamethasone) has been hypothesized to mitigate the systemic inflammatory response associated with CPB, but evidence of significant clinical benefit is lacking.[139] Steroids may reduce the incidence of atrial fibrillation and thus reduce the length of stay. Otherwise, aside from marginally reducing blood loss, they may cause hyperglycemia and metabolic acidosis and have not been shown to improve pulmonary function. The only other benefit has been an improvement in appetite.[140]

J. Preoperative prophylactic **antibiotics** must be administered before surgical incision. Vancomycin should be started within 2 hours of incision, and other antibiotics within 1 hour of incision. A first-generation cephalosporin, such as cefazolin, is commonly chosen because of its effectiveness against Gram-positive organisms. There is some evidence that overall infection rates may be lower with use of a second-generation cephalosporin, such as cefuroxime. Vancomycin is used if there is a severe allergy to penicillin or the cephalosporins and is often selected in patients undergoing valvular surgery because of its excellent efficacy against Gram-positive organisms. Since vancomycin provides poor Gram-negative coverage, the STS guidelines suggest that the addition of an aminoglycoside be considered to improve prophylaxis.[141] Vancomycin should not be used indiscriminately, however, to minimize the emergence of strains of vancomycin-resistant enterococci, a growing concern in intensive care units.

  K. Preoperative medications are ordered by the anesthesia service. Although some patients may benefit from receiving mild sedation "on-call" to the operating room, most patients are given midazolam by the anesthesiologist once the initial intravenous lines are inserted.

VII. Preoperative Orders and Checklist

Once the patient has been accepted for surgery, orders should be written to address general and patient specific concerns (tests, medications) before surgery. Standardized preprinted order sheets are helpful and can be individualized as necessary (Table 3.6 and Appendix 2). The evening before surgery, the covering physician/physician assistant/nurse practitioner should write a brief preoperative note summarizing essential information that should be reviewed before proceeding with the operation. Writing this note prevents important details from being overlooked (Table 3.7). For patients undergoing elective surgery, similar laboratory tests are ordered and the surgical team must take the responsibility of confirming that all of the requisite information has been reviewed, abnormalities addressed, and the information placed on the patient's office chart the night before admission to be available to the operating room when the patient arrives in the morning. The following should be noted:

  A. The planned operative procedure

  B. Indication for surgery

  C. Brief summary of the cardiac catheterization data

  D. Results of the laboratory data obtained

  E. Surgical note and **consent** in chart

  F. Anesthesia note and consent in chart

  G. Confirmation of blood bank cross-match and blood setup

  1. Guidelines for blood setup are shown in Table 3.8. One can generally determine the potential need for transfusion based on the patient's blood volume (which correlates with body size and usually with gender), and the preoperative hemoglobin level. More blood transfusions are commonly required during complex procedures requiring long durations of CPB, during which a large amount of crystalloid is usually given, increasing the necessity for blood transfusions to maintain a satisfactory hematocrit (>18–20% on pump).

  2. Other comorbid factors that increase the need for transfusion include older age, urgent or emergent operations, poor ventricular function, reoperations, an elevated INR, insulin-dependent diabetes, peripheral vascular disease, elevated creatinine, and an albumin <4 g/dL, consistent with poor nutrition.[142–145]

  H. Preoperative orders are written:

  1. Antibiotics: (always check for allergy)

  a. Cefazolin 1–2 g IV to be given in the operating room within 1 hour of incision. The dose should be weight-based.

  • The STS recommendation is to give 1 g to patients <60 kg and 2 g for patients >60 kg.[141]

Table 3.6 • Typical Preoperative Order Sheet

1. Admit to:_____

2. Surgery date:_____

3. Planned procedure:_____

4. Diagnostic Studies
   - ☐ CBC with differential
   - ☐ PT/INR   ☐ PTT
   - ☐ Electrolytes, BUN, creatinine, blood glucose
   - ☐ Liver function tests (bilirubin, AST, ALT, alkaline phosphatase, albumin)
   - ☐ TSH level
   - ☐ Lipid profile
   - ☐ Hemoglobin A1c level
   - ☐ Urinalysis and urine culture, if indicated
   - ☐ Electrocardiogram
   - ☐ Chest x-ray PA and lateral
   - ☐ Room air oxygen saturation by pulse oximetry; obtain arterial blood gas if <90%
   - ☐ Antibody screen   ☐ Crossmatch: _____ units PRBC
   - ☐ Carotid duplex studies
   - ☐ Bilateral digital radial artery studies
   - ☐ Bilateral venous mapping
   - ☐ Pulmonary function tests
   - ☐ Other: _____

5. Treatments/Assessments
   - ☐ Admission vital signs
   - ☐ Measure height and weight
   - ☐ NPO after midnight except sips of water with meds
   - ☐ Surgical clippers to remove hair at 5 AM morning of surgery from chest, legs and both groins
   - ☐ Hibiclens scrub to chest and legs night before and AM of surgery
   - ☐ Incentive spirometry teaching

6. Medications
   - ☐ Mupirocin 2% (Bactroban ointment): apply Q-tip nasal swabs the evening before and the morning of surgery
   - ☐ Chlorhexidine 0.12% (Peridex) gargle on-call to OR
   - ☐ Cefazolin   ☐ 1 g IV   ☐ 2 g IV – send to OR with patient
   - ☐ Vancomycin 15–20 mg/kg = _____ g IV – send to OR with patient
   - ☐ Discontinue clopidogrel immediately
   - ☐ Reduce aspirin to 81 mg daily if patient on a higher dose
   - ☐ Discontinue heparin at _____
   - ☐ Continue heparin drip into OR
   - ☐ Discontinue low-molecular-weight heparin after AM/PM dose on _____
   - ☐ Discontinue IIb/IIIa inhibitor at 3 AM prior to surgery
   - ☐ Other: _____

Table 3.7 • Preoperative Checklist

1. Planned operation:_____
2. Indication for surgery: _____
3. Brief summary of cardiac catheterization results
4. Lab results
   a. Electrolytes, BUN, creatinine, blood glucose
   b. PT, PTT, platelet count, CBC
   c. Urinalysis
   d. Chest x- ray
   e. Electrocardiogram
   f. Additional test results: carotid studies, PFTs, vein mapping
5. Surgical note and consent in chart
6. Anesthesia note and consent in chart
7. Confirmation of blood bank setup
8. Preoperative orders written

- Because antibiotic serum levels fall up to 50% on pump, an additional 1 g may be considered on pump or every 3–4 hours during surgery.

or

b. Vancomycin 15–20 mg/kg to be started within 2 hours of surgery but infused over at least 30 minutes to avoid hypotension and the "red-neck syndrome".[141,146]

- It usually does not need to be redosed on pump.
- The STS guidelines suggest that the addition of an aminoglycoside, such as gentamicin 4 mg/kg for 1–2 doses, should also be considered.[141]

Table 3.8 • Blood Setup Guidelines for Open-Heart Surgery

Procedure	PRBC Setup
Minimally invasive CABG without pump	Type and screen
Weight >70 kg and hematocrit >35%	One unit
Weight <70 kg or hematocrit <35%	Two units
Reoperations	Three units
Ascending aortic surgery	Three units
Descending aortic surgery	Six units
PRBC, packed red blood cells.	

2. Specific orders to stop medications listed in section VI, above.

3. Antiseptic scrub (chlorhexidine) with which to shower the night before and the morning of surgery. Preferably this should be applied several times rather than during a single shower.[147]

4. Mupirocin 2% (Bactroban) nasal ointment is effective in reducing nasal carriage of *Staph aureus* and can reduce the incidence of surgical-site infections with these organisms. In patients who are not nasal carriers, mupirocin has no benefit and may potentially increase the risk of infection from antibiotic-resistant organisms.[148–150] If polymerase chain reaction (PCR) testing is available, mupirocin administration can be limited to patients who test positive for MRSA carriage.[151,152] Otherwise, a routine policy of pre-, intra-, and a few days of postoperative nasal mupirocin can be recommended (one swab bid × 3 days).[141]

5. Chlorhexidine 0.12% (Peridex) mouthwash.

6. Skin preparation. This is best performed the morning of surgery, as it has been well documented that the closer the prep to the time of surgery, the lower the wound infection rate.[153] Use of clippers is preferable to shaving with a razor, which increases the risk of infection.

7. NPO after midnight.

8. Preoperative medications per anesthesia service.

I. For outpatients, it is important that documentation of a very brief updated history and physical exam be written in the medical record the day of surgery, indicating whether there has been any change since the patient's preoperative evaluation.

VIII. Risk Assessment and Informed Consent

A. General comments

1. An important element of the preoperative preparation for cardiac surgery is an assessment of the patient's surgical risk. Risk stratification can afford patients and their families insight into the **real** risk of complications and mortality. It can also increase the awareness of the healthcare team to the high-risk patient for whom more aggressive therapy in the perioperative period may be beneficial. Documentation in the chart of an informed-consent discussion is **mandatory** prior to any cardiac surgical procedure. This note should quantify in some fashion the estimated mortality risk, should list some of the more common complications of the operation being performed, and should address risks that may be unique to the individual patient.

2. Although public reporting of hospitals' and individual surgeons' mortality rates is becoming more commonplace, the correlation of mortality with quality of care is imprecise. Mortality rate is more commonly related to the underlying cardiac disease and comorbidities, and perhaps, most importantly, to patient selection. Nonetheless, the incidence of postoperative complications remains quite substantial, especially in older patient populations, and many are simply not preventable. Although the ability to predict and hopefully prevent postoperative complications may have some influence on overall mortality rates, it should have a significant impact on the patient's recovery and quality of life after surgery and may reduce hospital length of stay and costs.

B. **Risk stratification** is based on an assessment of four important interrelated categories of risk factors (Table 3.2).

1. **Patient demographics.** These include patient-related factors independent of disease, such as age, gender, and race.

2. **Patient-related comorbidities.** These refer to coexisting diseases that are not necessarily directly related to the cardiac disease, but can have significant impact on the patient's ability to recover from surgery. In fact, in most patients, mortality and complications are related to preexisting comorbidities, such as diabetes, renal dysfunction, cerebrovascular disease, and chronic obstructive pulmonary disease. These render the patient more susceptible to the insults of CPB or to complications from a low cardiac output state.

3. **Cardiac and procedure-related factors.** The clinical presentation (stable vs. acute coronary syndrome, recent MI, CHF), nature and extent of cardiac disease (isolated coronary artery disease, associated valve disease, pulmonary hypertension), and the degree of ventricular dysfunction are important considerations in determining operative risk. For the vast majority of patients at low to moderate risk, these factors generally do not raise the operative risk significantly. The extent of the planned operation raises the baseline risk, and reoperations nearly always double or triple the operative risk. Uncommon surgical situations, such as very recent myocardial infarction (within 24 hours), profound LV dysfunction (EF <20%), or cardiogenic shock with or without mechanical complications of infarction (ventricular septal rupture or papillary muscle rupture), are powerful risk factors for mortality. Postcardiotomy ventricular dysfunction can exacerbate organ system dysfunction related to preexisting comorbidities, such as chronic kidney disease, and may contribute to operative mortality.

4. **Preoperative status.** The immediate risk of death is greatest in patients requiring emergency surgery. Such patients usually have a "critical preoperative state" with unstable cardiac disease which may include ongoing ischemia, hemodynamic compromise (such as cardiogenic shock) that requires inotropes or IABP support, or even ongoing cardiopulmonary resuscitation.

C. **Preoperative predictors of operative mortality**

1. The risk factors for operative mortality have been analyzed in several large databases and numerous risk models have been designed.[154-160] These models can be used to objectively provide the patient with an individualized predicted mortality rate. The most common risk factors noted in these studies include, in approximate decreasing order of significance:

   a. Emergency surgery, which includes some of the powerful but fairly uncommon risk factors (cardiogenic shock, ongoing CPR)

   b. Renal dysfunction

   c. Reoperations

   d. Older age (>75–80)

   e. Poor ventricular function (EF <30%)

   f. Female gender

   g. Left main disease

   h. Other comorbidities, such as COPD, peripheral vascular disease, diabetes, and cerebrovascular disease

2. The calculation of an individual patient's operative risk can be performed with "bedside" or computerized models, most of which provide comparable risk assessment in patients at low to moderate risk.[154,155] The most common bedside models are the Parsonnet,[156] the Northern New England (NNE),[157] and the additive EuroSCORE models (Tables 3.9–3.11 and Figure 3.1).[158] These assign weights or points to each factor based on their odds ratio, which reflects the relative contribution of each factor to mortality in a validated model. The score derived from the weight of various factors can then be used to provide an "expected" mortality.

3. The computer software packages compatible with the STS database require extensive data entry and provide sophisticated risk modeling that allows for calculation of an expected mortality rate. This risk calculator is available on the STS website at www.sts.org.[159]

4. It has been suggested that the additive EuroSCORE tends to overestimate mortality in low-risk patients and underestimate it in high-risk patients compared with other risk models. A more sophisticated logistic EuroSCORE is a computerized model that is arguably more accurate than the additive EuroSCORE model in patients at high risk, with the divergence occurring above an estimated risk of 8–10%.[160–162] Both are available at www.euroscore.org/calc.html. Although this assessment of predicted mortality has been validated in Europe as well as in North America, other studies suggest that, in comparison with the STS model, the EuroSCORE tends to overestimate risks in CABG and valve patients and is inferior to the STS model in estimating mortality in high-risk aortic valve patients.[163–165]

D. **Preoperative predictors of postoperative morbidity**

1. Studies suggest that risk factors for morbidity are not necessarily comparable to those predicting increased mortality.[155,166] Nonetheless, complications are more common in elderly patients with preoperative anemia and comorbidities, such as stroke, COPD, CHF, and hypertension, and also with emergency operations and reoperations. Several models provide an estimated risk for certain complications based on preoperative factors. Specifically, the NNE database can provide an estimate of the risk of stroke and mediastinitis (Table 3.10),[157] while the STS database provides an estimated risk for stroke, reexploration for bleeding, mediastinitis, renal dysfunction, and prolonged ventilation.[159] Other studies have evaluated risk models for predicting the risks of respiratory failure (Figure 10.2, page 397)[58,167] and the need for dialysis (Figures 12.3 and 12.4, pages 593 and 594).[168,169] Although most factors are not modifiable, such as patient age, gender, redo status, urgency status, or the extent of cardiac disease, they do heighten awareness of the increased risk for postoperative complications. Thus, additional steps may be indicated to try to reduce their occurrence.

2. It is noteworthy that the overall incidence of complications following standard cardiac surgical procedures is quite high, approximating 40–50% in the STS database, when fairly common occurrences such as atrial fibrillation (AF) are included. Although AF is fairly benign, it does increase the risk of stroke and prolong the length of stay. In contrast, the less common complications tend to be associated with significant mortality. Although the results shown in Table 3.12

Table 3.9 • Preoperative Risk-Estimation Worksheet (Parsonnet)[156]

Risk Factor		Scoring	Value
Female gender		6	
Age	70–75	2.5	
	76–79	7	
	80 +	11	
CHF		2.5	
COPD (severe)		6	
Diabetes		3	
Ejection fraction	30–49%	6.5	
	<30%	8	
Hypertension	>140/90	3	
Left main disease	>50%	2.5	
Morbid obesity	>1.5 ideal body weight	1	
Preoperative IABP		4	
Reoperation	First	10	
	Second or subsequent	20	
Aortic valve replacement		0	
Mitral valve replacement		4.5	
CABG-valve		6	
Special situations			
		TOTAL	

Risk Values for Special Conditions

Cardiac		Hepatorenal	
Cardiogenic shock	12	Cirrhosis	12.5
Endocarditis, active	6.5	Dialysis dependency	13.5
Endocarditis, treated	0	Renal failure, acute or chronic	3.5
LV aneurysm resection	1.5		
Tricuspid valve	5	**Vascular**	
Pacemaker dependency	0		
Transmural acute MI < 48 h	4	Abdominal aortic aneurysm, asymptomatic	0.5
Ventricular septal defect, acute	12		
Ventricular tachycardia ventricular fibrillation, aborted sudden death	1	Carotid disease (bilateral or 100% unilateral occlusion)	2
		Peripheral vascular disease, severe	2.5

Pulmonary		Miscellaneous	
Asthma	1	Blood products refused	11
Preoperative endotracheal tube	4	Severe neurologic disorder (healed CVA, paraplegia)	5
Idiopathic thrombocytopenic purpura	12	PTCA or catheterization failure	5.5
Pulmonary hypertension (mean PA > 30)	11	Substance abuse	4.5

LV; left ventricular; CVA; cerebrovascular accident; PTCA; percutaneous transluminal coronary angioplasty; PAP; pulmonary arterial pressure.

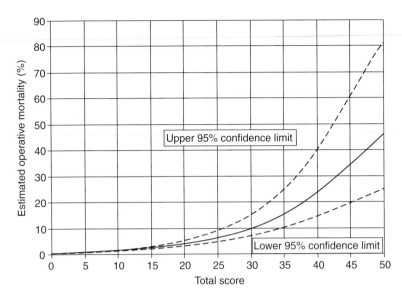

Figure 3.1 • The estimated mortality risk for patients using the preoperative risk-estimation worksheet shown in Table 3.9. (Modified with permission from Bernstein and Parsonnet, Ann Thorac Surg 2000;69:823–8)[156]

are somewhat dated and can no longer be obtained, the association of certain complications with a high mortality rate points out the significance of identifying and treating potentially modifiable factors.

E. **Measures to modify risk factors for operative mortality and morbidity**

  1. Recognizing preexisting organ system dysfunction or risk factors for their development is essential to reduce postoperative morbidity and mortality. This is especially important in elderly patients, who are more predisposed to renal dysfunction, ventilatory issues, stroke, bleeding, and atrial arrhythmias. Concern about the following complications should prompt specific measures to prevent their occurrence or minimize their impact if they occur.

  2. **Renal failure** that requires dialysis carries a mortality rate of nearly 50%. There are several models to predict the risks of postoperative acute kidney injury and the need for dialysis (Figures 12.1–12.4, pages 592–594).[168,169] Optimizing renal function before, during, and after surgery is critical in patients with preexisting renal dysfunction. Even if dialysis is not required, chronic kidney disease is associated with increased operative mortality and worse long-term survival (see Chapter 12).

  3. **Prolonged ventilation.** The STS database definition considers postoperative mechanical ventilation for over 24 hours – from the time the patient arrives in the ICU – to represent a postoperative complication. The operative mortality for patients requiring intubation for over 5 days is approximately 20%. Several risk models have been evaluated to predict the risk of postoperative prolonged ventilation.[58,167] In patients with compromised pulmonary function, aggressive

Table 3.10 • Preoperative Estimation of Risk of Mortality, Cerebrovascular Accident (CVA), and Mediastinitis for Patients Undergoing Coronary Artery Bypass Surgery (Northern New England Cardiovascular Disease Study Group)[157]

Patient Characteristic	Mortality Score	CVA Score	Mediastinitis Score
Age 60–69	2	3.5	0
Age 70–79	3	5	0
Age ≥80	5	6	0
Female sex	1.5	0	0
EF <40%	1.5	1.5	2
Urgent surgery	2	1.5	1.5
Emergent surgery	5	2	3.5
Prior CABG	5	1.5	0
PVD	2	2	0
Diabetes	0	0	1.5
Dialysis or creatinine >2	4	2	2.5
COPD	1.5	0	3.5
Obesity (BMI 31–36)	0	0	2.5
Severe obesity (BMI ≥37)	0	0	3.5

Perioperative Risk

Total Score	Mortality	CVA	Mediastinitis
0	0.4	0.3	0.4
1	0.5	0.4	0.5
2	0.7	0.7	0.6
3	0.9	0.9	0.7
4	1.3	1.1	1.1
5	1.7	1.5	1.5
6	2.2	1.9	1.9
7	3.3	2.8	3.0
8	3.9	3.5	3.5
9	6.1	4.5	5.8
10	7.7	≥6.5	≥6.5
11	10. 6		
12	13.7		
13	17.7		
14	>28.3		

Table 3.11 • EuroSCORE Risk Model (Additive risk model)[158]

Patient-related Factors	
Age: per 5 years above 60	1
Female	1
Chronic pulmonary disease	1
Extracardiac arteriopathy	2
Neurological dysfunction	2
Previous cardiac surgery	3
Creatinine >2.3 mg/dL	2
Active endocarditis	3
Critical preoperative state, including VT/VF, on ventilator, inotropes, IABP, urine output <10 mL/hr	3
Cardiac-related Factors	
Unstable angina	2
LV function: EF 30–50%	1
EF <30%	3
Recent MI <90 days	2
Pulmonary hypertension (PA >60)	2
Operation-related Factors	
Emergency	2
Other than isolated CABG	2
Surgery on thoracic aorta	3
Postinfarct VSD	4
Low risk: 0–2 points: estimated mortality = 1.3%	
Medium risk: 3–5 points: estimated mortality = 3%	
High risk: ≥6 points: estimated mortality = 11%	
Logistic risk model using the same point score can be found at www.euroscore.org/calc.html.	

Table 3.12 • Postoperative Complications of Coronary Bypass Surgery and Their Mortality Risks (STS database)*

Risk Variable	Incidence for First Operations	Risk Ratio	Mortality (%)
Multisystem failure	0.6	28.52	74.4
Cardiac arrest	1.3	29.63	64.1
Renal failure (dialysis)	0.8	17.61	47.6
Septicemia	0.9	13.92	38.6
Renal failure (no dialysis: creatinine >2.0)	2.8	13.53	30.6
Ventilated >5 days	5.5	10.73	21
Permanent stroke	1.5	10.35	28
Tamponade	0.3	8.25	25
Anticoagulation-related	0.4	8.23	25
Perioperative MI	1.2	6.64	19
GI complication	2.0	6.02	17
Reexploration for bleeding	2.1	4.53	13
Deep sternal infection	0.6	3.74	11

*Data obtained from STS database website in mid-1990s; data no longer available.

preoperative treatment of remediable conditions is essential. This may involve use of antibiotics for pulmonary infiltrates or bronchitis (and delay of surgery), bronchodilators for bronchospasm, diuresis for CHF, or even mechanical ventilation for hypoxemia or hypercarbia. Intraoperative management should entail judicious fluid administration, steps to reduce pulmonary artery pressures, steroids and bronchodilators for bronchospasm, and inotropic support if indicated. Postoperatively, aggressive diuresis as tolerated by hemodynamic performance, bronchodilators, early mobilization, and incentive spirometry are a few of the routine measures that can be utilized to minimize pulmonary morbidity (see Chapter 10).

4. Preexisting **cerebrovascular disease**, whether symptomatic or not, increases the risk of stroke.[96] Oftentimes, it is a marker for severe atherosclerosis, and most strokes are related to aortic manipulation rather than to preexisting carotid disease. Although the overall risk of permanent stroke is only 1–2%, this incidence is higher in elderly patients. Development of a permanent

perioperative stroke carries about a 25% mortality rate. Identifying carotid disease in patients at higher risk, using epiaortic imaging in the operating room to identify ascending aortic or arch atherosclerosis, using cerebral oximetry, maintaining a higher blood pressure on pump, or performing off-pump surgery, are a few examples of measures that should be considered in elderly patients to reduce the risk of stroke and neurocognitive dysfunction.

5. **Mediastinal bleeding** remains a concern after all cardiac operations, whether performed on- or off-pump. It may result from surgical bleeding sites, a coagulopathy, or a combination of both. A higher prevalence is noted following more complex operations, especially valve surgery. Meticulous attention to hemostasis remains imperative, especially in elderly patients with poor tissue quality. Bleeding may produce hemodynamic compromise from a low output state or tamponade and also increases the requirement for blood and blood component transfusions, which independently increase the risk of infection, respiratory failure, renal dysfunction, and mortality. Reoperation for bleeding and the development of tamponade carry significant mortality rates (about 13% and 25%, respectively).[170] Particular attention to modifying preoperative antiplatelet therapy or anticoagulants, use of antifibrinolytic drugs, and vigilance and patience in the operating room should minimize the risk of bleeding and its adverse consequences.

6. **Anticoagulation-related hemorrhage**, specifically delayed tamponade, is a potential complication of postoperative anticoagulation. Aspirin is routinely started within the first 24 hours after surgery once postoperative bleeding has tapered to a minimal level. Some surgeons use clopidogrel postoperatively, especially after OPCABs or CABG for NSTEMIs. Heparin may be given to patients with atrial fibrillation, mechanical valve prostheses until warfarin has achieved a therapeutic INR, or for VTE prophylaxis. The risk of delayed bleeding is heightened in patients receiving multiple antiplatelet or anticoagulant drugs, which may be indicated for several concurrent issues.[171] One must always weigh the risks and benefits of early anticoagulation and maintain constant vigilance for the early clinical signs of delayed tamponade. This is an easily correctable problem if identified. If not, it can be lethal.

7. **Deep sternal wound infections** (DSWI) occur in less than 1% of patients, but can be difficult to treat. They occasionally occur in critically ill patients in the ICU and thus are associated with a significant mortality rate (about 10–20%). Treating infections noted preoperatively, using perioperative mupirocin in nasal carriers of *Staph aureus*, administering prophylactic antibiotics appropriately in the operating room and continuing for no more than 48 hours, proper invasive line care, and strict control of intraoperative and postoperative hyperglycemia with an insulin protocol are essential in minimizing this problem. Unfortunately, it is highly unlikely that DSWIs can be entirely eliminated no matter how ideal the care provided.

References

1. Bybee KA, Powell BD, Valeti U, et al. Preoperative aspirin therapy is associated with improved postoperative outcomes in patients undergoing coronary artery bypass grafting. *Circulation* 2005;112 (Suppl I): I-286–92.

2. Dacey LJ, Munoz JJ, Johnson ER, et al. Effects of preoperative aspirin use on mortality in coronary artery bypass grafting patients. *Ann Thorac Surg* 2000;70:1986–90.

3. Cannon CP, Mehta SR, Aranki SF. Balancing the benefit and risk of oral antiplatelet agents in coronary artery bypass surgery. *Ann Thorac Surg* 2005;80:768–79.

4. Aranki SF, Body SC. Antiplatelet agents used for early intervention in acute coronary syndromes. *J Thorac Cardiovasc Surg* 2009;138:807–10. Additional tables with literature review available at www.jtcs.cnetjournals.org.

5. Ferraris VA, Ferraris SP, Moliterno DJ, et al. The Society of Thoracic Surgeons practice guideline series: aspirin and other antiplatelet agents during operative coronary revascularization (executive summary). *Ann Thorac Surg* 2005;79:1454–61.

6. Dunning J, Versteegh M, Fabbri A, et al. Guideline on antiplatelet and anticoagulation management in cardiac surgery. *Eur J Cardiothorac Surg* 2008;34:73–92.

7. Alghamdi AA, Moussa F, Fremes SE. Does the use of preoperative aspirin increase the risk of bleeding in patients undergoing coronary artery bypass graft surgery? Systematic review and meta-analysis. *J Card Surg* 2007;22:247–56.

8. Sun JC, Whitlock R, Cheng J, et al. The effect of pre-operative aspirin on bleeding, transfusion, myocardial infarction, and mortality in coronary artery bypass surgery: a systematic review of randomized and observational studies. *Eur Heart J* 2008;29:1057–71.

9. Kamran M, Ahmed A, Dar MI, Khan AB. Effect of aspirin on postoperative bleeding in coronary artery bypass grafting. *Ann Thorac Cardiovasc Surg* 2008;14:224–9.

10. Gulbins J, Malkoc A, Ennker IC, Ennker J. Preoperative platelet inhibition with ASA does not influence postoperative blood loss following coronary artery bypass grafting. *Thorac Cardiovasc Surg* 2009;557:18–21.

11. Gibbs NM, Weightman WM, Thackray NM, Michalopoulos N, Weidmann C. The effects of recent aspirin ingestion on platelet function in cardiac surgical patients. *J Cardiothorac Vasc Anesth* 2001;15:55–9.

12. Furukawa K, Ohteki H. Changes in platelet aggregation after suspension of aspirin therapy. *J Thorac Cardiovasc Surg* 2004;127:1814–5.

13. Suwalski G, Suwalski P, Filipiak KJ, Postula M, Majstrak F, Opolski G. The effect of off-pump coronary artery bypass grafting on platelet activation in patients on aspirin until surgery day. *Eur J Cardiothorac Surg* 2008;34:365–9.

14. Bednar F, Osmancik P, Vanek T, et al. Platelet activity and aspirin efficacy after off-pump compared with on-pump coronary artery bypass surgery: results from the prospective randomized trial (PRAGUE 11-Coronary Artery Bypass and REactivity of Thrombocytes (CABARET). *J Thorac Cardiovasc Surg* 2008;136:1054–60.

15. Velik-Salchner C, Maier S, Innerhofer P, et al. Point-of-care whole blood impedance aggregometry versus classical light transmission aggregometry for detecting aspirin and clopidogrel: the results of a pilot study. *Anesth Analg* 2008;107:1798–806.

16. Santilli F, Rocca B, De Cristofaro R, et al. Platelet cyclooxygenase inhibition by low-dose aspirin is not reflected consistently by platelet function assays. Implications for aspirin "resistance". *J Am Coll Cardiol* 2009;53:667–77.

17. Berger JS, Frye CB, Harshaw Q, Edwards FH, Steinhubl SR, Becker RC. Impact of clopidogrel in patients with acute coronary syndromes requiring coronary artery bypass surgery. A multicenter analysis. *J Am Coll Cardiol* 2008;52:1693–701.

18. Filsoufi F, Rahmanian PB, Castillo JG, Kahn RA, Fisher G, Adams DH. Clopidogrel treatment before coronary artery bypass graft surgery increases postoperative morbidity and blood product requirements. *J Cardiothorac Vasc Anesth* 2008;22:60–6.

19. von Heymann C, Redlich U, Moritz M, et al. Aspirin and clopidogrel taken until 2 days prior to coronary artery bypass graft surgery is associated with increased postoperative drainage loss. *Thorac Cardiovasc Surg* 2005;53:341–5.

20. Herman CR, Buth KJ, Kent BA, Hirsch GM. Clopidogrel increases blood transfusion and hemorrhagic complications in patients undergoing cardiac surgery. *Ann Thorac Surg* 2010;89:397–402.

21. Maltais S, Perrault LP, Do QB. Effect of clopidogrel on bleeding and transfusions after off-pump coronary artery bypass graft surgery: impact of discontinuation prior to surgery. *Eur J Cardiothorac Surg* 2008;34:127–31.

22. Vaccarino GN, Thierer J, Albertal M, et al. Impact of preoperative clopidogrel in off pump coronary artery bypass surgery: a propensity score analysis. *J Thorac Cardiovasc Surg* 2009;137:309–13.

23. Shim JK, Choi YS, Oh YJ, Bang SO, Yoo KJ, Kwak YL. Effects of preoperative aspirin and clopidogrel therapy on perioperative blood loss and blood transfusion requirements in patients undergoing off-pump coronary artery bypass graft surgery. *J Thorac Cardiovasc Surg* 2007;134:59–64.

24. Grines CL, Bonow RO, Casey DE Jr, et al. Prevention of premature discontinuation of dual antiplatelet therapy in patients with coronary artery stents. A science advisory from the American Heart Association, American College of Cardiology, Society for Cardiovascular Angiography and Interventions, American College of Surgeons, and American Dental Association, with Representation from the American College of Physicians. *Circulation* 2007;115:813–8; J Am Coll Cardiol 2007;49:734–9.

25. Airoldi F, Colombo A, Morici N, et al. Incidence and predictors of drug-eluting stent thrombosis during and after discontinuation of thienopyridine treatment. *Circulation* 2007;116:745–54.

26. Desai NR, Bhatt DL. The state of periprocedural antiplatelet therapy after recent trials. *JACC Cardiovasc Interv* 2010;3:571–83.

27. Wiviott SD, Braunwald E, McCabe CH, et al. Prasugrel versus clopidogrel in patients with acute coronary syndromes. *N Engl J Med* 2007;357:2001–15.

28. Wallentin L, Becker RC, Budaj A, et al. Ticagrelor versus clopidogrel in patients with acute coronary syndromes. *N Engl J Med* 2009;361:1045–57.

29. Harrington RA, Stone GW, McNulty S, et al. Platelet inhibition with cangrelor in patients undergoing PCI. *N Engl J Med* 2009;361:2318–29.

30. Kincaid EH, Monroe ML, Saliba DL, Kon ND, Byerly WG, Reichert MG. Effects of preoperative enoxaparin versus unfractionated heparin on bleeding indices in patients undergoing coronary artery bypass grafting. *Ann Thorac Surg* 2003;76:124–8.

31. Whitlock RP, Crowther MA, Warkentin TE, Blackall MH, Farrokhyar F, Teoh KHT. Warfarin cessation before cardiopulmonary bypass: lessons learned from a randomized controlled trial of oral vitamin K. *Ann Thorac Surg* 2007;84:103–9.

32. McDonald SB, Renna M, Spitznagel EL, et al. Preoperative use of enoxaparin increases the risk of postoperative bleeding and re-exploration in cardiac surgery patients. *J Cardiothorac Vasc Anesth* 2005;19:4–10.

33. Weitz JI, Hirsh J, Samama MM. New antithrombotic drugs. American College of Chest Physicians evidence-based clinical practice guidelines (8th edition). *Chest* 2008;133:234S–56S.

34. Kearon C, Hirsh J. Management of anticoagulation before and after elective surgery. *N Engl J Med* 1997;336:1506–11.

35. Ansell J, Hirsh J, Hylek E, Jacobson A, Crowther M, Palareti G. Pharmacology and management of the vitamin K antagonists. American College of Chest Physicians evidence-based clinical practice guidelines (8th edition). *Chest* 2008;133:160S–198S.

36. Chun R, Orser BA, Madan M. Platelet glycoprotein IIb/IIIa inhibitors: overview and implications for the anesthesiologist. *Anesth Analg* 2002;95:879–88.

37. Patrono C, Baigent C, Hirsh J, Roth G. Antiplatelet drugs. American College of Chest Physicians evidence-based clinical practice guidelines (8th edition). *Chest* 2008;133:199S–233S.

38. Bizzari F, Scolletta S, Tucci E, et al. Perioperative use of tirofiban hydrochloride (Aggrastat) does not increase surgical bleeding after emergency or urgent coronary artery bypass grafting. *J Thorac Cardiovasc Surg* 2001;122:1181–5.

39. Silvestry SC, Smith PK. Current status of cardiac surgery in the Abciximab-treated patient. *Ann Thorac Surg* 2000;70:S12–9.

40. Poullis M, Manning R, Haskard D, Taylor K. ReoPro removal during cardiopulmonary bypass using a hemoconcentrator. *J Thorac Cardiovasc Surg* 1999;117:1032–4.

41. Schafer AI. Effects of nonsteroidal anti-inflammatory drugs on platelet function and systemic hemostasis. *J Clin Pharmacol* 1995;35:209–19.

42. Mori TA, Beilin LJ, Burke V, Morris J, Ritchie J. Interactions between dietary fat, fish, and fish oils and their effects on platelet function in men at risk of cardiovascular disease. *Arterioscler Thromb Vasc Biol* 1997;17:279–86.

43. Larson MK, Ashmore JH, Harris KA, et al. Effects of omega-3 acid ethyl esters and aspirin, alone and in combination, on platelet function in healthy subjects. *Thromb Haemost* 2008;100:634–41.

44. Allman MA, Pena MM, Pang D. Supplementation with flaxseed oil versus sunflowerseed oil in healthy young men consuming a low fat diet: effects on platelet composition and function. *Eur J Clin Nutr* 1995;49:169–78.

45. Celestini A, Pulcinelli FM, Pignatelli P, et al. Vitamin E potentiates the antiplatelet activity of aspirin in collagen-stimulation platelets. *Haematologica* 2002;87:420–6.

46. Antiplatelet effects of herbal products. *Dermatol Nurs* 2002;14:207.

47. Valli G, Giardina EGV. Benefits, adverse effects, and drug interactions of herbal therapies with cardiovascular effects. *J Am Coll Cardiol* 2002;39:1083–95.

48. Freedman JE, Parker C., III, Li L, et al. Select flavonoids and whole juice from purple grapes inhibit platelet function and enhance nitric oxide release. *Circulation* 2001;103:2792–8.

49. Weiss S, Nyzio JB, Cines D, et al. Antiphospholipid syndrome: intraoperative and postoperative anticoagulation in cardiac surgery. *J Cardiothorac Vasc Anesth* 2008;22:735–9.

50. Gorki H, Malinovski V, Stanbridge RDL. The antiphospholipid syndrome and heart valve surgery. 2008;33:168–81.

51. Hogan WJ, McBane RD, Santrach PJ, et al. Antiphospholipid syndrome and perioperative hemostatic management of cardiac valvular surgery. *Mayo Clin Proc* 2000;75:971–6.

52. Spiess BD. Treating heparin resistance with antithrombin or fresh frozen plasma. *Ann Thorac Surg* 2008;85:2153–60.

53. Ad N, Henry L, Halpin L, et al. The use of spirometry testing prior to cardiac surgery may impact the Society of Thoracic Surgeons risk prediction score: a prospective study in a cohort of patients at high risk for chronic lung disease. *J Thorac Cardiovasc Surg* 2010;139:686–91.

54. Samuels LE, Kaufman MS, Morris RJ, Promisloff R, Brockman SK. Coronary artery bypass grafting in patients with COPD. *Chest* 1998;113:878–82.

55. Jacob B, Amoateng-Adjepong Y, Rasakulasuriar S, Manthous CA, Haddad R. Preoperative pulmonary function tests do not predict outcome after coronary artery bypass. *Conn Med* 1997;61:327–32.

56. Hulzebos EH, Van Meeteren NL, De Bie RA, Dagnelie PC, Helders PJ. Prediction of postoperative pulmonary complications on the basis of preoperative risk factors in patients who had undergone coronary artery bypass graft surgery. *Phys Ther* 2003;83:8–16.

57. Rady MY, Ryan T, Starr NJ. Early onset of acute pulmonary dysfunction after cardiovascular surgery: risk factors and clinical outcome. *Crit Care Med* 1997;25:1831–9.

58. Filsoufi F, Rahmanian PB, Castillo JG, Chikwe J, Adams DH. Logistic risk model predicting postoperative respiratory failure in patients undergoing valve surgery. *Eur J Cardiothorac Surg* 2008;34:953–9.

59. Nakagawa M, Tanaka H, Tsukuma H, Kishi Y. Relationship between the duration of the preoperative smoke-free period and the incidence of postoperative pulmonary complications after pulmonary surgery. *Chest* 2001;120:705–10.

60. Al-Sarraf N, Thalib L, Hughes A, Tolan M, Young V, McGovern E. Effect of smoking on short-term outcome of patients undergoing coronary artery bypass surgery. *Ann Thorac Surg* 2008;86:517–23.

61. Rajendran AJ, Pandurangi UM, Murali R, Gomathi S, Vijayan VK, Cherian KM. Pre-operative short-term pulmonary rehabilitation for patients of chronic obstructive pulmonary disease undergoing coronary artery bypass graft surgery. *Indian Heart J* 1998;50:531–4.

62. Jeong DS, Kim KH, Kim CY, Kim JS. Relationship between plasma B-type natriuretic peptide and ventricular function in adult cardiac surgery patients. *J Int Med Res* 2008;36:31–9.

63. Mueller C, Scholer A, Laule-Kilian K, et al. Use of B-type natriuretic peptide in the evaluation and management of acute dyspnea. *N Engl J Med* 2004;350:647–54.

64. Mickleborough LL, Maruyama H, Mohamed S, et al. Are patients receiving amiodarone at increased risk for cardiac operations? *Ann Thorac Surg* 1994;58:622–9.

65. Kaushik S, Hussain A, Clarke P, Lazar HL. Acute pulmonary toxicity after low-dose amiodarone therapy. *Ann Thorac Surg* 2001;72:1760–1.

66. An Y, Xiao YB, Zhong QJ. Open-heart surgery in patients with liver cirrhosis. *Eur J Cardiothorac Surg* 2007;31:1094–8.

67. Filsoufi F, Salzberg SP, Rahmanian PB, et al. Early and late outcome of cardiac surgery in patients with liver cirrhosis. *Liver Transpl* 2007;13:990–5.

68. Hayashida N Shoujima T, Teshima H, et al. Clinical outcome after cardiac operations in patients with cirrhosis. *Ann Thorac Surg* 2004;77:500–5.

69. Suman A, Barnes DS, Zein NN, Levinthal GN, Connor JT, Carey WD. Predicting outcome after cardiac surgery in patients with cirrhosis: a comparison of Child-Pugh and MELD Scores. *Clin Gastroenterol Hepatol* 2004;2:719–23.

70. Morisaki A, Hosono M, Sasaki Y, et al. Risk factor analysis in patients with liver cirrhosis undergoing cardiovascular operations. *Ann Thorac Surg* 2010;89:811–8.

71. Luciani N, Nasso G, Gaudino M, et al. Coronary artery bypass grafting in type II diabetic patients: a comparison between insulin-dependent and non-insulin-dependent patients at short- and mid-term follow-up. *Ann Thorac Surg* 2003;76:1149–54.

72. Marcheix B, Eynden FV, Demers P, Bouchard D, Cartier R. Influence of diabetes mellitus on long-term survival in systematic off-pump coronary artery bypass surgery. *Ann Thorac Surg* 2008;86:1181–8.

73. Singh SK, Desai ND, Petroff SD, et al. The impact of diabetic status on coronary artery bypass graft patency. Insights from the radial artery patency study. *Circulation* 2008;118(suppl 1):S222–5.

74. Hueb W, Gersh BJ, Costa F, et al. Impact of diabetes on five-year outcomes of patients with multivessel coronary artery disease. *Ann Thorac Surg* 2007;83:93–9.

75. Mohammadi S, Dagenais F, Mathieu P, et al. Long-term impact of diabetes and its comorbidities in patients undergoing isolated primary coronary artery bypass graft surgery. *Circulation* 2007;116(suppl I):I-220–5.

76. Halkos ME, Puskas JD, Lattouf OM, et al. Elevated preoperative hemoglobin A1c level is predictive of adverse events after coronary artery bypass surgery. *J Thorac Cardiovasc Surg* 2008;136:631–40.

77. Halkos ME, Lattouf OM, Puskas JD, et al. Elevated preoperative hemoglobin A1c is associated with reduced long-term survival after coronary artery bypass surgery. *Ann Thorac Surg* 2008;86:1431–7.

78. Alserius T, Anderson RE, Hammar N, Nordqvist T, Ivert T. Elevated glycosylated haemoglobin (HbA1c) is a risk marker in coronary artery bypass surgery. *Scand Cardiovasc J* 2008;42:392–8.

79. Savage EB, Grab JD, O'Brien SM, et al. Use of both internal thoracic arteries in diabetic patients increases deep sternal wound infection. *Ann Thorac Surg* 2007;83:1002–7.

80. Nakano J, Okabayashi H, Hanyu M, et al. Risk factors for wound infection after off-pump coronary artery bypass grafting: should bilateral internal thoracic arteries be harvested in patients with diabetes? *J Thorac Cardiovasc Surg* 2008;135:540–5.

81. Yamazaki K, Kato H, Tsujimoto S, Kitamura R. Diabetes mellitus, internal thoracic artery grafting, and the risk of an elevated hemidiaphragm after coronary artery bypass surgery. *J Cardiothorac Vasc Anesth* 1994;8:437–40.

82. Weiler JM, Gellhaus MA, Carter JG, et al. A prospective study of the risk of an immediate adverse reaction to protamine sulfate during cardiopulmonary bypass surgery. *J Allergy Clin Immunol* 1990;85:713–9.

83. Schmeltz LR, DeSantis AJ, Thiyagarajan V, et al. Reduction of surgical mortality and morbidity in diabetic patients undergoing cardiac surgery with a combined intravenous and subcutaneous insulin glucose management strategy. *Diabetes Care* 2007;30:823–8.

84. Swenne CL, Lindholm C, Borowiec J, Schnell AE, Carlsson M. Peri-operative glucose control and development of surgical wound infections in patients undergoing coronary artery bypass graft. *J Hosp Infect* 2005;61:201–12.

85. Halkos ME, Puskas JD, Lattouf OM, Kilgo P, Guyton RA, Thourani VH. Impact of preoperative neurologic events on outcomes after coronary artery bypass grafting. *Ann Thorac Surg* 2008;86:504–10.

86. Redmond JM, Greene PS, Goldsborough MA, et al. Neurologic injury in cardiac surgical patients with a history of stroke. *Ann Thorac Surg* 1996;61:42–7.

87. Durand DJ, Perler BA, Roseborough GS, et al. Mandatory versus selective preoperative carotid screening: a retrospective analysis. *Ann Thorac Surg* 2004;78:159–66.

88. Denton TA, Trento L, Cohen M, et al. Radial artery harvesting for coronary bypass operations: neurologic complications and their potential mechanisms. *J Thorac Cardiovasc Surg* 2001;121:951–6.

89. Siminelakis S, Karfis E, Anagnostopolous C, Toumpoulis I, Katsaraki A, Drossos G. Harvesting radial artery and neurologic complications. *J Card Surg* 2004;19:505–10.

90. Ikizler M, Ozkan S, Dernck S, et al. Does radial artery harvesting for coronary revascularization cause neurological injury in the forearm and hand? *Eur J Cardiothorac Surg* 2005;28:421–4.

91. Shah SA, Chark D, Williams J, et al. Retrospective analysis of local sensorimotor deficits after radial artery harvesting for coronary artery bypass grafting. *J Surg Res* 2007;139:203–8.

92. Quenot JP, Thiery N, Barbar S. When should stress ulcer prophylaxis be used in the ICU? *Curr Opin Crit Care* 2009;15:139–43.

93. Yasny JS, Silvay G. The value of optimizing dentition before cardiac surgery. *J Cardiothorac Vasc Anesth* 2007;21:587–91.

94. Terezhalmy GT, Safadi TJ, Longworth DL, Muehrcke DD. Oral disease burden in patients undergoing prosthetic heart valve implantation. *Ann Thorac Surg* 1997;63:402–4.

95. D'Agostino RS, Svensson LG, Neumann DJ, Balkhy HH, Williamson WA, Shahian DM. Screening carotid ultrasonography and risk factors for stroke in coronary artery surgery patients. *Ann Thorac Surg* 1996;62:1714–23.

96. Hirotani T, Kameda T, Kumamoto T, Shirota S, Yamano M. Stroke after coronary artery bypass grafting in patients with cerebrovascular disease. *Ann Thorac Surg* 2000;70:1571–6.

97. Cywinski JB, Koch CG, Krajewski LP, Smedira N, Li L, Starr NJ. Increased risk associated with combined carotid endarterectomy and coronary artery bypass graft surgery: a propensity-matched comparison with isolated coronary artery bypass graft surgery. *J Cardiothorac Vasc Anesth* 2006;20:796–802.

98. Ricotta JJ, Wall LP, Blackstone E. The influence of concurrent carotid endarterectomy on coronary bypass: a case-controlled study. *J Vasc Surg* 2005;41:397–401.

99. Borger MA, Fremes SE, Weisel RD, et al. Coronary bypass and carotid endarterectomy: does a combined approach increase risk? A meta-analysis. *Ann Thorac Surg* 1999;68:14–21.

100. Akins CW, Hilgenberg AD, Vlahakes GJ, et al. Late results of combined carotid and coronary surgery using actual versus actuarial methodology. *Ann Thorac Surg* 2005;80:2091–7.

101. Kolh PH, Comte L, Tchana-Sato V, et al. Concurrent coronary and carotid artery surgery: factors influencing perioperative outcome and long-term results. *Eur Heart J* 2006;27:49–56.

102. Timaran CH, Rosero EB, Smith ST, Valentine RJ, Modrall JG, Clagett GP. Trends and outcomes of concurrent carotid revascularization and coronary bypass. *J Vasc Surg* 2008;48:355–60.

103. Versaci F, Reimers B, Del Giudice C, et al. Simultaneous hybrid revascularization by carotid stenting and coronary artery bypass grafting: the SHARP study. *JACC Cardiovasc Interv* 2009;2:393–401.

104. Chu D, Bakaeen FG, Wang XL, et al. The impact of peripheral vascular disease on long-term survival after coronary artery bypass graft surgery. *Ann Thorac Surg* 2008;86:1175–80.

105. Sinclair MC, Singer RL, Manley NJ, Montesano RM. Cannulation of the axillary artery for cardiopulmonary bypass: safeguards and pitfalls. *Ann Thorac Surg* 2003;75:931–4.

106. Bell ML, Grunwald GK, Baltz JH, et al. Does preoperative hemoglobin independently predict short-term outcomes after coronary artery bypass graft surgery? *Ann Thorac Surg* 2008;86:1415–23.

107. Kulier A, Levin J, Moser R, et al. Impact of preoperative anemia on outcome in patients undergoing coronary artery bypass grafting. *Circulation* 2007;116:471–9.

108. Ereth MH, Nuttall GA, Orszulak TA, Santrach PJ, Cooney WP IV, Oliver WC Jr. Blood loss from coronary angiography increases transfusion requirements for coronary artery bypass graft surgery. *J Cardiothorac Vasc Anesth* 2000;14:177–81.

109. Dacey LJ, DeSimone J, Braxton JH, et al. Preoperative white blood cell count and mortality and morbidity after coronary artery bypass grafting. *Ann Thorac Surg* 2003;76:760–4.

110. Newall N, Grayson AD, Oo AY, et al. Preoperative white blood cell count is independently associated with higher perioperative cardiac enzyme release and increased 1-year mortality after coronary artery bypass grafting. *Ann Thorac Surg* 2006;81:583–90.

111. Albert AA, Beller CJ, Walter JA, et al. Preoperative high leukocyte count: a novel risk factor for stroke after cardiac surgery. *Ann Thorac Surg* 2003;75:1550–7.

112. Warkentin TE, Crowther MA. When is HIT really HIT? *Ann Thorac Surg* 2007;83:21–3.

113. Warkentin TE, Greinacher A, Koster A, Lincoff AM. Treatment and prevention of heparin-induced thrombocytopenia. American College of Chest Physicians evidence-based clinical practice guidelines (8th edition). *Chest* 2008;133:340S–380S.

114. Cooper WA, O'Brien SM, Thourani VH, et al. Impact of renal dysfunction on outcomes of coronary artery bypass surgery: results from the Society of Thoracic Surgeons National Adult Cardiac Database. *Circulation* 2006;113:1063–70.

115. Brown JR, Cochran RP, MacKenzie TA, et al. Long-term survival after cardiac surgery is predicted by estimated glomerular filtration rate. *Ann Thorac Surg* 2008;86:4–11.

116. Martino E, Bartalen L, Bogazzi F, Braverman LE. The effects of amiodarone on the thyroid. *Endocr Rev* 2001;22:240–54.

117. Piga M, Serra A, Boi F, Tanda ML, Martino E, Mariotti S. Amiodarone-induced thyrotoxicosis. A review. *Minerva Endocrinol* 2008;33:213–28.

118. Fox AA, Shernan SK, Collard CD, et al. Preoperative B-type natriuretic peptide is an independent predictor of ventricular dysfunction and mortality after primary coronary artery bypass grafting. *J Thorac Cardiovasc Surg* 2008;136:452–61.

119. Pedrazzini GB, Masson S, Latini R, et al. Comparison of brain natriuretic peptide plasma levels versus logistic EuroSCORE in predicting in-hospital and late postoperative mortality in patients undergoing aortic valve replacement for symptomatic aortic stenosis. *Am J Cardiol* 2008;102:749–54.

120. van Straten AHM, Soliman Hamad M, van Zundert AJ, et al. Preoperative C-reactive protein levels to predict early and late mortalities after coronary artery bypass surgery: eight years of follow-up. *J Thorac Cardiovasc Surg* 2009;138:954–8.

121. Karkouti K, McCluskey S. Pro: preoperative autologous blood donation has a role in cardiac surgery. *J Cardiothorac Vasc Anesth* 2003;17:121–5.

122. Alghamdi AA, Albanna MJ, Guru V, Brister SJ. Does the use of erythropoietin reduce the risk of exposure to allogeneic blood transfusion in cardiac surgery? A systematic review and meta-analysis. *J Card Surg* 2008;21:320–6.

123. Yazicioğlu L, Eryilmaz S, Şirlak M, et al. Recombinant human erythropoietin administration in cardiac surgery. *J Thorac Cardiovasc Surg* 2001;122:741–5.

124. Johnson RG, Thurer RL, Kruskall MS, et al. Comparison of two transfusion strategies after elective operations for myocardial revascularization. *J Thorac Cardiovasc Surg* 1992;104: 307–14.

125. Murphy GH, Angelini GD. Indications for blood transfusion in cardiac surgery. *Ann Thorac Surg* 2006;82:2323–34.

126. Society of Thoracic Surgeons Blood Conservation Guideline Task Force, Ferraris VA, Ferraris SP, Saha SP, et al. Perioperative blood transfusion and blood conservation in cardiac surgery: the Society of Thoracic Surgeons and the Society of Cardiovascular Anesthesiologists clinical practice guideline. *Ann Thorac Surg* 2007;83(5 suppl):S27–86.

127. Ferguson TB, Coombs LP, Peterson ED. Preoperative beta-blocker use and mortality and morbidity following CABG surgery in North America. *JAMA* 2002;287:2221–7.

128. Augoustides JGT. Angiotensin blockade and general anesthesia: so little known, so far to go. *J Cardiothorac Vasc Anesth* 2008;22:177–9.

129. Raja SG, Fida N. Should angiotensin converting enzyme inhibitors/angiotensin II receptor antagonists be omitted before cardiac surgery to avoid postoperative vasodilation? *Interact Cardiovasc Thorac Surg* 2008;7:470–5.

130. Miceli A, Capoun R, Fino C, et al. Effects of angiotensin-converting enzyme inhibitor therapy on clinical outcome in patients undergoing coronary artery bypass grafting. *J Am Coll Cardiol* 2009;54:1778–84.

131. Arora P, Rajagopalam S, Ranjan R, et al. Preoperative use of angiotensin-converting enzyme inhibitors/angiotensin receptor blockers is associated with increased risk for acute kidney injury after cardiovascular surgery. *Clin J Am Soc Nephrol* 2008;3:1266–73.

132. Benedetto U, Sciarretta S, Roscitano A, et al. Preoperative angiotensin-converting enzyme inhibitors and acute kidney injury after coronary artery bypass grafting. *Ann Thorac Surg* 2008;86:1160–5.

133. Mitchell LB, Exner DV, Wyse DG, et al. Prophylactic oral amiodarone for the prevention of arrhythmias that begin early after revascularization, valve replacement, or repair: PAPABEAR: a randomized controlled trial. *JAMA* 2005;294:3093–100.

134. Lazar HL. Should all patients receive statins before cardiac surgery: are more data necessary? *J Thorac Cardiovasc Surg* 2006;131:520–2.

135. Liakopoulos OJ, Choi YH, Kuhn EW, et al. Statins for prevention of atrial fibrillation after cardiac surgery: a systematic literature review. *J Thorac Cardiovasc Surg* 2009;138:678–86.

136. Liakopoulos OJ, Choi YH, Haldenwang PL, et al. Impact of preoperative statin therapy on adverse postoperative outcomes in patients undergoing cardiac surgery: a meta-analysis of over 30,000 patients. *Eur Heart J* 2008;29:1548–59.

137. Takagi H, Kawai N, Umemoto T. Preoperative statin therapy reduces postoperative all-cause mortality in cardiac surgery: a meta-analysis of controlled studies. *J Thorac Cardiovasc Surg* 2009;137:e52–3.

138. Katznelson R, Djaiani GN, Borger MA, et al. Preoperative use of statins is associated with reduced early delirium rates after cardiac surgery. *Anesthesiology* 2009;110:67–73.

139. Whitlock RP, Chan S, Devereaux PJ, et al. Clinical benefit of steroid use in patients undergoing cardiopulmonary bypass: a meta-analysis of randomized trials. *Eur Heart J* 2008;29:2592–600.

140. Halvorsen P, Raeder J, White PF, et al. The effect of dexamethasone on side effects after coronary revascularization procedures. *Anesth Analg* 2003;96:1578–83.

141. Engelman R, Shahian D, Shemin R, et al. The Society of Thoracic Surgeons practice guideline series: antibiotic prophylaxis in cardiac surgery, Part II: Antibiotic choice. *Ann Thorac Surg* 2007;83:1569–76.

142. Ranucci M, Pazzaglia A, Bianchini C, Bozzetti G, Isgrò G. Body size, gender, and transfusions as determinants of outcome after coronary operations. *Ann Thorac Surg* 2008;85:481–7.

143. Moskowitz DM, Klein JJ, Shander A, et al. Predictors of transfusion requirements for cardiac surgical procedures at a blood conservation center. *Ann Thorac Surg* 2004;77:626–34.

144. Parr KG, Patel MA, Dekker R, et al. Multivariate predictors of blood product use in cardiac surgery. *J Cardiothorac Vasc Anesth* 2003;17:176–81.

145. Arora RC, Légaré JF, Buth KJ, Sullivan JA, Hirsch GM. Identifying patients at risk of intraoperative and postoperative transfusion in isolated CABG: toward selective conservation strategies. *Ann Thorac Surg* 2004;78:1547–55.

146. Rybak MJ, Lomaestro B, Rotschafer JC, et al. Vancomycin therapeutic guidelines: a summary of consensus recommendations from the Infectious Diseases Society of America, the American Society of Health-System Pharmacists, and the Society of Infectious Diseases Pharmacists. *Clin Infect Dis* 2009;49:325–7.

147. Kaiser AB, Kernodle DS, Barg NL, Petracek MR. Influence of preoperative showers on staphylococcal skin colonization: a comparative trial of antiseptic skin cleansers. *Ann Thorac Surg* 1988;45:35–8.

148. Muñoz P, Hortal J, Giannella M, et al. Nasal carriage of S. aureus increases the risk of surgical site infection after major heart surgery. *J Hosp Infect* 2008;68:25–31.

149. Tom TSM, Kruse MW, Reichman RT. Update: methicillin-resistant Staphylococcus aureus screening and decolonization in cardiac surgery. *Ann Thorac Surg* 2009;88:695–702.

150. Kallen AJ, Wilson CT, Larson RJ. Perioperative intranasal mupirocin for the prevention of surgical-site infections: systematic review of the literature and meta-analysis. *Infect Control Hosp Epidemiol* 2005;26:916–22.

151. Jog S, Cunningham R, Cooper S, et al. Impact of preoperative screening for methicillin-resistant Staphylococcus aureus by real-time polymerase chain reaction in patients undergoing cardiac surgery. *J Hosp Infect* 2008;69:124–30.

152. Shrestha NK, Banbury MK, Weber M, et al. Safety of targeted perioperative mupirocin treatment for preventing infections after cardiac surgery. *Ann Thorac Surg* 2006;81:2183–8.

153. Ko W, Lazenby WD, Zelano JA, Isom OW, Krieger KH. Effects of shaving methods and intraoperative irrigation on suppurative mediastinitis after bypass operations. *Ann Thorac Surg* 1992;53:301–5.

154. Granton T, Cheng D. Risk stratification models for cardiac surgery. *Semin Cardiothorac Vasc Anesth* 2008;12:167–74.

155. Geissler HJ, Hölzl P, Marohl S, et al. Risk stratification in heart surgery: comparison of six score systems. *Eur J Cardiothorac Surg* 2000;17:400–6.

156. Bernstein AD, Parsonnet V. Bedside estimation of risk as an aid for decision-making in cardiac surgery. *Ann Thorac Surg* 2000;69:823–8.

157. O'Connor GT, Plume SK, Olmstead EM, et al. Multivariate prediction of in-hospital mortality associated with coronary artery bypass graft surgery. Northern New England Cardiovascular Disease Study Group. *Circulation* 1992;85:2110–8.

158. Nashef SAM, Roques F, Michel P, Gauducheau E, Lemeshow S, Salamon R, EuroSCORE study group. European system for cardiac operative risk evaluation (EuroSCORE). *Eur J Cardiothorac Surg* 1999;16:9–13.

159. Edwards FH, Grover FL, Shroyer ALW, Schwartz M, Bero J. The Society of Thoracic Surgeons national cardiac surgery database: current risk assessment. *Ann Thorac Surg* 1997;63:903–8.

160. Gogbashian A, Sedrakyan A, Treasure T. EuroSCORE: a systematic review of international performance. *Eur J Cardiothorac Surg* 2004;25:695–700.

161. Michel P, Roques F, Nashef SAM, the EuroSCORE project group. Logistic or additive EuroSCORE for high-risk patients? *Eur J Cardiothorac Surg* 2003;23:684–7.

162. Shanmugam G, West M, Berg G. Additive and logistic EuroSCORE performance in high risk patients. *Interact Cardiovasc Thorac Surg* 2005;4:299–303.

163. Gummert JF, Funkat A, Osswald B, et al. EuroSCORE overestimates the risk of cardiac surgery: results from the national registry of the German Society of Thoracic and Cardiovascular Surgery. *Clin Res Cardiol* 2009;98:363–9.

164. Wendt D, Osswald BR, Kayser K, et al. Society of Thoracic Surgeons score is superior to the EuroSCORE determining mortality in high risk patients undergoing isolated aortic valve replacement. *Ann Thorac Surg* 2009;88:468–75.

165. Nashef SA, Roques F, Michel P, Gauducheau E, Lemeshow S, Salamon R. Validation of European system for cardiac operative risk evaluation (EuroSCORE) in North American cardiac surgery. *Eur J Cardiothorac Surg* 2002;22:101–5.

166. Ferraris VA, Ferraris SP. Risk factors for postoperative morbidity. *J Thorac Cardiovasc Surg* 1996;111:731–41.

167. Reddy SLC, Grayson AD, Griffiths EM, Pullan DM, Rashid A. Logistic risk model for prolonged ventilation after adult cardiac surgery. *Ann Thorac Surg* 2007;84:528–36.

168. Mehta RH, Grab JD, O'Brien SM, et al. Bedside tool for predicting the risk of postoperative dialysis in patients undergoing cardiac surgery. *Circulation* 2006;114:2208–16.

169. Thakar CV, Arrigain S, Worley S, Yared JP, Paganin EP. A clinical score to predict acute renal failure after cardiac surgery. *Am J Soc Nephrol* 2005;16:162–8.

170. Ranucci M, Bozzetti G, Ditta A, Cotza M, Carboni G, Ballotta A. Surgical reexploration after cardiac operations: why a worse outcome? *Ann Thorac Surg* 2008;86:1557–62.

171. Jones HU, Mulestein JB, Jones KW, et al. Early postoperative use of unfractionated heparin or enoxaparin is associated with increased surgical re-exploration for bleeding. *Ann Thorac Surg* 2005;80:519–22.

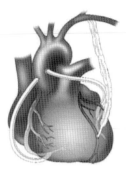

CHAPTER 4

Cardiac Anesthesia

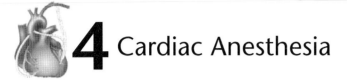

4 Cardiac Anesthesia

Although excellence in pre- and postoperative care can often make the difference between an uneventful and a complicated recovery, the care provided in the operating room usually has the most significant impact on patient outcome. Performing a technically proficient, complete, and expeditious operation is only one component of this phase. Refinements in anesthetic techniques and monitoring, cardiopulmonary bypass (CPB), and myocardial protection have enabled surgeons to operate successfully on extremely ill patients with far advanced cardiac disease and multiple comorbidities. Use of off-pump modalities to avoid CPB is particularly useful in patients at high risk because of associated comorbidities. Minimally invasive approaches, including robotic surgery, may lessen the trauma of a surgical procedure, expediting surgical recovery. Many patients previously considered inoperable will now survive the operative period to provide a challenge to postoperative care. This chapter will describe anesthesia considerations in cardiac surgery, including monitoring, transesophageal echocardiography (TEE), use of anesthetic agents, and bleeding and anticoagulation-related issues. It will also discuss anesthetic considerations related to CPB and the immediate postbypass period.

I. Preoperative Visit

   A. A preoperative visit by the cardiac anesthesiologist is essential before all operations. This provides an opportunity to review the patient's history, perform a relevant examination, and explain the techniques of monitoring and postoperative ventilatory support. This evaluation should identify any potential problems that might require further workup or could influence intraoperative management.

   1. History: cardiac symptoms, significant comorbidities, previous anesthetic experiences, surgical procedures, allergies, medications, and recent use of steroids

   2. Examination: heart, lungs, intubation concerns (loose teeth, ability to open mouth, laxity of jaw)

   B. The anesthesiologist should instruct the patient on which medications to continue up to the time of surgery, which ones to stop, and which ones to take in modified doses. Specifically, he/she should tell the patient to:

   1. Continue all antihypertensive and antianginal medications up to and including the morning of surgery. Exceptions include angiotensin-converting enzyme (ACE) inhibitors and angiotensin receptor blockers (ARBs), which should be withheld the morning of surgery to reduce the risk of low systemic resistance in the perioperative period.[1]

Manual of Perioperative Care in Adult Cardiac Surgery, 5th Edition. By Robert M. Bojar.
Published 2011 by Blackwell Publishing Ltd.

2. Withhold insulin or oral hypoglycemic medications the morning of surgery. Blood glucose should be obtained on arrival in the operating room and checked frequently during surgery with coverage provided by intravenous insulin.

3. Follow the surgeon's recommendations for cessation of anticoagulants and antiplatelet agents. Warfarin should be stopped at least 4 days before surgery so that the INR will normalize before surgery. Aspirin can be stopped 3–5 days before valvular surgery without coronary disease and in truly elective CABGs. However, aspirin 81 mg daily should be continued in most coronary patients and should have little impact on perioperative bleeding.[2,3] Clopidogrel and prasugrel should be stopped for 5–7 days before elective surgery, but may need to be continued or stopped for a shorter period of time in patients with recently placed drug-eluting stents.[4] Unfractionated heparin may be continued into the operating room for patients with critical coronary disease, but otherwise can be stopped about 4 hours before surgery. The last dose of low-molecular-weight heparin should be given 18–24 hours before surgery, and the patient should not receive fondaparinux for at least 48 hours before surgery.[5] IIb/IIIa inhibitors (eptifibatide and tirofiban) should be stopped at least 4 hours prior to surgery.[6]

C. Informed consent should be obtained for anesthesia management including the insertion of monitoring lines, with a discussion of potential complications.

II. Preoperative Medications

These are usually not given before the patient is brought into the operating room. Once the initial intravenous lines are inserted, low doses of midazolam (1–4 mg IV) can be given to reduce the patient's anxiety and produce amnesia to allow for the safe insertion of additional monitoring lines without producing hemodynamic stress. Prophylactic antibiotics should be given within 1 hour of skin incision (starting 2 hours beforehand for vancomycin).[7]

III. Intraoperative Monitoring and Transesophageal Echocardiography

A. Patients undergoing cardiac surgical procedures are extensively monitored. Hemodynamic alterations and myocardial ischemia that occur during the induction of anesthesia, in the prebypass period, during CPB, and following resumption of cardiac activity can have significant adverse effects on myocardial function and recovery. It should be noted that even though both hypertension and tachycardia can increase myocardial oxygen demand, an increase in heart rate results in more myocardial ischemia at an equivalent increase in oxygen demand.[8]

B. Standard monitoring in the operating room consists of a five-lead ECG system, noninvasive blood pressure cuff, a radial (and occasionally femoral) arterial line, pulse oximetry, an end-tidal CO_2 measurement, a Swan-Ganz pulmonary artery (PA) catheter, cerebral oximetry, and a urinary Foley catheter to measure urine output and core body temperature (Figure 4.1).

1. For uncomplicated coronary artery bypass surgery performed on- or off-pump in patients with normal or mildly depressed ventricular function, use of a central venous pressure (CVP) monitoring line instead of a PA catheter can provide an adequate assessment of filling pressures.[9–12]

2. Specially designed Swan-Ganz catheters can be used to obtain continuous cardiac outputs and mixed venous oxygen saturations. Arterial pulse wave monitoring

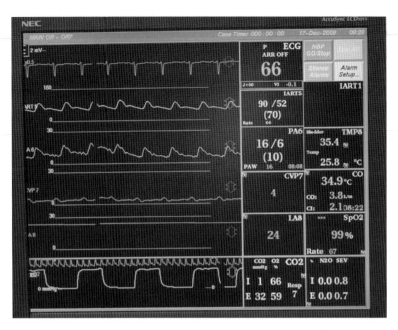

Figure 4.1 • Display monitor in the operating room. From top to bottom are displays of one ECG lead, the arterial pressure, pulmonary artery and central venous pressures from the Swan-Ganz catheter, an additional module for a second pressure tracing (initially the retrograde cardioplegia pressure and later a second arterial tracing, usually from the femoral artery), pulse oximetry, and capnography. The first column on the right gives the heart rate, digital readouts of pressures (phasic and mean pressures), capnography values, and the FIO$_2$. In the far right column are displays of the systemic, myocardial, and pulmonary artery temperatures, cardiac output values, SaO$_2$ by pulse oximetry, and doses of inhalational gases being administered.

devices, such as the Vigileo/FloTrac device (Edwards Lifesciences), can also be used to obtain continuous cardiac outputs.[13,14] These devices are invaluable during off-pump surgery and are helpful in patients in whom a Swan-Ganz catheter cannot be placed (tricuspid valve surgery) or when thermodilution cardiac outputs are unreliable (moderate-to-severe tricuspid regurgitation).[15] Transesophageal echocardiography (TEE) is routine in most centers and is cost-effective in providing useful information that may alter the operative approach.[16,17] There should be provisions to perform epiaortic scanning to assess for ascending aortic atherosclerosis, which may also influence conduct of the operation.[18–20]

C. **Swan-Ganz pulmonary artery catheters** are usually placed before the induction of anesthesia, especially if left ventricular (LV) dysfunction is present, but they may be placed after induction and intubation, especially in the anxious patient. These catheters are used to measure right (CVP) and left-sided filling pressures (pulmonary artery diastolic [PAD] and pulmonary capillary wedge [PCW] pressures), and obtain thermodilution cardiac outputs. Despite the nearly universal use of these catheters to carefully monitor patients and provide objective data on cardiac performance in the pre- and postbypass periods, it has not been demonstrated that they influence the outcome of cardiac surgery.

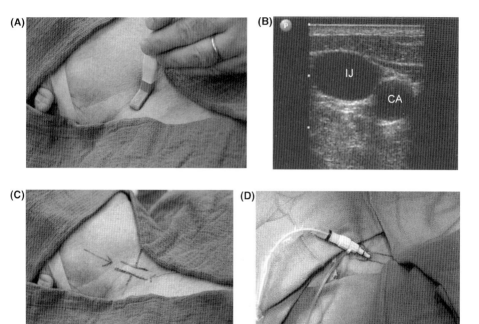

Figure 4.2 • (A) Use of an echo probe to identify the location of the internal jugular vein. (B) Echo image of the neck identifies the location and size of the internal jugular vein (IJ) and its relationship to the carotid artery (CA). (C) The site is marked, and (D) the catheter is placed.

1. The catheter is usually inserted through an 8.5 Fr introducer placed into the internal jugular vein or, less commonly, the subclavian vein. Ultrasound-guided access, using an echo probe on the neck to identify the internal jugular vein, is very helpful in facilitating line placement (Figure 4.2). The introducer sheath contains one side port that provides central venous access for the infusion of vasoactive medications and potassium. Multilumen introducers, such as the 8.5 Fr and 9 Fr high-flow advanced venous access (AVA) devices (Edwards Lifesciences and Arrow), can be used to provide additional venous access in patients with poor arm veins and limited peripheral access. A manifold with multiple stopcocks is attached to the side port of the introducer or to one of the additional ports of the AVA through which all medications are administered.

2. The catheter is passed into the right atrium, and the balloon at the catheter tip is inflated. The catheter is advanced through the right ventricle (RV) and pulmonary artery (PA) into the pulmonary capillary wedge (PCW) position as confirmed by pressure tracings (Figure 4.3). The PA tracing should reappear when the balloon is deflated. **Note:** Caution is essential in passing the catheter through the right ventricle in patients with left bundle branch block (LBBB), in whom complete heart block might occur. In this situation, unless provisions for urgent pacing are available (temporary pacing wires, external pads), it is best to wait until the chest is open before advancing the catheter so that the surgeon can directly pace the heart if necessary.[21]

3. The proximal port of the Swan-Ganz catheter (30 cm from the tip) is used for CVP measurements from the right atrium and for fluid injections to determine the

mmHg

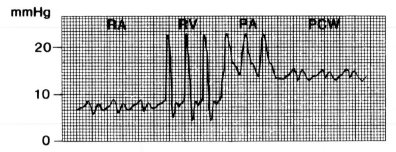

Figure 4.3 • Swan-Ganz catheter pressures. Intracardiac pressures are recorded from the distal (PA) port as the catheter is passed through the right atrium (RA), right ventricle (RV), and pulmonary artery (PA), into the pulmonary capillary wedge (PCW) position.

cardiac output. Care must be exercised when injecting sterile fluid for cardiac outputs to prevent bolusing of vasoactive medications that might be running through the CVP port. **Note:** One must *never* infuse anything through this port if the catheter has been pulled back so that the tip lies in the right atrium and the CVP port lies outside the patient! This might not be noticed, because the catheter is usually placed through a sterile sheath that allows for advancement or withdrawal of the catheter. This concept must always be kept in mind when critical medications, such as heparin prior to cannulation, are being administered.

4. The distal port should always be transduced and displayed on a monitor to allow for detection of catheter advancement into the permanent wedge position, which could result in pulmonary artery injury. Balloon inflation ("wedging" of the catheter) is rarely necessary during surgery. Medications should never be given through the distal PA port.

5. A variety of Swan-Ganz catheters are available that provide additional functions.

   a. Some catheters contain additional ports for the placement of right atrial and ventricular pacing wires, which is helpful during minimally invasive surgery when access to the heart is limited.

   b. Other catheters have been modified for assessment of continuous cardiac outputs and mixed venous oxygen saturations (SvO_2) by fiberoptic oximetry (Figure 4.4). These catheters are invaluable during off-pump surgery to evaluate

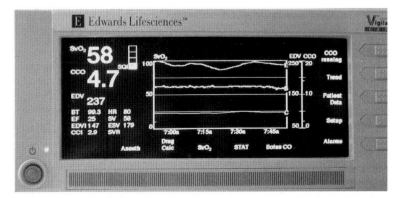

Figure 4.4 • Continuous cardiac output monitor display.

the patient's hemodynamic status, and may contribute to a therapeutic maneuver in many patients.[22] Oximetric catheters are also helpful in patients with tricuspid regurgitation, in whom thermodilution technology tends to underestimate the cardiac output. In these patients, the Vigileo/FloTrac cardiac output monitoring system is invaluable.

    c. Volumetric Swan-Ganz catheters use thermodilution to determine a right ventricular ejection fraction from which the right ventricular end-diastolic and end-systolic volumes can be determined.[23] This is particularly valuable in patients with pulmonary hypertension and compromised right ventricular function.

6. The primary concerns during insertion of a PA catheter are arterial puncture, arrhythmias during passage through the right ventricle, and potential heart block in patients with preexisting LBBB. Other complications of Swan-Ganz catheters are noted on page 292.

7. **Pulmonary artery perforation** is a very serious complication.[24–26] It may occur during insertion of the catheter or during the surgical procedure when hypothermia causes the catheter to become rigid. Since a cold, stiff catheter may advance into the lung when the heart is manipulated, it is advisable to pull it back slightly during CPB to prevent perforation and then readvance it after CPB. Migration of the catheter into the wedge position may be evident by loss of pulse pressure in the PA waveform before or after bypass or by a very high PA pressure measurement on bypass when the heart is decompressed.

    a. If perforation occurs, blood will appear in the endotracheal tube. The goals of management are to maintain gas exchange and arrest the hemorrhage. Positive end-expiratory pressure (PEEP) should be applied to the ventilator circuit. If the degree of hemoptysis is not severe, it may abate once CPB is terminated and protamine is administered.

    b. If the airway is compromised by bleeding, CPB should be resumed with venting of the pulmonary artery. Bronchoscopy is then performed with placement of a bronchial blocker or a double-lumen endotracheal tube that can provide differential lung ventilation. The pleural space should be entered to evaluate the problem. If application of PEEP or occluding the hilar vessels does not control the bleeding, pulmonary resection may be required. Use of femoral artery–femoral venous extracorporeal membrane oxygenation (ECMO) may control bleeding by lowering the PA pressures, but does require persistent heparinization.[27] Because of the risk of recurrence, pulmonary angiography and embolization may be considered once the bleeding is controlled.

D. **Intraoperative TEE** has become routine in most cardiac surgical centers.[16,17,28–30] The probe is placed after the patient is anesthetized and before heparinization. TEE provides an analysis of regional and global right and left ventricular function, is very sensitive in detecting ischemia,[31] and identifies the presence of valvular pathology or intracardiac masses (Table 4.1 and Figures 2.16–2.19, pages 108–111). Color flow and pulsed wave Doppler are used to analyze valvular function or suspected shunts. Although TEE may image the aorta for atheromatous disease, epiaortic imaging provides better visualization of the ascending aorta and arch when there are significant concerns about atheromatous disease. After bypass, TEE can be used

Table 4.1 • Specific Uses of Intraoperative Echocardiography

Pre-bypass	Identify or confirm preoperative pathology (see Table 2.3, page 113)
	Epiaortic imaging for aortic atherosclerosis in ascending aorta, arch and descending aorta
	Intracardiac thrombus (LA appendage, LV apex)
During Off-Pump Surgery	Regional wall motion abnormalities
Post-bypass Coronary disease	Regional dysfunction (incomplete/inadequate revascularization)
Valve surgery	Presence of intracardiac air on weaning from CPB
	RV and LV function (circumflex artery entrapment after MVR, coronary ostial obstruction after AVR)
	Valve regurgitation from paravalvular leak or inadequate repair
	Outflow tract obstruction after MV repair or replacement
	Obstruction to prosthetic leaflet opening or closing
	Residual stenosis after commissurotomy
VSD closure	Residual VSD
IABP	Location of device relative to aortic arch
All patients	Evaluation of iatrogenic aortic dissection

to assess ventricular function, the presence of intracardiac air, and the competency of valvular repairs and replacements. An individual trained in performing and reading TEE, whether a cardiac anesthesiologist or a cardiologist, is essential to optimize its usefulness. Before the probe is placed, consideration must be given to contraindications to TEE placement that could produce catastrophic complications, such as hypopharyngeal, proximal or distal esophageal perforation or bleeding, which are noted in fewer than 0.1% of patients.[32–35] TEE must be used cautiously or avoided in patients with prior esophageal surgery or with known esophageal pathology, such as strictures, Schatzki's ring, or esophageal varices.

1. Multiplane TEE allows for rotation of the probe through 180 degrees, thus affording excellent images of the heart in multiple views. The probe is advanced up and down the esophagus and then into the stomach for transgastric views. The tip of the probe can be flexed in four different directions, and the shaft of the probe can also be rotated. The American Society of Echocardiography and the Society of Cardiovascular Anesthesiologists have defined 20 standard views for a routine examination (Figure 4.5).[29] The best views during cardiac surgery include the following:

   a. In the mid-upper esophagus, rotation of the probe allows for visualization of the aortic valve and proximal ascending aorta in short- and long-axis views (Figure 4.6).

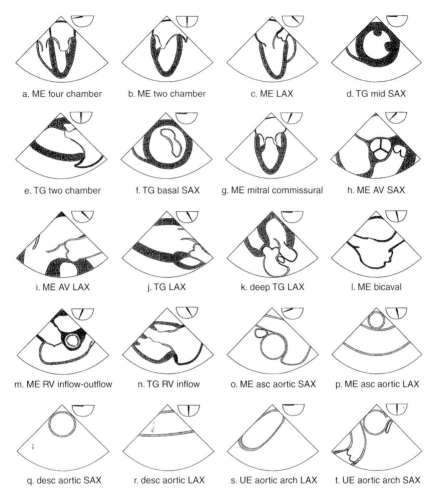

a. ME four chamber　　b. ME two chamber　　c. ME LAX　　d. TG mid SAX

e. TG two chamber　　f. TG basal SAX　　g. ME mitral commissural　　h. ME AV SAX

i. ME AV LAX　　j. TG LAX　　k. deep TG LAX　　l. ME bicaval

m. ME RV inflow-outflow　　n. TG RV inflow　　o. ME asc aortic SAX　　p. ME asc aortic LAX

q. desc aortic SAX　　r. desc aortic LAX　　s. UE aortic arch LAX　　t. UE aortic arch SAX

Figure 4.5 • Recommended views for intraoperative transesophageal echocardiography. (Reproduced with permission from Shanewise et al., *Anesth Analg* 1999;89:870–84.)[29]

    b. In the mid-lower esophagus, the standard views can be obtained by rotating the probe through 135 degrees. With progressive rotation, these views include a four-chamber view (0 degrees), a long-axis two-chamber view (90 degrees), and a long-axis view of the LV outflow tract (130–150 degrees) (Figure 4.7).

    c. With the probe anteflexed in the transgastric views, the three standard views are the short-axis view of the RV and LV (0 degrees), the longitudinal two-chamber LV view (70–90 degrees), and the LV outflow tract (110–135 degrees) (Figure 4.8).

2. During **on-pump coronary artery surgery**, prebypass TEE will provide a baseline analysis of regional and global ventricular function. The midpapillary long- and short-axis views are best to assess most regions of the left ventricle.

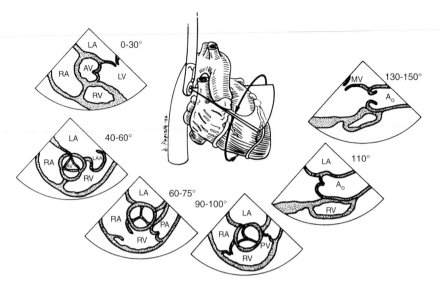

Figure 4.6 • Mid-upper esophageal echocardiographic imaging of the aortic valve. Rotation of the probe allows for visualization of the aortic valve and proximal ascending aorta in short- and long-axis views. (Reproduced with permission from Roelandt J, Pandian NG, eds., *Multiplane Transesophageal Echocardiography*. Churchill Livingstone, 1996.)

The ability of the heart muscle to thicken is consistent with viability, whereas areas of thinned-out muscle represent infarcted areas. Following bypass, slight improvement in previously ischemic zones may be noted, especially with inotropic stimulation. These areas of hypokinesis may represent stunned or hibernating myocardium that have contractile reserve and may gradually recover function after revascularization. The new onset of hypokinesis raises the specter of hypoperfusion from an anastomotic or graft problem, incomplete revascularization, or inadequate myocardial protection. The new onset of mitral regurgitation (MR) may reflect loading conditions but could indicate ischemia.

3. During **off-pump surgery**, the midesophageal windows are best for assessing RV and LV function and the presence of MR. Baseline views are obtained. During vessel occlusion, TEE should assess for the acute development of regional LV dysfunction or acute MR during construction of left-sided grafts and for RV dysfunction during right coronary grafting. The transgastric views are not helpful when the heart is elevated out of the chest.[36–38] The development and persistence of a new regional wall motion abnormality after a graft is completed suggest a flow problem, usually at the anastomosis. However, the latter may occur even in the absence of a regional wall motion abnormality.

4. In **minimally invasive** access procedures (usually aortic or mitral valve surgery), TEE can confirm the location of the retrograde coronary sinus catheter since it

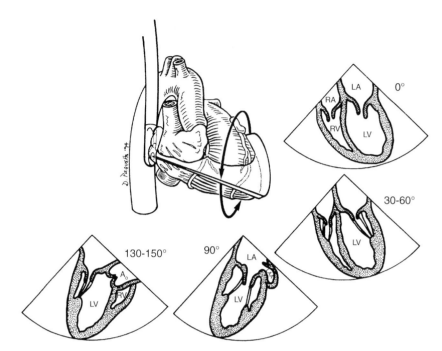

Figure 4.7 • Mid-lower esophageal echocardiographic imaging. Standard views can be obtained by rotating the probe through 135 degrees. With progressive rotation, these views include a four-chamber view (0 degrees), a long-axis two-chamber view (90 degrees), and a long-axis view of the LV outflow tract (130–150 degrees). (Reproduced with permission from Roelandt J, Pandian NG, eds., *Multiplane Transesophageal Echocardiography*. Churchill Livingstone, 1996.)

cannot be palpated by the surgeon. It can also visualize the intracardiac location of a long venous catheter placed via the femoral vein. Upon weaning from bypass, TEE is essential to identify intracardiac air and to assess valve competence.

5. **Aortic valve surgery.** In aortic valve operations, the best TEE views are obtained from the mid to upper esophagus (Figure 4.6) and can provide several important pieces of information to the surgeon:

   a. Quantify the degree of aortic stenosis by planimetry and by continuous wave and pulsed wave Doppler flow analysis. These permit assessment of transvalvular pressure gradients, and, using the continuity equation, provide calculation of the aortic valve area.

   b. Quantify the degree of aortic regurgitation using color flow and continuous wave Doppler analysis. If moderate to severe, this will contraindicate delivery of antegrade cardioplegia into the aortic root.

   c. Assess the degree of left ventricular hypertrophy and its nature (concentric, septal).

   d. Assess annular and aortic root size.

   e. Identify the presence of systolic and/or diastolic dysfunction, which may influence filling pressures and pharmacologic management coming off pump.

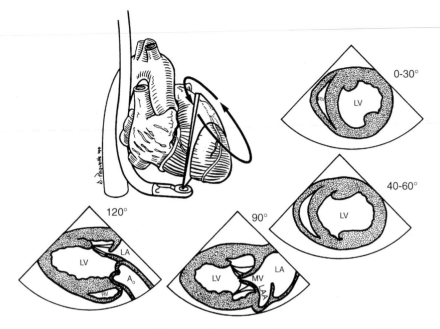

Figure 4.8 • Transgastric views. With the probe anteflexed in the transgastric position, the standard views are the short-axis view of the RV and LV (0 degrees), the longitudinal two-chamber LV view (90 degrees), and the LV outflow tract (120 degrees). (Reproduced with permission from Roelandt J, Pandian NG, eds., *Multiplane Transesophageal Echocardiography.* Churchill Livingstone, 1996.)

    f. After bypass, TEE should initially be used to identify intracardiac air and ventricular function. It is then used to assess opening and closing of valve leaflets and identify paravalvular leaks. Competence of homografts, autografts (Ross procedure), and the native aortic valve in a valve-sparing procedure can be confirmed. Rarely, an unusual finding may be demonstrated, such as a ventricular septal defect or an aorto-left atrial fistula.

    g. Three-dimensional echo imaging is being evaluated as a means of assessing anatomic and functional changes after transcatheter aortic valve implantation.[39,40]

  6. Mitral valve surgery. The best visualization of the mitral valve is from the lower and midesophagus.

    a. Prebypass assessment should confirm the valvular pathology and identify the mechanism of MR (e.g., a flail leaflet and the direction of the regurgitant jet) (Figure 2.16, page 109). However, in some patients with MR, it is not uncommon to note a discrepancy in the degree of MR between preoperative and intraoperative TEE due to alteration in loading conditions. The left atrial appendage should be evaluated for the presence of thrombus.

   b. During weaning from bypass, TEE is helpful in identifying intracardiac air. After termination of bypass it should be used to assess the competence of valve repairs, identify paravalvular leaks after mitral valve replacement (MVR) (Figure 4.9), and assess LV and RV function. Occasionally, the TEE will reveal an unsuspected finding such as:

   i. Systolic anterior motion (SAM) of the anterior mitral valve leaflet obstructing the LV outflow tract (after valve repairs or MVR with retention of the anterior leaflet)

   ii. Evidence of valve dysfunction with a trapped or obstructed leaflet

   iii. Aortic valve regurgitation after a difficult mitral valve operation (due to suture entrapment of an aortic valve cusp or distortion of the aortic annulus from placement of too small a mitral valve).

   c. Three-dimensional echocardiography has significantly improved imaging of the mitral valve with precise identification of valve pathology and has allowed for refinement of reparative techniques (Figure 2.20, page 112).[41,42]

7. The diagnosis of **an aortic dissection** can be confirmed by TEE once the patient is anesthetized (Figure 2.18, page 111). It not only identifies the intimal flap, but can also determine whether aortic regurgitation is present, mandating aortic valve resuspension or replacement. If a large pericardial effusion is present, groin cannulation may be necessary for the emergent institution of CPB before opening the pericardium. TEE can also identify flaps in cases of iatrogenic dissections at the cannulation or clamp sites.

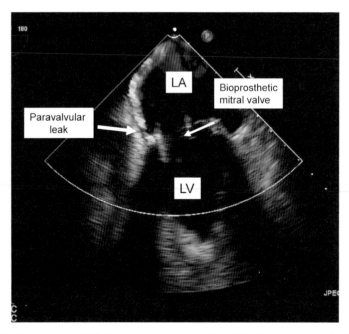

Figure 4.9 • Postoperative TEE showing a paravalvular leak following tissue mitral valve replacement.

8. In **thoracic aortic surgery**, TEE is useful in assessing cardiac performance and intracardiac volume status during the period of clamping and after unclamping, when PA pressures tend to be elevated out of proportion to preload. This may influence fluid and pharmacologic management.[43] Positioning of an endograft for thoracic aortic repairs, including traumatic aortic tears, type B dissections, and thoracic aortic aneurysms, is usually confirmed by fluoroscopy, and the TEE probe should usually be pulled out to avoid interference with the x-ray beam.

IV. Anesthetic Considerations for Various Types of Heart Surgery

A. Anesthetic management must be individualized, taking into consideration the patient's age, comorbidities, the nature and extent of coronary or valvular disease, the degree of left ventricular dysfunction, and plans for early extubation. These factors will determine which medications should be selected to avoid myocardial depression, tachycardia, or bradycardia, or to counteract changes in vasomotor tone. Generally, a balanced anesthetic technique using a combination of narcotics and potent inhalational agents is used for all open-heart surgery to minimize myocardial depression. Specific anesthetic concerns for various disease processes are presented in this section.

B. **Coronary artery bypass surgery**

1. Factors that increase myocardial oxygen demand, such as tachycardia and hypertension, must be prevented in the prebypass period, especially during the induction of anesthesia. Hypotension, often resulting from the vasodilating effects of narcotics, anxiolytics (midazolam), and sedatives (propofol), should be counteracted with fluids and α-agents since hypotension is more likely to produce ischemia than hypertension.

2. Detection and treatment of ischemia is critical in the prebypass period. TEE is the most sensitive means of detecting ischemic regional wall motion abnormalities and can be recommended for all cardiac cases. Ischemia may also be manifested by an elevation in the pulmonary artery pressures or by ST segment changes in the ECG leads. Aggressive management with nitroglycerin, β-blockers (esmolol), and narcotics can usually control prebypass ischemia.[44] If not, prompt initiation of CPB may be necessary.

3. Narcotic/sedative regimens are the standard for coronary surgery, especially in patients with left ventricular dysfunction. Use of low-dose fentanyl or sufentanil, inhalational anesthetics, and propofol or dexmedetomidine at the conclusion of surgery allow for early postoperative extubation. Use of the short-acting narcotic remifentanil along with a volatile inhalational anesthetic with rapid onset and offset of effect, such as sevoflurane or desflurane, allows for "ultra fast tracking" with extubation in the operating room or upon arrival in the ICU.[45–51]

4. Anesthetic techniques for **off-pump surgery** (OPCAB) commonly involve use of a continuous cardiac output Swan-Ganz catheter with in-line mixed venous oxygen saturation monitoring. Tilting of the operating room table (Trendelenburg position and to the right) to augment cardiac filling, judicious fluid administration, antiarrhythmic therapy (lidocaine/magnesium), α-agents (phenylephrine) and inotropes (epinephrine/milrinone), and, on occasion, insertion of an intra-aortic

balloon pump (IABP) may be used. Use of a warming system, especially the Kimberly-Clark warming system (formerly the Arctic Sun temperature management system), is helpful in preventing hypothermia during OPCAB surgery.[52] The essential elements of a successful off-pump operation include a patient surgeon who uses good judgment in deciding when off-pump surgery is feasible and when conversion to CPB or right-heart assist is necessary, an anesthesiologist who is experienced and comfortable with off-pump surgery, and a qualified, actively involved first assistant. See section IX (pages 212–215) for a more detailed discussion of anesthesia for off-pump surgery.

5. MIDCAB procedures may involve internal thoracic artery takedown either with direct vision or with endoscopic or robotic assistance. The anastomosis to the left anterior descending artery (LAD) is then performed through a small thoracotomy incision, but can also be performed robotically. One-lung anesthesia is generally used. With use of stabilization platforms, it is not necessary to slow the heart down pharmacologically. Robotic coronary surgery can be performed off-pump or on-pump with groin cannulation.

C. **Left ventricular aneurysms** (LVAs). Anesthetic drugs that cause myocardial depression must be avoided because of the association of LVAs with significant left ventricular dysfunction. Swan-Ganz monitoring is important in optimizing preload and contractility before and after bypass. TEE is the most sensitive means of detecting the presence of LV thrombus and provides an excellent assessment of ventricular wall thickness and motion (akinesia, hypokinesia, and dyskinesia noted with aneurysms).

D. **Ventricular septal defects** are usually operated upon on an emergent basis when the patient is in cardiogenic shock, usually on inotropic support and an IABP. Thus, myocardial depression must be avoided. Systemic hypertension may increase the shunt and should be prevented.

E. **Aortic valve surgery**

1. **Aortic stenosis.** The induction of anesthesia is a critical period for patients with aortic stenosis. The left ventricle is generally hypertrophied and stiff with evidence of diastolic dysfunction. Avoidance of hypovolemia, myocardial depression, vasodilation, tachycardia, or dysrhythmias is important, as all of these can lower the cardiac output precipitously. An α-agent, such as phenylephrine or norepinephrine, is particularly valuable in supporting systemic resistance. Atrial fibrillation (AF) developing before the initiation of bypass is often associated with profound hypotension, and cardioversion may be necessary. The best TEE views of the aortic valve are obtained in the midesophageal short- and long-axis views.

2. **Aortic regurgitation.** The hemodynamic goals in the prebypass period are to maintain satisfactory preload and avoid bradycardia and hypertension. Vasodilation may be beneficial, but hypotension may reduce the diastolic perfusion pressure and precipitate ischemia. The transgastric long-axis view with color Doppler is best for assessing aortic regurgitation.

3. **Transcatheter aortic valve implantation** can be performed through a transfemoral or transapical approach (Figure 1.12, page 26). Both are performed under general anesthesia, anticipating extubation at the conclusion of the procedure. Intravenous access and monitoring should take into consideration the possible

need to emergently initiate CPB. TEE is essential in assessing annulus size, aortic pathology, left ventricular function, and the presence of MR. It is then used along with fluoroscopy to appropriately position the introducing catheter for balloon deployment to inflate the stented valve. This is performed at a time of minimal cardiac ejection induced by rapid ventricular pacing with transient cessation of ventilation. These maneuvers usually result in hypotension and arrhythmias, which can be minimized by initiation of vasopressor therapy just prior to pacing. After the valve is inflated, TEE can be used to assess for any aortic regurgitation or aortic dissection.[53]

F. Hypertrophic obstructive cardiomyopathy. Measures that produce hypovolemia or vasodilation must be avoided because they increase the outflow tract gradient. Volume infusions should be used to maintain preload, with the use of α-agents to maintain systemic resistance. Use of β-blockers and calcium channel blockers to reduce heart rate and contractility are beneficial in the immediate preoperative and prebypass periods. Inotropic drugs with predominantly β-adrenergic effects could provoke the gradient and must be avoided.

G. Mitral valve surgery

1. **Mitral stenosis.** Attention should be paid to maintaining preload, reducing heart rate, and preventing an increase in pulmonary vascular resistance (PVR).

   a. Preload must be adjusted judiciously to ensure adequate left ventricular filling across the stenotic valve while simultaneously avoiding excessive fluid administration that could lead to pulmonary edema. In patients with severe pulmonary hypertension and right ventricular dysfunction, a volumetric (RVEF) Swan-Ganz catheter is valuable in the assessment of right ventricular volumes and ejection fractions. The PA diastolic pressure may overestimate the left atrial pressure, and placement of a left atrial line for monitoring post-bypass may be considered. Balloon inflation ("wedging") of a PA catheter should be avoided or performed with a minimal amount of balloon inflation in patients with pulmonary hypertension because of the increased risk of PA rupture.

   b. The heart rate should be reduced to prolong the diastolic filling period. For patients in atrial fibrillation, small doses of esmolol or diltiazem can be used to control a rapid ventricular response. Cardiac output is usually marginal in patients with mitral stenosis and can be further compromised if the ventricular rate is excessively slow.

   c. Factors that can increase the PVR must be avoided. Preoperative sedation can induce hypercarbia and should not be given. Hypoxemia, hypercarbia, acidosis, and nitrous (not nitric) oxide should be avoided in the operating room. The PVR can be reduced with systemic vasodilators (propofol) or nonspecific pulmonary vasodilators (usually nitroglycerin) before bypass. Following bypass, RV support is best achieved using inotropic agents that can produce pulmonary vasodilation (usually milrinone). In patients with severe pulmonary hypertension and RV dysfunction, inhaled nitric oxide, epoprostenol (Flolan), or iloprost (Ventavis) can be used. Nesiritide may reduce the PA pressures most likely because of its lusitropic effects. A further discussion of the postoperative management of mitral valve surgery and the management of RV dysfunction is noted on pages 317–318, 327–328, and 452–457.

2. Mitral regurgitation

a. Measures that can increase pulmonary artery pressure, such as hypoxemia, hypercarbia, acidosis, and nitrous oxide, should be avoided. Preoperative sedation should be light or avoided altogether.

b. In the prebypass period, adequate preload must be maintained to ensure forward output. Systemic hypertension should be avoided, because the increased resistance to outflow will usually worsen MR. If the patient has ischemic MR or a borderline cardiac output, use of systemic vasodilators or an IABP will improve forward flow.

c. TEE is invaluable in identifying the precise anatomic cause for mitral regurgitation and in evaluating the surgical result. Three-dimensional TEE is especially helpful in these patients. TEE is performed once the patient is anesthetized. Occasionally, there is a discrepancy between preoperative and intraoperative studies due to alterations in systemic resistance and loading conditions. Elevating the blood pressure with α-agents may increase the amount of regurgitation in patients with moderate ischemic MR and aid in the decision to repair the valve during coronary bypass surgery. Midesophageal and transgastric long-axis views with rotation of the probe can evaluate the mitral valve quite precisely.

d. Measures noted above to decrease PA pressures should be used before or after bypass to optimize RV function.

H. Maze procedure for atrial fibrillation

1. The cut-and-sew Cox-Maze procedure to eliminate atrial fibrillation has been replaced by devices that produce comparable transmural ablation lines using radiofrequency, cryo-, or high-intensity focused ultrasound (HIFU) energy. A left atrial Maze procedure is most commonly performed as a concomitant procedure with mitral valve surgery (Figures 1.25 and 1.26, pages 56 and 57).

2. Bilateral pulmonary vein isolation (PVI) with resection and oversewing of the left atrial appendage is an appropriate procedure for patients with paroxysmal AF. This operation can be performed as an adjunct to any cardiac procedure or as an isolated operation. Surgery for lone AF may be performed through a sternotomy incision or through bilateral thoracoscopic ports. This requires repositioning of the patient with the operated side elevated about 30 degrees and use of one-lung anesthesia to allow the surgeon better exposure to isolate the pulmonary veins.

3. During the procedure, the patient is loaded with IV amiodarone which is then continued orally for several months. Other anesthetic considerations pertain to the specific lesion for which surgery is being performed if the Maze procedure is an adjunct.

I. Tricuspid valve disease

1. Maintenance of an elevated CVP is essential to achieve satisfactory forward flow in tricuspid stenosis. A Swan-Ganz PA catheter can be placed for monitoring of left-sided pressures in patients with tricuspid regurgitation, although cardiac output determinations are of little value. The FloTrac monitor can provide adequate cardiac output measurements based on the arterial line pulse wave. A Swan-Ganz catheter is usually pulled back out of the field during tricuspid valve surgery and then can be advanced through a repaired tricuspid valve or a bioprosthetic valve replacement.

2. Normal sinus rhythm provides better hemodynamics than atrial fibrillation, although the latter is frequently present. Slower heart rates are preferable for tricuspid stenosis and faster heart rates for tricuspid regurgitation.

3. Functional tricuspid regurgitation usually results from RV dilatation and dysfunction secondary to increased RV afterload from pulmonary hypertension. RV dysfunction is not uncommon once valve competence has been restored and this is exacerbated by suboptimal RV protection during cardioplegic arrest. Inotropes that can also lower the PVR (milrinone, dobutamine, and rarely isoproterenol) or selective pulmonary vasodilators may be required.

4. Patients with hepatic congestion often have impaired liver function that can affect the synthesis of clotting factors. A coagulopathy may develop after CPB, necessitating use of multiple blood component transfusions (especially fresh frozen plasma and cryoprecipitate) to control bleeding.

J. Endocarditis

1. Anesthetic management is dictated by the hemodynamic derangements associated with the particular valve involved. TEE is invaluable in identifying vegetations and regurgitant lesions, and may occasionally demonstrate involvement of additional valves that was not appreciated on preoperative studies.

2. Patients with aortic valve endocarditis may develop heart block from involvement of the conduction system by periannular infection. This may require preoperative placement of a transvenous pacing wire.

3. Ongoing sepsis may produce refractory hypotension on pump despite use of α-agents. Vasopressin may be necessary to maintain the blood pressure.

K. Aortic dissections

1. Maintenance of hemodynamic stability and especially avoidance of hypertension are critical to prevent aortic rupture, especially during the induction of anesthesia and line insertion. Use of a Swan-Ganz catheter is important to optimize perioperative hemodynamics. Its insertion can be delayed until after intubation to minimize the stress response.

2. Most patients require emergency surgery and should be considered to have a full stomach. A modified rapid-sequence induction should be performed to minimize the risk of aspiration while ensuring hemodynamic stability.

3. TEE is useful in localizing the site of the intimal tear and the proximal (and occasionally the distal) extent of the dissection, the degree of aortic regurgitation, and the presence of a hemopericardium. Because the diagnosis of an aortic dissection is usually obtained by a contrast CT scan, TEE is best performed once the patient has been anesthestized. If the diagnosis is in doubt, it may be elected to perform the TEE in an awake patient. In this situation, TEE must be performed **very cautiously** with light sedation for fear of precipitating hypertension, rupture, and then tamponade.

4. Repair of type A dissections is performed during a period of deep hypothermic circulatory arrest (DHCA). The head is packed in ice, and medications may be given to potentially provide additional cerebral protection (see section L.1, below). Use of a temperature management system is important.

5. Repair of type B dissections via an open approach requires a period of descending aortic cross-clamping. Because less collateral flow is present in patients with

dissections than with atherosclerotic aneurysms, the risk of paraplegia is greater. Left-heart bypass may reduce the risk of paraplegia.[54] A cerebrospinal fluid (CSF) drainage catheter should be placed before the patient is anesthetized. Proximal hypertension must be controlled during application of the cross-clamp, but should not be so low as to compromise spinal cord perfusion. A CSF drain is also useful if an endovascular stent procedure is performed for a complicated type B dissection.[55]

L. Ascending aortic and arch aneurysms

1. Aneurysms limited to the ascending aorta are repaired on CPB with application of an aortic cross-clamp. If they extend more distally or the arch is extensively involved, a period of DHCA at 18–20 °C core temperature is used. This usually ensures a lower nasopharyngeal or tympanic temperature, which correlates best with brain temperature. At this point, it is inferred that there is EEG silence with a bispectral analysis (BIS) reading of 0. This should provide about 45 minutes of safe arrest time and minimize the risk of neurologic insult.

2. Adjuncts to improve cerebral protection include selective antegrade or retrograde cerebral perfusion, and packing the head in ice.[56] Administration of methyl-prednisolone 30 mg/kg, magnesium 1 g, and occasionally thiopental or pentobarbital 5–10 mg/kg may be considered, but evidence of any benefit is unclear.[57,58] Some groups prefer to use cold cerebral perfusion techniques to protect the brain while maintaining the body at only moderate hypothermia (21–28 °C).[59]

3. Profound hypothermia and warming are associated with a coagulopathy. Platelets, fresh frozen plasma, and cryoprecipitate are helpful in achieving hemostasis. Supplemental use of warming devices is beneficial in warming the patient and preventing temperature afterdrop.

M. Descending aortic and thoracoabdominal aneurysms (TAA)

1. Arterial monitoring lines are inserted in the right radial and femoral arteries to monitor proximal and distal pressures during the period of aortic cross-clamping. The femoral line is valuable when left-heart bypass techniques are used.

2. A Swan-Ganz catheter is important to monitor filling pressures during the period of cross-clamping. TEE is helpful in evaluating myocardial function and often demonstrates a hypovolemic left ventricular chamber despite elevated pulmonary artery pressures when the cross-clamp is removed. Ensuring adequate intravascular volume will reduce the risk of "declamping shock" upon release of the aortic cross-clamp.

3. One-lung anesthesia using a double-lumen or Univent tube with a bronchial blocker improves operative exposure.

4. Control of proximal hypertension is essential during the cross-clamp period to minimize the adverse effects of increased afterload on LV function. However, lowering the pressure too much can reduce renal and spinal cord perfusion and increase the CSF pressure. Therefore, additional steps should be taken to minimize the risk of distal ischemic injury during aortic cross-clamping. This should include use of CSF drainage, distal perfusion, or consideration of other techniques such as cold renal perfusion, epidural cooling or use of DHCA.[60–63] Fenoldopam 0.03–0.1 μg/kg/min might be helpful in reducing the occurrence of acute kidney injury with TAA surgery.[64]

5. Endovascular stent placement is performed under general anesthesia. A femoral cutdown is performed, and the stent is placed either directly through the femoral

artery or through a side graft in patients with extensive aortoiliac disease. The landing zones are located by fluoroscopy.

N. Implantable cardioverter-defibrillator (ICD) placement

1. ICD implantation is usually performed in an electrophysiology laboratory under moderate sedation with propofol, allowing the patient to breathe spontaneously. When ventricular fibrillation is induced, deepening the level of sedation and assisted ventilation usually suffice. This requires close nursing or anesthesia attendance and careful monitoring. Most patients have markedly depressed ventricular function, and provisions for cardiac resuscitation (personnel and equipment) should be immediately available. External defibrillator pads should be placed for rescue defibrillation.

2. Medications that could be potentially arrhythmogenic, such as the catecholamines, must be avoided. Antiarrhythmic medications are continued unless there are plans for an electrophysiology study, which is usually performed with the patient off medications.

O. Cardioversion

1. Awake patients requiring emergency cardioversion in the ICU are generally hemodynamically unstable and should be given extremely light sedation prior to being cardioverted (1–2.5 mg of midazolam or 2–5 mg morphine). If the patient is still anesthetized and sedated, an increase in the infusion rate of propofol may be considered.

2. Patients requiring less urgent cardioversion for hemodynamic compromise or undergoing elective cardioversion (usually after TEE confirmation of absence of left atrial appendage thrombus) should receive a brief general anesthetic with propofol (50–100 mg) for the procedure.[65] Alternatively, etomidate (10–20 mg bolus) can be used, although it may produce myoclonus in nearly 50% of patients, which can cause ECG interference, making synchronized cardioversion very difficult. Anesthesia stand-by is recommended to provide airway support during the short period of sedation.

P. Surgery for pericardial disease

1. Pericardial drainage of a large pericardial effusion or tamponade is often performed urgently or emergently. In the immediate postoperative period, emergent exploration through a full sternotomy incision may be carried out in the ICU if tamponade is associated with severe hypotension or cardiac arrest. Otherwise, emergency exploration is carried out in the operating room. Most patients still have a Swan-Ganz catheter and satisfactory venous access in place, and there is little time for insertion of additional lines. Patients are generally in a low cardiac output state, and blood pressure is dependent on adequate preload, increased heart rate, and increased sympathetic tone. Volume infusions and β-agents are beneficial in maintaining hemodynamic stability. The patient should be prepped and draped before the administration of additional anesthetic agents. There is generally striking hemodynamic improvement once the pericardial blood is evacuated.

2. In less emergent situations, drainage is usually indicated for hemodynamically significant effusions. This may be accomplished by a pericardiocentesis performed in the cath lab with local anesthesia, depending on the size and location of the effusion. If this cannot be accomplished, the procedure is performed in the operating room. A

large bore central venous line should be inserted. A subxiphoid incision can be made under local anesthesia with moderate sedation, but more commonly is done under general anesthesia. Since blood pressure is similarly dependent on adequate preload, heart rate and increased sympathetic tone, agents that produce vasodilation, bradycardia, or myocardial depression must be avoided. Since loss of sympathetic tone can be catastrophic in a patient with tamponade physiology, prepping and draping of the patient should be considered before the induction of anesthesia.

3. TEE is invaluable in identifying the size and hemodynamic effects of an effusion. With limited surgical approaches, such as a subxiphoid window or thoracoscopy, TEE can identify whether the effusion has been adequately drained.

4. After resolution of tamponade, filling pressures generally fall, blood pressure increases, and a brisk diuresis occurs. Depending on the duration of tamponade, some patients may require transient inotropic support after the fluid is removed.

5. Patients with chronic constrictive pericarditis are usually in a chronic, compensated low cardiac output state. It is similarly essential to avoid hypovolemia, vasodilation, bradycardia or myocardial depression. After the constricted heart is decorticated, filling pressures may transiently fall, but many patients develop a low output state associated with right ventricular dilatation and will require inotropic support. Inadequate decortication may be evident when a fluid challenge that restores the preoperative filling pressures fails to increase cardiac output. Pulmonary edema may develop if the surgeon decorticates the right ventricle while the left ventricle remains constricted.

V. Induction and Maintenance of Anesthesia

A. Cardiac anesthesia is provided by a combination of medications including induction agents, anxiolytics, amnestics, analgesics, muscle relaxants, and inhalational anesthetics.

B. Induction agents include propofol, etomidate, thiopental, ketamine, or a benzodiazepine. Most commonly, anesthesia is induced with a combination of propofol, a narcotic, and a neuromuscular blocker to provide muscle relaxation and prevent chest wall rigidity that is associated with high-dose narcotic inductions. Succinylcholine is a depolarizing agent with rapid onset that can be used during rapid-sequence inductions or in patients with difficult airways. Although rarely used, ketamine given with a benzodiazepine is very useful in patients with compromised hemodynamics or tamponade. Ketamine does not produce myocardial depression, and its dissociative effects and sympathetic stimulant properties that produce hypertension and tachycardia are attenuated by use of a benzodiazepine.[66]

C. Subsequently, anesthesia is maintained by additional dosing of narcotics and muscle relaxants in combination with an anxiolytic (midazolam or propofol) and an inhalational agent (Tables 4.2 and 4.3). Bispectral electroencephalographic monitoring (BIS) can be used during on- and off-pump surgery to titrate and minimize the amount of medication required to maintain adequate anesthesia (a level around 55–60) while minimizing hemodynamic alterations and preventing awareness.[67,68] This is useful during bypass, when hemodilution increases the effective volume of distribution of anesthetic medications and may necessitate redosing. The dose and selection of anesthetic agents must provide adequate anesthesia and analgesia during surgery, but may be modified to allow for extubation in the operating room, or, more frequently, several hours after arrival in the ICU.

Table 4.2 • Hemodynamic Effects of Commonly Used Anesthetic Agents

	HR	Contractility	SVR	Net Effect on BP
Induction Agents				
Thiopental	↑	↓	↓	↓
Propofol	↓	↓	↓↓	↓↓
Etomidate	↔	↔	↔	↔
Anxiolytics				
Midazolam	↑	↔	↓	↓
Propofol	↓	↓	↓	↓
Lorazepam	↔	↔	↓	↓
Narcotics				
Fentanyl	↓	↔	↓	↓
Sufentanil	↓	↔	↓	↓
Alfentanil	↓	↔	↓	↓
Remifentanil	↓	↔	↓	↓
Muscle Relaxants				
Pancuronium	↑	↔	↔	↑
Vecuronium	↔	↔	↔	↔
Atracurium	↔	↔	↓	↓
Cisatracurium	↔	↔	↔	↔
Rocuronium	↔	↔	↔	↔
Succinylcholine	↑↓	↓	↔	↑↓

HR, heart rate; SVR, systemic vascular resistance; BP, blood pressure.

D. Commonly used narcotics include low-dose fentanyl, sufentanil, or remifentanil.[45–48] Low-dose fentanyl and sufentanil have a duration of action of 1–4 hours and allow patients to awaken within hours of completion of the operation. Remifentanil is a very short-acting narcotic with a duration of action of only 10 minutes. It is beneficial in shorter operations and allows for very early awakening and extubation.

E. Midazolam has an elimination half-life of over 10 hours in patients undergoing cardiac surgery. Therefore, its use is best limited to the prebypass period. Propofol is usually given at the termination of CPB and continued in the ICU. Propofol can be used to control postbypass hypertension because of its strong vasodilator properties. When the patient is stable, the propofol is turned off and the patient is allowed to awaken.

F. Inhalational agents provide muscle relaxation and unconsciousness, with variable effects on myocardial depression. Agents commonly used include sevoflurane, desflurane, and isoflurane. They are generally given during CPB to maintain anesthesia and reduce blood pressure, and allow for use of lower doses of intravenous

Table 4.3 • Dosages and Metabolism of Commonly Used Anesthetic Agents

	Usual Dosage	Duration of Action
Induction Agents		
Thiopental	3–5 mg/kg	5–10 min
Propofol	1–3 mg/kg → 10–100 μg/kg/min	2–8 min
Etomidate	0.2–0.4 mg/kg → 5–10 μg/kg/min	3–8 min
Anxiolytics		
Propofol	25–75 μg/kg/min	up to 20 min
Midazolam	2.5–5 mg IV q2h or 1–4 mg/h	up to 10 h
Lorazepam	1–4 mg q4h or 0.02–0.05 mg/kg	4–6 h
Narcotics		
Fentanyl	5–10 μg/kg → 1–5 μg/kg	1–4 h
Sufentanil	1 μg/kg → 0.25–0.75 μg/kg/h	1–4 h
Alfentanil	50–75 μg/kg → 0.5–3 μg/kg/min	1–1.6 h
Remifentanil	1 μg/kg → 0.05–2 μg/kg/min	10 min
Muscle Relaxants		
Pancuronium	0.1 mg/kg → 0.01 mg/kg q1h	180–240 min[a]/0–60 min[b]
Vecuronium	0.1 mg/kg → 0.01 mg/kg q30–45 min	45–90 min[a]/25–40 min[b]
Atracurium	0.3–0.5 mg/kg → 0.2–0.4 mg/kg/h	30–45 min[a]/15–30 min[b]
Cisatracurium	0.15 mg/kg → 0.03 mg/kg q20–50 min	60 min
Rocuronium	0.6–1.2 mg/kg IV → 10 μg/kg/min	30–60 min
Succinylcholine	1 mg/kg	5–10 min

[a] After initial intubating dose
[b] After repeat dose

medications, although they provide no analgesia. Desflurane and sevoflurane have less lipid solubility with a rapid onset of action and are quickly reversible, allowing for early extubation.[49–51] Nitrous oxide is contraindicated in that it reduces the amount of oxygen that can be delivered and it also may increase pulmonary artery pressures.

G. Muscle relaxants are given throughout the operation to minimize patient movement and suppress shivering during hypothermia. Adequate muscle relaxation might reduce some of the paraspinal muscle soreness often noted after surgery due to sternal retraction. Most neuromuscular blockers have minimal effect on myocardial function or blood pressure other than atracurium, which tends to lower the blood pressure (Tables 4.2 and 4.3).

1. **Pancuronium** (Pavulon) is the most commonly used neuromuscular blocker. It increases both heart rate and blood pressure and mitigates narcotic-induced bradycardia and hypotension. **Atracurium** (Tracrium) and **vecuronium** (Norcuron) do not undergo renal elimination and may be selected in patients with renal insufficiency. These drugs do not have vagolytic properties. **Rocuronium** (Zemuron) and **cisatracurium** (Nimbex) are short-acting neuromuscular blockers with rapid onset of action that can be used if very early extubation is planned.

2. Although some centers reverse muscle relaxants at the end of the operation to expedite extubation, this may prove detrimental if the patient becomes agitated and develops hemodynamic alterations. A conservative approach is to observe the patient in the ICU for several hours, during which time most of the neuromuscular blockade dissipates, and extubation can then be achieved. **Adequate sedation must be maintained in the ICU while a patient remains pharmacologically paralyzed**.

H. Dexmedetomidine (Precedex) is an α_2-adrenergic agonist with numerous properties, including sedation, analgesia, anxiolysis, and sympatholysis. However, it lacks an amnesic effect. During surgery, it can be used to reduce the dosage of other medications, allowing for early, comfortable extubation. It may also reduce shivering and myocardial ischemia. The most beneficial use of dexmedetomidine is to aid in ventilatory weaning when agitation and patient–ventilator dyssynchrony occur as the patient is weaned off propofol. It is given as a loading dose of 1 µg/kg over 10 minutes followed by a continuous infusion of 0.2–0.7 µg/kg/h.[69–72]

VI. General Prebypass Considerations (Table 4.4)

A. Prior to the commencement of surgery, the anesthesiologist is responsible for the safe insertion of monitoring lines, avoidance or treatment of hemodynamic or ischemic changes during the induction of anesthesia and intubation, and the placement and initial interpretation of the TEE. In addition, the anesthesiologist is responsible for:

1. The administration of prophylactic antibiotics starting within 1 hour of surgery (cephalosporins) or within 2 hours (vancomycin)

2. Placing external defibrillator pads (over the midaxillary line and back) for reoperations

3. Ensuring that positioning of the head and arms is safe (with nursing)

4. Ensuring adequate functioning of the cerebral oximetry pads (with perfusion)

B. Avoidance of ischemia prior to initiating bypass is critical for all types of heart surgery. Identification of ischemic ECG changes, elevation in filling pressures, or regional wall motion abnormalities on TEE requires prompt attention. Manipulation of the heart by the surgeon for cannula placement, blood loss during redo dissections, ongoing blood loss from leg incisions, and atrial fibrillation during atrial cannulation are a few of the potential insults that must be addressed. Judicious use of fluids and α-agents to counteract vasodilation and hypotension, β-blockers or additional anesthetic agents for hypertension or tachycardia, and nitroglycerin for ischemia must be selected appropriately to maintain stable hemodynamics. In the prebypass period, fluids are usually administered in the form of crystalloid, but excessive infusions in vasodilated

Table 4.4 • Anesthetic Considerations Prior to Cardiopulmonary Bypass
1. Line insertion and monitoring
2. Antibiotics prior to skin incision
3. External defibrillator pads for reoperations
4. Selection of medications for "balanced anesthesia" and plans for early extubation
5. Endotracheal intubation
6. Transesophageal echocardiography
7. Antifibrinolytic drug administration
8. Insertion of coronary sinus catheter or vents in minimally invasive surgery
9. Maintaining hemodynamics and avoiding or treating ischemia
10. Monitoring and treatment of abnormal cerebral oximetry
11. Heparinization for CPB

patients and those with significant preoperative anemia should be avoided. During any form of minimally invasive surgery, the limited exposure prevents the surgeon from directly visualizing most of the heart, reinforcing the importance of the anesthesiologist in using appropriate monitoring to identify and address abnormalities to ensure a stable perioperative course.

C. **Transesophageal echocardiography** should be performed after intubation and line placement to provide a baseline assessment of regional wall motion abnormalities and identify known or overlooked valvular pathology. In minimally invasive cases, it is used to identify the placement of coronary sinus catheters and pulmonary artery vents and the positioning of long venous lines into the right atrium.

D. **Autologous blood withdrawal** before the institution of bypass protects platelets from the damaging effects of CPB. The quality of this blood is excellent, with only slight activation of platelets, and it has been demonstrated to preserve red cell mass and reduce transfusion requirements.[73–75] It can be considered in patients for whom the calculated hematocrit on pump will remain adequate after withdrawal of 1–2 units of blood with nonheme fluid replacement.

E. **Steroids** might be considered to mitigate the systemic inflammatory response to CPB and possibly to reduce the incidence of atrial fibrillation.[76,77] Although steroids administered before CPB reduce the generation of inflammatory markers, evidence of any clinical benefit is weak.[78] Use of high doses of methylprednisolone (30 mg/kg) has been associated with hyperglycemia and metabolic acidosis.[78] Dexamethasone 1 mg/kg has been associated with hyperglycemia, transient subclinical organ system damage, as well as more pronounced pulmonary dysfunction.[79] Other studies have shown little clinical benefit other than an improvement in emetic symptoms or appetite.[80,81]

F. **Antifibrinolytic drugs** have been demonstrated to reduce perioperative blood loss in cardiac operations. They should be used for all on-pump procedures and may be of benefit in off-pump cases as well.[82–86] Most protocols include giving the first dose at the time of skin incision or before heparinization, giving a dose in the pump prime, and administering a constant infusion throughout the operation.

1. **ε-aminocaproic acid** (EACA or Amicar) is an inexpensive medication that has antifibrinolytic properties, and it may also preserve platelet function by inhibiting the conversion of plasminogen to plasmin. It is primarily effective in reducing bleeding when given prophylactically, with questionable benefit if given only for postoperative bleeding with suspected fibrinolysis.[87]

   a. One common regimen is to give 5 g after the induction of anesthesia, 5 g on pump, and 1 g/h during the procedure. Twice this dose is commonly used in patients weighing over 100 kg.

   b. A pharmacokinetic study showed that the clearance of ε-aminocaproic acid decreases and the volume of distribution increases during CPB. To maintain a plasma level of 260 μg/mL, an alternative weight-based protocol of a 50 mg/kg load over 20 minutes followed by a maintenance infusion of 25 mg/kg/h has been described.[88]

   c. Few adverse clinical effects have been noted with use of ε-aminocaproic acid. There is no increased risk of stroke.[89] Although a subtle degree of renal tubular dysfunction may occur, as demonstrated by an increase in urine β_2-microglobulin levels, a 10 g dose was not shown to alter creatinine clearance.[90]

2. **Tranexamic acid** (TA) has similar properties to EACA, inhibiting fibrinolysis at a serum concentration of 10 μg/mL, and reducing plasmin-induced platelet activation at a level of 16 μg/mL.[91,92] It has been shown to reduce perioperative blood loss in on- and off-pump surgery.[93] There are a variety of dosing protocols that have been recommended, but all have generally been designed to achieve a TA level >20 μg/mL. These include:

   a. 10 mg/kg over 20 minutes followed by a 1 mg/kg/h infusion (the most common regimen)[91,92]

   b. 10 mg/kg load, 40 mg/2 L pump prime (50 mg for a 2.5 L circuit), and an infusion rate of 2 mg/kg/h with a reduction in rate for a serum creatinine >1.5 mg/dL[94]

   c. 100 mg/kg given before CPB[95]

3. **Aprotinin** is a serine protease inhibitor that was found to be extremely effective in reducing perioperative bleeding in most cardiac procedures. It exhibited antifibrinolytic effects, preserved platelet function, and inhibited kallikrein, producing an antiinflammatory effect. Despite numerous reports that confirmed its safety, a few observational studies suggested that aprotinin increased the risk of renal dysfunction, stroke, myocardial infarction, and long-term mortality.[96] Although most of these criticisms have been refuted, and despite widespread popular use because of its tremendous benefits, aprotinin was withdrawn from the market in November 2007.

G. **Anticoagulation for cardiopulmonary bypass**

1. Anticoagulation is essential during CPB to minimize the generation of thrombin and fibrin monomers caused by interaction of blood with a synthetic interface. Unfractionated heparin (UFH) is universally used because it is an effective anticoagulant and is reversible with protamine. In contrast, other anticoagulants that could be used for CPB, such as the direct thrombin inhibitors bivalirudin and argatroban, are not reversible.[97,98]

2. **Heparin dosing.** Heparin inhibits the coagulation system by binding to antithrombin III, inactivating primarily thrombin and factor Xa. Inactivation of

thrombin prevents fibrin formation and also inhibits thrombin-induced activation of platelets and factors V, VIII, and XI. A baseline activated clotting time (ACT) should be drawn after the operation has commenced and before systemic heparinization. One study recommended that the initial ACT should be drawn through the introducer sheath prior to placing a heparin-coated PA catheter which may artificially elevate the baseline ACT.[99] A small dose of heparin (5000 units = 50 mg) is given before division of the internal thoracic artery or radial artery. The most common practice is to administer an empiric total dose of 2.5–4 mg/kg of heparin prior to cannulation for CPB. Porcine heparin is associated with a lower risk of heparin antibody formation than bovine heparin and is therefore recommended.[100]

3. **Heparin monitoring** is performed using a number of systems that measure the ACT.

   a. This widely used test qualitatively assesses the anticoagulant effect of heparin, but does not measure or necessarily correlate with heparin concentrations. There is great variability in patient response to heparin, and the ACT can be affected by hypothermia, hemodilution, and to a lesser degree by thrombocytopenia. Nonetheless, due to its simplicity and overall safety, achieving and maintaining a satisfactory ACT (>480 seconds but >300–350 seconds in biocompatible circuits) throughout the pump run is acceptable and universally utilized.[101] ACTs should be monitored every 20–30 minutes during bypass (or prior to bypass if there is a significant delay after initial heparinization) and additional heparin given as necessary.

   b. Because of individual patient variability in response to heparin, anticoagulation can also be assessed by calculating dose-response curves using the Medtronic Hepcon or Hemochron RxDx systems. These measure circulating levels of heparin (desired level is >2.7 units/mL), determine the appropriate amount of heparin to achieve a desired ACT, and calculate the dose of protamine required to neutralize the heparin. Achieving patient-specific heparin levels more effectively suppresses hemostatic system activation than standard dosing based on ACT alone and may contribute to less bleeding after protamine neutralization. Whether these systems indicate that more or less heparin is necessary in individual patients, their use is generally associated with less perioperative blood loss.[102–104] During cases involving DHCA, maintenance of blood heparin concentrations, rather than ACTs, has been shown to preserve the coagulation system better.[105]

   c. Use of heparin-bonded circuits to reduce the inflammatory response has reduced the requisite level of heparinization to minimize activation of the coagulation system.[73,106] However, underanticoagulation results in thrombin generation, which then triggers platelet activation, resulting in clotting within the bypass circuit. ACTs around 350 seconds are acceptable in routine coronary operations, but higher levels are recommended for more complex surgery.

   d. During off-pump surgery, the optimal ACT is not known. Using 2.5 mg/kg of heparin to achieve a target ACT >250 seconds appears to be acceptable, producing minimal thrombin generation, activation of the coagulation system, and fibrinolysis. This ACT level is not associated with an increased risk of thrombotic complications.[107,108]

   e. An alternative means of assessing anticoagulation is the high-dose thrombin time. This correlates better with heparin concentration and is not affected by temperature or hemodilution.[109]

4. **Heparin resistance** is present when a heparin dose of 5 mg/kg fails to raise the ACT to an adequate level (>400 seconds). This is usually caused by antithrombin III (AT III) deficiency and is relatively uncommon. However, it it is more likely to occur in patients on preoperative heparin, intravenous nitroglycerin, or an IABP, with elevated platelet counts, and in patients with infective endocarditis.[110,111] If additional heparin does not elevate the ACT, AT III must be given, either as fresh frozen plasma or in a commercially available pooled product of AT III (Thrombate III), which provides 500 IU per vial.[112] Precise dosing of this product is difficult because baseline levels of AT III are unknown in most cases and are most likely higher than levels noted in the rare patient with a hereditary antithrombin deficiency. The amount needed is calculated as (desired − baseline AT III level) × weight (kg) divided by 1.4. For example, to reach 120% of normal levels (which is recommended) in a 70 kg man with a baseline level 80% of normal would require $[(120 − 80)/1.4] × 70 = 2000$ IU.

5. **Heparin-induced thrombocytopenia (HIT)** is a condition associated with the development of platelet factor 4 (PF4)−heparin complex antibodies that bind to platelets triggering arterial and venous thrombosis.[113] A fall of >50% in platelet count following heparinization is noted in most patients with HIT, but other potential etiologies for thrombocytopenia must be considered (especially the use of glycoprotein IIb/IIIa inhibitors). If HIT is not identified and appropriately dealt with by using alternative anticoagulation regimens during surgery, it may be associated with life-threatening postoperative complications.

   a. Most patients have been exposed to heparin for catheterization, and heparin-PF4 antibodies are detected by ELISA testing prior to surgery in 5−19% of patients in various studies.[114–117] However, only a minority of these patients actually have HIT-causing antibodies and are susceptible to thrombotic complications that can be avoided by using alternative anticoagulation.[118] The presence of antibodies alone is arguably not associated with an increased thrombotic risk, but may be associated with other adverse outcomes, independent of the occurrence of HIT.[114–116]

   b. The benefit of assessing for the presence of preoperative heparin-PF4 antibodies is not defined. Some experts believe there is no role for testing for preoperative antibodies in the absence of thrombocytopenia, thrombosis, or a known history of HIT.[113] However, if thrombocytopenia or thrombosis is present, it is important to document whether the heparin-PF4 antibodies that may be present do in fact activate platelets. PF4-dependent ELISA tests may be positive in the absence of platelet-activating IgG antibodies. The presence of these antibodies can be confirmed with the highest specificity by functional washed platelet activation assays, including the serotonin release assay (SRA) and the heparin-induced platelet activation (HIPA) assay. The stronger the test result, the greater the risk of HIT.[118]

   c. If surgery is not urgent, it is best to wait 3 months before performing surgery. Antibodies usually clear in less than 3 months, at which time UFH can be used safely during surgery if the washed platelet activation assay is negative.

   d. When surgery is necessary on a more urgent basis and either acute HIT or subacute HIT (recovery from thrombocytopenia but a positive washed platelet activation assay) is present, use of UFH alone increases the risk of rapid-onset HIT. Therefore, an alternate anticoagulation regimen is indicated (Table 4.5).

e. **Direct thrombin inhibitors**[113]

　i. **Bivalirudin** is a synthetic hirudin analog that is a direct thrombin inhibitor and the drug of choice for anticoagulation. It has a rapid onset of action and a half-life of 25 minutes. It is primarily metabolized by proteolytic cleavage with only 20% renal elimination, so slight modification is necessary in patients with renal dysfunction. It cannot be reversed, but it can be eliminated by hemofiltration and plasmapheresis. Studies comparing bivalirubin with UFH for cardiac surgery (on- and off-pump) in patients without HIT have shown comparable outcomes.[119–122] Attention must be paid to avoidance of blood stagnation, which will cause nonenzymatic degradation of bivalirudin causing clotting, and of use of cardiotomy suction to minimize activation of the coagulation cascade.

- Dosing for on-pump surgery: 1 mg/kg bolus, 50 mg in pump prime, then 2.5 mg/kg/h infusion. The infusion rate may be increased in increments of 0.1–0.5 mg/kg/h to maintain the ACT >2.5 times baseline.
- Dosing for off-pump surgery: 0.75 mg/kg bolus, then 1.75 mg/kg/h to maintain an ACT >300 seconds.

　ii. **Lepirudin** is a recombinant hirudin analog that is a direct thrombin inhibitor. It has a slow onset of action and a long half-life of 60–80 minutes in patients with normal renal function. It is contraindicated in patients with renal dysfunction because it is primarily excreted by the kidneys. Because of its long half-life and the absence of a pharmacologic antidote (although it can be eliminated by hemofiltration), it is not an ideal choice for use during surgery. Anticoagulation efficacy is monitored by an ecarin clotting time (ECT), attempting to achieve a level of 400–450 seconds. This corresponds to a hirudin level >4 μg/mL. The recommended dosing regimen is 0.25 mg/kg before CPB, 0.2 mg/kg in pump prime, and a continuous infusion of 0.5 mg/min. It should be discontinued 15–30 minutes before the anticipated end of CPB.

　iii. **Argatroban** is a direct thrombin inhibitor that has a half-life of about 45 minutes. It is primarily metabolized by the liver with about 25% excretion by the kidneys and thus would be preferable (at least to lepirudin) in patients with renal dysfunction. It is monitored by the ACT, aiming for a level of 300–400 seconds. For on-pump surgery, a few case reports recommend a bolus dose of 0.1–0.4 mg/kg followed by a continuous infusion of 5–40 μg/kg/min. For off-pump surgery, one recommended dose is 2.5 μg/kg/min to achieve an ACT of twice baseline.[123]

f. An alternative to use of a direct thrombin inhibitor is administration of UFH in the usual dose along with drugs that inhibit platelet activation, such as the prostacyclin analogs and IIb/IIIa inhibitors.

　i. **Epoprostenol** is given in a dose of 5 ng/kg/min and increased by 5 ng/kg/min increments every 5 minutes (observing for systemic hypotension) up to 25 ng/kg/min, following which a heparin bolus is given. After protamine administration, the dose is weaned in 5 ng/kg decrements.[124]

Table 4.5 • Thrombin Inhibitors for Anticoagulation During Cardiopulmonary Bypass in Patients with Heparin-Induced Thrombocytopenia

Drug	Half-life	Metabolism	Monitoring	Dosing for CPB
Bivalirudin	25 min	Metabolic > Renal	ACT	1 mg/kg bolus, 50 mg in pump, then 2.5 mg/kg/h
Lepirudin	80 min	Renal	ECT	0.25 mg/kg bolus, 0.2 mg/kg in pump, then 0.5 mg/min
Argatroban	45 min	Hepatic > Renal	ACT	0.1–0.4 mg/kg bolus, then 5–40 μg/kg/min
Danaparoid	24 hours	Renal	Factor Xa levels	125 U/kg bolus, 3 U/kg in pump, then 7 U/kg/h

ACT, activating clotting time; ECT, ecarin clotting time

ii. **Iloprost** can be given starting at a dose of 3 ng/kg/min with a doubling of dose every 5 minutes to a dose determined by preoperative *in vitro* testing. The usual dose required is 6–24 ng/kg/min.[125]

iii. The short-acting glycoprotein IIb/IIIa inhibitor **tirofiban** can be given as a 10 μg/kg bolus 10 minutes prior to administration of standard-dose heparin, followed by 0.15 μg/kg/min, to be stopped 1 hour before the anticipated conclusion of CPB. Generally, 80% of the antiplatelet effect dissipates within 4 hours. Thus, bleeding may persist for a period of time after CPB has terminated, for which recombinant factor VIIa has been found beneficial.[126]

g. **Danaparoid** sodium is a heparinoid that inhibits factor Xa, resulting in inhibition of thrombin generation. It has low cross-reactivity with anti-heparin antibodies (about 10%). It has a long half-life (24 hours), undergoes renal metabolism, requires monitoring of factor Xa levels to assess its effectiveness, and its effects are not reversible. Thus, it is invariably associated with significant intraoperative bleeding and is not an ideal drug to use. The recommended dosing protocol is 125 anti-factor Xa units/kg IV bolus, 3 units/kg in the pump prime, then 7 units/kg/h to be stopped 45 minutes before the anticipated conclusion of CPB. For off-pump surgery, a dose of 40 anti-factor Xa units/kg is adequate.[113] It is not approved for use in the United States.

VII. Considerations During Cardiopulmonary Bypass (Table 4.6)

A. Virtually all valve surgery and most coronary bypass surgery is performed using CPB. The essential components of the CPB circuit are discussed in Chapter 5. Basically, the blood drains by gravity or with vacuum assist from the right atrium into a reservoir, is oxygenated, cooled or warmed, and then returned to the patient through an arterial cannula usually placed in the ascending aorta. The same principles apply during minimally invasive surgery, although the cannulation sites may vary (see pages 233–240). Desired hemodynamic and laboratory values during bypass are noted in Table 5.2 (page 241).

B. The lungs are not ventilated during bypass as oxygenation occurs within the oxygenator and carbon dioxide is eliminated by the gas flow into the oxygenator (the sweep rate). Although studies have suggested that the efficacy of gas exchange

---

Table 4.6 • *Anesthetic Considerations During Bypass (With Perfusionist)*

1. Use of vasopressor drugs to support systemic blood pressure
2. Administration of adjunctive drugs to optimize renal perfusion (nesiritide/fenoldopam)
3. Maintain adequate level of anesthesia with inhalational anesthetics or drugs
4. Monitor cerebral oximetry
5. Sample blood for ACTs
6. Readministration of antibiotics (cephalosporin) either when going on pump or at 4-hour intervals
7. Maintain blood glucose <180 mg/dL with IV insulin infusion

post-pump is improved if the lungs remain inflated during CPB, this is not a common practice.[127,128] Arterial blood gases are measured to ensure that the oxygenator is providing adequate oxygenation and that CO_2 extraction is sufficient. Venous oxygen saturation is measured to determine if the systemic flow rate is adequate (>65–70%). If in-line monitoring is not available, studies should be repeated every 15–20 minutes.

C. Systemic hypothermia is utilized to varying degrees during on-pump surgery as a means of organ protection during a period of nonphysiologic, nonpulsatile flow at lower mean pressures.[129] Cooling is initiated soon after CPB is started and warming is commenced based on the amount of additional surgery required in anticipation of achieving near-normothermia when CPB is terminated. Overwarming the patient to greater than 37 °C should be avoided because of the risk of neurologic damage.[130] Temperature afterdrop is uncommon when mild-to-moderate hypothermia (>30 °C) is used, and warming devices are not necessary. In contrast, these devices are very helpful in preserving body temperature upon warming from deeper hypothermia. A warming device should be used for blood and blood-product transfusions which may be given at a rapid rate.

D. The serum level of antibiotics falls approximately 30–50% at the time of initiation of CPB and an additional dose of a cephalosporin should be considered at that time. Alternatively, a second dose can be given 3–4 hours after the initial dose.[7] An additional dose of vancomycin is not necessary.

E. The optimal mean blood pressure during CPB to maintain adequate organ system perfusion is controversial. It has been shown that cerebral blood flow is more dependent on blood pressure than on flow rate.[131,132] The brain is able to maintain cerebral blood flow by autoregulation until the pressure falls below 40 mm Hg, but this response is inadequate in diabetic and hypertensive patients, in whom a higher pressure must be maintained. Systemic pressures are subject to a number of variables.

   1. Hypotension may be related to hemodilution, use of preoperative vasodilators (ACE inhibitors, ARBs, calcium channel blockers, and amiodarone), vasodilation during rewarming, and autonomic dysfunction. It may also result from inadequate systemic flow rates, impairment of venous drainage, aortic regurgitation, the administration of cardioplegia, and during return of large amounts of cardiotomy-suctioned blood into the circulation.

   2. Hypertension may be related to vasoconstriction with hypothermia, inadequate levels of anesthesia and analgesia, elevation in endogenous catecholamine levels, and alterations in acid-base balance and blood gas exchange.

   3. Although a higher mean blood pressure (around 80 mm Hg) might reduce some of the neurocognitive changes seen after bypass, the standard management is to maintain a mean blood pressure around 65 mm Hg using vasodilators (narcotics or inhalational anesthetics) or vasopressors (phenylephrine, norepinephrine, or vasopressin) as long as flow rates are adequate. A venous oxygen saturation exceeding 65% generally indicates that the systemic flow rate is satisfactory, although there may be differences in regional flow (i.e., less to the kidneys and splanchnic circulation). The venous saturation tends to be higher during systemic hypothermia due to lower oxygen extraction, and may decrease significantly during rewarming, necessitating an increase in flow rates.

F. Cerebral oximetry, usually using the Somanetics INVOS monitoring system, is an essential element of intraoperative care. It uses near-infrared technology to assess regional cerebral oxygen saturations (rSO_2) from bifrontal sensing pads placed on the patient's forehead (Figure 4.10). A reduction in rSO_2 greater than 20% may be associated with adverse neurologic outcomes and should be treated. Prior to bypass, steps to increase the systemic pressure or the PCO_2 will improve cerebral blood flow. The rSO_2 tends to fall during initiation of bypass from hemodilution and a reduction in systemic pressures, and then fall again during rewarming, even with an increase in systemic flow rates. Modifications of flow rate, blood pressure, PCO_2, or the

(A)

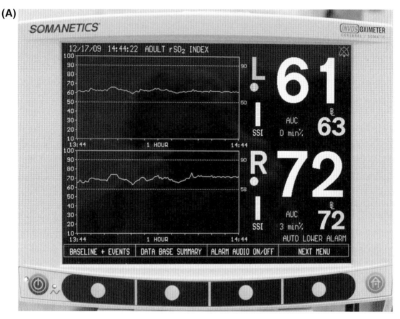

(B)

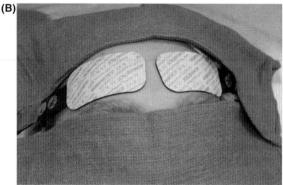

Figure 4.10 • (A) The Somanetics INVOS cerebral oximeter. This device uses near-infrared spectroscopy to measure the regional saturation of predominantly venous blood directly in the brain through optical sensors placed on the right and left sides of the forehead (B).

hematocrit may be beneficial. Marked cerebral desaturation (unless caused by a poorly adherent sensor) may be associated with brain malperfusion from cannula malplacement, aortic dissection, oxygenator or other pump-related failures, air embolism, anaphylactic reactions (such as protamine), or monitoring problems. Although interventions to improve rSO_2 should inituitively reduce the adverse effects of desaturation, few studies have documented improvements in clinical outcome.[133,134]

G. Blood glucose tends to be elevated due to the hormonal stress response to surgery and CPB with insulin resistance. The infusion of insulin to maintain blood glucose <180–200 mg/dL during surgery has not been shown to reduce inotropic requirements or the occurrence of arrhythmias, but may reduce the incidence of neurocognitive dysfunction and other adverse outcomes, including death.[135–138] Overly aggressive protocols to maintain blood glucose <100 mg/dL during surgery may increase the risk of stroke and death.[139]

H. Measures to optimize renal function should be considered in patients with preoperative renal dysfunction (creatinine >1.4 mg/dL or GFR <60 mL/min), especially in diabetic, hypertensive patients. The primary considerations should be maintaining a higher mean perfusion pressure (around 80 mm Hg), keeping the pump run as short as possible, or avoiding it entirely with off-pump techniques. Pharmacologic means to optimize renal perfusion may include nesiritide (0.01 µg/kg/min), fenoldopam (0.03–0.1 µg/kg/min) or sodium bicarbonate (3 mL/kg load, followed by 1 mL/kg/h of a 150 mEq/L mix).[140–142] Although both renal-dose dopamine (3 µg/kg/min) and furosemide may increase urine output during CPB, neither has been found to be renoprotective.[143] In fact, furosemide has actually been shown to increase the incidence of postoperative renal dysfunction. However, the major cause of postoperative renal dysfunction is a low output state, so maintenance of satisfactory hemodynamics at the termination of CPB is essential so that any intraoperative renal insults are transient.

I. When the cross-clamp is removed, lidocaine (100 mg) and magnesium (1–2 g) may be given to reduce the incidence of atrial and ventricular arrhythmias.[144] Ventricular fibrillation tends to occur when the heart is maintained at cold temperatures during the period of cardioplegic arrest and usually requires defibrillation, although spontaneous conversion to a sinus mechanism may occur.

J. Administration of perioperative amiodarone reduces the incidence of postoperative atrial fibrillation. If not started preoperatively,[145] one protocol involves initiation of therapy with a 150 mg bolus intraoperatively, followed by a 24-hour intravenous infusion and then conversion to oral therapy. This should also be used in patients undergoing Maze procedures for ablation of atrial fibrillation.

VIII. Termination of Bypass and Reversal of Anticoagulation (Table 4.7)

A. Once the cardiac portion of the operation has been completed, the lungs are ventilated and pacing is initiated, if necessary. Just prior to weaning bypass, calcium chloride 1 g may be given to increase systemic vascular resistance (SVR) and provide some initial inotropic support.

B. Inotropic medications should be started before terminating bypass if it is anticipated that hemodynamic support may be necessary. This should be considered in patients with preexisting LV dysfunction, prebypass ischemia, recent infarction, suboptimal

---

Table 4.7 • Anesthetic Considerations at the Conclusion of CPB

When Terminating Bypass

1. Establish pacing as indicated
2. Resume mechanical ventilation
3. TEE to identify intracardiac air and assess ventricular function
4. Initiate pharmacologic therapy to support cardiac function and blood pressure as identified by TEE and Swan-Ganz catheter assessments

After Terminating Bypass

1. TEE to assess ventricular function and valve issues (native valves, repairs, replacements); identify residual air
2. Adjustment of pharmacologic support based on systemic blood pressure, TEE, and Swan-Ganz catheter measurements
3. Protamine administration
4. Use of blood and/or blood-component therapy as indicated (point-of-care testing)

---

or incomplete revascularization, left ventricular hypertrophy, and long cross-clamp times. If an α-agent (phenylephrine, norepinephrine) was necessary on pump to support systemic pressure, it will usually be required for a brief period of time after CPB is terminated.

C. Bypass is weaned by gradually reducing the venous return to the CPB circuit, increasing intravascular volume in the patient, and reducing the arterial flow rate.

D. **Arterial blood pressure** monitoring in the radial artery is commonly inconsistent with the central aortic pressure due to the presence of peripheral vasodilation. Measurement of the central aortic pressure using a stopcock on the aortic line is very helpful in sorting out discrepancies. If this problem persists for more than 10–15 minutes, it is helpful to insert a femoral arterial monitoring line.

E. **TEE** is utilized as the patient is being weaned from bypass and after bypass is terminated (Table 4.1) to:

1. Identify intracardiac air. This is essential in valvular heart procedures or any procedure in which the left side of the heart has been entered (including venting). It is particularly valuable during minimally invasive procedures, in which exposure to the heart for deairing is limited.

2. Assess regional and global ventricular function and loading conditions. TEE is the only means of assessing intravascular volume directly. The volume-pressure relationship is altered by decreased ventricular compliance after cardioplegic arrest, so higher filling pressures measured with the Swan-Ganz catheter are usually necessary to achieve adequate intravascular volume. The TEE assessment of ventricular volume should be correlated with pressure measurements to determine optimal filling pressures for subsequent management. TEE is invaluable in determining whether hypotension should be treated by volume infusions, inotropic medications, or α-agents.

3. Detect paravalvular leaks, obstructed valve leaflets, or the competence of a valve repair.

F. In most patients with satisfactory cardiac function, fluid administration to optimize preload is usually sufficient to obtain adequate hemodynamic parameters. Initially, filling pressures are increased by transfusing volume from the pump. After protamine administration, the blood remaining in the pump circuit is processed through the cell-saving device into bags and reinfused into the patient. If this is not immediately available, a colloid is often chosen to maintain intravascular volume. Albumin is preferable to hetastarch compounds, which have been shown to increase bleeding and transfusion requirements.[146] Even the rapidly degradable low-molecular-weight hetastarch compounds have been shown to impair fibrin formation and clot strength and should be avoided.[147]

G. If hemodynamic performance is not ideal, the anesthesiologist must work in concert with the surgeon in assessing myocardial function and the need for inotropes. Visual inspection of the heart, assessment of serial cardiac outputs and filling pressures with a Swan-Ganz catheter, and TEE imaging can be used to assess ventricular function and identify potential problems.

1. Inotropic support is usually initiated with a catecholamine, such as epinephrine (1–2 µg/min) or dobutamine (5–10 µg/kg/min). If cardiac performance remains unsatisfactory, milrinone is extremely helpful in unloading the heart and providing inotropic support. Its preemptive use just prior to terminating bypass has been suggested as a means of ameliorating postoperative deterioration in cardiac performance and oxygen transport, and reducing the need for catecholamine support.[148]

2. If the patient has a satisfactory cardiac output and good ventricular function on TEE, but has persistent hypotension ("vasoplegic" state), increasing doses of norepinephrine or phenylephrine are indicated. If the patient remains refractory to these medications, a bolus of 1 unit of vasopressin may be sufficient to "turn the corner". It may be necessary to continue vasopressin as an infusion of 0.01–0.07 units/min to maintain vascular tone.

3. If the patient has persistent hypotension or a low cardiac output state for more than a minute or so, reinstitution of CPB to reperfuse the heart at a low workload will frequently result in improved ventricular function. This will also allow time to sort out the nature of the problem. In most situations, time and patience are all that is required to allow the heart to recover on bypass as additional inotropic support is initiated. Remediable problems that might be encountered include:

a. Air embolism down the right coronary artery may cause RV dysfunction and hypotension, necessitating a brief period of resumption of bypass to resolve. This is not an uncommon phenomenon after mitral valve surgery.

b. A new regional wall motion abnormality may suggest a technical problem with graft flow (kinking, twisting, anastomotic problem) that can be remedied. In mitral valve surgery, it might suggest circumflex artery entrapment if associated with lateral ECG changes. After aortic valve surgery or Bentall procedures, it might suggest impairment of coronary ostial flow by the valve prosthesis or by kinking of the proximal coronary arteries, respectively.

c. A paravalvular leak or impairment in mechanical valve leaflet motion may require additional surgery.

4. If the heart still does not function well after being rested on bypass or after use of multiple pharmacologic agents, insertion of an IABP is usually necessary. When all of the above fail, consideration should be given to use of a circulatory assist device in appropriate candidates (see pages 478–494).

H. Protamine is a polycationic peptide administered to counteract the effects of heparin and is usually given in a 0.5:1 to 1:1 mg/mg ratio to the dose of heparin to return the ACT to baseline. The ACT may remain elevated from residual heparin effect, for which small (50 mg) additional doses of protamine may be given. This is helpful if the patient is transfused with several bags of cell-saver blood, which does contain a small amount of heparin. However, the ACT may also be elevated in patients with significant thrombocytopenia or a coagulopathy despite complete neutralization of heparin. Thus, additional protamine administered for an elevated ACT may not return it to baseline. Although moderate thrombocytopenia has not been shown to increase the ACT in patients with normally functioning platelets, it does seem to increase it when associated with platelet dysfunction after bypass.[149]

1. The systems that perform heparin-protamine titration tests measure heparin levels in the bloodstream and determine the appropriate dose of protamine necessary to neutralize the remaining heparin. This usually results in less protamine being administered than empiric dosing based on the heparin dose.[104,105] This may restore platelet responsiveness to thrombin and attenuate platelet α-granule secretion, resulting in less bleeding.[150] Thus, these systems should prevent the unnecessary use of protamine to correct an abnormal ACT that is not attributable to excessive heparin. In fact, excessive protamine (exceeding a 1.3:1 ratio to the heparin dose in one study[151] and 2.6:1 in another[152]) activates platelets and may elevate the ACT, thus serving as an anticoagulant that can cause more bleeding!

2. "Heparin rebound" may occur when heparin reappears in the bloodstream after protamine neutralization. This is more likely to occur in patients who have received large doses of heparin during bypass and is more common in obese patients.[153] This may occur because the half-life of protamine is only about 5 minutes and it has nearly completely disappeared from the bloodstream within 20 minutes.[154] An elevated ACT or PTT commonly reflects this phenomenon and can be reversed with additional doses of protamine.

3. Intravenous administration of protamine may cause histamine release from the lungs, contributing to a decrease in systemic resistance and blood pressure, an effect not seen with intra-arterial injection. Nonetheless, studies have shown no hemodynamic advantage to intravenous vs. intra-arterial administration of protamine.[155]

I. Protamine reactions are unusual and are often unpredictable, although they have been noted with greater frequency in patients taking NPH insulin, those with fish or medication allergies, those with prior protamine exposure, and men who have had vasectomies. Awareness of the possibility of a protamine reaction, with a prompt therapeutic response if it occurs, is essential because protamine reactions are associated with increased perioperative mortality.[156–158]

1. **Type I.** Systemic hypotension from rapid administration (entire neutralizing dose after CPB given within 3 minutes). This is caused by a histamine-related reduction in systemic and pulmonary vascular resistance. It can be avoided by infusing the protamine over a 10–15 minute period and should be reversible with α-agent support.

2. **Type II.** Anaphylactic or anaphylactoid reaction resulting in hypotension, tachycardia, bronchospasm, flushing, and pulmonary edema.

   a. IIA. Idiosyncratic IgE- or IgG-mediated anaphylactic reaction. Release of histamine, leukotrienes, and kinins produces a systemic capillary leak causing hypotension and pulmonary edema. This tends to occur within the first 10 minutes of administration.

   b. IIB. Immediate nonimmunologic anaphylactoid reaction.

   c. IIC. Delayed reactions, usually occurring 20 minutes or more after the protamine infusion has been started, probably related to complement activation and leukotriene release, producing wheezing, hypovolemia, and noncardiogenic pulmonary edema from a pulmonary capillary leak.

3. **Type III.** Catastrophic pulmonary vasoconstriction (CPV) manifested by elevated PA pressures, systemic hypotension from peripheral vasodilation, decreased left atrial pressures, right ventricular dilatation, and myocardial depression. This reaction tends to occur about 10–20 minutes after the protamine infusion has started. One proposed mechanism involves activation of complement by the heparin–protamine complex that triggers leukocyte aggregation and release of liposomal enzymes that damage pulmonary tissue leading to pulmonary edema. Activation of the arachidonic acid pathway produces thromboxane which constricts the pulmonary vessels. Pulmonary vasoconstriction usually abates after about 10 minutes.[159]

4. Prevention of protamine reactions is usually not possible. Skin testing has not proved of any value. In patients considered at high risk, type II reactions might be attenuated by the prophylactic use of histamine blockers (ranitidine 150 mg IV, diphenhydramine 50 mg IV) and steroids (hydrocortisone 100 mg IV). This common practice has not been shown clinically to be of much benefit.

5. Treatment of protamine reactions involves correction of hemodynamic abnormalities that are identified. They must be differentiated from other conditions that can cause hemodynamic deterioration, such as hypoperfusion, air embolism, poor myocardial protection, or valve dysfunction. Measures must be taken to support systemic blood pressure while reversing pulmonary vasoconstriction if it is also present. Preparations to reinstitute cardiopulmonary bypass are frequently necessary. The following options may be effective:

   a. Calcium chloride 500 mg IV to increase systemic resistance and provide some inotropic support

   b. α-agents (phenylephrine, norepinephrine) to support systemic resistance

   c. β-agents for inotropic support that can also reduce pulmonary resistance (low-dose epinephrine, dobutamine, milrinone, inamrinone)

   d. Readily available drugs to reduce preload and pulmonary pressures (nitroglycerin)

   e. Aminophylline for wheezing

   f. Readministration of heparin to reverse the protamine reaction by reducing heparin–protamine complex size

   g. Steroids (hydrocortisone 100 mg IV)

   h. Methylene blue (1 mg/kg) might be beneficial because of the possible involvement of nitric oxide in the pathogenesis of CPV.[160]

J. Alternatives to reverse anticoagulation. Although simply not reversing heparin and administering clotting factors may suffice in ameliorating the bleeding caused by residual heparin, other measures have been evaluated to reverse heparin effect without use of protamine. These include use of heparinase I, recombinant platelet factor 4, and heparin removal devices. However, none has shown enough promise to reach clinical applicability.[161–163] Interestingly, platelet factor 4 has been shown to reverse the effects of low-molecular-weight heparin, which is incompletely accomplished by protamine.[164]

K. Treatment of coagulopathy. A meticulous operation and routine use of antifibrinolytic drugs should result in minimal postoperative bleeding in most patients undergoing cardiac surgery. However, a coagulopathy of varying degrees is probably present in all patients after CPB. Generally, the longer the duration of CPB, the more profound the degree of systemic hypothermia, and the more blood transfusions required on pump, the greater the coagulopathy. Furthermore, preoperative medications, especially antiplatelet drugs, have adverse effects on hemostasis.

1. Most groups treat coagulopathies in the operating room by the "shotgun approach". This entails the empiric administration of additional protamine for an elevated ACT, and transfusion of platelets, fresh frozen plasma, and occasionally cryoprecipitate. It is best to prioritize these products based on suspicion of the hemostatic defect while awaiting the results of coagulation studies. For example, platelet transfusions should be given first to patients on aspirin or clopidogrel or with uremia; fresh frozen plasma should be considered first for patients on preoperative warfarin, with hepatic dysfunction, or when multiple transfusions are given on pump; and uremic patients might benefit from desmopressin (see page 366). Cryoprecipitate is helpful in improving platelet function, especially when the fibrinogen level is low. Recombinant factor VIIa is particularly effective in achieving hemostasis when the coagulopathy is severe.[165]

2. Although this particular approach will usually stem the "coagulopathic tide", it is more scientific and cost-effective to use point-of-care testing to assess the specific hemostatic defect and direct care accordingly.[109] Systems are available to measure the PT, PTT, and platelet count, and several are capable of measuring platelet function as well. The thromboelastogram is a valuable test that evaluates the entire clotting process and is very effective in the bleeding patient in identifying the exact hemostatic defect that needs to be addressed (Figure 9.1, page 360).

3. Further comments on the prevention, assessment, and management of mediastinal bleeding are found in Chapter 9.

IX. Anesthetic Considerations During Off-Pump Coronary Surgery (Table 4.8)[166]

A. **Monitoring considerations**

1. In contrast to on-pump surgery, off-pump surgery via a median sternotomy requires that the heart provide adequate systemic perfusion at all times. Hemodynamics may be compromised by positioning of the heart, myocardial ischemia, ventricular arrhythmias, bleeding, and valvular regurgitation.

Table 4.8 • Key Elements of Anesthetic Management of Off-Pump Surgery

1. Continuous cardiac output and mixed venous oxygen monitoring
2. Transesophageal echocardiography
3. Antifibrinolytic drugs
4. Low-level heparinization with ACT >250 seconds
5. Short-acting anesthetic agents
6. Maintenance of systemic normothermia with use of warming devices
7. Arrhythmia prophylaxis with lidocaine and magnesium
8. Availability of pacing capability
9. Maintenance of hemodynamics with fluid, α-agents, and inotropes
10. Patience and emotional support for the surgeon!

---

2. To assess for myocardial ischemia and dysfunction when the heart is positioned at unorthodox angles, more intensive monitoring is required than for on-pump surgery. Swan-Ganz catheters that provide in-line continuous cardiac output and mixed venous oxygen saturation are very beneficial. These will dictate whether volume infusion or pharmacologic management is indicated. Pulse contour analysis using the Vigileo/FloTrac or the PulseCO system (LiDCO, Aspect Medical Systems) attached to the radial artery catheter can also provide accurate cardiac output measurements during heart displacement when TEE imaging may be suboptimal.[167] Simply maintaining an adequate blood pressure and heart rate pharmacologically may not suffice and often will provide no premonitory indication that the heart is becoming ischemic and subject to precipitous deterioration into ventricular fibrillation.

3. TEE is helpful is assessing for the development of regional wall motion (RWM) abnormalities during construction of an anastomosis that may be indicative of acute ischemia. The anesthesiologist should be well trained in TEE and must immediately communicate any problem to the surgeon. Steps can then be taken to resolve the problem, often with the placement of a shunt to improve flow.[168] During vessel occlusion, TEE should assess for the acute development of regional LV dysfunction or acute MR during construction of left-sided grafts and for RV or inferior wall dysfunction during right-sided grafting. If RWM abnormalities persist after the graft is completed, a technical problem with the anastomosis should be suspected. The midesophageal windows are best for assessing RV and LV function. The transgastric views are not helpful when the heart is elevated out of the chest. TEE will lead to modifications of the surgical strategy in a significant number of patients.[169]

B. **Anesthetic agents** are similar to those used for on-pump surgery, although shorter-acting medications may be selected depending on plans for extubation. Although patients can be extubated in the operating room, a more common practice is to use propofol for sedation at the end of surgery and for several hours in the ICU before considering extubation.

C. **Heparinization** is essential during off-pump surgery during vessel occlusion, and the extrinsic coagulation system is still activated by release of tissue factor. The requisite amounts of heparin and minimally acceptable ACT levels have not been delineated. Usually about 2–2.5 mg/kg of heparin suffices to raise the ACT to >250 seconds, with significant patient variability. There have been concerns about the prothrombotic tendency noted after OPCAB, since the hemodilution, platelet dysfunction, and fibrinolysis associated with CPB may not be seen.[107,170–172] This prothrombotic tendency may be related to the procoagulant activity of platelets or to activation of fibrinogen and other acute-phase reactants that result from the surgery. However, this recommended dose of heparin is not associated with significant thrombin generation, activation of the coagulation system, or fibrinolysis, and has not been associated with graft closure problems.

D. **Antifibrinolytic therapy** primarily with tranexamic acid, has been to shown to minimize bleeding in OPCAB surgery.[93] Although the blood is not subject to contact activation in an extracorporeal circuit, heparinization does induce fibrinolysis, and antifibrinolytic agents may be beneficial without causing a hypercoagulable state. Amicar can also be used with the same anticipated benefit.

E. **Patient temperature** tends to drift during open-chest procedures, but should be maintained as close to normothermia as possible to prevent arrhythmias, bleeding, and subsequent shivering in the ICU. The ambient room temperature must be raised into the low-70s°F and some form of warming blanket should be considered. These include a sterile Bair Hugger (Arizant) and heat-emitting devices, such as the Kimberly-Clark temperature management system.[173] The endovascular Thermogard system (Alsius Corporation) has also been used effectively in optimizing intraoperative temperature control during OPCAB.[174] All fluids must be warmed as they are being administered.[175]

F. **Maintenance of hemodynamics.** During cardiac positioning, the patient is placed in Trendelenburg position and the operating room table is rotated to the right. Deep pericardial sutures are placed to aid with retraction. Apical suction devices can also be used to rotate the heart cephalad and to the right. Central venous and PA pressures increase in the head-down position, and care must be taken not to administer too much fluid and increase these pressures even more. Transducer location may need to be adjusted to ensure accuracy. The possibility of producing cerebral edema should be kept in mind.

1. Magnesium and lidocaine should be given to increase the arrhythmic threshold.

2. Blood pressure should be maintained in the 120–140 mm Hg systolic range to optimize coronary perfusion, especially collateral flow. This can be done with some fluid administration, but usually with liberal administration of α-agents.

3. Atrial pacing wires may be placed if there is a concern about bradycardia developing with heart positioning. Transesophageal pacing may be utilized. Induced bradycardia is not essential with use of current stabilizing devices. However, tachycardia should be controlled. Ventricular pacing cables should be immediately available in case heart block develops. Coronary shunting may be helpful during bypass of the right coronary artery, during which there may be compromise of flow to the AV node, producing heart block.

4. Detection of ischemia can be difficult, since the ECG and TEE can be difficult to interpret in the translocated heart. A reduction in the SvO_2 is one of the first signs of the struggling heart. Intracoronary shunting or aortocoronary shunting during

construction of an anastomosis ameliorates distal ischemia. Upon the first suspicion of ventricular dysfunction, the surgeon should be informed immediately so that a shunt may be placed, if not done so prophylactically, to try to minimize ischemia.

5. If inotropic support is required, low-dose epinephrine is given first, and then milrinone may be given if more support is needed. In high-risk cases, such as severe left main disease, a prophylactic IABP may be helpful. Unless there is a strong indication for OPCAB, such as severe comorbidities, immediate conversion to an on-pump procedure may be a wise decision if instability persists.

G. **Blood loss** can be insidious during OPCAB if proximal and distal vessel control are suboptimal, especially if the proximal vessel does not have a critical stenosis. Blood should be scavenged into a cell saver and retransfused to the patient. Not infrequently, a significant amount of blood drains into the left pleural space and is scavenged during these operations.

H. **Proximal anastomoses** are usually performed last. During construction of proximal anastomoses with a side-clamp, the systolic blood pressure should be reduced to 90–100 mm Hg systolic to reduce the risk of aortic injury and atheroembolism. However, induced hypotension may increase the risk of renal dysfunction, and distal coronary perfusion through vein grafts is compromised until all grafts are sewn to the aorta and the clamp is removed. Thus, the patient may become unstable at this time. Induced hypotension is not necessary if an aortic sealing device, such as the HEARTSTRING proximal seal system (Maquet Cardiovascular), is used during the construction of proximal anastomoses.

I. Protamine is given in a 1:1 ratio to heparin. Bleeding should be minimal if the anastomoses are hemostatic. Pacing wires should be placed on the atrium and ventricle, chest tubes are placed, and the chest is closed.

X. Anesthetic Considerations with Endoscopic and Robotic Techniques for CABG

A. Coronary operations performed through limited thoracotomy incisions are less extensive than those performed through sternotomy incisions and do not result in much cardiac manipulation. Robotics can be used for internal thoracic artery (ITA) takedowns as well as for construction of coronary anastomoses and can be performed through small ports. Anastomoses may be performed with clips or distal anastomotic connector devices. However, despite endoscopic/robotic ITA takedown, many surgeons will hand-sew the anastomosis through a small thoracotomy incision.

B. Intubation for one-lung anesthesia improves surgical exposure with small thoracotomy incisions. The limited exposure to the heart and avoidance of CPB mandate adequate monitoring for ischemia, comparable to that noted above for OPCABs. Similarly, pacing capabilities using Swan-Ganz pacing catheters and use of body warmers to maintain normothermia are important. Because these operations are less invasive, anesthetic agents should be given to allow for early extubation, with appropriate provision of analgesia because of the pain associated with thoracotomy incisions.

XI. Anesthetic Considerations During Minimally Invasive Valve Procedures

A. Minimally invasive valve surgery is performed through small incisions (ministernotomy, thoracotomy) but requires use of CPB. Depending on the exposure, arterial and venous cannulation may be performed directly through the incision or through the femoral vessels. Additional venous drainage may be accomplished by cannulation of the internal jugular vein by the anesthesiologist. This requires careful attention to clamping and unclamping of this catheter to prevent inadvertent (and potentially exsanguinating) drainage. Aortic clamping can be performed through the operative field or via a separate incision, but can also be accomplished with an endoballoon ("endoclamp") placed through the femoral artery.

B. TEE is essential in these procedures to assist in the positioning of catheters since limited exposure prevents the surgeon from palpating their location. These include placing a retrograde cardioplegia catheter into the coronary sinus and advancing a catheter into the pulmonary artery for venting. TEE can also identify the placement of a long venous drainage line placed into the heart from the femoral vein. If an endoballoon is used for aortic occlusion, TEE is required to identify its exact location so as to avoid impingement on the aortic valve proximally and the innominate artery distally. TEE is especially beneficial in evaluating for air prior to termination of CPB, since direct deairing maneuvers are not possible. Use of carbon dioxide flooding may minimize air entrapment.[176] Robotic surgery is primarily approved for mitral valve repairs, so TEE is important in assessing the quality of the repair.

C. With thoracotomy procedures, one-lung anesthesia is important in the pre- and postbypass periods to improve exposure to the heart and great vessels.

D. In cases where there is little exposure to place pacing wires on the heart, use of a PA catheter through which pacing wires can be placed ("paceport" SG catheter) is helpful, although external pacing pads could also be used.

E. Cases involving a prolonged period of CPB, especially if accomplished by retrograde perfusion from a femoral artery, may result in ischemia/reperfusion injury to the leg, potentially resulting in a compartment syndrome of the lower extremity. The anesthesiologist should remind the surgeon to evaluate the patient's calves at the conclusion of surgery for tenseness. Although edema is common after a long case, there should be a low threshold for measuring compartment pressures if the leg has been ischemic for over 4–6 hours. If significantly elevated, a fasciotomy should be considered to prevent muscle necrosis.

References

1. Raja SG, Fida N. Should angiotensin converting enzyme inhibitors/angiotensin II receptor antagonists be omitted before cardiac surgery to avoid postoperative vasodilation? *Interact Cardiovasc Thorac Surg* 2008;7:470–5.

2. Sun JC, Whitlock R, Cheng J, et al. The effect of pre-operative aspirin on bleeding, transfusion, myocardial infarction, and mortality in coronary artery bypass surgery: a systematic review of randomized and observational studies. *Eur Heart J* 2008;29:1057–71.

3. Ferraris VA, Ferraris SP, Moliterno DJ, et al. The Society of Thoracic Surgeons practice guideline series: aspirin and other antiplatelet agents during operative coronary revascularization (executive summary). *Ann Thorac Surg* 2005;79:1454–61.

4. Grines CL, Bonow RO, Casey DE Jr, et al. Prevention of premature discontinuation of dual antiplatelet therapy in patients with coronary artery stents: a science advisory from the American Heart Association, American College of Cardiology, Society for Cardiovascular Angiography and Interventions, American College of Surgeons, and American Dental Association, with representation from the American College of Physicians. *Circulation* 2007;115:813–8 and *J Am Coll Cardiol* 2007;49:734–9.

5. Kincaid EH, Monroe ML, Saliba DL, Kon ND, Byerly WG, Reichert MG. Effects of preoperative enoxaparin versus unfractionated heparin on bleeding indices in patients undergoing coronary artery bypass grafting. *Ann Thorac Surg* 2003;76:124–8.

6. Chun R, Orser BA, Madan M. Platelet glycoprotein IIb/IIIa inhibitors: overview and implications for the anesthesiologist. *Anesth Analg* 2002;95:879–88.

7. Engelman R, Shahian D, Shemin R, et al. The Society of Thoracic Surgeons practice guideline series. Antibiotic prophylaxis in cardiac surgery, part II: Antibiotic choice. *Ann Thorac Surg* 2007;83:1569–76.

8. Loeb HS, Saudye A, Croke RP, Talano JV, Klodnycky ML, Gunnar RM. Effects of pharmacologically-induced hypertension on myocardial ischemia and coronary hemodynamics in patients with fixed coronary obstruction. *Circulation* 1978;57:41–6.

9. Djaini G, Karski J, Yudin M, et al. Clinical outcomes in patients undergoing elective coronary artery bypass graft surgery with and without utilization of pulmonary artery-generated data. *J Cardiothorac Vasc Anesth* 2006;20:307–10.

10. Resano FG, Kapetanakis EI, Hill PC, Haile E, Corso PJ. Clinical outcomes of low-risk patients undergoing beating-heart surgery with or without pulmonary artery catheterization. *J Cardiothorac Vasc Anesth* 2006;20:300–6.

11. Stewart RD, Psyhojos T, Lahey SJ, Levitsky S, Campos CT. Central venous catheter use in low-risk coronary artery bypass grafting. *Ann Thorac Surg* 1998;66:1306–11.

12. Schwann TA, Zacharias A, Riordan CJ, Durham SJ, Engoren M, Habib RH. Safe, highly selective use of pulmonary artery catheters in coronary artery bypass grafting: an objective patient selection method. *Ann Thorac Surg* 2002;73:1394–402.

13. Zimmermann A, Kufner C, Hofbauer S, et al. The accuracy of the Vigileo/FloTrac continuous cardiac output monitor. *J Cardiothorac Vasc Anesth* 2008;22:388–93.

14. Mehta Y, Chand RK, Sawhney R, Bhise M, Singh A, Trehan N. Cardiac output monitoring: comparison of a new arterial pressure waveform analysis to the bolus thermodilution technique in patients undergoing off-pump coronary artery bypass surgery. *J Cardiothorac Vasc Anesth* 2008;22:394–9.

15. Balik M, Pachl J, Hendl J. Effect of the degree of tricuspid regurgitation on cardiac output measurements by thermodilution. *Intensive Care Med* 2002;28:1117–21.

16. Eltzschig HK, Rosenberger P, Löffler M, Fox JA, Aranki SF, Shernan SK. Impact of intraoperative transesophageal echocardiography on surgical decisions in 12,566 patients undergoing cardiac surgery. *Ann Thorac Surg* 2008;85:845–52.

17. Minhaj M, Patel K, Muzic D, et al. The effect of routine intraoperative transesophageal echocardiography on surgical management. *J Cardiothorac Vasc Anesth* 2007;21:800–4.

18. Rosenberger P, Shernan SK, Löffler M, et al. The influence of epiaortic ultrasonography on intraoperative management in 6051 cardiac surgical patients. *Ann Thorac Surg* 2008;85:548–53.

19. Reeves ST, Glas KE, Eltzschig H, et al. Guidelines for performing a comprehensive epicardial echocardiography examination: recommendations of the American Society of Echocardiography and the Society of Cardiovascular Anesthesiologists. *Anesth Analg* 2007;105:22–9.

20. Whitley WS, Glas KE. An argument for routine ultrasound screening of the thoracic aorta in the cardiac surgery population. *Semin Cardiothorac Vasc Anesth* 2008;12:290–7.

21. Wadsworth R, Littler C. Cardiac standstill, pulmonary artery catheterisation and left bundle branch block. *Anaesthesia* 1996;51:97.

22. Vedrinne C, Bastien O, De Varax R, et al. Predictive factors for usefulness of fiberoptic pulmonary artery catheter for continuous oxygen saturation in mixed venous blood monitoring in cardiac surgery. *Anesth Analg* 1997;85:2–10.

23. Perings SM, Perings C, Kelm M, Strauer BE. Comparative evaluation of thermodilution and gated blood pool method for determination of right ventricular ejection fraction at rest and during exercise. *Cardiology* 2001;95:161–3.

24. Mullerworth MH, Angelopoulos P, Couyant MA, et al. Recognition and management of catheter-induced pulmonary artery rupture. *Ann Thorac Surg* 1998;66:1242–5.

25. Bossert T, Gummert JF, Bittner HB, et al. Swan-Ganz catheter-induced severe complications in cardiac surgery: right ventricular perforation, knotting, and rupture of the pulmonary artery. *J Card Surg* 2006;21:292–5.

26. Abreu AR, Campos MA, Krieger BP. Pulmonary artery rupture induced by a pulmonary artery catheter: a case report and review of the literature. *J Intensive Care Med* 2004;19:291–6.

27. Bianchini R, Melina G, Benedetto U, et al. Extracorporeal membrane oxygenation for Swan-Ganz induced intraoperative hemorrhage. *Ann Thorac Surg* 2007;83:2213–4.

28. Schneider AT, Hsu TL, Schwartz SL, Pandian NG. Single, biplane, multiplane, and three-dimensional transesophageal echocardiography. Echocardiographic–anatomic correlations. *Cardiol Clinics* 1993;11:361–87.

29. Shanewise JS, Cheung AT, Aronson S, et al. ASE/SCA guidelines for performing a comprehensive intraoperative multiplane transesophageal echocardiography examination: Recommendations of the American Society of Echocardiography Council for Intraoperative Echocardiography and the Society of Cardiovascular Anesthesiologists Task Force for certification in perioperative transesophageal echocardiography. *Anesth Analg* 1999;89:870–84.

30. Oh JK, Seward JB, Tajik AJ. *The Echo Manual*, 3rd edition. Philadelphia: Lippincott Williams & Wilkins, 2007.

31. Koide Y, Keehn L, Nomura T, Long T, Oka Y. Relationship of regional wall motion abnormalities detected by biplane transesophageal echocardiography and electrocardiographic changes in patients undergoing coronary artery bypass graft surgery. *J Cardiothorac Vasc Anesth* 1996;10:719–27.

32. Kallmeyer IJ, Collard CD, Fox JA, Body SC, Shernan SK. The safety of intraoperative transesophageal echocardiography: a case series of 7200 cardiac surgical patients. *Anesth Analg* 2001;92:1126–30.

33. Lennon MJ, Gibbs NM, Weightman WM, Leber J, Ee HC, Yusoff IF. Transesophageal echocardiography-related gastrointestinal complications in cardiac surgical patients. *J Cardiothorac Vasc Anesth* 2005;19:141–5.

34. Piercy M, McNicol L, Dinh DT, Story DA, Smith JA. Major complications related to the use of transesophageal echocardiography in cardiac surgery. *J Cardiothorac Vasc Anesth* 2009;23:62–5.

35. Min JK, Spencer KT, Furlong KT, et al. Clinical features of complications from transesophageal echocardiography: a single-center case series of 10,000 consecutive examinations. *J Am Soc Echocardiogr* 2005;18:925–9.

36. Shanewise JS, Zaffer R, Martin RP. Intraoperative echocardiography and minimally invasive cardiac surgery. *Echocardiography* 2002;19:579–82.

37. Wang J, Filipovic M, Rudzitis A, et al. Transesophageal echocardiography for monitoring segmental wall motion during off-pump coronary artery bypass surgery. *Anesth Analg* 2004;99:965–73.

38. Morganstern J, Kanchuger M. Pro: all off-pump coronary artery bypass graft surgeries should include intraoperative transesophageal echocardiography assessment. *J Cardiothorac Vasc Anesth* 2008;22:625–8.

39. Scohy TV, Soliman OI, Lecomte PV, et al. Intraoperative real time three-dimensional transesophageal echocardiographic measurement of hemodynamic, anatomic, and function changes after aortic valve replacement. *Echocardiography* 2009;26:96–9.

40. Bouzas-Mosquera A, Alvarez-Garcia N, Ortiz-Vázquez E, Cuenca-Castillo JJ. Images in cardiothoracic surgery: role of real-time 3-dimensional transesophageal echocardiography in transcatheter aortic valve implantation. *Eur J Cardiothorac Surg* 2009;35:909.

41. Grewal J, Mankad S, Freeman WK, et al. Real-time three-dimensional transesophageal echocardiography in the intraoperative assessment of mitral valve disease. *J Am Soc Echocardiogr* 2009;22:34–41.

42. Jungwirth B, Mackensen GB. Real-time 3-dimensional echocardiography in the operating room. *Semin Cardiothorac Vasc Anesth* 2008;12:248–64.

43. Iafrati MD, Gordon G, Staples MH, et al. Transesophageal echocardiography for hemodynamic management of thoracoabdominal aneurysm repair. *Am J Surg* 1993;166:179–85.

44. Zangrillo A, Turi S, Creszenzi G, et al. Esmolol reduces perioperative ischemia in cardiac surgery: a meta-analysis of randomized controlled studies. *J Cardiothorac Vasc Anesth* 2009;23:625–32.

45. Myles PS, McIlroy D. Fast-track cardiac anesthesia: choice of anesthetic agents and techniques. *Semin Cardiothorac Vasc Anesth* 2005;9:5–16.

46. Lison S, Schill M, Conzen P. Fast-track cardiac anesthesia: efficacy and safety of remifentail versus sufentanil. *J Cardiothorac Vasc Anesth* 2007;21:35–40.

47. Guggenberger H, Schroeder TH, Vonthein R, Dieterich HJ, Shernan SK, Eltzschig HK. Remifentanil or sufentanil for coronary surgery: comparison of postoperative respiratory impairment. *Eur J Anaesthesiol* 2006;23:832–40.

48. Lena P, Balarac N, Arnulf JJ, Bigeon JY, Tapia M, Bonnet F. Fast-track coronary artery bypass grafting surgery under general anesthesia with remifentanil and spinal analgesia with morphine and clonidine. *J Cardiothorac Vasc Anesth* 2005;19:49–53.

49. Hemmerling T, Olivier JF, Le N, Prieto I, Bracco D. Myocardial protection by isoflurane vs. sevoflurane in ultra-fast-track anaesthesia for off-pump aortocoronary bypass grafting. *Eur J Anaesthesiol* 2008;25:230–6.

50. Landoni G, Biondi-Zoccai GGL, Zangrillo A, et al. Desflurane and sevoflurane in cardiac surgery: a meta-analysis of randomized clinical trials. *J Cardiothorac Vasc Anesth* 2007;21:502–11.

51. Delphin E, Jackson D, Gubenko Y, et al. Sevoflurane provides earlier tracheal extubation and assessment of cognitive recovery than isoflurane in patients undergoing off-pump coronary artery bypass surgery. *J Cardiothorac Vasc Anesth* 2007;21:690–5.

52. Grocott HP, Mathew JP, Carver EH, et al. A randomized controlled trial of the Arctic Sun Temperature Management System versus conventional methods for preventing hypothermia during off-pump cardiac surgery. *Anesth Analg* 2004;98:298–302.

53. Billings FT 4th, Kodali SK, Shanewise JS. Transcatheter aortic valve implantation: anesthetic considerations. *Anesth Analg* 2009;108:1453–62.

54. Shimokawa T, Horiuchi K, Ozawa N, et al. Outcome of surgical treatment in patients with acute type B aortic dissection. *Ann Thorac Surg* 2008;86:103–7.

55. Hnath JC, Mehta M, Taggert JB, et al. Strategies to improve spinal cord ischemia in endovascular thoracic aortic repair: outcomes of a prospective cerebrospinal fluid drainage protocol. *J Vasc Surg* 2008;48:836–40.

56. Apostolakis E, Shuhaiber JH. Antegrade or retrograde cerebral perfusion as an adjunct during hypothermic circulatory arrest for aortic arch surgery. *Expert Rev Cardiovasc Ther* 2007;5:1147–61.

57. Dewhurst AT, Moore SJ, Liban JB. Pharmacologic agents as cerebral protectants during deep hypothermic circulatory arrest in adult thoracic aortic surgery. *Anaesthesia* 2002;57:1016–21.

58. Schubert S, Stoltenburg-Didinger G, Wehsack A, et al. Large-dose pretreatment with methylprednisolone fails to attenuate neuronal injury after deep hypothermic circulatory arrest in neonatal piglet model. *Anesth Analg* 2005;101:1311–8.

59. Minatoya K, Ogino H, Matsuda H, et al. Evolving selective cerebral perfusion for aortic arch replacement: high flow rate with moderate hypothermic circulatory arrest. *Ann Thorac Surg* 2008;86:1827–31.

60. Safi HJ, Miller CC 3rd, Huynh TT, et al. Distal aortic perfusion and cerebrospinal fluid drainage for thoracoabdominal and descending thoracic aortic repair: ten years of organ protection. *Ann Surg* 2003;238:372–80.

61. Black JH, Davidson JK, Cambria RP. Regional hypothermia with epidural cooling for prevention of spinal cord ischemic complications after thoracoabdominal aortic surgery. *Semin Thorac Cardiovasc Surg* 2003;15:345–52.

62. Lemaire SA, Jones MM, Conklin LD, et al. Randomized comparison of cold blood and cold crystalloid renal perfusion for renal protection during thoracoabdominal aortic aneurysm repair. *J Vasc Surg* 2009;49:11–9.

63. Fehrenbacher JW, Hart DW, Huddleston E, Siderys H, Rice C. Optimal end-organ protection for thoracic and thoracoabdominal aneurysm repair using deep hypothermic circulatory arrest. *Ann Thorac Surg* 2007;83:1041–6.

64. Sheinbaum R, Ignacio C, Safi HJ, Estrera A. Contemporary strategies to preserve renal function during cardiac and vascular surgery. *Rev Cardiovasc Med* 2003;4(suppl 1):S21–8.

65. Hullander RM, Leivers D, Wingler K. A comparison of propofol and etomidate for cardioversion. *Anesth Analg* 1993;77:690–4.

66. Dhadphale PR, Jackson AP, Alseri S. Comparison of anesthesia with diazepam and ketamine vs. morphine in patients undergoing heart-valve replacement. *Anesthesiology* 1979;51:200–3.

67. Puri GD, Murthy SS. Bispectral index monitoring in patients undergoing cardiac surgery under cardiopulmonary bypass. *Eur J Anaesthesiol* 2003;20:451–6.

68. Muralidhar K, Banakal S, Murthy K, Garg R, Rani GR, Dinesh R. Bispectral index-guided anaesthesia for off-pump coronary artery bypass grafting. *Ann Card Anaesth* 2008;11:105–10.

69. Carollo DS, Nossaman BD, Ramadhyani U. Dexmedetomidine: a review of clinical applications. *Curr Opin Anaesthesiol* 2008;21:457–61.

70. Doufas AG, Lin CM, Suleman MI, et al. Dexmedetomidine and meperidine additively reduce shivering threshold in humans. *Stroke* 2003;34:1218–23.

71. Herr DL, Sum-Ping STJ, England M. ICU sedation after coronary artery bypass graft surgery: dexmedetomidine-based versus propofol-based sedation regimens. *J Cardiothorac Vasc Anesth* 2003;17:576–84.

72. Riker RR, Shehabi Y, Bokesch PM, et al. Dexmedetomidine vs midazolam for sedation of critically ill patients: a randomized trial. *JAMA* 2009;301:489–99.

73. Society of Thoracic Surgeons Blood Conservation Tast Force, Ferraris VA, Ferraris SP, Saha SP, et al. Perioperative blood transfusion and blood conservation in cardiac surgery: the Society of Thoracic Surgeons and the Society of Cardiovascular Anesthesiologists clinical practice guideline. *Ann Thorac Surg* 2007;83(5 suppl):S27–86.

74. Ramnath AN, Naber HR, de Boer A, Leusink JA. No benefit of intraoperative whole blood sequestration and autotransfusion during coronary artery bypass grafting: results of a randomized clinical trial. *J Thorac Cardiovasc Surg* 2003;125:1432–7.

75. Flom-Halvorsen HI, Øvrum E, Øystese R, Brosstad F. Quality of intraoperative autologous blood withdrawal for retransfusion after cardiopulmonary bypass. *Ann Thorac Surg* 2003;76:744–8.

76. Whitlock RP, Chan S, Devereaux PJ, et al. Clinical benefit of steroid use in patients undergoing cardiopulmonary bypass: a meta-analysis of randomized trials. *Eur Heart J* 2008;29:2592–600.

77. Halonen J, Halonon P, Jarvinen O, et al. Corticosteroids for the prevention of atrial fibrillation after cardiac surgery. A randomized controlled trial. *JAMA* 2007;297:1562–7.

78. Bourbon A, Vionnet M, Leprince P, et al. The effect of methylprednisolone treatment on the cardiopulmonary bypass-induced systemic inflammatory response. *Eur J Cardiothorac Surg* 2004;26:932–8.

79. Morariu AM, Loef BG, Aarts LP, et al. Dexamethasone: benefit and prejudice for patients undergoing on-pump coronary artery bypass grafting: a study on myocardial, pulmonary, renal, intestinal, and hepatic injury. *Chest* 2005;128:2677–87.

80. Sobieski MA 2nd, Graham JD, Pappas PS, Tatooles AJ, Slaughter MS. Reducing the effects of the systemic inflammatory response to cardiopulmonary bypass: can single dose steroids blunt systemic inflammatory response syndrome? *ASAIO J* 2008;54:203–6.

81. Halvorsen P, Raeder J, White PF, et al. The effect of dexamethasone on side effects after coronary revascularization procedures. *Anesth Analg* 2003;96:1578–83.

82. Henry DA, Carless PA, Moxey AJ, et al. Anti-fibrinolytic use for minimising perioperative allogenic blood transfusion. *Cochrane Database Syst Rev* 2007;4:CD001886.

83. Umscheid CA, Kohl BA, Williams K. Antifibrinolytic use in adult cardiac surgery. *Curr Opin Hematol* 2007;14:455–67.

84. McIlroy DR, Myles PS, Phillips LE, Smith JA. Antifibrinolytics in cardiac surgical patients receiving aspirin: a systematic review and meta-analysis. *Br J Anaesth* 2009;102:168–78.

85. Henry D, Carless P, Fergusson D, Laupacis A. The safety of aprotinin and lysine-derived antifibrinolytic drugs in cardiac surgery: a meta-analysis. *CMAJ* 2009;180:183–93.

86. Chauhan S, Gharde P, Bisoi A, Kale S, Kiran U. A comparison of aminocaproic acid and tranexamic acid in adult cardiac surgery. *Ann Card Anaesth* 2004;7:40–3.

87. Ray MJ, Hales MM, Brown L, O'Brien MF, Stafford EG. Postoperatively administered aprotinin or epsilon aminocaproic acid after cardiopulmonary bypass has limited benefit. *Ann Thorac Surg* 2001;72:521–6.

88. Butterworth J, James RL, Lin Y, Prielipp RC, Hudspeth AS. Pharmacokinetics of epsilon-aminocaproic acid in patients undergoing aortocoronary bypass surgery. *Anesthesiology* 1999;90:1624–35.

89. Bennett-Guerrero E, Spillane WF, White WD, et al. Epsilon aminocaproic acid administration and stroke following coronary artery bypass graft surgery. *Ann Thorac Surg* 1999;67:1283–7.

90. Stafford-Smith M, Phillips-Bute B, Reddan DN, Black J, Newman MF. The association of epsilon-aminocaproic acid with postoperative decrease in creatinine clearance in 1502 coronary bypass patients. *Anesth Analg* 2000;91:1085–90.

91. Fiechtner BK, Nuttall GA, Johnson ME, et al. Plasma tranexamic acid concentrations during cardiopulmonary bypass. *Anesth Analg* 2001;92:1131–6.

92. Mengistu AM, Röhm KD, Boldt J, Mayer J, Suttner SW, Piper SN. The influence of aprotinin and tranexamic acid on platelet function and postoperative blood loss in cardiac surgery. *Anesth Analg* 2008;107:391–7.

93. Murphy GJ, Mango E, Lucchetti V, et al. A randomized trial of tranexamic acid in combination with cell salvage plus a meta-analysis of randomized trials evaluating tranexamic acid in off-pump coronary artery bypass grafting. *J Thorac Cardiovasc Surg* 2006;132:475–80.

94. Nuttall GA, Gutierrez MC, Dewey JD, et al. A preliminary study of a new tranexamic acid dosing schedule for cardiac surgery. *J Thorac Cardiovasc Surg* 2008;22:230–5.

95. Karski JM, Dowd NP, Joiner R, et al. The effect of three different doses of tranexamic acid on blood loss after cardiac surgery with mild systemic hypothermia (32°C). *J Cardiothorac Vasc Anesth* 1998;12:642–6.

96. Mangano DT, Tudor IC, Dietzel L. Multicenter Study of Perioperative Ischemia Research group; Ischemia Research and Education Foundation. The risk associated with aprotinin in cardiac surgery. *N Engl J Med* 2006;354:353–65.

97. Warkentin TE. Anticoagulation for cardiopulmonary bypass: is a replacement for heparin on the horizon? *J Thorac Cardiovasc Surg* 2006;131:515–6.

98. Yavari M, Becker RC. Anticoagulant therapy during cardiopulmonary bypass. *J Thromb Thrombolysis* 2008;26:218–28.

99. Haering JH, Maslow AD, Parker RA, Lowenstein E, Comunale ME. The effect of heparin-coated pulmonary artery catheters on activated coagulation time in cardiac surgical patients. *J Cardiothorac Vasc Anesth* 2000;14:260–3.

100. Francis JL, Palmer GJ 3rd, Moroose R, Drexler A. Comparison of bovine and porcine heparin in heparin antibody formation after cardiac surgery. *Ann Thorac Surg* 2003;75:17–22.

101. Slight RD, Buell R, Nzewi OC, McClelland DBL, Mankad PS. A comparison of activated coagulation time-based techniques for anticoagulation during cardiac surgery with cardiopulmonary bypass. *J Cardiothorac Vasc Anesth* 2008;22:47–52.

102. Despotis GJ, Joist JH, Hogue CW Jr, et al. The impact of heparin concentration and activated clotting time monitoring on blood conservation. A prospective, randomized evaluation in patients undergoing cardiac operation. *J Thorac Cardiovasc Surg* 1995;110:46–54.

103. Despotis GJ, Joist JH, Hogue CW Jr, et al. More effective suppression of hemostatic system activation in patients undergoing cardiac surgery by heparin dosing based on heparin blood concentrations rather than ACT. *Thromb Haemost* 1996;76:902–8.

104. Runge M, Møller CH, Steinbrüchel DA. Increased accuracy in heparin and protamine administration decreases bleeding: a pilot study. *J Extra Corpor Technol* 2009;41:10–4.

105. Shirota K, Watanabe T, Takagi Y, Ohara Y, Usui A, Yasuura K. Maintenance of blood heparin concentration rather than activated clotting time better preserves the coagulation system in hypothermic cardiopulmonary bypass. *Artif Organ* 2000;24:49–56.

106. Mangoush O, Purkayastha S, Haj-Yahia S, et al. Heparin-bonded circuits versus nonheparin-bonded circuits: an evaluation of their effect on clinical outcomes. *Eur J Cardiothorac Surg* 2007;31:1058–69.

107. Cartier R, Robitaille D. Thrombotic complications in beating heart operations. *J Thorac Cardiovasc Surg* 2001;121:920–2.

108. Englberger L, Immer FF, Eckstein FS, Berdat PA, Haeberli A, Carrel TP. Off-pump coronary artery bypass operation does not increase procoagulant and fibrinolytic activity: preliminary results. *Ann Thorac Surg* 2004;77:1560–6.

109. Shore-Lesserson L. Point-of-care coagulation monitoring for cardiovascular patients: past and present. *J Cardiothorac Vasc Anesth* 2002;16:99–106.

110. Dietrich W, Spannagl M, Schramm W, Vogt W, Barankay A, Richter JA. The influence of preoperative anticoagulation on heparin response during cardiopulmonary bypass. *J Thorac Cardiovasc Surg* 1991;102:505–14.

111. Ranucci M, Isgrò G, Cazzaniga A, Soro G, Menicanti L, Frigiola A. Predictors for heparin resistance in patients undergoing coonary artery bypass grafting. *Perfusion* 1999;14:437–42.

112. Spiess BD. Treating heparin resistance with antithrombin or fresh frozen plasma. *Ann Thorac Surg* 2008;85:2153–60.

113. Warkentin TE, Greinacher A, Koster A, Lincoff A. Treatment and prevention of heparin-induced thrombocytopenia. American College of Chest Physicians evidence-based clinical practice guidelines (8th edition). *Chest* 2008;133:340S–380S.

114. Bennett-Guerrero E, Slaughter TF, White WD, et al. Preoperative anti-PF4/heparin antibody level predicts adverse outcome after cardiac surgery. *J Thorac Cardiovasc Surg* 2005;130:1567–72.

115. Kress DC, Aronson S, McDonald ML, et al. Positive heparin-platelet factor 4 antibody complex and cardiac surgical outcomes. *Ann Thorac Surg* 2007;83:1737–43.

116. Everett BM, Yeh R, Foo SY, et al. Prevalence of heparin/platelet factor 4 antibodies before and after cardiac surgery. *Ann Thorac Surg* 2007;83:592–7.

117. Bauer TL, Arepally G, Konkle BA, et al. Prevalence of heparin-associated antibodies without thrombosis in patients undergoing cardiopulmonary bypass surgery. *Circulation* 1997;95:1242–6.

118. Greinacher A, Levy JH. HIT happens: diagnosing and evaluating the patient with heparin-induced thrombocytopenia. *Anesth Analg* 2008;107:356–8.

119. Merry AF, Raudkivi PJ, Middleton NG, et al. Bivalirudin versus heparin and protamine in off-pump coronary artery bypass surgery. *Ann Thorac Surg* 2004;77:925–31.

120. Dyke CM, Aldea G, Koster A, et al. Off-pump coronary artery bypass with bivalirudin for patients with heparin-induced thrombocytopenia or antiplatelet factor four/heparin antibodies. *Ann Thorac Surg* 2007;84:836–9.

121. Dyke CM, Smedira NG, Koster A, et al. A comparison of bivalirudin to heparin with protamine reversal in patients undergoing cardiac surgery with cardiopulmonary bypass: The EVOLUTION-ON study. *J Thorac Cardiovasc Surg* 2006;131:533–9.

122. Koster A, Dyke CM, Aldea G, et al. Bivalirudin during cardiopulmonary bypass in patients with preivous or acute heparin-induced thrombycytopenia and heparin antibodies: Results of CHOOSE-ON Trial. *Ann Thorac Surg* 2007;83:572–7.

123. Smith AI, Stroud R, Damiani P, Vaynblat M. Use of argatroban for anticoagulation during cardiopulmonary bypass in a patient with heparin allergy. *Eur J Cardiothorac Surg* 2008;34:1113–4.

124. Mertzlufft F, Kuppe H, Koster A. Management of urgent high-risk cardiopulmonary bypass with heparin-induced thrombocytopenia type II and coexisting disorders of renal function: use of heparin

and epoprostenol combined with on-line monitoring of platelet function. *J Cardiothorac Vasc Anesth* 2000;14:304–8.

125. Palatianos GM, Foroulis CN, Vassili MI, et al. Preoperative detection and management of immune heparin-induced thrombocytopenia in patients undergoing heart surgery with Iloprost. *J Thorac Cardiovasc Surg* 2004;127:548–54.

126. Durand M, Lecompte T, Hacquard M, Carteaux JP. Heparin-induced thrombocytopenia and cardiopulmonary bypass: anticoagulation with unfractionated heparin and the glycoprotein IIb/IIIa inhibitor tirofiban and successful use of rFVIIa for post-protamine bleeding due to persistent platelet blockade. *Eur J Cardiothorac Surg* 2008;34:687–9.

127. Ng CSH, Arifi AA, Wan S, et al. Ventilation during cardiopulmonary bypass: impact on cytokine response and cardiopulmonary function. *Ann Thorac Surg* 2008;85:154–62.

128. Loeckinger A, Kleinsasser A, Lindner KH, Margreiter J, Keller C, Hoermann C. Continuous positive airway pressure at 10 cm H$_2$O during cardiopulmonary bypass improves postoperative gas exchange. *Anesth Analg* 2000;91:522–7.

129. Campos JM, Paniagua P. Hypothermia during cardiac surgery. *Best Pract Res Clinical Anaesthesiol* 2008;22:695–709.

130. Nussmeier NA. Management of temperature during and after cardiac surgery. *Tex Heart Inst J* 2005;32:472–6.

131. Schwartz AE, Sandhu AA, Kaplon RJ, et al. Cerebral blood flow is determined by arterial pressure and not cardiopulmonary bypass flow rate. *Ann Thorac Surg* 1995;60:165–70.

132. Schwartz AE. Regulation of cerebral blood flow during hypothermic cardiopulmonary bypass. Review of experimental results and recommendations for clinical practice. *CVE* 1997;2:133–7.

133. Murkin JM, Adams SJ, Novick RJ, et al. Monitoring brain oxygen saturation during coronary bypass surgery: a randomized, prospective study. *Anesth Analg* 2007;104:51–8.

134. Slater JP, Guarino T, Stack J, et al. Cerebral oxygen desaturation predicts cognitive decline and longer hospital stay after cardiac surgery. *Ann Thorac Surg* 2009;87:36–44.

135. Groban L, Butterworth J, Legault C, Rogers AT, Kon ND, Hammon JW. Intraoperative insulin therapy does not reduce the need for inotropic or antiarrhythmic therapy after cardiopulmonary bypass. *J Cardiothorac Vasc Anesth* 2002;16:405–12.

136. Gandhi GY, Nuttall GA, Abel MD, et al. Intraoperative hyperglycemia and perioperative outcomes in cardiac surgical patients. *Mayo Clin Proc* 2005;80:862–6.

137. Puskas F, Grocott HP, White WD, Mathew JP, Newman MF, Bar-Yosef S. Intraoperative hyperglycemia and cognitive decline after CABG. *Ann Thorac Surg* 2007;84:1467–73.

138. Butterworth J, Wagenknecht LE, Legault C, et al. Attempted control of hyperglycemia during cardiopulmonary bypass fails to improve neurologic or neurobehavioral outcomes in patients without diabetes mellitus undergoing coronary artery bypass grafting. *J Thorac Cardiovasc Surg* 2005;130:1319–25.

139. Gandhi GY, Nuttall GA, Abel MD, et al. Intensive intraoperative insulin therapy versus conventional glucose management during cardiac surgery: a randomized trial. *Ann Intern Med* 2007;146:233–43.

140. Chen HH, Sundt TM, Cook DJ, Heublein DM, Burnett JC Jr. Low dose nesiritide and the preservation of renal function in patients with renal dysfunction undergoing cardiopulmonary-bypass surgery: a double-blind placebo controlled pilot study. *Circulation* 2007;116(11 suppl):I-134–8.

141. Landoni G, Biondi-Zoccai GG, Marino G, et al. Fenoldopam reduces the need for renal replacement therapy and in-hospital death in cardiovascular surgery: a meta-analysis. *J Cardiothorac Vasc Anesth* 2008;22:27–33.

142. Haase M, Haase-Fielitz A, Bellomo R, et al. Sodium bicarbonate to prevent increases in serum creatinine after cardiac surgery: a pilot double-blind randomized controlled trial. *Crit Care Med* 2009;37:39–47.

143. Lassnigg A, Donner E, Grubhofer G, Presterl E, Druml W, Hiesmayr M. Lack of renoprotective effects of dopamine and furosemide during cardiac surgery. *J Am Soc Nephrol* 2000;11:97–104.

144. Wilkes NJ, Mallett SV, Peachey T, Di Salvo C, Walesby R. Correction of ionized magnesium during cardiopulmonary bypass reduces the risk of postoperative cardiac arrhythmia. *Anesth Analg* 2002;95:828–34.

145. Mitchell LB, Exner DV, Wyse DG, et al. Prophylactic oral amiodarone for the prevention of arrhythmias that begin early after revascularization, valve replacement, or repair: PAPABEAR: a randomized controlled trial. *JAMA* 2005;294:3093–100.

146. Knutson JE, Deering JA. Hall FW, et al. Does intraoperative hetastarch administration increase blood loss and transfusion requirements after cardiac surgery? *Anesth Analg* 2000;90:801–7.

147. Schramko AA, Suojaranta-Ylinen T, Kuitunen AH, Kukkonen SI, Niemi TT. Rapidly degradable hydroxyethyl starch solutions impair blood coagulation after cardiac surgery: a prospective randomized trial. *Anesth Analg* 2009;108:30–6.

148. Kikura M, Sato S. The efficacy of preemptive milrinone or amrinone therapy in patients undergoing coronary artery bypass grafting. *Anesth Analg* 2002;94:22–30.

149. Ammar T, Fisher CF, Sarier K, Coller BS. The effects of thrombocytopenia on the activated coagulation time. *Anesth Analg* 1996;83:1185–8.

150. Shigeta O, Kojima H, Hiramatsu Y, et al. Low-dose protamine based on heparin-protamine titration method reduces platelet dysfunction after cardiopulmonary bypass. *J Thorac Cardiovasc Surg* 1999;118:354–60.

151. Mochizuki T, Olson PJ, Szlam F, Ramsay JG, Levy JH. Protamine reversal of heparin affects platelet aggregation and activated clotting time after cardiopulmonary bypass. *Anesth Analg* 1998;87:781–5.

152. McLaughlin KE, Dunning J. In patients post cardiac surgery do high doses of protamine cause increased bleeding? *Interact Cardiovasc Thorac Surg* 2003;2:424–6.

153. Gravlee GP, Rogers AT, Dudas LM, et al. Heparin management protocol for cardiopulmonary bypass influences postoperative heparin rebound but not bleeding. *Anesthesiology* 1992;76: 393–401.

154. Butterworth J, Lin YA, Prielipp RC, Bennett J, Hammon JW, James RL. Rapid disappearance of protamine in adults undergoing cardiac operation with cardiopulmonary bypass. *Ann Thorac Surg* 2002;74:1589–95.

155. Milne B, Rogers K, Cervenko F, Salerno T. The haemodynamic effects of intraaortic versus intravenous administration of protamine for reversal of heparin in man. *Can Anaesth Soc J* 1983;30:347–51.

156. Nybo M, Madsen JS. Serious anaphylactic reactions due to protamine sulfate: a systematic literature review. *Basic Clin Pharmacol Toxicol* 2008;103:192–6.

157. Kimmel SE, Sekeres MA, Berlin JA, Ellison N, DiSesa VJ, Strom BL. Risk factors for clinically important adverse events after protamine administration following cardiopulmonary bypass. *J Am Coll Cardiol* 1998;32:1916–22.

158. Kimmel SE, Sekeres M, Berlin JA, Ellison N. Mortality and adverse events after protamine administration in patients undergoing cardiopulmonary bypass. *Anesth Analg* 2002;94:1402–8.

159. Hiong YT, Tang YK, Chui WH, Das SR, A case of catastrophic pulmonary vasoconstriction after protamine administration in cardiac surgery: role of intraoperative transesophageal echocardiography. *J Cardiothorac Vasc Anesth* 2008;22:727–31.

160. Viaro F, Dalio MB, Evora PR. Catastrophic cardiovascular adverse reactions to protamine are nitric oxide/cyclic guanosine monophosphate dependent and endothelium mediated: should methylene blue be the treatment of choice? *Chest* 2002;122:1061–6.

161. Stafford-Smith M, Lefrak EA, Qazi AG, et al. Efficacy and safety of heparinase I versus protamine in patients undergoing coronary artery bypass grafting with and without cardiopulmonary bypass. *Anesthesiology* 2005;103:229–40.

162. Mixon TA, Dehmer GJ. Recombinant platelet factor 4 for heparin neutralization. *Semin Thromb Hemost* 2004;30:369–77.

163. Zwischenberger JB, Tao W, Deyo DJ, Vertrees RA, Alpard SK, Shulman G. Safety and efficacy of a heparin removal device: a prospective randomized preclinical outcomes study. *Ann Thorac Surg* 2001;71:270–7.

164. Fiore MM, Mackie IM. Mechanism of low-molecular-weight heparin reversal by platelet factor 4. *Throm Res* 2009;124:149–55.

165. Warren O, Mandal K, Hadjianastassiou V, et al. Recombinant activated factor VII in cardiac surgery: a systematic review. *Ann Thorac Surg* 2007;83:707–14.

166. Michelsen LG, Horswell S. Anesthesia for off-pump coronary artery bypass grafting. *Semin Thorac Cardiovasc Surg* 2003;15:71–82.

167. Missant C, Rex S, Wouters PF. Accuracy of cardiac output measurements with pulse contour analysis (PulseCO) and Doppler echocardiography during off-pump coronary artery bypass grafting. *Eur J Anaesthesiol* 2008;25:243–8.

168. Bergsland J, Lingaas PS, Skulstad H, et al. Intracoronary shunt prevents ischemia in off-pump coronary artery bypass surgery. *Ann Thorac Surg* 2009;87:54–60.

169. Gurbuz AT, Hecht ML, Arsian AH. Intraoperative transesophageal echocardiography modifies strategy in off-pump coronary artery bypass grafting. *Ann Thorac Surg* 2007;83:1035–40.

170. Tanaka KA, Thourani VH, Williams WH, et al. Heparin anticoagulation in patients undergoing off-pump and on-pump bypass surgery. *J Anesth* 2007;21:297–303.

171. Englberger L, Streich M, Tevaearai H, Carrel TP. Different anticoagulation strategies in off-pump coronary artery bypass operations: a European study. *Interact Cardiovasc Thorac Surg* 2008;7:378–82.

172. Casati V, Gerli C, Franco A, et al. Activation of coagulation and fibrinolysis during coronary surgery: on-pump versus off-pump techniques. *Anesthesiology* 2001;95:1103–9.

173. Zangrillo A, Pappalardo F, Talò G, et al. Temperature management during off-pump coronary artery bypass graft surgery: a randomized clinical trial on the efficacy of a circulating water system versus a forced-air system. *J Cardiothorac Vasc Anesth* 2006;20:788–92.

174. Allen GS. Intraoperative temperature control using the Thermogard system during off-pump coronary artery bypass grafting. *Ann Thorac Surg* 2009;87:284–8.

175. Jeong SM, Hahm KD, Jeong YB, Yang HS, Choi IC. Warming of intravenous fluids prevents hypothermia during off-pump coronary artery bypass graft surgery. *J Cardiothorac Vasc Anesth* 2008;22:67–70.

176. Webb WR, Harrison LH Jr, Helmcke FR, et al. Carbon dioxide field flooding minimizes residual intracardiac air after open heart operations. *Ann Thorac Surg* 1997;64:1489–91.

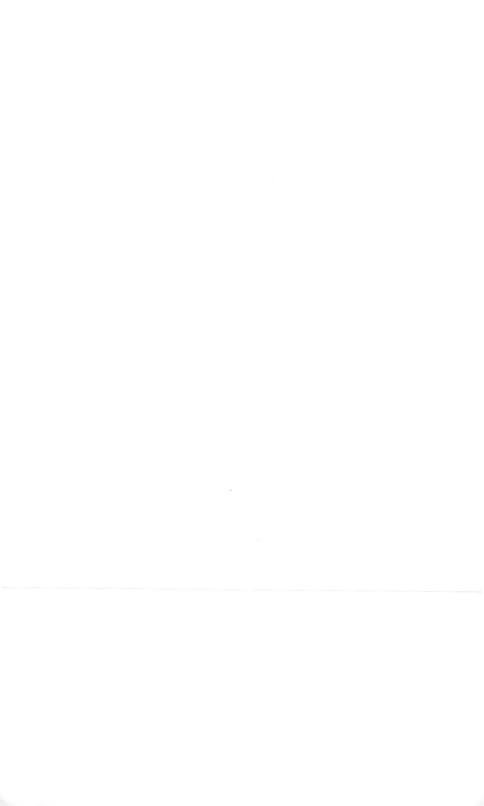

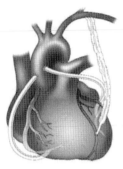

CHAPTER 5

Cardiopulmonary Bypass

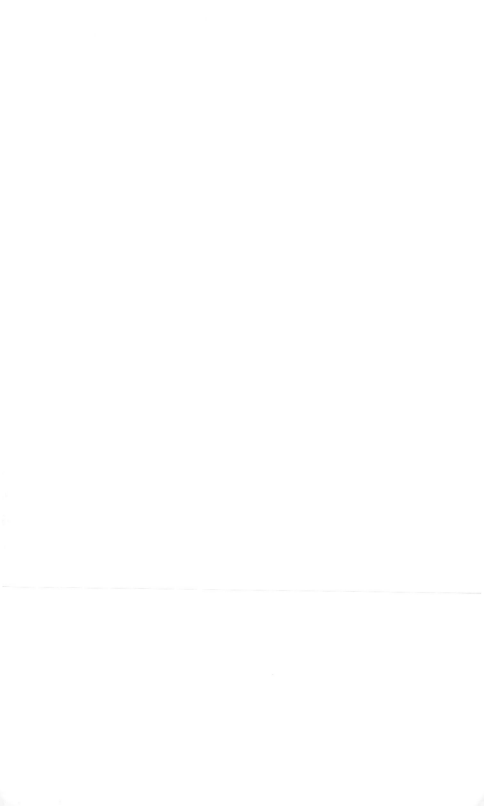

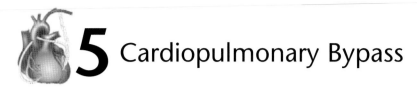

5 Cardiopulmonary Bypass

Extracorporeal circulation has evolved into a remarkably safe means of providing systemic perfusion during open-heart surgery. Modifications of the extracorporeal circuit have enabled surgeons to use a variety of surgical approaches for open-heart procedures while minimizing some of the adverse effects of cardiopulmonary bypass (CPB). Concerns about the impact of CPB on organ system function, especially neurocognitive function, have encouraged many surgeons to utilize off-pump techniques for coronary surgery, although the advantages are controversial. Catheter-based interventions for coronary disease are well established, and the role of transcatheter valve placement is being assessed. However, the vast majority of both coronary and valve procedures are performed on CPB, so it is important to review the technology and physiologic concepts of CPB in cardiac surgery.

I. General Comments

A. Cardiopulmonary bypass involves an extracorporeal circuit that provides oxygenated systemic blood flow when the heart and lungs are not functional. CPB is accompanied by normovolemic hemodilution and nonpulsatile flow.

B. The contact of blood with the extracorporeal circuit results in the activation of numerous cascades, including the kallikrein, coagulation, and complement systems.[1-5] Among the consequences of this contact are thrombin generation, the release of proinflammatory cytokines, and a systemic inflammatory response. Endothelial-based reactions, including platelet adhesion, aggregation, and activation, as well as leukocyte adhesion and activation have been implicated in myocardial reperfusion damage, pulmonary and renal dysfunction, neurocognitive changes, and a generalized capillary leak. Fortunately, adverse effects of this inflammatory response are not clinically significant in most patients. However, in patients requiring long pump runs or in those with significant hemodynamic compromise following surgery, this systemic inflammatory response may persist for days, leading to multiple organ system compromise.

C. Use of membrane oxygenators, biocompatible circuits, centrifugal pumps, and intraoperative steroids, minimal use of red cell transfusions, avoidance of cardiotomy suction, and arguably the use of leukocyte filters may reduce the inflammatory effects of CPB, but have not had a significant impact on clinical outcomes.[6-22]

D. Despite adequate heparinization, the bypass circuit is a potent activator of the coagulation system with generation of factor Xa and thrombin that contribute to the inflammatory response and potentially to ischemia/reperfusion injury.[5] A coagulopathy may develop from activation of platelets and the fibrinolytic system, as well as from dilution of clotting factors and platelets during bypass.

II. The Cardiopulmonary Bypass Circuit

A. The extracorporeal circuit consists of polyvinylchloride (PVC) tubing and polycarbonate connectors. Circuits coated with the Carmeda BioActive surface, heparin (Duraflo II), Trillium biopassive surface coating, or poly(2-methoxyethylacrylate) (PMEA) have been shown to improve biocompatibility, with reduced complement, leukocyte, and platelet activation, and less release of proinflammatory mediators.[15–22]

    1. Although these circuits may reduce bleeding, atrial fibrillation (which may be inflammatory-mediated), and the degree of pulmonary dysfunction, permitting earlier extubation and shortening the hospital length of stay, other clinical benefits of their antiinflammatory properties are modest. Studies have not shown that these circuits decrease thrombin generation, which is a marker of coagulation system activation and a trigger of endothelial cell dysfunction. Use of centrifugal pumps, reduced priming volumes, and avoidance of cardiotomy suction need to be used along with biocompatible circuits to minimize blood activation during CPB.[15]

    2. Although it is controversial whether use of lower levels of heparin with these coated circuits may be associated with less postoperative bleeding, an adequate level of heparinization is still required to minimize activation of the coagulation system, thrombin generation, and fibrinolysis.[23–26] This is especially important since there is little correlation between activated clotting times (ACTs) and the level of thrombin markers. Acceptable ACTs are probably >350 seconds for a low-risk CABG or valve surgery with an anticipated short pump time, and >400 seconds for more complex surgery.

B. The pump is primed with a balanced electrolyte solution, such as Lactated Ringer's, Normosol, or Plasmalyte, although normal saline may be used in patients with chronic kidney disease to reduce the potassium load. The average priming volume is approximately 1500 mL. A colloid, usually albumin, is commonly added to the pump prime to increase oncotic pressure and reduce fluid requirements, thus decreasing extravascular lung water. It may also ameliorate bleeding by delaying fibrinogen absorption and reducing platelet activation.[27] Albumin is preferable to high-molecular-weight heta-starches, which have been associated with increased perioperative bleeding.[28] In fact, hetastarch has also been shown to increase the risk of bleeding complications following OPCAB.[29] In 2004, the US Food and Drug Administration (FDA) issued a warning about use of hetastarch (Hespan) during surgery.[30]

C. Miniaturized circuits with lower priming volumes minimize hemodilution and reduce the blood–artificial surface interface, possibly minimizing the inflammatory response. These systems also allow for centrifugation of shed blood before retransfusion to reduce blood activation and lipid embolism. Studies have demonstrated improved clinical outcomes, with decreased transfusion rates, lower troponin release, a reduced incidence of neurologic damage and atrial fibrillation, and a shorter duration of ventilation.[31–35] The decrease in the inflammatory response may be equivalent to that seen during off-pump surgery.[31] However, these circuits do lower the safety margins for volume loss and air emboli, and make weaning and termination of bypass more difficult because of low volume reserve in the system.

D. Venous blood drains by gravity from the right atrium or vena cavae into a cardiotomy reservoir bag, passes through an oxygenator attached to a heater/cooler unit, and is returned to the arterial system through a filter using either a roller or a centrifugal pump (Figure 5.1).

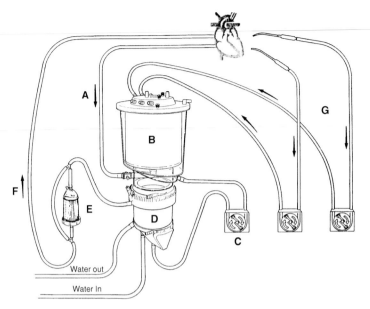

Figure 5.1 • The basics of an extracorporeal circuit. Blood drains by gravity through the venous lines (A) into a cardiotomy reservoir (B), is pumped using a roller head (C) (or preferentially a centrifugal pump) through the oxygenator/heat exchanger (D) and arterial line filter (E) back into the arterial circuit (F). Additional suction lines (G) can be used for intracardiac venting and scavenging of blood from the operative field.

1. In a closed reservoir system, which contains a collapsible bag, air passing through the venous lines can be vented through ports at the top of the bag. In a hard shell open system, air can potentially get entrained into the oxygenator if the cardiotomy volume is too low, so low-volume alarms must be utilized and keen attention paid to reservoir volumes.

2. Active venous drainage using vacuum assist or kinetic assist (with a centrifugal pump) can be used to augment venous drainage. This is valuable during minimally invasive procedures or when small venous catheters are utilized.[36,37] The least amount of negative pressure necessary to augment drainage should be used, although a pressure up to −60 mm Hg is acceptable. Use of vacuum assist may produce hemolysis, but more importantly, one must consider the possibility of venous air entrainment and undetected air microembolism when this technique is utilized.[38–43] Excessive vacuum may pull air retrograde through the oxygenator membrane, causing depriming of a centrifugal pump. It has been suggested that aggressive monitoring for gaseous emboli on both the venous and arterial side be utilized to minimize these risks.[42] However, with appropriate attention to detail, vacuum assist may not increase air microembolism or the neurologic risk.[43]

E. Systemic flow is provided by either a roller pump or a centrifugal pump, but is nonpulsatile with both systems unless additional technology is utilized to provide pulsatile flow. Roller pumps are pressure-insensitive and can pressurize the arterial line in the face of outflow obstruction. Centrifugal pumps are afterload-sensitive, such that they will reduce flow if the outflow is obstructed. Studies have indicated that centrifugal pumps might cause less blood trauma than roller pumps, but the inflammatory response and effects on perioperative bleeding are fairly similar with both types of pumps.[6,44]

F. Suction lines return extravasated blood (mostly from the pericardium) to the cardiotomy reservoir to conserve blood and blood elements and to maintain pump volume.

1. Despite the nearly universal use of these suction lines, the benefits of blood salvage into the pump may be offset by the adverse effects of the aspirated blood. Studies have shown that blood in contact with tissue factor in the pericardium is replete with fat and procoagulant and proinflammatory mediators, such as complement and cytokines. Thus, aspirated blood is a significant activator of coagulation, causing increased generation of thrombin and complement that promotes inflammation, and is a major cause of hemolysis.[45−49] Cytokines may contribute to increased perioperative bleeding and neurologic sequelae.

2. Elimination of cardiotomy suction may reduce thrombin generation, platelet activation, and the systemic inflammatory response.[50] Use of cell-saving devices to aspirate and wash shed blood can preserve red cells while eliminating many of these inflammatory mediators and removing fat from the blood, but centrifugation does remove coagulation factors and platelets from the blood.[51−54] Notably, return of cardiotomy suction into the circuit usually causes systemic hypotension, most likely because of the high levels of inflammatory mediators present.[55]

G. An additional suction line can be connected to an intracardiac vent, draining blood from the left ventricle or other cardiac chamber into the reservoir by active suctioning by a roller pump head. These lines are useful in providing ventricular decompression and/or improving surgical exposure. Active root venting is commonly used upon termination of cardiopulmonary bypass in valve cases to evacuate ejected air.

H. Oxygen and compressed air pass into the oxygenator from a blender which regulates oxygen concentration by adjusting the FIO_2 and also determines the gas flow by adjusting a "sweep rate". The sweep rate is generally maintained slightly less than the systemic flow rate to eliminate CO_2 from the blood to achieve a desired value (generally around 40–50 mm Hg). To minimize blood activation, the oxygenator may be coated with heparin or Trillium to improve biocompatibility.[56]

I. The pump setup includes a separate heat exchanger for cardioplegia delivery. Tubes of differing diameters are passed through the same roller pump head, delivering a preselected ratio of pump volume to cardioplegia solution (such as 4:1). The final mixture then passes through this heat exchanger for delivery of cold or warm cardioplegia. Pressure monitoring of infusion pressure is essential, especially for retrograde delivery, which generally provides about 200 mL/min of flow at a pressure that should not exceed 40 mm Hg to prevent coronary sinus rupture. Very high line pressures indicate obstruction to flow, either because the line is clamped or because the cardioplegia catheter is obstructed. A low line pressure generally indicates misplacement of the catheter, either back into the right atrium or from perforation of the coronary sinus. Microplegia systems (such as the Quest MPS system) minimize the volume of crystalloid vehicle required during cardioplegia delivery. It mixes the essential cardioplegia contents (primarily potassium and magnesium) with the blood in a specified ratio that is then delivered to the heart. This allows for a large amount of cardioplegia to be delivered with minimal hemodilution.

J. Additional features of the CPB circuit may include the following:

    1. In-line monitoring of arterial and venous blood gases, electrolytes, hematocrit, and temperatures at multiple sites simultaneously. The last of these is useful during deep hypothermia cases.

    2. A direct connection to the cell-saving device, through which excess volume can be directed during the pump run. After CPB is terminated, this allows for centrifugation and "cell-washing" of pump contents for reinfusion into the patient.

    3. An arterial line filter (usually 40 μm), which is essential to remove microemboli before blood is returned to the patient. Microemboli may consist of air, blood or platelet microaggregates, or other particulate matter. Fat microemboli are found in abundance in cardiotomy suction and can be removed by 20 μm filters. Unfortunately, large emboli may become fractionated before reaching the arterial line filter, and may not be completely removed. Venous line filtration can also be used to optimize removal of gaseous microemboli.[57]

    4. Recirculation lines to allow for venting of air and to prevent stagnation of blood. This is essential during circulatory arrest cases and when direct thrombin inhibitors are used for anticoagulation in patients with heparin-induced thrombocytopenia.

    5. Hemofilters or hemoconcentrators, which can be placed in the circuit to remove excessive volume in patients with preexisting fluid overload or renal dysfunction. Modified ultrafiltration (MUF) at the end of the pump run can hemoconcentrate the pump contents by pumping blood from the arterial cannula through the concentrator for retransfusion through the venous cannula into the right atrium.[58]

K. A detailed checklist must be utilized by the perfusionist before every case to make sure that no detail is overlooked. The patient's life is dependent on the perfusionist and proper function of the heart–lung machine. Accurate record keeping during bypass is essential (Figures 5.2 and 5.3).

III. Cannulation for Bypass

    A. **Arterial cannulation** is usually accomplished by placement of a cannula in the ascending aorta just proximal to the innominate artery (Figure 5.4). Cannula size is determined by the anticipated flow rate for the patient based on body surface area, so as to minimize line pressure and shear forces (Table 5.1).

        1. Cannula designs have been modified in a variety of ways to minimize shear forces and jet effects on the aortic wall (Figure 5.5). Some have end holes and some have multiple side holes through which blood exits at lower velocity (Soft-Flow and dispersion cannulas).[59] The latter might theoretically reduce the risk of cerebral embolization, especially to the left hemisphere.[60] A cannula with a small distal net has been designed to trap embolic material upon aortic unclamping, and this has been shown to reduce the risk of stroke (Embol-X).[61] Distal arch cannulation with placement of the tip of the cannula beyond the left subclavian artery has been proposed as a means of reducing cerebral emboli in patients with severe ascending aortic atherosclerosis.[62]

        2. Steps to prevent systemic embolization, primarily to the brain, are imperative when CPB is used during surgery. Although gaseous microembolization can be addressed by improvements in CPB technology, cannulation and clamping are the primary causes of atheroembolism and stroke.[63] Although most surgeons palpate the

☐ Patient chart reviewed and assessed
☐ Heart-Lung machine properly plugged in; all batteries checked and operational
☐ Centrifugal pump in correct position and properly mounted
☐ Hand cranks available
☐ All pump tubing connections correct and tightened
☐ MPS machine properly set up and primed, correct ratio, KCL, MgSO4 and temps
☐ Cardioplegia tubing placement in correct direction in pump head raceway and occlusions checked and set
☐ Adequate tubing clamps available
☐ Sweep gas line attached to oxygenator / FIO2 and gas flow selected
☐ Fluotec checked and filled with Isoflourane
☐ Scavenger line prepared
☐ Venous sat. monitor, battery checked
☐ Venous sat. probe attached and checked for proper functioning and positioning
☐ Pump cart available with adequate supply of drugs, solutions, syringes, needles, filters, etc.
☐ Centrifugal pump flow probe attched properly
☐ Oxygen analyzer calibrated and battery checked
☐ Connections to table lines properly made and checked, A-V Loop primed
☐ Heater/Cooler connected and primed and properly set
☐ Ice in room and added to appropriate heater/cooler
☐ Cardioplegia solution prepared and correct for surgeon
☐ Hepcon machine set up, with adequate supplies and patient data entered
☐ Baseline ACT performed and heparin dose calculated/reported to anesthesiologist
☐ Heparin given by anesthesiologist
☐ Adequate post-heparin ACT achieved
☐ Arterial and venous lines properly clamped
☐ Cardiotomy reservoir set up and vented
☐ Pump suction and vent line placed correctly in pump head
☐ Occlusions properly checked and set
☐ Blood gas analyzer shift Q.C. completed

Signature: _____   Date: _____

DISPOSABLES	MANUFACTURER	LOT #
Oxygenator:		
Cardioplegia:		
Tubing Pack:		
Cell Saver:		
Hemoconcentrator:		

Figure 5.2 • Pre-bypass checklist.

ascending aorta to assess for the presence of atherosclerotic plaque and calcification, this is a very insensitive means of detecting plaque. Transesophageal echocardiography (TEE) may identify protruding atheromas, but epiaortic imaging is the gold standard for identifying plaque and may lead to modification of the surgical approach.[64]

3. If ascending aortic cannulation is not feasible, an alternative cannulation site must be sought. Femoral artery cannulation, either percutaneously or via cutdown, is feasible if there is minimal aortoiliac atherosclerosis and the TEE

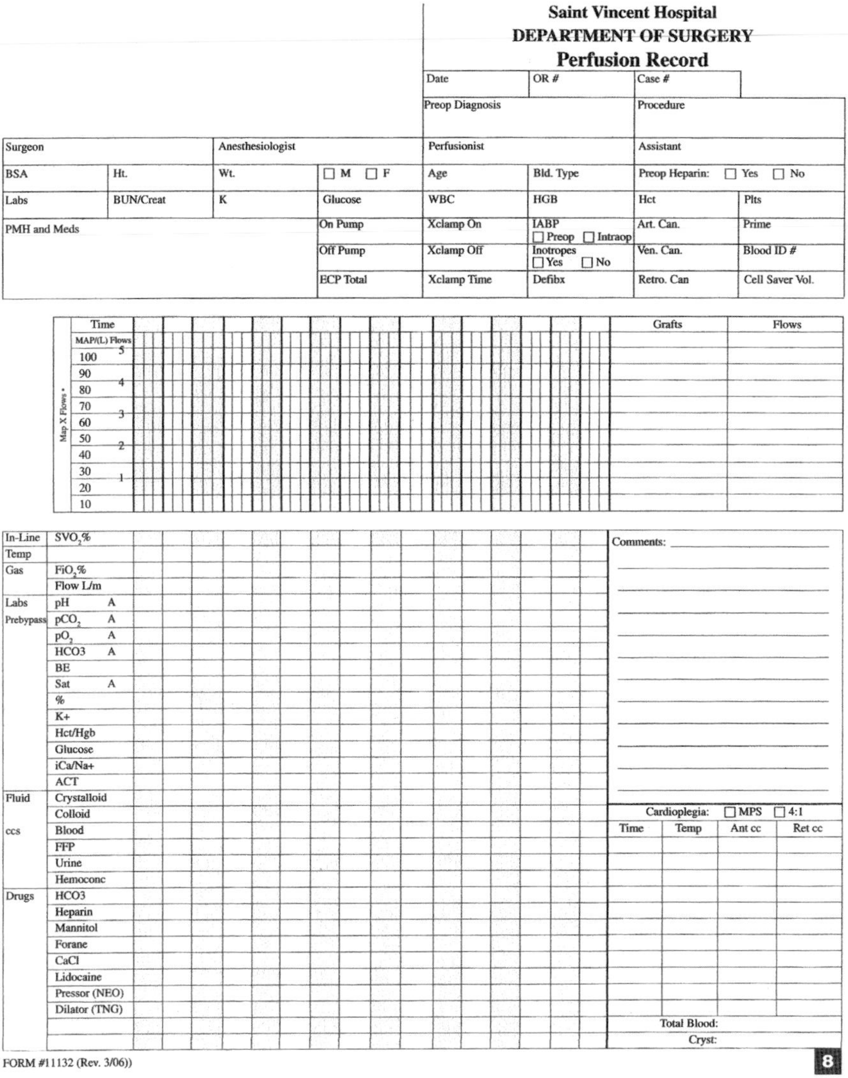

Saint Vincent Hospital
DEPARTMENT OF SURGERY
Perfusion Record

Date	OR #	Case #
Preop Diagnosis		Procedure

Surgeon		Anesthesiologist		Perfusionist		Assistant	

BSA	Ht.	Wt.	☐ M ☐ F	Age	Bld. Type	Preop Heparin: ☐ Yes ☐ No	
Labs	BUN/Creat	K	Glucose	WBC	HGB	Hct	Plts

PMH and Meds	On Pump	Xclamp On	IABP ☐ Preop ☐ Intraop	Art. Can.	Prime
	Off Pump	Xclamp Off	Inotropes ☐ Yes ☐ No	Ven. Can.	Blood ID #
	ECP Total	Xclamp Time	Defibx	Retro. Can	Cell Saver Vol.

Time					Grafts	Flows
MAP/(L) Flows						

Map X Flows chart:
100 — 5
90
80 — 4
70
60 — 3
50
40 — 2
30
20 — 1
10

		Comments:
In-Line	SVO₂%	
Temp		
Gas	FiO₂%	
	Flow L/m	
Labs	pH A	
Prebypass	pCO₂ A	
	pO₂ A	
	HCO3 A	
	BE	
	Sat A	
	%	
	K+	
	Hct/Hgb	
	Glucose	
	iCa/Na+	
	ACT	
Fluid	Crystalloid	
	Colloid	Cardioplegia: ☐ MPS ☐ 4:1
ccs	Blood	Time	Temp	Ant cc	Ret cc
	FFP	
	Urine	
	Hemoconc	
Drugs	HCO3	
	Heparin	
	Mannitol	
	Forane	
	CaCl	
	Lidocaine	
	Pressor (NEO)	
	Dilator (TNG)	
		Total Blood:
		Cryst:

FORM #11132 (Rev. 3/06)) — 8

Figure 5.3 • Typical perfusion record.

does not demonstrate significant descending aortic atherosclerosis which could produce retrograde cerebral embolization and stroke. Femoral cannulation also runs the risk of a retrograde dissection. Satisfactory flow into the cannula must be assured before connecting the cannula to the CPB circuit. After decannulation, distal flow must be confirmed after the femoral arteriotomy has been repaired.

4. Although central cannulation can be accomplished in many types of minimally invasive surgery, femoral arterial cannulation is commonly used and is required

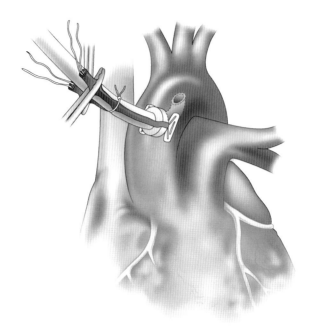

Figure 5.4 • Arterial cannulation. The arterial cannula is placed amidst two pursestrings in the ascending aorta just proximal to the innominate artery. The outflow should be directed into the arch, not into the innominate artery.

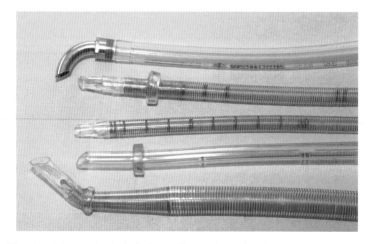

Figure 5.5 • Arterial cannulas include (top to bottom): Medtronic DLP 20 Fr curved metal cannula, Sarns Terumo 7 Fr Soft-Flow cannula with multiple side holes, Medtronic 20 Fr EOPA cannula with end and side holes, Medtronic DLP 22 Fr straight arch cannula, and Medtronic 22 mm 3D select cannula.

Table 5.1 • Flow Rates and Desired Cannula Sizes

BSA	Venous		Arterial		Flow L/min
	Bicaval (Fr)	2 or 3 Stage (Fr)	French	Metric	
1.3	26 & 28		18 Fr	6.5 mm (Curved)	3.1
1.4		29/37 29/29/29			3.4
1.5	28 & 30				3.6
1.6					3.8
1.7	30 & 32		20 Fr (EOPA)		4.1
1.8					4.3
1.9	32 & 34	32/40 29/37/37			4.6
2.0					4.8
2.1				7–8 mm (Soft-Flow)	5.0
2.2					5.3
2.3	34 & 36	36/46 29/46/37	22/24 Fr (Select 3D)		5.5
2.4					5.8
2.5					6.0
2.6					6.2

Note that smaller venous cannulas can be used when vacuum-assisted drainage is employed. BSA, body surface area (m^2).

during robotic valvular surgery. In these patients, it is imperative to assess the patient's iliofemoral system prior to surgery to identify whether femoral artery cannulation will be feasible. Furthermore, when a long duration of CPB is anticipated (complex minimally invasive or robotic surgery), there is an increased risk of a lower-extremity compartment syndrome from ischemia/reperfusion injury.[65–67] In these situations, one should place the cannula percutaneously without a distal snare or consider cannulating through a sidearm graft sewn to the femoral artery to ensure distal flow. Alternatively, one could place cannulas for both proximal retrograde and distal perfusion.[68,69]

5. If femoral cannulation is not feasible, or in patients requiring surgery of the ascending aorta and arch, cannulation of the distal subclavian/axillary artery is an excellent alternative (Figure 5.6). This may be performed directly through an arteriotomy or preferably through an 8 mm sidearm graft anastomosed to the

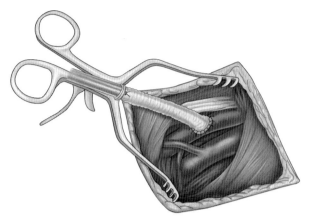

Figure 5.6 • Axillary artery cannulation. An 8 mm side graft is sewn to the distal subclavian/axillary artery, into which the cannula is placed and secured in position.

vessel, which provides distal arm circulation during bypass. With snaring of the proximal innominate artery, axillary cannulation allows for selective antegrade brain perfusion during deep hypothermic circulatory arrest (DHCA). In these cases, additional cannulation of the left carotid artery may also be considered.[70–73]

6. Either femoral or axillary arterial cannulation should be immediately available when there is concern about potential cardiac, aortic, or graft damage during resternotomy or for patients with ruptured ascending aortic aneurysms or aortic dissections with hemopericardium. The artery should be exposed and occasionally may need to be cannulated, either for immediate initiation of bypass if problems are encountered after sternotomy or rarely to initiate bypass and systemic cooling before the sternotomy is performed, depending on the anatomy.

B. **Venous drainage** for most open-heart surgery is accomplished with a double- or triple-stage cavoatrial cannula (Figure 5.7). This is placed through the right atrial appendage or right atrial free wall with the distal end situated in the inferior vena cava (IVC) (Figure 5.8A). Blood drains from the IVC through several apertures near the end and from the right atrium through additional side holes. These catheters are used for most procedures that do not require opening of the right heart. The triple-stage cannula provides excellent flow and allows for use of a smaller outer-diameter cannula, especially with vacuum-assisted drainage.

1. Mitral valve surgery may be accomplished using a double- or triple-staged cannula or with bicaval cannulation, although the latter is required if a biatrial transseptal approach is planned. Tricuspid valve surgery always requires bicaval cannulation with placement of caval snares around the cannulas to prevent air entry into the venous lines. A cannula may be placed directly into the superior vena cava (SVC) or passed through the right atrial appendage into the SVC. The IVC cannula is placed through a pursestring suture low in the right atrial free wall (Figure 5.8B).

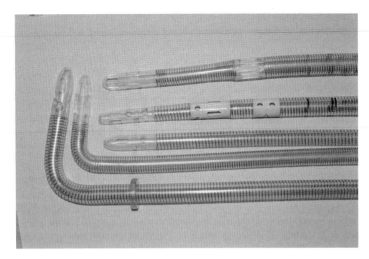

Figure 5.7 • Venous cannulas include (top to bottom): Medtronic 32/40 double-stage cavoatrial cannula, RMI 29/37/37 triple-stage cannula, RMI 30 Fr straight "lighthouse" tipped cannula, and short DLP 32 Fr and long RMI 36 Fr right-angle cannulas.

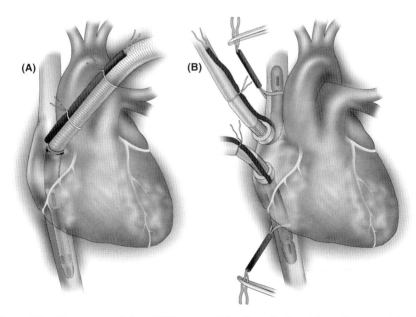

Figure 5.8 • Venous cannulation. (A) The cavoatrial catheter is placed through a pursestring in the right atrial appendage. The tip consists of multiple side holes and is placed into the inferior vena cava (IVC). The "basket" lies in the mid-atrium and drains flow from the superior vena cava (SVC) and coronary sinus through multiple holes 9 cm back from the tip for dual-stage cannulas and 6 and 11 cm from the tip for triple-stage cannulas. (B) Bicaval cannulation. The SVC cannula may be placed directly into the SVC or via the right atrial appendage. The IVC cannula is placed through a pursestring low on the right atrial free wall.

2. Femoral venous cannulation is used in robotic and minimally invasive cases and may be supplemented by a 16 Fr venous line placed into the internal jugular vein. The femoral catheter is 50 cm long and is passed through the femoral vein to lie within the right atrium to ensure adequate venous drainage. Shorter venous catheters can be used, if necessary. Exposure of the femoral vein or even cannulation and establishment of CPB may also be used in high-risk situations of hemodynamic instability or redo surgery.

3. Femoral arterial and venous cannulation have been used to systemically warm patients presenting with profound accidental hypothermia and can be used in emergency situations, such as cardiac arrest, to establish an extracorporeal membrane oxygenation (ECMO) circuit.

C. Figure 5.9 provides an illustration of cannulation and clamping for a routine on-pump coronary bypass operation.

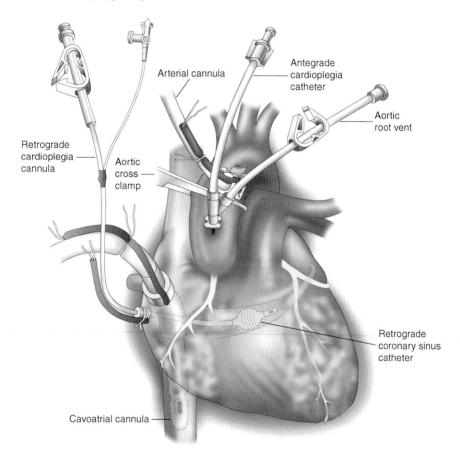

Figure 5.9 • Cannulation and clamping during a routine on-pump coronary bypass operation. Note aortic and venous cannulation, antegrade and retrograde cardioplegia catheters, and the aortic cross-clamp just proximal to the aortic cannulation site.

IV. Initiation and Conduct of Cardiopulmonary Bypass (Table 5.2)

A. **Heparin management**. Anticoagulation is essential to minimize thrombin formation within the extracorporeal circuit. Heparin is administered in a dose of 3–4 mg/kg for uncoated circuits with monitoring of its anticoagulant effect by the activated clotting time (ACT). A blood sample is drawn 3–5 minutes after heparin administration and should achieve an ACT > 480 seconds. Patients with heparin resistance may require more heparin or other blood products to achieve adequate anticoagulation (see page 247). For heparin-coated circuits, a level of >350 seconds is generally acceptable. Because of patient variability in response to heparin and the effects of hypothermia and hemodilution on the ACT, an individual dose-response curve can be generated using the Medtronic Hepcon system, which calculates the precise amount of heparin necessary to achieve a specified ACT. This may reduce heparin over- or underdosing and has been shown to reduce thrombin generation, fibrinolysis, and neutrophil activation.[74] During off-pump surgery, the ACT should reach 250 seconds because coronary arteries are occluded during the procedure. Although rarely used, the high-dose thrombin time correlates better with heparin concentration than the ACT and is not affected by temperature or hemodilution.

B. In a patient with documented **heparin-induced thrombocytopenia (HIT)**, an alternative means of anticoagulation must be sought. One approach is simultaneous administration of antiplatelet medications (glycoprotein IIb/IIIa inhibitors, prostaglandin analogs) with heparin during bypass. Alternatively, direct thrombin

Table 5.2 • Desired Values on Pump	
1. ACT	>480 seconds >350 seconds for biocompatible circuits
2. Systemic flow rates	2–2.5 L/min/m^2 at 37 °C 1.7–2.0 (low flow) or 2.0–2.5 L/min/m^2 (high flow) at 30 °C
3. Systemic blood pressure	50–70 mm Hg
4. Arterial blood gases	PO_2 > 250 torr, PCO_2 40–50 torr with pH 7.40 Deep hypothermia: α–stat pH 7.40 measured at 37 °C pH–stat pH 7.40 at systemic temperature
5. SVO$_2$	>70%
6. Hematocrit	>20%
7. Blood glucose	100–180 mg/dL

inhibitors, such as bivalirudin, lepirudin or argatroban, can be used to avoid heparin entirely. This issue is discussed in more detail on pages 201–204.

C. **Retrograde autologous priming (RAP)** can be used to reduce the hemodilutional effects of the priming solution and maintain a higher hematocrit on pump. The crystalloid prime is back-drained from the venous line into the bypass circuit and aspirated into the cell saver before initiating bypass. Simultaneously, an α-agent is given to maintain systemic pressure. Often an infusion of albumin is necessary to minimize the reduction in circulating volume, although, to some degree, this may offset the benefits of a reduced priming volume on maintaining a higher hematocrit. Retrograde autologous priming does maintain a higher oncotic pressure during the pump run and has been shown to minimize the accumulation of extravascular lung water and postoperative weight gain. It is probably most beneficial in small patients with low blood volumes and low hematocrits. Although the impact of RAP on clinical outcomes is not significant, it may reduce the overall number of transfusions required.[75–78]

D. **Systemic pressures and flows**. When pump flow is initiated, the patient's pulsatile perfusion is replaced by nonpulsatile flow. The blood pressure initially decreases from hemodilution with a reduction in blood viscosity. It should then be maintained between 50 and 70 mm Hg during the pump run. It may transiently decrease during cardioplegia delivery (probably from potassium delivery into the systemic circulation), from return of large volumes of cardiotomy suction (from inflammatory mediators), and during rewarming (from vasodilation). Blood pressure may rise due to vasoconstriction from hypothermia, and from dilution of narcotics by the pump prime.

1. The systemic flow rate is calculated based on the patient's body surface area and modified by the degree of hypothermia and the venous oxygen saturation (SvO_2). It should also take into account the degree of anemia, which can influence whole-body oxygen delivery. The flow rate should exceed $2 \, L/min/m^2$ at normothermia and can be reduced to $1.5–1.7 \, L/min/m^2$ at $30\,°C$ with "low flow" bypass. Flow needs to be increased during rewarming, when increased metabolism usually decreases the SvO_2. Low-flow bypass during moderate hypothermia has been shown to improve myocardial protection, reduce collateral flow improving exposure, reduce hemolysis, and reduce fluid requirements without any compromise in tissue perfusion.[79]

2. The optimal flow rate should be based on an assessment of adequate oxygen delivery. Means of assessing this include the venous oxygen saturation, blood lactate levels, and in-line monitoring of CO_2 production.[80] The latter two together may be the best way of predicting anaerobic metabolism, which is not assessed by the venous oxygen saturation. Nonetheless, in most practices, as long as the venous oxygen saturation exceeds 70%, the flow rate is considered to be adequate, although this may not reflect regional flow.[81]

   a. For example, at normothermia, the brain and kidney autoregulate to maintain perfusion as the flow rate is reduced at the expense of skeletal muscle and splanchnic flow. However, renal blood flow is determined primarily by the systemic flow rate, and can be adversely affected during hypothermia, which impairs renal autoregulation.[82] Due to concerns that the combination of hemodilution and a lower flow rate may reduce the mean arterial pressure below the autoregulatory threshold and compromise organ system function, there are proponents of using "high flow" ($2-2.4\,L/min/m^2$) rather than "low flow" bypass during hypothermia.[83] One study demonstrated that renal function was not affected by using lower target blood pressures on CPB ($< 60\,mm$ Hg vs. $60-69\,mm$ Hg vs. $>70\,mm$ Hg), alth-ough urine output was less at the lower pressures.[84] However, other factors, such as older age and longer CPB times, were associated with acute kidney injury.

   b. Some studies have demonstrated that a low hematocrit ($< 21\%$ or even $< 25\%$) may adversely affect renal function and increase mortality.[85-87] However, maintenance of adequate systemic oxygen delivery by increasing the systemic flow rate may offset the deleterious effects of a low hematocrit.[88]

3. One of the primary concerns with CPB is maintenance of adequate cerebral oxygenation, which is determined by both blood pressure and systemic flow rate. Cerebral autoregulation allows for maintenance of cerebral blood flow down to a mean arterial pressure as low as $40-50\,mm$ Hg, but autoregulation may be inadequate in hypertensive or diabetic patients, in whom it may be desirable to maintain a higher pressure.[89] In fact, some studies have shown that cerebral oxygenation is impaired at this level even if the flow rate is satisfactory, so the blood pressure must be maintained at an adequate level regardless of the flow rate, usually using vasopressors, such as phenylephrine, norepinephrine, or vasopressin.[90] This may improve cerebral oxygenation but reduce flow to other regions, specifically the kidneys and splanchnic viscera.

4. The adequacy of cerebral oxygenation during CPB is usually assessed by cerebral oximetry using bifrontal sensors with near-infrared spectroscopy (Somanetics INVOS cerebral oximeter) (Figure 4.10, page 206). The regional cerebral oxygen saturation (rSO_2) tends to fall during initiation of bypass and during rewarming, even with an increase in systemic flow. The rSO_2 promptly detects problems with arterial desaturation even before it is evident by pulse oximetry.[91] Studies have demonstrated that oxygen desaturation is associated with an increased incidence of neurocognitive changes.[92] If the oxygen satura-tion falls more than 20% below baseline or below 40%, an intervention is recommended to restore cerebral blood flow. Before initiating bypass, an increase in blood pressure or an elevation in PCO_2 will be effective in increasing cerebral blood flow. Once on bypass, modifications of flow rate, blood pressure, PCO_2 or the hematocrit are beneficial. This technology may also alert the cardiac surgical team to potential catastrophes associated with brain malperfu-sion from cannula malplacement, dissections, oxygenator or other pump-related failures, air embolism, anaphylactic reactions (such as protamine), monitoring problems, etc. Although interventions to improve rSO_2 should intuitively reduce the adverse effects of desaturation, few studies have documented improvements in clinical outcome.[92]

E. Both the **hematocrit** (HCT) on pump and the systemic flow rate determine the amount of oxygen delivery to the body. Hemodilution from the pump prime commonly reduces oxygen delivery by 25% as estimated from the following equation:

$$\text{Predicted HCT on pump} = \frac{(70 \times kg \times \text{preop HCT}/100)}{(70 \times kg) + \text{prime volume} + \text{IV fluids pre-CPB}}$$

where $70 \times kg$ equals the blood volume and $70 \times kg \times$ preop HCT is the RBC volume.

1. Hemodilution reduces blood viscosity and improves microcirculatory flow, but at the extremes of hemodilution there is a significant reduction in oncotic pressure that increases fluid requirements. This can exacerbate the systemic inflammatory response and capillary leak, causing substantial tissue edema. This may contribute to cerebral edema, papilledema, and ischemic optic neuropathy, and can lead to respiratory compromise, among other adverse effects.[93]

2. Very low hematocrits on pump have been associated with increased mortality and an increase in the incidence of renal dysfunction, stroke, and prolonged mechanical ventilation.[85–87,94] Generally, the lower acceptable limit of hematocrit on pump has been considered to be 18%, and one study noted the lowest risk of renal dysfunction occurred with a hematocrit of 21–24%.[85] The association of low hematocrit with adverse effects is presumably on the basis of inadequate oxygen delivery, causing ischemic organ system injury. Increasing the systemic flow rate to improve oxygen delivery may offset the consequences of profound anemia,[95] but transfusing patients to hematocrits over 24% offers little advantage during bypass and may prove deleterious because of immunomodulatory effects and other potential adverse organ system sequelae of transfusions.[96]

F. **Temperature management**. The systemic temperature may be maintained at normothermia or at varying degrees of hypothermia depending on the surgeon's preference and the operative procedure. Most surgeons use moderate hypothermia to provide some organ system protection during nonpulsatile perfusion and also in the event that a temporary problem arises with surgery (need to reduce flow to place sutures) or with perfusion (impaired drainage, low blood pressure, air embolism, pump head failure, oxygenator failure, etc.). Although the rate of rewarming may affect neurocognitive outcome, no conclusive advantage of using either normothermic or hypothermic bypass has been established in terms of inflammatory activation, perioperative hemostasis, or neurocognitive outcome.[97,98]

G. **Gas exchange**. Oxygenation and elimination of CO_2 are determined by the sweep rate, which is adjusted on the blender. Most oxygenators are not stressed until the flow rate exceeds 7 L/min, which should be adequate for even a 175 kg patient. The PO_2 should be maintained above 250 torr in the event of a temporary reduction in flow or pump malfunction, and can be monitored in-line or by intermittent blood gases every 30 minutes. Inhalational anesthetics, such as sevoflurane, desflurane, or isoflurane, are administered through the blender and must be scavenged via the oxygenator.

H. **Ventilation**. Upon initiation of full flow on bypass, ventilation is stopped. Several studies have suggested that ventilation during bypass may improve pulmonary function and gas exchange with less release of inflammatory mediators, but this is not a common practice.[99,100]

I. **pH management**. With progressive hypothermia, CO_2 production decreases and pH normally rises. With mild or moderate hypothermia, pH is generally maintained between 7.40 and 7.50 by adjusting the sweep rate and maintaining the PCO_2 around 40–50 torr. Evidence of metabolic acidosis on pump may be a sign of inadequate tissue oxygenation despite normal blood gases. Regional hypoperfusion, especially of the splanchnic bed, may be contributory to this problem. In fact, lactate release with levels greater than 4 mmol/L during reperfusion is predictive of an increased risk of complications and death.[101,102] During deep hypothermia, two pH management strategies can be used. With pH-stat, the pH is temperature-corrected and maintained at 7.40 by adding a mixture of O_2 and CO_2 ("Carbogen") to the circuit. With this strategy, there is an increase in cerebral blood flow with a potentially increased risk of cerebral microembolism. In contrast, with α-stat, the pH is maintained at 7.40 measured at 37 °C (i.e., not temperature-corrected). Cerebral blood flow is autoregulated and coupled to cerebral oxygen demand. The latter strategy is preferred during DHCA cases.[103,104]

J. **Medications** to maintain anesthesia or control blood pressure are given into a sampling manifold that flows into the venous reservoir. Other medications that may be given by the perfusionist into the circuit during bypass include mannitol, insulin, sodium bicarbonate, calcium chloride, magnesium sulfate, antibiotics, vasopressors, and inotropes.

K. Intermittent measurements of serum potassium, glucose, and hematocrit should be performed in addition to arterial and venous blood gases and ACTs. This should be performed using point-of-care machines in the operating room (Figure 5.10). An

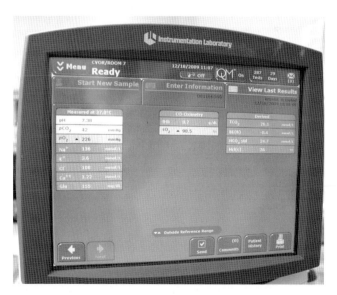

Figure 5.10 • Point-of-care testing machine available to the perfusionist to obtain arterial blood gases, electrolytes, glucose levels, oxygen saturations, and hematocrit levels.

elevated potassium may necessitate a change in the composition or frequency of cardioplegia delivery and may require administration of diuretics or insulin for control. An elevated glucose is related to increased levels of endogenous epinephrine and insulin resistance and may be associated with an increased risk of neurologic injury.[2] Blood glucose should generally be maintained at a level below 180 mg/dL, but excessively stringent control (glucose <100 mg/dL) may be more harmful than beneficial.[105–108]

V. Terminating Bypass

A. Before terminating bypass, the patient should be warmed toward normothermia (to at least 36 °C). Overwarming the patient with inflow temperatures greater than 38 °C should be avoided to avoid protein denaturation and potential cerebral damage. If significant hypothermia is used, the gradient between the arterial and venous return temperatures should be no more than 10–12 °C to minimize the formation of gaseous emboli. The rate of rewarming may also affect neurocognitive outcome.[109]

B. Once the heart is ready to come off bypass, the lungs are ventilated, taking care to identify the course of the internal thoracic artery (ITA) to avoid stretching of the pedicle. Pacing is initiated, if necessary. Calcium chloride 1 g may be given prior to coming off bypass to provide an increase in systemic vascular resistance and some inotropic support. The heart is filled by restricting venous return as bypass flow is reduced and turned off. Active root venting is used in cases of intracardiac entry (primarily valve operations) to evacuate any ejected air.

C. Cardiac performance is assessed by incorporating visual assessment with echocardiographic imaging, filling pressures, and cardiac output measurements. Inotropic support should be considered for marginal cardiac performance. Low systemic resistance is common and α-agents may be necessary to improve the blood pressure.

D. On rare occasions, the patient may manifest "vasoplegia", a condition of profound peripheral vasodilation despite adequate cardiac output. It is more frequently seen in patients on preoperative ACE inhibitors or ARBs, as well as those on amiodarone, which may be associated with α- and β-receptor blockade. If moderate doses of norepinephrine or phenylephrine are insufficient to combat the low systemic resistance, an infusion of vasopressin 0.01–0.07 units/min is usually successful in restoring the blood pressure.[110] Methylene blue (1–2 mg/kg) has also been used in this situation.[111,112] Terlipressin is a synthetic vasopressin analog available in Europe that is similarly useful in vasoplegic patients.[113,114]

E. When the patient is stable, protamine is administered to reverse heparin effect and should return the ACT to normal. The dosage is commonly based on a 1 : 1 mg:mg ratio to the administered heparin, although with use of the Hepcon system, which measures heparin levels, a heparin–protamine titration test can be used to determine the actual heparin concentration in the blood and the precise dose of protamine needed to reverse its effects. Protamine reactions are uncommon, but can be life-threatening (see pages 210–211). They require immediate attention, occasionally requiring reinstitution of bypass after additional administration of heparin.

F. The suction lines are turned off once the protamine administration has started. The venous line is usually removed first and drained into the cardiotomy reservoir. Blood may then be transfused through the arterial cannula as needed to maintain filling pressures. Once the aorta is decannulated and the patient is stable, the pump contents are drained into a cell-saving device, centrifuged, and made available in bags for the anesthesiologist to transfuse as necessary.

G. The cannulation sites are secured. Hemostasis is then achieved and the chest is closed.

VI. Potential Problems Encountered During Cardiopulmonary Bypass (Table 5.3)

A. Inadequate ACT from standard doses of heparin usually results from antithrombin (AT III) deficiency. Antithrombin is a major inhibitor of thrombin and factors Xa and IXa, and its deficiency leads to hypercoagulable states. The basis for anticoagulation with heparin is the rapid activation of antithrombin inhibitory activity. Antithrombin deficiency results in resistance to treatment with heparin and is noted most frequently in patients maintained preoperatively on heparin therapy or intravenous nitroglycerin or those with high platelet counts.[115] Additional administration of 1–2 mg/kg of heparin will usually achieve an adequate ACT. If not, antithrombin can be provided by transfusion of fresh frozen plasma or, if available, by a commercial AT III product (Thrombate III), which provides 500 units per vial.[116] Because preoperative AT III levels are rarely known, the exact dose required to reach 120% of normal, which is recommended, can only be estimated. Studies have shown successful elevation of the ACT using a wide dosage range of AT III doses to as high as 75 IU/kg.[116,117] The calculation of the amount needed equals the (desired − baseline AT III level) × weight (kg) divided by 1.4. For example, to reach 120% of normal levels in a 70 kg man with a baseline level that is 80% of normal would require [(120 − 80)/1.4] × 70 = 2000 IU (or 28 U/kg); if the baseline level is 50% of normal, 3500 units (50 U/kg) should be given.

Table 5.3 • Potential Problems on Pump

1. Inadequate heparinization (low ACT)
2. Inadequate venous drainage
3. Ventricular distention
4. Air entry into the venous lines
5. Inadequate systemic pressure
6. Inadequate systemic oxygenation
7. High arterial line pressure
8. Inadequate retrograde cardioplegia delivery
9. Systemic or coronary air embolism
10. Cold agglutinins

B. Inadequate venous drainage will be detected by the surgeon as a distended right heart and by the perfusionist as a drop in the blood level in the venous reservoir (which should trigger a low-volume alarm with use of hard shell reservoirs) with inability to maintain systemic flow rates. It may result from an airlock in the venous line, kinking of the line on the field or close to the reservoir, inadvertent clamping of the venous line, retraction of the heart impeding flow into the venous cannula, or malposition of the venous cannula (either being too far in or not far in enough). Inadequate venous drainage not only warms the heart during systemic hypothermia, potentially compromising myocardial protection, but it may adversely affect the organs that are not drained well. A high central venous pressure (CVP) may indicate impaired SVC drainage and can produce cerebral edema. More commonly, drainage from the IVC is impaired, which could result in renal impairment or hepatic or splanchnic congestion with significant fluid sequestration in the bowel. In this situation, the surgeon may note that the right atrium is well drained but the perfusionist notes a distinct reduction in venous return. Simply readjusting the depth of the IVC line usually resolves this issue. Rarely, when the SVC or IVC is snared with a tourniquet, the catheter may have inadvertently pulled back into the atrium, compromising virtually all flow into the venous lines.

C. Distention of the heart on bypass is indicative of poor venous drainage, aortic valve insufficiency, or tremendous collateral flow. It may stretch the ventricular fibers producing myocardial injury, increase PA pressures producing pulmonary barotrauma, or increase ventricular warming impairing myocardial protection. The cause of distention should be remedied, either by readjusting the venous lines and/or by placing a vent, either in the left ventricle or in the pulmonary artery.

D. Air entry into the venous lines usually arises from the venous cannulation site or the retrograde cardioplegia site, and can be controlled by an additional suture around the catheter. Rarely, it may result from inadvertent damage to the IVC or from an atrial septal defect. Air entrapment with use of vacuum assist can result in arterial gaseous embolization.[38–41]

E. Inadequate systemic pressures have been incriminated as the cause of multisystem organ dysfunction, including neurocognitive changes, renal failure, and splanchnic hypoperfusion. Whether low-flow or high-flow CPB is optimal for organ system protection is controversial, but a minimum pressure of 50–60 mm Hg should be maintained unless it is desired to intentionally maintain a higher pressure (e.g., the patient with significant uncorrected carotid disease or the hypertensive, diabetic patient with preexisting renal dysfunction). Phenylephrine or norepinephrine is commonly used on pump to maintain systemic pressures, accepting the transient dips that occur with cardioplegia infusion or reinfusion of shed blood aspirated through the cardiotomy suckers. However, adequate flow rates must be maintained, because α-agents will shunt blood away from the muscles and splanchnic circulation. Occasionally, in the patient on numerous antihypertensive medications, including ACE inhibitors, ARBs, amiodarone, and/or calcium channel blockers, a state of refractory hypotension exists. This state of autonomic dysfunction or "vasoplegia" may require the infusion of vasopressin to maintain blood pressure.[110] On rare occasions, methylene blue 1–2 mg/kg may be used to maintain blood pressure.[111,112]

F. **Inadequate systemic oxygenation** occurring on pump may result from failure of the oxygenator or oxygen blender, or disconnection from an oxygen source. It might also result from a catastrophic aortic dissection or malperfusion syndrome. Evidence of cerebral oxygen desaturation is first evident by cerebral oximetry, then by pulse oximetry, and eventually by systemic venous oxygen desaturation. Problems with the pump should be immediately recognizable by a change in the color of the blood in the arterial return line. A reduction in systemic oxygen delivery can be mitigated by improving the systemic flow rates and increasing the hematocrit. Mild systemic hypothermia can provide some element of organ system protection during the period of poor oxygenation as emergency steps are being taken by the perfusionist to correct the problem. On rare occasions, when the patient is no longer on pump, this may result from the anesthesiologist failing to provide ventilation to the patient (usually after the surgeon has asked that the lungs not be ventilated to improve exposure).

G. **High arterial line pressure** measured by the perfusionist is a potentially alarming situation. With pressurized roller pumps, this could result in a catastrophic line disconnection. With centrifugal pumps, which are afterload-sensitive, unsafe high line pressures should not occur because the pump head automatically reduces flow. A high line pressure caused by a high flow rate through a small cannula should not occur if the appropriately sized cannula is selected. For example, a 20 Fr curved-tip cannula may provide up to 5 L/min flow at acceptable line pressures, but excessive shear force with higher line pressures may be noted at higher flow rates. In contrast, a 7 or 8 mm Sarns Soft-Flow or Medtronic EOPA cannula can flow more than 6 L/min without producing high line pressures. Malposition of the tip of the aortic cannula, kinking or clamping of the line, or an aortic dissection can also account for a high line pressure. When a dissection occurs, the high line pressure is accompanied by very low systemic pressures, and mandates immediate cessation of pump flow and relocation of the arterial inflow cannula.

H. **Inadequate retrograde cardioplegia delivery** may produce inadequate myocardial protection. Low retrograde cardioplegia line pressures may be associated with rupture of the coronary sinus, a left SVC, or catheter displacement back into the right atrium.[118,119] High line pressures may be noted in patients with a small coronary sinus, impingement of the end of the catheter on the sinus wall, inadvertent clamping of the catheter, or kinking of the cardioplegia line or catheter. Placement too far into the sinus may reduce flow to the right ventricle and impair its protection. Filling of the posterior descending vein suggests that the right ventricle is being adequately protected, but this may not always be the case.

I. **Systemic or coronary air embolism** is always a possibility upon termination of bypass when there has been intracardiac entry, but its occurrence during bypass is a catastrophic problem.

1. Careful attention to deairing of the left heart chambers is important when there has been intracardiac entry (valve surgery) or active intracardiac or root venting. Ventilating the lungs, restricting venous return, and/or stopping vent return should be performed to evacuate air prior to closing the left atrium, left ventricle, or aorta. Needle aspiration of the left ventricle should be performed after aortic valve surgery. Carbon dioxide flooding of the field may minimize the amount of air retained during intracardiac procedures.[120] Active root venting upon termination of bypass

is mandatory to evacuate any ejected air, but it is not uncommon for some air to pass down the right coronary artery or an aortocoronary venous bypass graft and cause right ventricular dysfunction upon weaning from bypass. This problem usually resolves quickly, but bypass should be reinstituted if hemodynamics are compromised. TEE monitoring is the best means of identifying retained air as the heart is weaned from bypass.

2. Systemic air embolism occurring during CPB is usually related to inattention to the venous reservoir level in open circuits with delivery of air through a roller pump head. It may also occur with use of vacuum-assisted drainage. Air embolism may also occur on bypass when the aorta is not clamped and air trapped in the left heart is ejected when the pressure generated by the left ventricle exceeds that in the aorta. Significant air embolism requires cessation of bypass with immediate venting of air from the aorta with a needle or through a stopcock on the aortic line and then removal of air from the bypass circuit. Ventilation with 100% oxygen, steep Trendelenburg position, and retrograde SVC perfusion should be used to try to eliminate air from the cerebral circulation. Steroids, barbiturates, and reinstitution of bypass with deep hypothermia may also reduce the degree of cerebral injury.[121,122]

3. Systemic air embolism may occur if there is air entry into the inflow drainage lines of an assist device, because there is no reservoir or means available for venting or filtration of the air. The air will fragment and be pumped back into the arterial system.

J. **Cold-reactive autoimmune diseases** are rarely detected preoperatively but may result in red cell agglutination and hemolysis on bypass at cold temperatures. This may be noted in the bypass or cardioplegia circuit.[123]

1. Cold hemagglutinin disease is caused by an IgM autoimmune antibody that causes red cell agglutination and hemolysis at cold temperatures. This may cause microvascular thrombosis that may contribute to myocardial infarction, renal failure, or other organ system failure. Since less than 1% of patients have cold agglutinins, screening is not routinely performed, and it rarely poses a problem during bypass because hemodilution lowers antibody titers. However, should antibody titers be measured and be in high concentration ($> 1:1000$), agglutination will occur at warmer temperatures.

2. If high-titer agglutinins are present, systemic hypothermia and cold blood cardioplegia must be avoided. Either warm cardioplegia or cold crystalloid cardioplegia after an initial normothermic flush can be used. Even better would be performance of off-pump coronary bypass surgery or on-pump beating- or fibrillating-heart surgery.

3. De novo discovery of cold agglutinins may occur on-pump by detecting agglutination and sedimentation in the blood cardioplegia heat exchanger or any stagnant line containing blood. It has also been identified when the retrograde cardioplegia line develops high pressure due to obstruction from agglutination. In these circumstances, the patient should be warmed back to normothermia, and crystalloid cardioplegia used to flush out the coronary arteries.

4. Paroxysmal cold hemoglobinuria (PCH) is an autoimmune disease in which a nonagglutinating IgG antibody binds to red cells in the cold causing hemolysis. It should be managed in a similar fashion.[124]

VII. Special Types of Extracorporeal Circulation

A. **Deep hypothermic circulatory arrest** (DHCA) is used primarily in situations when the aorta cannot be clamped to perform an aortic anastomosis.

1. Indications for DHCA include:

   a. Severe aortic atherosclerosis or calcification (porcelain aorta for aortic valve replacement) (Figure 2.9, page 100)

   b. Avoidance of aortic wall damage and improved distal anastomosis (type A dissections)

   c. Clamp placement too close to a planned suture line – ascending aortic or hemiarch repairs, arch repair, proximal descending thoracic aneurysms

   d. Complex descending thoracic aortic surgery to improve anastomotic exposure while providing neuroprotection for the brain and/or spinal cord

   e. Resection of IVC tumors

2. With traditional DHCA, the patient is cooled systemically to 18 °C to achieve electroencephalographic (EEG) silence. The temperature is measured at multiple sites, including the tympanic membrane, nasopharynx, bladder and/or rectum, with the presumption that this will ensure uniform cooling of the cerebral cortex. Since an EEG is usually not performed, surgeons rely on clinical studies that have shown that about 45 minutes of DHCA at 18 °C is safe in minimizing cerebral damage.[125] The head is packed in ice, and methylprednisolone 20 mg/kg is also given. The arterial line is clamped and blood is drained from the circulation, taking care not to allow air entry in the lines.

3. Near-infrared spectroscopy usually shows an increase in rSO_2 as the patient is cooled systemically, but it usually falls during the first 5 minutes of DHCA. If the rSO_2 has not reached a steady state > 90% of baseline despite reaching the desired temperature, a few additional minutes of cooling may be beneficial.[126]

4. Measures that may extend the acceptable period of DHCA include antegrade or retrograde cerebral perfusion.

   a. **Antegrade cerebral perfusion** (ACP) provides flow into the arch vessels during the period of circulatory arrest and provides oxygenated blood to the brain. This may allow for use of higher systemic temperatures at the time when DHCA is initiated without an added risk of cerebral damage.[127]

      i. Axillary artery cannulation with occlusion of the proximal innominate artery can provide flow to the right side of the brain, and, through the circle of Willis, to the left side. It may be augmented by a catheter placed into the left common carotid artery (LCCA).[128] Generally, infusing arterial blood at a rate of 10 mL/kg at a pressure of 50 mm Hg appears to give the best protection.[129]

      ii. If the patient is undergoing aortic arch reconstruction, use of a trifurcation graft sewn to the arch vessels can minimize the time when there is no cerebral perfusion and can potentially shorten the duration of DHCA. The brain can then be perfused and the patient warmed while the distal aortic anastomosis is performed. The proximal end of the trifurcation graft is then sewn off the proximal aortic graft (Figure 1.23, page 53).[130]

    b. Retrograde cerebral perfusion (RCP) provides oxygenated, cold blood into the SVC at a flow rate up to 500 mL/min and a pressure of up to 20 mm Hg. Studies suggest that this is not effective in providing nutrients to the brain, but can maintain cerebral hypothermia. Although this is an effective technique for neuroprotection, it is probably best used when the duration of DHCA will not be prolonged much beyond 45 minutes. RCP is beneficial in flushing air and debris out of the cerebral vessels.[131,132]

  5. Extensive cooling and rewarming are often associated with a coagulopathy that may require blood-product transfusions. Warming generally takes twice as long as cooling, and the gradient between the arterial inflow and the patient's temperature should be no more than $10-12\,°C$ to prevent generation of gaseous emboli.

  6. When bypass flow is reinstituted, care must be taken to eliminate any air or atherosclerotic debris from the arterial tree.

B. Left-heart bypass for thoracic aortic surgery

  1. Impairment of blood supply to the lower body is inherent to any aortic procedure involving descending aortic cross-clamping. The greatest risks are those of paraplegia and renal dysfunction. Left-heart bypass entails drainage of oxygenated blood from the left side of the heart and returning it more distally in the arterial tree (Figure 5.11).[133,134]

  2. Inflow to a centrifugal pump may come from the left atrium or preferentially from the inferior pulmonary vein, which may be associated with fewer complications.[135] The blood is returned either to the femoral artery or to the distal aorta below the lowest clamp in patients with limited disease (such as traumatic tears or Crawford type I aneurysms (Figure 1.22, page 51). The blood does not pass through an oxygenator, although one can be placed in the circuit to improve oxygenation during one-lung anesthesia.[136]

  3. Minimal heparinization is necessary for this setup (about 5000 units to achieve an ACT of 250 seconds), which is beneficial in trauma cases or cases requiring extensive dissection. Flow rates of up to 3 L/min can be used, with monitoring of lower-extremity mean pressures in the femoral artery that should approximate 50 mm Hg. Drainage should not be so excessive as to compromise antegrade flow from the heart to the brain.

C. Assisted right-heart bypass for off-pump surgery. During manipulation of the heart for off-pump surgery, especially with hypertrophied hearts, there may be compromise of right ventricular filling. Several devices have been designed that provide right-heart assist by draining blood from the right atrium and pumping it into the pulmonary artery during these procedures.[137]

D. Perfusion-assisted direct coronary artery bypass (PADCAB). During off-pump surgery, there is compromise of distal flow during temporary vessel occlusion required for construction of an anastomosis. This may lead to a subtle or severe degree of ischemia and potential myocardial necrosis. Intracoronary or aortocoronary shunts can be used to provide distal perfusion when constructing the anastomosis, either routinely or if there is evidence of ischemia.[138] PADCAB provides perfusion-assisted flow at a designated pressure (usually 120 mm Hg) that is independent of the systemic blood pressure. Additionally, medications such as nitroglycerin can be administered in the perfusate to provide coronary vasodilation. Placing a small

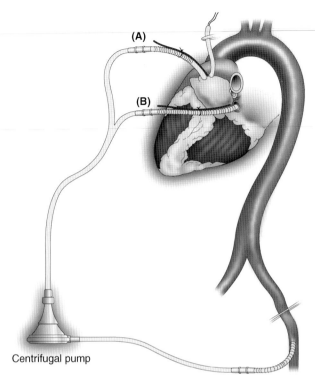

Centrifugal pump

Figure 5.11 • Left-heart bypass setup. Inflow to the pump comes from either the left atrial appendage (A) or the left inferior pulmonary vein (B). Blood is then returned by a centrifugal pump to the femoral artery or to the distal aorta in cases of limited disease, such as traumatic tears of the aorta.

catheter directly into the coronary artery allows for distal perfusion as the anastomosis is being constructed. Subsequently, flow can be directed through 2–3 mm cannulas placed into the conduits until the proximal anastomoses are performed. A comparative study of no shunting, passive shunting, and active perfusion showed that myocardial protection (measured by troponin levels) and performance was superior with active perfusion.[139]

E. **Extracorporeal membrane oxygenation (ECMO)** is a means of providing a prolonged period of cardiopulmonary bypass. It is applicable to patients with severe hypoxemic respiratory failure as well as those with severe myocardial dysfunction associated with hypoxemia. The latter requires arteriovenous access, with the arterial line usually placed through a side graft sewn to the femoral artery to ensure distal perfusion of the leg, and venous cannulas in the femoral and/or jugular vein. Either arteriovenous or venovenous access can be used in the patient with respiratory failure. The system should include a centrifugal pump, a heparin-coated circuit to minimize systemic heparinization requirements, a specially designed membrane oxygenator capable of providing several days to weeks of support without producing cellular destruction, and a warming unit. One ECMO system produced by Maquet Cardiopulmonary includes the QUADROX PLS oxygenator, ROTAFLOW RF 32 centrifugal pump, and the HU 35 Heater unit (see www. maquet.com). ECMO is discussed in more detail on pages 483–484.[140]

F. **Ventricular assist devices (VADs)** consist of extracardiac circuits and pumps that provide hemodynamic support to patients with severe ventricular dysfunction. This may be noted with postinfarction or postcardiotomy cardiogenic shock, or in patients with end-stage heart failure. These devices may be used as a bridge to recovery or transplantation, or for destination therapy in patients with end-stage heart failure who are not transplant candidates. They function solely for hemodynamic support since they do not provide oxygenation. Use of assist devices is discussed more extensively on pages 478–494.

References

1. Levy JH, Tanaka KA. Inflammatory response to cardiopulmonary bypass. *Ann Thorac Surg* 2003;75: S715–20.

2. Shann KG, Likosky DS, Murkin JM, et al. An evidence-based review of the practice of cardiopulmonary bypass in adults: a focus on neurologic injury, glycemic control, hemodilution, and the inflammatory response. *J Thorac Cardiovasc Surg* 2006;132:283–90.

3. Elahi MM, Yii M, Matata BM. Significance of oxidants and inflammatory mediators in blood of patients undergoing cardiac surgery. *J Cardiothorac Vasc Anesth* 2008;22:455–67.

4. Edmunds LH, Coleman RW. Thrombin during cardiopulmonary bypass. *Ann Thorac Surg* 2006;82:3215–22.

5. Raivio P, Lassila R, Petäjä J. Thrombin in myocardial ischemia-reperfusion during cardiac surgery. *Ann Thorac Surg* 2009;88:318–25.

6. Baufreton C, Intrator L, Jansen PGM, et al. Inflammatory response to cardiopulmonary bypass using roller or centrifugal pumps. *Ann Thorac Surg* 1999;67:972–7.

7. DioDato CP, Likosky DS, DeFoe GR, et al. Cardiopulmonary bypass recommendations in adults: the northern New England experience. *J Extra Corpor Technol* 2008;40:16–20.

8. Whitlock RP, Chan S, Devereaux PJ, et al. Clinical benefit of steroid use in patients undergoing cardiopulmonary bypass: a meta-analysis of randomized trials. *Eur Heart J* 2008;29:2592–600.

9. Kilger E, Weis F, Briegel J, et al. Stress doses of hydrocortisone reduce severe systemic inflammatory response syndrome and improve early outcome in a risk group of patients after cardiac surgery. *Crit Care Med* 2003;31:1068–74.

10. Senay S, Toraman F, Gunaydin S, Kilercik M, Karabulut H, Alhan C. The impact of allogenic red cell transfusion and coated bypass circuit on the inflammatory response during cardiopulmonary bypass: a randomized study. *Interact Cardiovasc Thorac Surg* 2009;8:93–9.

11. Boodram S, Evans E. Use of leukocyte-depleting filters during cardiac surgery with cardiopulmonary bypass: a review. *J Extra Corpor Technol* 2008;40:27–42.

12. Warren O, Alexiou C, Massey R, et al. The effects of various leukocyte filtration strategies in cardiac surgery. *Eur J Cardiothorac Surg* 2007;31:665–76.

13. Warren OJ, Tunnicliffe CR, Massey RM, et al. Systemic leukofiltration does not attenuate pulmonary injury after cardiopulmonary bypass. *ASAIO J* 2008;54:78–88.

14. Leal-Noval SR, Amaya R, Herruzo A, et al. Effects of a leukocyte depleting arterial line filter on perioperative morbidity in patients undergoing cardiac surgery: a controlled randomized trial. *Ann Thorac Surg* 2005;80:1394–400.

15. Ranucci M, Balduini A, Ditta A, Boncilli A, Brozzi S. A systematic review of biocompatible cardiopulmonary bypass circuits and clinical outcome. *Ann Thorac Surg* 2009;87:1311–9.

16. Jensen E, Andréasson S, Bengtsson A, et al. Influence of two different perfusion systems on inflammatory response in pediatric heart surgery. *Ann Thorac Surg* 2003;75:919–25.

17. Mangoush O, Purkayastha S, Haj-Yahia S, et al. Heparin-bonded circuits versus nonheparin-bonded circuits: an evaluation of their effect on clinical outcomes. *Eur J Cardiothorac Surg* 2007;31:1058–69.

18. Svenmaker S, Häggmark S, Jansson E, et al. Use of heparin-bonded circuits in cardiopulmonary bypass improves clinical outcome. *Scand Cardiovasc J* 2002;36:241–6.

19. Ikuta T, Fujii H, Shibata T, et al. A new poly-2-methoxyethylacrylate-coated cardiopulmonary bypass circuit possesses superior platelet preservation and inflammatory suppression efficacy. *Ann Thorac Surg* 2004;77:1678–83.

20. Hoel TN, Videm V, Baksaas ST, Mollnes TE, Brosstad F, Svennevig JL. Comparison of a Duraflo II-coated cardiopulmonary bypass circuit and a trillium-coated oxygenator during open-heart surgery. *Perfusion* 2004;19:177–84.

21. Kutay V, Noyan T, Ozcan S, Melek Y, Ekim H, Yakut C. Biocompatibility of heparin-coated cardiopulmonary bypass circuits in coronary patients with left ventricular dysfunction is superior to PMEA-coated circuits. *J Card Surg* 2006;21:572–7.

22. Ask A, Holt D, Smith L. *In vivo* comparison of FDA-approved surface-modifying additives and poly-2-methoxyethylacrylate circuit surfaces coatings during cardiopulmonary bypass. *J Extra Corpor Technol* 2006;38:27–32.

23. Mirow N, Zittermann A, Koertke H, et al. Heparin-coated extracorporeal circulation in combination with low dose systemic heparinization reduces early postoperative blood loss in cardiac surgery. *J Cardiovasc Surg (Torino)* 2008;49:277–84.

24. Kuitunen AH, Heikkilä LJ, Salmenperä MT. Cardiopulmonary bypass with heparin-coated circuits and reduced systemic anticoagulation. *Ann Thorac Surg* 1997;63:438–44.

25. Øvrum E, Brosstad F, Holen EA, Tangen G, Abdelnoor M. Effects on coagulation and fibrinolysis with reduced versus full systemic heparinization and heparin-coated cardiopulmonary bypass. *Circulation* 1995;92:2579–84.

26. Kumano H, Suehiro S, Hattori K, et al. Coagulofibrinolysis during heparin-coated cardiopulmonary bypass with reduced heparinization. *Ann Thorac Surg* 1999;68:1252–6.

27. Kaplan M, Cimen S, Demirtas MM. Effects of different pump prime solutions on postoperative fluid balance and hemostasis. *Chest* 2001;120:172S.

28. Wilkes MM, Navickis RJ, Sibbald WJ. Albumin versus hydroxyethyl starch in cardiopulmonary bypass surgery: a meta-analysis of postoperative bleeding. *Ann Thorac Surg* 2001;72:527–34.

29. Hecht-Dolnik M, Barkan H, Taharka A, Loftus J. Hetastarch increases the risk of bleeding complications in patients after off-pump coronary bypass surgery: a randomized clinical trial. *J Thorac Cardiovasc Surg* 2009;138:703–11.

30. Haynes GR, Havidich JE, Payne KJ. Why the Food and Drug Administration changed the warning label for hetastarch. *Anesthesiology* 2004;101:560–1.

31. Formica G, Broccolo F, Martino A, et al. Myocardial revascularization with miniaturized extracorporeal circulation versus offpump: evaluation of systemic and myocardial inflammatory response in a prospective randomized study. *J Thorac Cardiovasc Surg* 2009;137:1206–12.

32. Willcox TW, Mitchell SJ, Gorman DF. Venous air in the bypass circuit: a source of arterial line emboli exacerbated by vacuum-assisted drainage. *Ann Thorac Surg* 1999;68:1285–9.

33. Zangrillo A, Garozzo FA, Biondi-Zoccai G, et al. Miniaturized cardiopulmonary bypass improves short-term outcome in cardiac surgery: a meta-analysis of randomized controlled studies. *J Thorac Cardiovasc Surg* 2010;139:1162–9.

34. Issitt RW, Mulholland JW, Oliver MD, et al. Aortic surgery using total miniaturized cardiopulmonary bypass. *Ann Thorac Surg* 2008;86:627–31.

35. Nollert G, Schwabenland I, Maktav D, et al. Miniaturized cardiopulmonary bypass in coronary artery bypass surgery: marginal impact on inflammation and coagulation but loss of safety margins. *Ann Thorac Surg* 2005;80:2326–32.

36. Colangelo N, Torracca L, Lapenna E, Moriggia S, Crescenzi G, Alfieri O. Vacuum-assisted venous drainage in extrathoracic cardiopulmonary bypass management during minimally invasive cardiac surgery. *Perfusion* 2006;21:361–5.

37. Murai N, Cho M, Okada S, et al. Venous drainage method for cardiopulmonary bypass in single-access minimally invasive cardiac surgery: siphon and vacuum-assisted drainage. *J Artif Organs* 2005;8:91–4.

38. Cirri S, Negri L, Babbini M, et al. Haemolysis due to active venous drainage during cardiopulmonary bypass: comparison of two different techniques. *Perfusion* 2001;16:313–8.

39. LaPietra A, Grossi EA, Pua BB, et al. Assisted venous drainage presents the risk of undetected air microembolism. *J Thorac Cardiovasc Surg* 2000;120:856–63.

40. Willcox TW, Mitchell SJ, Gorman DF. Venous air in the bypass circuit: a source of arterial line emboli exacerbated by vacuum-assisted drainage. *Ann Thorac Surg* 1999;68:1285–9.

41. Jegger D, Tevaearai HT, Mueller XM, Horisberger J, von Segesser LK. Limitations using the vacuum-assist venous drainage technique during cardiopulmonary bypass procedures. *J Extra Corpor Technol* 2003;35:207–11.

42. Wang S, Undar A. Vacuum-assisted venous drainage and gaseous microemboli in cardiopulmonary bypass. *J Extra Corpor Technol* 2008;40:249–56.

43. Carrier M, Cyr A, Voisine P, et al. Vacuum-assisted venous drainage does not increase the neurological risk. *Heart Surg Forum* 2002;5:285–8.

44. Scott DA, Silbert BS, Blyth C, O'Brien J, Santamaria J. Blood loss in elective coronary artery surgery: a comparison of centrifugal versus roller pump heads during cardiopulmonary bypass. *J Cardiothorac Vasc Anesth* 2001;15:322–5.

45. Fabre O, Vincentelli A, Corseaux D, et al. Comparison of blood activation in the wound, active vent, and cardiopulmonary bypass circuit. *Ann Thorac Surg* 2008;86:537–42.

46. Westerberg M, Bengstsson A, Jeppsson A. Coronary surgery without cardiotomy suction and autotransfusion reduces the postoperative systemic inflammatory response. *Ann Thorac Surg* 2004;78:54–9.

47. Tabuchi N, de Hann J, Boonstra PW, van Oeveren W. Activation of fibrinolysis in the pericardial cavity during cardiopulmonary bypass. *J Thorac Cardiovasc Surg* 1993;106:828–33.

48. Johnell M, Elgue G, Larsson R, Larsson A, Thelin S, Siegbahn A. Coagulation, fibrinolysis, and cell activation in patients and shed mediastinal blood during coronary artery bypass grafting with a new heparin-coated surface. *J Thorac Cardiovasc Surg* 2002;124:321–32.

49. De Somer F, Van Belleghem Y, Caes F, et al. Tissue factor as the main activator of the coagulation system during cardiopulmonary bypass. *J Thorac Cardiovasc Surg* 2002;123:951–8.

50. Aldea GS, Soltow LO, Chandler WL, et al. Limitation of thrombin generation, platelet activation, and inflammation by elimination of cardiotomy suction in patients undergoing coronary artery bypass grafting treated with heparin-coated circuits. *J Thorac Cardiovasc Surg* 2002;123:742–55.

51. Carrier M, Denault A, Lavoie J, Perrault LP. Randomized controlled trial of pericardial blood processing with a cell-saving device on neurologic markers in elderly patients undergoing coronary artery bypass surgery. *Ann Thorac Surg* 2006;82:51–5.

52. Marcheix B, Carrier M, Martel C, et al. Effect of pericardial blood processing on postoperative inflammation and the complement pathways. *Ann Thorac Surg* 2008;85:530–5.

53. Kaza AK, Cope JT, Fiser SM, et al. Elimination of fat microemboli during cardiopulmonary bypass. *Ann Thorac Surg* 2003;75:555–9.

54. Jewell AE, Akowuah EF, Suvarna SK, Braidley P, Hopkinson D, Cooper G. A prospective randomised comparison of cardiotomy suction and cell saver for recycling shed blood during cardiac surgery. *Eur J Cardiothorac Surg* 2003;23:633–6.

55. Westerberg M, Gäbel J, Bengtsson A, Sellgren J, Eidem O, Jeppsson A. Hemodynamic effects of cardiotomy suction blood. *J Thorac Cardiovasc Surg* 2006;131:1352–7.

56. Vanden Eynden F, Carrier M, Ouellet S, et al. Avecor Trillium oxygenator versus noncoated Monolyth oxygenator: a prospective randomized controlled study. *J Card Surg* 2008;23:288–93.

57. De Somer F. Impact of oxygenator characteristics on its capability to remove gaseous microemboli. *J Extra Corpor Technol* 2007;39:271–3.

58. Boodhwani M, Hamilton A, de Varennes B, et al. A multicenter randomized controlled trial to assess the feasibility of testing modified ultrafiltration as a blood conservation technology in cardiac surgery. *J Thorac Cardiovasc Surg* 2010;139:701–6.

59. Grooters RK, Ver Steeg DA, Stewart MJ, Thieman KC, Schneider RF. Echocardiographic comparison of the standard end-hole cannula, the soft-flow cannula, and the dispersion cannula during perfusion into the aortic arch. *Ann Thorac Surg* 2003;75:1919–23.

60. Weinstein GS. Left hemispheric strokes in coronary surgery: implications for end-hole aortic cannulas. *Ann Thorac Surg* 2001;71:128–32.

61. Sobielski MA 2nd, Pappas PS, Tatooles AJ, Slaughter MS. Embol-X intra-aortic filtration system: capturing particulate emboli in the cardiac surgery patient. *J Extra Corpor Technol* 2005;37:222–6.

62. Borger MA, Taylor RL, Weisel RD, et al. Decreased cerebral emboli during distal aortic arch cannulation: a randomized clinical trial. *J Thorac Cardiovasc Surg* 1999;118:740–5.

63. Slaughter MS, Sobieski MA, Tatooles AJ, Pappas PS. Reducing emboli during cardiac surgery: does it make a difference? *Artif Organs* 2008;32:880–4.

64. Djaiani G, Ali M, Borger MA, et al. Epiaortic scanning modifies planned intraoperative surgical management but not cerebral embolic load during coronary artery bypass surgery. *Anesth Analg* 2008;106:1611–8.

65. Gates JD, Bichell DP, Rizzo RJ, Couper GS, Donaldson MC. Thigh ischemia complicating femoral vessel cannulation for cardiopulmonary bypass. *Ann Thorac Surg* 1996;61:730–3.

66. James T, Friedman SG, Scher L, Hall M. Lower extremity compartment syndrome after coronary artery bypass. *J Vasc Surg* 2002;36:1069–70.

67. Alameddine AK. Lower limb ischemia with compartment syndrome related to femoral artery cannulas. *Ann Thorac Surg* 1997;64:884–5.

68. Vander Salm TJ. Prevention of lower extremity ischemia during cardiopulmonary bypass via femoral cannulation. *Ann Thorac Surg* 1997;63:251–2.

69. Hendrickson SC, Glower DD. A method for perfusion of the leg during cardiopulmonary bypass via femoral cannulation. *Ann Thorac Surg* 1998;65:1807–8.

70. Sinclair MC, Singer RL, Manley NJ, Montesano RM. Cannulation of the axillary artery for cardiopulmonary bypass: safeguards and pitfalls. *Ann Thorac Surg* 2003;75:931–4.

71. Etz CD, Plestis KA, Kari FA, et al. Axillary cannulation significantly improves survival and neurologic outcome after atherosclerotic aneurysm repair of the aortic root and ascending aorta. *Ann Thorac Surg* 2008;86:441–7.

72. Ogino H, Sasaki H, Minatoya K, et al. Evolving arch surgery using integrated antegrade selective cerebral perfusion: impact of axillary artery perfusion. *J Thorac Cardiovasc Surg* 2008;136:641–8.

73. Malvindi PG, Scrascia G, Vitale N. Is unilateral antegrade cerebral perfusion equivalent to bilateral cerebral perfusion for patients undergoing aortic arch surgery? *Interact Cardiovasc Thorac Surg* 2008;7:891–7.

74. Koster A, Fischer T, Praus M, et al. Hemostatic activation and inflammatory response during cardiopulmonary bypass. Impact of heparin management. *Anesthesiology* 2002;97:837–41.

75. Rosengart TK, DeBois W, O'Hara M, et al. Retrograde autologous priming for cardiopulmonary bypass. A safe and effective means of decreasing hemodilution and transfusion requirements. *J Thorac Cardiovasc Surg* 1998;115:426–39.

76. Eising GP, Pfauder M, Niemeyer M, et al. Retrograde autologous priming: is it useful in elective on-pump coronary artery bypass surgery? *Ann Thorac Surg* 2003;75:23–7.

77. Murphy GS, Szokol KW, Nitsun M, et al. Retrograde autologous priming of the cardiopulmonary bypass circuit: safety and impact on postoperative outcomes. *J Cardiothorac Vasc Anesth* 2006;20:156–61.

78. Saczkowski RS, Bernier PL, Tchervenkov CI, Arellano R. Retrograde autologous priming and allogeneic blood transfusions in adults: a meta-analysis. *Interact Cardiovasc Thorac Surg* 2008;8:373–6.

79. DiNardo JA, Wegner JA. Pro: low-flow cardiopulmonary bypass is the preferred technique for patients undergoing cardiac surgical procedures. *J Cardiothorac Vasc Anesth* 2001;15:649–51.

80. De Somer F. What is the optimal flow rate and how to validate this. *J Extra Corpor Technol* 2007;39:278–80.

81. Boston US, Slater JM, Orszulak TA, Cook DJ. Hierarchy of regional oxygen delivery during cardiopulmonary bypass. *Ann Thorac Surg* 2001;71:260–4.

82. Andersson LG, Bratteby LE, Ekroth R, et al. Renal function during cardiopulmonary bypass: influence of pump flow and systemic blood pressure. *Eur J Cardiothorac Surg* 1994;8:597–602.

83. Cook DJ. Con: low-flow cardiopulmonary bypass is not the preferred technique for patients undergoing cardiac surgical procedures. *J Cardiothorac Vasc Anesth* 2001;15:652–4.

84. Sirvinskas E, Andrejaitiene J, Raliene L, et al. Cardiopulmonary bypass management and acute renal failure: risk factors and prognosis. *Perfusion* 2008;23:323–7.

85. Karkouti K, Beattie WS, Wijeysundera DN, et al. Hemodilution during cardiopulmonary bypass is an independent risk factor for acute renal failure in adult cardiac surgery. *J Thorac Cardiovasc Surg* 2005;129:391–400.

86. Habib RH, Zacharias A, Schwann TA, et al. Role of hemodilutional anemia and transfusion during cardiopulmonary bypass in renal injury after coronary revascularization: implications on operative outcome. *Crit Care Med* 2005;33:1749–56.

87. Habib RH, Zacharias A, Schwann TA, Riordan DJ, Durham SJ, Shah A. Adverse effects of low hematocrit during cardiopulmonary bypass in the adult: should current practice be changed? *J Thorac Cardiovasc Surg* 2003;125:1438–50.

88. Ranucci M, Romitti F, Isgrò G, et al. Oxygen delivery during cardiopulmonary bypass and acute renal failure after coronary operations. *Ann Thorac Surg* 2005;80:2213–20.

89. Croughwell N, Lyth M, Quill TJ, et al. Diabetic patients have abnormal cerebral autoregulation during cardiopulmonary bypass. *Circulation* 1990;82(5 Suppl):IV-407–12.

90. Schwartz AE, Sandhu AA, Kaplon RJ, et al. Cerebral blood flow is determined by arterial pressure and not cardiopulmonary bypass flow rate. *Ann Thorac Surg* 1995;60:165–70.

91. Tobias JD. Cerebral oximetry monitoring with near infrared spectroscopy detects alterations in oxygenation before pulse oximetry. *J Intensive Care Med* 2008;23:384–8.

92. Slater JP, Guarino T, Stack J, et al. Cerebral oxygen desaturation predicts cognitive decline and longer hospital stay after cardiac surgery. *Ann Thorac Surg* 2009;87:36–45.

93. Kalyani SD, Miller NR, Dong LM, Baumgartner WA, Alejo DE, Gilbert TB. Incidence of and risk factors for perioperative optic neuropathy after cardiac surgery. *Ann Thorac Surg* 2004;78:34–7.

94. Ranucci M, Conti D, Castelvecchio S, et al. Hematocrit on cardiopulmonary bypass and outcome after coronary surgery in nontransfused patients. *Ann Thorac Surg* 2010;89:11–8.

95. Ranucci M. Perioperative renal failure: hypoperfusion during cardiopulmonary bypass? *Semin Cardiothorac Vasc Anesth* 2007;11:265–8.

96. Speiss BD. Blood transfusions: the silent epidemic. *Ann Thorac Surg* 2001;72:S1832–7.

97. Engelman RM, Pleet AB, Rousou JA, et al. Influence of cardiopulmonary bypass perfusion temperature on neurologic and hematologic function after coronary artery bypass grafting. *Ann Thorac Surg* 1999;67:1547–56.

98. Gaudino M, Zamparelli R, Andreotti F, et al. Normothermia does not improve postoperative hemostasis nor does it reduce inflammatory activation in patients undergoing primary isolated coronary artery bypass. *J Thorac Cardiovasc Surg* 2002;123:1092–100.

99. Ng CSH, Arifi AA, Wan S, et al. Ventilation during cardiopulmonary bypass: impact on cytokine response and cardiopulmonary function. *Ann Thorac Surg* 2008;85:154–62.

100. Gabriel EA, Fagionato Locali R, Katsumi Matsuoka P, et al. Lung perfusion during cardiac surgery with cardiopulmonary bypass: is it necessary? *Interact Cardiovasc Thorac Surg* 2008;7:1089–95.

101. Demers P, Elkouri S, Martineau R, Couturier A, Cartier R. Outcome with high blood lactate levels during cardiopulmonary bypass in adult cardiac operation. *Ann Thorac Surg* 2000;70:2082–6.

102. Ranucci M, De Toffol B, Isgrò G, Romitti F, Conti D, Vicentini M. Hyperlactatemia during cardiopulmonary bypass: determinants and impact on postoperative outcome. *Crit Care* 2006;10:R167.

103. Patel RL, Turtle MR, Chambers DJ, James DN, Newman S, Venn GE. Alpha-stat acid–base regulation during cardiopulmonary bypass improves neuropsychological outcome in patients undergoing coronary artery bypass grafting. *J Thorac Cardiovasc Surg* 1996;111:1267–79.

104. Dahlbacka S, Alaoja H, Mäkelä J, et al. Effects of pH management during selective antegrade cerebral perfusion on cerebral microcirculation and metabolism: alpha-stat versus pH-stat. *Ann Thorac Surg* 2007;84:847–56.

105. Gandhi GY, Nuttall GA, Abel MD, et al. Intensive intraoperative insulin therapy versus conventional glucose management during cardiac surgery: a randomized trial. *Ann Intern Med* 2007;146:233–43.

106. Gandhi GY, Nuttall GA, Abel MD, et al. Intraoperative hyperglycemia and perioperative outcome in cardiac surgery patients. *Mayo Clin Proc* 2005;80:862–6.

107. Knapik P, Nadziakiewicz P, Urbanska E, Saucha W, Herdynska M, Zembala M. Cardiopulmonary bypass increases postoperative glycemia and insulin consumption after coronary surgery. *Ann Thorac Surg* 2009;87:1859–65.

108. Doenst T, Wijeysundera D, Karkouti K, et al. Hyperglycemia during cardiopulmonary bypass is an independent risk factor for mortality in patients undergoing cardiac surgery. *J Thorac Cardiovasc Surg* 2005;130:1144–50.

109. Grigore AM, Grocott HP, Mathew JP, et al. The rewarming rate and increased peak temperature alter neurocognitive outcome after cardiac surgery. *Anesth Analg* 2002;94:4–10.

110. Tayama E, Ueda T, Shojima T, et al. Arginine vasopressin is an ideal drug after cardiac surgery for the management of low systemic vascular resistant hypotension concomitant with pulmonary hypertension. *Interact Cardiovasc Thorac Surg* 2007;6:715–9.

111. Leyh RG, Kofidis T, Struber M, et al. Methylene blue: the drug of choice for catecholamine-refractory vasoplegia after cardiopulmonary bypass? *J Thorac Cardiovasc Surg* 2003;125:1426–31.

112. Shanmugam G. Vasoplegic syndrome – the role of methylene blue. *Eur J Cardiothorac Surg* 2005;28:705–10.

113. Kunstyr J, Lincova D, Mourad M, et al. A retrospective analysis of Terlipressin infusion in patients with refractory hypotension after cardiac surgery. *J Cardiovasc Surg (Torino)* 2008;49:381–7.

114. Singer M. Arginine vasopressin vs. terlipressin the treatment of shock states. *Best Pract Res Clin Anaesthesiol* 2008;22:359–68.

115. Ranucci M, Ingrò G, Cazzaniga A, Soro G, Menicanti L, Frigiola A. Predictors for heparin resistance in patients undergoing coronary artery bypass grafting. *Perfusion* 1999;14:437–42.

116. Spiess BD. Treating heparin resistance with antithrombin or fresh frozen plasma. *Ann Thorac Surg* 2008;85:2153–60.

117. Avidan MS, Levy JH, van Aken H, et al. Recombinant human antithrombin III restores heparin responsiveness and decreases activation of coagulation in heparin-resistant patients during cardiopulmonary bypass. *J Thorac Cardiovasc Surg* 2005;130:107–13.

118. Langenberg CJ, Pietersen HG, Geskes G, Wagenmakers AJM, Soeters PB, Durieux M. Coronary sinus catheter placement. Assessment of placement criteria and cardiac complications. *Chest* 2003;124:1259–65.

119. Economopoulos GC, Michalis A, Palatianos GM, Sarris GE. Management of catheter-related injuries to the coronary sinus. *Ann Thorac Surg* 2003;76:112–6.

120. Webb WR, Harrison LH Jr, Helmcke FR, et al. Carbon dioxide field flooding minimizes residual intracardiac air after open heart operations. *Ann Thorac Surg* 1997;64:1489–91.

121. Mills NL, Ochsner JL. Massive air embolism during cardiopulmonary bypass. *J Thorac Cardiovasc Surg* 1980;80:708–17.

122. Guy TS, Kelly MP, Cason B, Tseng E. Retrograde cerebral perfusion and delayed hyperbaric oxygen for massive air embolism during cardiac surgery. *Interact Cardiovasc Thorac Surg* 2008;8:382–3.

123. Atkinson VP, Soeding P, Horne G, Tatoulis J. Cold agglutinins in cardiac surgery: management of myocardial protection and cardiopulmonary bypass. *Ann Thorac Surg* 2008;85:310–1.

124. Kuypson AP, Warner JJ, Telen MJ, Milano CA. Paroxysmal cold hemoglobinuria and cardiopulmonary bypass. *Ann Thorac Surg* 2003;75:579–81.

125. Svensson LG, Crawford ES, Hess KR, et al. Deep hypothermia with circulatory arrest: determinants of stroke and early mortality in 656 patients. *J Thorac Cardiovasc Surg* 1993;106:19–28.

126. Tobias JD, Russo P, Russo J. Changes in near infrared spectroscopy during deep hypothermic circulatory arrest. *Ann Card Anaesth* 2009;12:17.

127. Minatoya K, Ogino H, Matsuda H, et al. Evolving selective cerebral perfusion for aortic arch replacement: high flow rate with moderate hypothermic circulatory arrest. *Ann Thorac Surg* 2008;86:1827–31.

128. Malvindi PG, Scrascia G, Vitale N. Is unilateral antegrade cerebral perfusion equivalent to bilateral cerebral perfusion for patients undergoing aortic arch surgery? *Interact Cardiovasc Thorac Surg* 2008;7:891–7.

129. Halstead JC, Meier M, Wurm M, et al. Optimizing selective cerebral perfusion: deleterious effects of high perfusion pressures. *J Thorac Cardiovasc Surg* 2008;135:784–91.

130. Spielvogel D, Etz CD, Silovitz D, Lansman SL, Griepp RB. Aortic arch replacement with a trifurcated graft. *Ann Thorac Surg* 2007;83:S791–5.

131. Barnard J, Dunning J, Grossebner M, Bittar MN. In aortic arch surgery is there any benefit in using antegrade cerebral perfusion or retrograde cerebral perfusion as an adjunct to hypothermic circulatory arrest? *Interact Cardiovasc Thorac Surg* 2004;3:621–30.

132. Estrera AL, Miller CC 3rd, Lee TY, Shah P, Safi HJ. Ascending and transverse aortic arch repair: the impact of retrograde cerebral perfusion. *Circulation* 2008;118(14 Suppl):S160–6.

133. Coselli JS, LeMaire SA. Left heart bypass reduces paraplegia rates after thoracoabdominal aortic aneurysm repair. *Ann Thorac Surg* 1999;67:1931–4.

134. Szwerc MF, Benckhart DH, Lin JC, et al. Recent clinical experience with left heart bypass using a centrifugal pump for repair of traumatic aortic transection. *Ann Surg* 1999;230:484–90.

135. Karmy-Jones R, Carter Y, Meissner M, Mulligan MS. Choice of venous cannulation for bypass during repair of traumatic rupture of the aorta. *Ann Thorac Surg* 2001;71:39–41.

136. Leach WR, Sundt TM 3rd, Moon MR. Oxygenator support for partial left-heart bypass. *Ann Thorac Surg* 2001;72:1770–1.

137. Mathison M, Buffolo E, Jatene AD, et al. Right heart circulatory support facilitates coronary artery bypass without cardiopulmonary bypass. *Ann Thorac Surg* 2000;70:1083–5.
138. Bergsland J, Lingaas PS, Skulstad H, et al. Intracoronary shunt prevents ischemia in off-pump coronary artery bypass surgery. *Ann Thorac Surg* 2009;87:54–60.
139. Vassiliades TA Jr, Nielsen JL, Lonquist JL. Coronary perfusion methods during off-pump coronary artery bypass: results of a randomized clinical trial. *Ann Thorac Surg* 2002;74:S1383–9.
140. Ailawadi G, Zacour RK. Cardiopulmonary bypass/extracorporeal membrane oxygenation/left heart bypass: indications, techniques, and complications. *Surg Clin North Am* 2009;89:781–96.

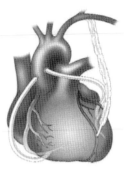

CHAPTER 6

Myocardial Protection

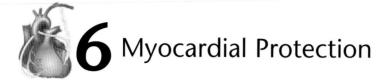

6 Myocardial Protection

Optimizing clinical outcomes in cardiac surgery depends upon the performance of a technically proficient operation without incurring myocardial damage during the procedure. Adherence to this principle is imperative, whether a minimally invasive approach, robotic surgery, off-pump surgery, or conventional surgery through a median sternotomy is performed. With the widespread application of percutaneous coronary interventions, patients requiring surgical revascularization tend to have severe coronary disease and more impaired ventricular function, requiring optimal myocardial preservation. The same holds true for patients undergoing valvular surgery, who are increasingly elderly and are commonly undergoing reoperations or complex multivalvular operations. In most of these cases, the surgeon must conscientiously apply the well-developed principles of cardioplegic arrest to minimize ischemia/reperfusion injury, which contributes to postischemic myocardial dysfunction. This will optimize both the short- and long-term results of surgery. In some situations, modifications of traditional approaches to myocardial protection with cardioplegia may prove beneficial.

I. Types of Myocardial Protection (Table 6.1)

A. **Cardioplegia** is used to arrest the heart after application of an aortic cross-clamp that interrupts the coronary circulation. Aortic cross-clamping without the use of cardioplegia results in anaerobic metabolism and depletion of myocardial energy stores. Thus, without a reduction in myocardial metabolism, either by hypothermia or by chemical cardiac arrest, aortic occlusion producing ischemic arrest for more than 15–20 minutes would result in severe myocardial dysfunction.

B. **Off-pump coronary artery bypass surgery** (OPCAB) is performed without cardiopulmonary bypass (CPB) and thus on a beating heart. The need to provide myocardial protection is limited, because, in the absence of ongoing ischemia, only the region subtended by the artery being bypassed should be in ischemic jeopardy. If ischemia develops, as evidenced by ECG changes or ventricular dysfunction, intracoronary shunting or aortocoronary shunting can be used to provide distal flow until the anastomosis is completed.[1,2] Additional support using miniaturized CPB systems or right ventricular assist can be used in high-risk off-pump cases.[3–5]

C. **On-pump beating-heart surgery** for coronary bypass grafting can be performed without aortic cross-clamping, using stabilizing OPCAB platforms to allow for the construction of distal anastomoses on a beating heart while the pump provides systemic flow. Because of the lower oxygen demand of the empty beating heart, ischemia should be better tolerated than standard OPCAB, but shunting techniques can still be used to

Manual of Perioperative Care in Adult Cardiac Surgery, 5th Edition. By Robert M. Bojar.
Published 2011 by Blackwell Publishing Ltd.

Table 6.1 • Options for Myocardial Protection
1. Off-pump surgery
a. Intraluminal shunting
b. Aortocoronary shunting
c. Perfusion-assisted shunting
d. Ischemic preconditioning
2. On-pump surgery
a. Cardioplegic arrest (antegrade/retrograde)
b. On-pump beating heart
c. Hypothermic fibrillatory arrest
d. Intermittent ischemic arrest
e. Redo AVR with patent ITA – cold retrograde blood or blood cardioplegia
3. Minimally invasive on-pump surgery
a. Cardioplegic arrest with direct clamping or endoclamp balloon
b. On-pump beating heart
c. Hypothermic fibrillatory arrest
AVR, aortic valve replacement; ITA, internal thoracic artery

optimize protection. This technique should be considered when safe aortic clamping cannot be performed (usually in a calcified or severely atherosclerotic aorta) or when the risk of arresting the heart is considered very high due to ongoing ischemia or severe ventricular dysfunction.[6] It may be beneficial in protecting hypertrophied hearts during valve surgery.[7] It can also be used for intracardiac operations, such as resection of a left ventricular aneurysm or surgical ventricular restoration, allowing the surgeon to palpate the border zone between viable muscle and scar tissue better than if the heart were arrested.

D. **Hypothermic fibrillatory arrest** is a variant of the "empty beating heart" approach. It can be used for coronary surgery, with the aorta remaining unclamped and the distal anastomoses performed on a cold vented fibrillating heart with high perfusion pressures. This technique provides less than ideal protection, especially in the hypertrophied heart, and is not commonly used for coronary surgery.[8] Stabilizing platforms can be used if necessary to optimize exposure. In cases where aortic cross-clamping is difficult, such as minimally invasive cases for valve surgery, or for closure of atrial septal defects, this technique can be used to avoid air ejection during the procedure.

E. Both on-pump beating-heart and fibrillating-heart techniques have been applied to patients undergoing valve surgery, especially with minimally invasive approaches.

1. Aortic valve surgery can be performed on a fibrillating heart, especially in redo cases with a patent internal thoracic artery graft, using retrograde tepid or cold blood or blood cardioplegia with systemic hypothermia for myocardial protection.[9–12]

2. Mitral valve surgery can be performed with these techniques as long as there is no aortic insufficiency, especially in minimally invasive surgery where access to the aorta may be difficult.[13–17]

F. **Intermittent ischemic arrest** involves multiple short periods of cross-clamping during mild systemic hypothermia to perform each distal anastomosis. Conceptually, this is a violation of the principle of preserving the heart by inducing diastolic arrest during the period of aortic cross-clamping. However, the heart is able to tolerate these brief periods of ischemia without adverse sequelae.[18,19]

G. **Ischemic preconditioning** refers to a phenomenon in which a transient reduction in blood flow to myocardial tissue enables it to tolerate a subsequent longer period of ischemia. The ideal application of this concept is in off-pump surgery, because, in the absence of collateral flow, there is obligatory transient ischemia with occlusion of a target vessel that might be lessened by ischemic preconditioning.[20] Studies suggest that this technique reduces troponin leakage, myocardial dysfunction, and arrhythmias during surgery using cardioplegic arrest, but not with intermittent cross-clamping with a fibrillating heart.[21–23]

H. **Ischemic postconditioning** involves the administration of medications at the time of initial reperfusion when the aortic cross-clamp is removed to modify ischemia/reperfusion damage. Use of adenosine 1.5 mg/kg has been shown to reduce troponin leakage postoperatively.[24]

II. Principles of Cardioplegia[25,26] (Table 6.2)

A. Prompt **diastolic arrest** of the heart is achieved using a delivery solution containing about 20–25 mEq/L of potassium chloride (KCl). The potassium may be added to a crystalloid solution which is administered undiluted ("crystalloid cardioplegia") or it may be concentrated in a smaller bag of crystalloid solution and administered in a mixture with blood in varying ratios (most commonly 4:1 blood) ("blood cardioplegia"). Systems are available that add the potassium directly to blood to minimize hemodilution (so-called "miniplegia"). Although no clinical advantages are evident with the miniplegia system, the lack of hemodilution and its low cost make it an attractive alternative.[27–29]

1. **Crystalloid cardioplegia** (CCP) provides little substrate and no oxygen to the heart during the period of ischemic arrest. It functions primarily by arresting the heart at cold temperatures. It can be oxygenated by bubbling oxygen through the solution, but this is not a common practice.

2. **Blood cardioplegia** (BCP) solutions provide oxygen, natural buffering agents, antioxidants, and free-radical scavengers. Standard supplemental additives to these solutions include other buffers to achieve an alkaline pH (THAM), citrate-phosphate-dextrose (CPD) or double-dextrose (CP2D) to lower the level of calcium, and occasionally drugs to maintain slight hyperosmolarity (mannitol). The cardioplegia mixture passes through a separate heater/cooler system in the extracorporeal circuit, with the infusion rate and pressure controlled by the perfusionist.

3. The oxygen demand of the heart is reduced nearly 90% by simply arresting the heart at normothermia, so maintenance of arrest during the cross-clamp period is essential (Figure 6.1). This is accomplished by readministering the solution every 15–20 minutes to deliver potassium and wash out metabolic by-products. A low-potassium solution (12–15 mEq/L) is used to maintain the arrest while avoiding an excess potassium load. The high-potassium solution should be readministered if the heart resumes any activity. Cold blood alone can be given retrograde into the coronary sinus as an alternative to

Table 6.2 • Principles and Composition of Cardioplegia

Principle	Composition
1. Prompt diastolic arrest	KCl 20–25 mEq/L
2. Buffering	THAM, bicarbonate
3. Reduction of calcium levels	Citrate-phosphate-dextrose (CPD) or double-dextrose (CP2D)
4. Adequate delivery	Antegrade ± retrograde administration
5. Temperature	Cold vs. tepid vs. warm
6. Substrate additives to optimize myocardial metabolism or prevent cell damage	Aspartate-glutamate Na^+- H^+ exchange inhibitors Insulin Magnesium L-arginine Calcium-channel blockers

THAM, tromethamine

subsequent doses of cardioplegia to optimize tissue oxygenation and metabolism while minimizing the potassium load. This is adequate as long as the heart remains arrested. It is especially beneficial in patients with renal dysfunction, who are predisposed to the development of hyperkalemia.

4. Clinical studies generally suggest that blood cardioplegia provides superior myocardial protection to crystalloid cardioplegia, with less troponin release and better hemodynamic performance post-pump. However, the rate of myocardial infarction has not been shown to differ.[30–33] The advantage of blood cardioplegia is probably most evident in patients with acute ischemia and more advanced left ventricular dysfunction, especially if given both antegrade and retrograde. However, myocardial protection remains suboptimal even with blood cardioplegia in hypertrophied hearts.[34]

5. Polarized arrest using a potassium channel opener, such as nicorandil, has been investigated as an alternative to the depolarized arrest induced by potassium. This has been shown to attenuate the elevation of intracellular calcium and may improve contractile function compared with standard potassium arrest.[35,36] Investigative studies have also shown benefits of non-depolarizing cardioplegia solutions that contain adenosine, adenosine-lidocaine, lidocaine-magnesium, and adenosine-lidocaine-magnesium (adenocaine).[37–40]

B. **Temperature.** Before the development of cardioplegia solutions, myocardial protection was provided entirely by systemic and topical hypothermia. It only seemed logical that administering cardioplegia at a cold temperature would be a significant factor in decreasing myocardial metabolism. However, the reduction in myocardial metabolism attributable to hypothermia is actually quite insignificant compared with that achieved

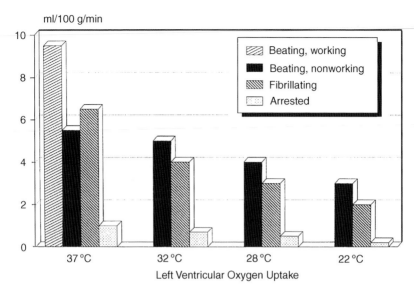

Figure 6.1 • Myocardial oxygen demand (mvO_2). Notice that the most significant decrease in mvO_2 occurs with the induction of the arrested state, and secondarily by the production of hypothermia. (Adapted with permission from Buckberg et al., *J Thorac Cardiovasc Surg* 1977;73:87–94.)

by diastolic arrest (Figure 6.1). Nonetheless, systemic hypothermia, supplemented by topical cold (not iced) saline and topical cooling devices that surround the left ventricle and protect the phrenic nerve from cold injury, are routinely used in patients receiving cold cardioplegia.

1. Some surgeons monitor myocardial temperatures with the presumption that adequate hypothermia (<15 °C) of the myocardium is providing satisfactory myocardial protection. However, in clinical practice, only one site is usually selected for monitoring (usually the left ventricular apex or septum), and there is commonly a significant discrepancy between the temperatures of different areas of the left ventricle, and especially between the left and right ventricles. It should be understood that temperature monitoring provides only a relative assessment of the degree of myocardial protection.[41] A more scientific means of doing so can be accomplished using a pH probe. The development of significant acidosis caused by a derangement in myocardial metabolism is indicative of poor protection.[42]

2. Use of intermittent "tepid" blood cardioplegia (whether at 32 °C or 20 °C) allows the heart to utilize more oxygen and glucose than a colder heart.[43] It may provide better metabolic and functional recovery than cold cardioplegia, with improved long-term results. Optimizing its benefits may require administration through both antegrade and retrograde routes, especially in hypertrophied hearts.[44–46]

3. Since enzymatic and cellular reparative processes function better at normothermia, some surgeons use "warm cardioplegia" for myocardial protection, with excellent

results.[47] However, because of the tendency for the heart to resume electrical activity at normothermia, this must be given continuously or with only short periods of interruption to protect the heart. An ischemic time of 15 minutes between repeat administrations is considered safe, and one study showed that supplementing cardioplegia with magnesium could safely extend this time to 25 minutes.[48] When given continuously, it can obscure the operative field. To minimize hemodilution from excessive cardioplegia administration, the "miniplegia" system that simply adds potassium or other substances (magnesium) to the blood is useful. One study of patients undergoing CABG compared intermittent antegrade delivery of warm vs. tepid cardioplegia and showed superior protection with the former, but no retrograde cardioplegia was delivered to these patients.[49]

4. Warm cardioplegia can also be used as an adjunct to cold cardioplegia when given just after aortic cross-clamping (warm induction) or just prior to removing the cross-clamp ("hot shot").

    a. **Warm induction** involves administering 500 mL of warm cardioplegia immediately after aortic cross-clamping. Studies suggest that this may be beneficial in actively ischemic hearts with energy depletion by providing a brief period of time during which oxygen can be used to repair cell damage and replace energy stores. More recent studies noted a benefit in all patients undergoing CABG that might be enhanced by enriching the solution with glutamate and aspartate.[50,51]

    b. Terminal warm blood cardioplegia (so-called "**hot shot**") is commonly given just before removal of the aortic cross-clamp, because it has been shown to improve myocardial metabolism.[52,53] The heart tends to remain asystolic for several minutes after removal of the aortic cross-clamp, during which time the heart is able to "repair" cellular processes or replenish energy stores while the oxygen demand is low. However, a study of patients with left ventricular hypertrophy undergoing aortic valve replacement did not show any clinical benefit of using "hot shot".[54] Another study compared standard "hot shot" with a modified reperfusion solution including aspartate and glutamate, and found no difference in clinical outcome.[55]

C. **Route of delivery**. Cardioplegia is initially administered antegrade into the aortic root, and then may be given retrograde through a catheter placed into the coronary sinus (see Figure 5.9 on page 240 and Figure 6.2).

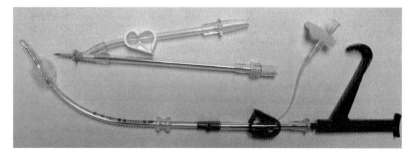

Figure 6.2 • (Top) Antegrade cardioplegia catheter with a side port for venting. (Bottom) A 14 Fr retrograde catheter with self-inflating balloon for measuring coronary sinus pressures.

1. The efficacy of antegrade cardioplegia (ACP) delivery may be compromised by severe coronary artery stenosis and is often dependent on collateral flow.[56,57] In addition, in patients with more than mild aortic regurgitation, sufficient root distention may not be achieved and ACP administration will be ineffective. In that situation, the initial dose must be given retrograde, and, if an aortic valve replacement is being performed, it may be supplemented by an infusion of antegrade cardioplegia directly into the coronary ostia once the aortotomy incision has been performed. ACP can be cumbersome and time-consuming to readminister during aortic valve operations. During mitral valve procedures, it is imperative to eliminate air from the aortic root when antegrade cardioplegia is readministered.

2. Retrograde cardioplegia (RCP) is easy to administer, either intermittently or continuously, and does not interrupt the flow of an operation. It is helpful in reducing the risk of atheroembolism from patent yet diseased saphenous vein grafts at reoperation. It generally provides excellent myocardial protection, although the efficiency of protection of the right ventricle and the posterior left ventricle is always of concern.[57,58] Careful monitoring of coronary sinus pressure during the administration of retrograde cardioplegia is essential: if it is too high (> 50 mm Hg), coronary sinus rupture can occur; if it is too low (< 20 mm Hg), there is usually a problem with catheter malposition or coronary sinus rupture.[59] A variety of catheters have been designed to prevent retrograde flow of cardioplegia into the right atrium and to optimize flow to the right ventricle and posterior wall of the left ventricle.[60,61] Transesophageal echocardiography is helpful in locating the position of the coronary sinus catheter, especially in minimally invasive cases during which the surgeon cannot feel the coronary sinus or when the catheter is placed by the anesthesiologist through the internal jugular vein.

3. Studies that have analyzed the distribution of cardioplegia solutions suggest that the routes of delivery should be complementary, not exclusive. Contrast echo studies have shown that perfusion of the left ventricle is better with warm antegrade delivery than retrograde delivery, and that delivery to the right ventricle is poor with either approach, especially if there is right coronary artery occlusion. However, the latter may be improved by constructing the right coronary graft first and infusing cardioplegia down that graft.[57,62,63] Use of combined antegrade/retrograde cardioplegia appears to provide the best protection and can be recommended for all cases.[64,65] Cold RCP is generally given intermittently, although continuous cold RCP may improve ventricular performance with reduced myocardial ischemia compared with intermittent administration.[66] However, tepid or warm cardioplegia should be given as continuously as possible.

4. Administration of simultaneous antegrade/retrograde cardioplegia usually involves administration down completed vein grafts at the same time as coronary sinus delivery. Despite concerns that this can be disruptive to myocardial cell homeostasis, with increased water accumulation in extracellular and intracellular compartments, this has not been demonstrated to jeopardize myocardial energy metabolism, especially when given for brief periods of time.[67]

D. **Cardioplegia additives.** Studies evaluating the benefits of a variety of cardioplegia additives that might potentially be cardioprotective by ameliorating ischemia/reperfusion injury have shown variable results. These additives include Na^+-H^+ exchange inhibitors (cariporide), insulin, adenosine, magnesium, lidocaine, N-acetylcysteine (intravenously or in the cardioplegia solution), and Krebs cycle intermediates (aspartate and glutamate).[40,68–76] Of particular interest is pexelizumab, a C5 complement inhibitor that has been shown to reduce the incidence of myocardial infarction and death after CABG.[77,78] Other medications given intravenously, including insulin, esmolol, and aminophylline, may also reduce myocardial injury after cardioplegia arrest and improve LV function.[79,80]

E. **Modified reperfusion**. Just prior to removal of the cross-clamp, the administration of a modified cardioplegia solution given under specific conditions has been shown to improve myocardial function.[25,26] Such controlled reperfusion, with or without substrate enhancement, such as aspartate and glutamate, should provide a low potassium load (8–10 mEq/L), CPD or CP2D to limit calcium influx, and hyperosmolarity, and should be given at low pressures (<50 mm Hg) over several minutes. Such a regimen may only be beneficial in high-risk cases.[81,82]

III. Cardioplegia Strategy

Numerous comparative studies have been done to elucidate the best cardioplegia strategy. These have evaluated the distribution of cardioplegia solutions, examined levels of cardiac-specific enzymes such as troponin, or assessed hemodynamic performance, use of inotropes, rates of infarction, or mortality. There are so many variables that can influence outcomes that it is very difficult to conclude which method of myocardial protection is truly superior in influencing surgical results. However, excellent myocardial protection can be obtained with numerous strategies that adhere to the generally accepted principles of cardioplegia delivery.

A. Most studies suggest that in low-risk cases, multidose cold crystalloid, cold, tepid, or warm blood cardioplegia, whether given antegrade and/or retrograde, all produce relatively comparable clinical results. In general, protection of the right ventricle is suboptimal with all strategies, especially in patients with right coronary artery disease. A combined ACP/RCP cold or tepid blood cardioplegia seems to be best for high-risk patients, and can be recommended for all operations.

B. A proposal for blood cardioplegia strategy is as follows:

1. Use warm induction for severely ischemic hearts only.

2. Induce cardioplegic arrest with about 500 mL of antegrade infusion (warm, cold, or tepid); then complete the initial dose by administering cardioplegia retrograde. This is especially important in patients with severe coronary artery disease. If temperature monitoring is used for cold cardioplegia, it should be maintained at less than 20 °C.

3. For valve surgery, after the initial antegrade dose, use either continuous warm retrograde cardioplegia or intermittent cold retrograde blood cardioplegia with a low-potassium solution every 20 minutes. If aortic insufficiency is present, administer cardioplegia retrograde, and if there is a large right coronary artery, consider direct antegrade administration into the right coronary ostium.

4. For redo aortic valve surgery in patients with a patent internal thoracic artery (ITA), the ITA pedicle may be left unclamped. Systemic hypothermia to at least 28 °C with use of cold retrograde blood or blood cardioplegia should provide adequate myocardial protection.

5. For coronary surgery, perform the right coronary graft first and administer low-potassium cardioplegia down that graft simultaneously with retrograde

cardioplegia for all subsequent administrations. Antegrade delivery, of course, cannot be delivered down pedicled grafts and is best avoided in free grafts (mammary or radial artery) to avoid the potential adverse impact of graft manipulation and hyperkalemia on endothelial function.

6. If warm retrograde cardioplegia is used, it should be run as continuously as possible as long as it does not interfere with exposure. A high-potassium solution should be used if there is return of cardiac activity.

7. Administer cardioplegia down each saphenous vein bypass graft as it is completed along with additional retrograde cardioplegia. Concomitant administration down all completed grafts along with retrograde cardioplegia might be helpful (Figure 6.3).

8. Administer 500 mL of "hot shot" retrograde just prior to removal of the cross-clamp. If retrograde cardioplegia is not used, give this into the aortic root at a pressure that does not exceed 50–80 mm Hg after ensuring that there is no air in the aortic root.

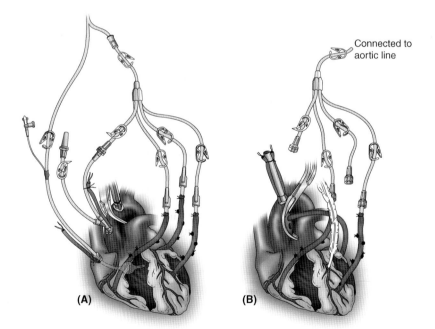

Figure 6.3 • (A) Technique of administering cardioplegia simultaneously down the completed vein grafts and the retrograde cannula. If proximal anastomoses are done during the cross-clamp period, cardioplegia is usually given retrograde, but can be delivered into the aortic root and down the completed grafts after de-airing the root. (B) Blood can be delivered off the aortic line during construction of the proximal anastomoses if they are performed with a side-clamp on the aorta.

9. In circulatory arrest cases for aortic root and arch surgery, cardioplegia should be administered either directly into the coronary ostia or retrograde at the time that circulatory arrest is initiated.

10. Careful adherence to the basic principles of cardioplegia (maintaining arrest and multidosing, in particular) should allow surgeons to patiently yet expeditiously perform even the most complex, time-consuming operations without worrying about poor myocardial protection.

References

1. Bergsland J, Lingaas PS, Skulstad H, et al. Intracoronary shunt prevents ischemia in off-pump coronary artery bypass surgery. *Ann Thorac Surg* 2009;87:54–60.

2. Vassiliades TA Jr, Nielsen JL, Lonquist JL. Coronary perfusion methods during off-pump coronary artery bypass: results of a randomized clinical trial. *Ann Thorac Surg* 2002;74:S1383–9.

3. Reber D, Fritz M, Tossios P, et al. Beating-heart coronary artery bypass grafting using a miniaturized extracorporeal circulation system. *Heart Surg Forum* 2008;111:E276–80.

4. Lundell DC, Crouch JD. A miniature right heart support system improves cardiac output and stroke volume during beating heart posterior/lateral coronary artery bypass grafting. *Heart Surg Forum* 2003;6:302–6.

5. Lima LE, Jatene F, Buffolo E, et al. A multicenter initial clinical experience with right heart support and beating heart coronary surgery. *Heart Surg Forum* 2001;4:60–4.

6. Ferrari E, Stalder N, von Segesser LK. On-pump beating heart coronary surgery for high risk patients requiring emergency multiple coronary artery bypass grafting. *J Cardiothorac Surg* 2008;3:38–43.

7. Wang J, Liu H, Xiang B, et al. Keeping the heart empty and beating improves preservation of hypertrophied hearts for valve surgery. *J Thorac Cardiovasc Surg* 2006;132:1314–20.

8. Akins CW. Noncardioplegic myocardial preservation for coronary revascularization. *J Thorac Cardiovasc Surg* 1984;88:174–81.

9. Bar-El Y, Kophit A, Cohen O, Kertzman V, Milo S. Minimal dissection and continuous retrograde cardioplegia for aortic valve replacement in patients with a patent left internal mammary artery graft. *J Heart Valve Dis* 2003;12:454–7.

10. Battellini R, Rastan AJ, Fabricius A, Moscoso-Luduena M, Lachmann N, Mohr FW. Beating heart aortic valve replacement after previous coronary artery bypass surgery with a patent internal mammary artery graft. *Ann Thorac Surg* 2007;83:1206–9.

11. Reber D, Fritz M, Bojara W, Marks P, Laczkovics A, Tossios P. Aortic valve replacement after previous coronary artery bypass grafting: experience with a simplified approach. *J Cardiovasc Surg* 2007;48:73–7.

12. Byrne JG, Karavas AN, Filsoufi F, et al. Aortic valve surgery after previous coronary artery bypass grafting with functioning internal mammary artery grafts. *Ann Thorac Surg* 2002;73:779–84.

13. Cicekcioglu F, Tutun U, Babaroglu S, et al. Redo valve surgery with on-pump beating heart technique. *J Cardiovasc Surg (Torino)* 2007;48:513–8.

14. Gersak B, Sutlic Z. Aortic and mitral valve surgery on the beating heart is lowering cardiopulmonary bypass and aortic cross clamp time. *Heart Surg Forum* 2002;5:182–6.

15. Salerno TA, Panos AL, Tian G, Deslauriers R, Calcaterra D, Ricci M. Surgery for cardiac valves and aortic root without cardioplegic arrest ("beating heart"): experience with a new method of myocardial perfusion. *J Card Surg* 2007;22:459–64.

16. Loulmet DF, Patel NC, Jennings JM, Subramanian VA. Less invasive intracardiac surgery performed without aortic clamping. *Ann Thorac Surg* 2008;85:1551–5.

17. Umakanthan R, Leacche M, Petracek MR, et al. Safety of minimally invasive mitral valve surgery without aortic cross-clamp. *Ann Thorac Surg* 2008;85:1544–9.

18. Raco L, Mills E, Millner RJ. Isolated myocardial revascularization with intermittent aortic crossclamping: experience with 800 cases. *Ann Thorac Surg* 2002;73:1436–40.

19. Alex J, Ansari J, Guerrero R, et al. Comparison of the immediate post-operative outcome of two different myocardial protection strategies: antegrade-retrograde cold St. Thomas blood cardioplegia versus intermittent cross-clamp fibrillation. *Interact Cardiovasc Thorac Surg* 2003;2:584–8.

20. Laurikka J, Wu ZK, Iisalo P, et al. Regional ischemic preconditioning enhances myocardial performance in off-pump coronary artery bypass grafting. *Chest* 2002;121:1183–9.

21. Walsh SR, Tang TY, Kullar P, et al. Ischaemic preconditioning during cardiac surgery: a systematic review and meta-analysis of perioperative outcomes in randomised clinical trials. *Eur J Cardiothorac Surg* 2008;34:985–94.

22. Ji B, Liu M, Wang G, Feng W, Lu F, Shengshou H. Evaluation by cardiac troponin I: the effect of ischemic preconditioning as an adjunct to intermittent blood cardioplegia on coronary artery bypass grafting. *J Card Surg* 2007;22:394–400.

23. Codispoti M, Sundaramoorthi T, Saad RA, Reid A, Sinclair C, Mankad P. Optimal myocardial protection strategy for coronary artery bypass grafting without cardioplegia: prospective randomised trial. *Interact Cardiovasc Thorac Surg* 2006;5:217–21.

24. Jin ZX, Zhou JJ, Xin M, et al. Postconditioning the human heart with adenosine in heart valve replacement surgery. *Ann Thorac Surg* 2007;83:2066–72.

25. Buckberg GD, Beyersdorf F, Allen BS, Robertson JM. Integrated myocardial management: background and initial application. *J Card Surg* 1995;10:68–89.

26. Cohen G, Borger MA, Weisel RD, Rao V. Intraoperative myocardial protection: current trends and future perspectives. *Ann Thorac Surg* 1999;68:1995–2001.

27. El-Hamamsy I, Stevens LM, Pellerin M, et al. A prospective randomized study of diluted versus non-diluted cardioplegia (minicardioplegia) in primary coronary artery bypass surgery. *J Cardiovasc Surg (Torino)* 2004;45:101–6.

28. Hayashi Y, Ohtani M, Hiraishi T, Kobayashi Y, Nakamura T. "Initial, continuous and intermittent bolus" administration of minimally-diluted blood cardioplegia supplemented with potassium and magnesium for hypertrophied hearts. *Heart Lung Circ* 2006;15:325–31.

29. Petrucci O, Wilson Vieira R, do Carmo RM, Martins de Oliveira PP, Antunes N, Marcolino Braile D. Use of (all-blood) miniplegia versus crystalloid cardioplegia in an experimental model of acute myocardial ischemia. *J Card Surg* 2008;23:361–5.

30. Jacob S, Kallikourdis A, Sellke F, Dunning J. Is blood cardioplegia superior to crystalloid cardioplegia? *Interact Cardiovasc Thorac Surg* 2008;7:491–8.

31. Guru V, Omura J, Alghamdi A, Weisel R, Fremes SE. Is blood superior to crystalloid cardioplegia? A meta-analysis of randomized clinical trials. *Circulation* 2006;114(1 Suppl):I-331–8.

32. Fallouh HB, Chambers DJ. Is blood versus crystalloid cardioplegia relevant? Significantly improved protection may require new cardioplegic concepts! *Interact Cardiovasc Thorac Surg* 2008;7:1162–3.

33. Dar MI. Cold crystalloid versus warm blood cardioplegia for coronary artery bypass surgery. *Ann Thorac Cardiovasc Surg* 2005;11:382–5.

34. Ascione R, Caputo M, Gomes WJ, et al. Myocardial injury in hypertrophic hearts of patients undergoing aortic valve surgery using cold or warm blood cardioplegia. *Eur J Cardiothorac Surg* 2002;21:440–6.

35. Steensrud T, Nordhaug D, Elvenes OP, Korvald C, Sørlie DG. Superior myocardial protection with nicorandil cardioplegia. *Eur J Cardiothorac Surg* 2003;23:670–7.

36. Takarabe K, Okazaki Y, Higuchi S, Murayama J, Natsuaki M, Itoh T. Nicorandil attenuates reperfusion injury after long cardioplegic arrest. *Asian Cardiovasc Thorac Ann* 2007;15:204–9.

37. Jakobsen O, Stenberg TA, Losvik O, Ekse S, Sørlie DG, Ytrebø LM. Adenosine instead of supranormal potassium in cardioplegia solution preserves endothelium-derived hyperpolarization factor-dependent vasodilation. *Eur J Cardiothorac Surg* 2008;33:18–24.

38. Sloots KL, Vinten-Johansen J, Dobson GP. Warm nondepolarizing adenosine and lidocaine cardioplegia: continuous versus intermittent delivery. *J Thorac Cardiovasc Surg* 2007;133:1171–8.

39. Yamaguchi S, Watanabe G, Tomita S, Tabata S. Lidocaine-magnesium blood cardioplegia was equivalent to potassium blood cardioplegia in left ventricular function of canine heart. *Interact Cardiovasc Thorac Surg* 2007;6:172–6.

40. O'Rullian JJ, Clayson SE, Peragallo R. Excellent outcomes in a case of complex re-do surgery requiring prolonged cardioplegia using a new cardioprotective approach: adenocaine. *J Extra Corpor Technol* 2008;40:203–5.

41. Dearani JA, Axford TC, Patel MA, Healey NA, Lavin PT, Khuri SF. Role of myocardial temperature measurement in monitoring the adequacy of myocardial protection during cardiac surgery. *Ann Thorac Surg* 2001;72:S2235–44.

42. Khabbaz KR, Feng J, Boodhwani M, Clements RT, Bianchi C, Sellke FW. Nonischemic myocardial acidosis adversely affects microvascular and myocardial function and triggers apoptosis during cardioplegia. *J Thorac Cardiovasc Surg* 2008;135:139–46.

43. Badak MI Gurcun U, Discigil B, Boga M, Ozkisacik EA, Alayunt DA. Myocardium utilizes more oxygen and glucose during tepid cardioplegic infusion in arrested heart. *Int Heart J* 2005;46:219–29.

44. Mallidi HR, Sever J, Tamariz M, et al. The short-term and long-term effects of warm or tepid cardioplegia. *J Thorac Cardiovasc Surg* 2003;125:711–20.

45. Bezon E, Choplain JN, Khalifa AA, Numa H, Salley N, Barra JA. Continuous retrograde blood cardioplegia ensures prolonged aortic cross-clamping without increasing the operative risk. *Interact Cardiovasc Thorac Surg* 2006;5:403–7.

46. Fujii T, Watanabe Y, Shiono N, et al. Limitations of retrograde continuous tepid blood cardioplegia for myocardial remodeling. *Ann Thorac Cardiovasc Surg* 2006;12:397–403.

47. Salerno TA. Warm heart surgery: reflections on the history of its development. *J Card Surg* 2007;22:257–9.

48. Casalino S, Tesler UF, Novelli E, et al. The efficacy and safety of extending the ischemic time with a modified cardioplegic technique for coronary artery surgery. *J Card Surg* 2008;23:444–9.

49. Sirvinskas E, Nasvytis L, Raliene L, Vaskelyte J, Toleikis A, Trumbeckaite S. Myocardial protective effect of warm blood, tepid blood, and cold crystalloid cardioplegia in coronary artery bypass grafting surgery. *Croat Med J* 2005;46:879–88.

50. Ji B, Liu M, Liu F, et al. Warm induction cardioplegia and reperfusion dose influence the occurrence of post CABG TnI level. *Interact Cardiovasc Thorac Surg* 2006;5:67–70.

51. Wallace AW, Ratcliffe MB, Nosé PS, et al. Effect of induction and reperfusion with warm substrate-enriched cardioplegia on ventricular function. *Ann Thorac Surg* 2000;70:1301–7.

52. Teoh KH, Christakis GT, Weisel RD, et al. Accelerated myocardial metabolic recovery with terminal warm blood cardioplegia. *J Thorac Cardiovasc Surg* 1986;91:888–95.

53. Caputo M, Dihmis WC, Bryan AJ, Suleiman MS, Angelini GD. Warm blood hyperkalaemic reperfusion ("hot shot") prevents myocardial substrate derangement in patients undergoing coronary artery bypass surgery. *Eur J Cardiothorac Surg* 1998;13:559–64.

54. Ascione R, Suleiman SM, Angelini GD. Retrograde hot-shot cardioplegia in patients with left ventricular hypertrophy undergoing aortic valve replacement. *Ann Thorac Surg* 2008;85:454–8.

55. Edwards R, Treasure T, Hossein-Nia M, Murday A, Kantidakis GH, Holt DW. A controlled trial of substrate-enhanced, warm reperfusion ("hot shot") versus simple reperfusion. *Ann Thorac Surg* 2000;69:551–5.

56. Aronson S, Jacobsohn E, Savage R, Albertucci M. The influence of collateral flow on the antegrade and retrograde distribution of cardioplegia in patients with an occluded right coronary artery. *Anesthesiology* 1998;89:1099–107.

57. Honkonen EL, Kaukinen L, Pehkonen EJ, Kaukinen S. Myocardial cooling and right ventricular function in patients with right coronary artery disease: antegrade vs. retrograde cardioplegia. *Acta Anaesthesiol Scand* 1997;41:287–96.

58. Kouerinis IA, Manopoulos CG, Zografos GC, et al. Retrograde cardioplegia in CABG: is it really useful? The microcirculation and a capillary unit model. *Med Sci Monit* 2006;12:RA265–8.

59. Langenberg CJ, Pietersen HG, Geskes G, Wagenmakers AJM, Soeters PB, Durieux M. Coronary sinus catheter placement. Assessment of placement criteria and cardiac complications. *Chest* 2003;124:1259–65.

60. Cerillo A, Storti S, Haxhiademi D, et al. The double balloon cannula: a means to prevent backward flow of retrograde cardioplegia to the right atrium. *Interact Cardiovasc Thorac Surg* 2006;5:289–93.

61. Matsui Y, Shimura S, Suto Y, Sasaki S. Occluding the junction of the middle cardiac vein in retrograde cardioplegia: a new retrograde cannula for optimizing retrograde cardioplegic delivery. *Surg Today* 2007;37:89–92.

62. Borger MA, Wei KS, Weisel RD, et al. Myocardial perfusion during warm antegrade and retrograde cardioplegia: a contrast echo study. *Ann Thorac Surg* 1999;68:955–61.

63. Allen BS, Winkelmann JW, Hanafy H, et al. Retrograde cardioplegia does not adequately perfuse the right ventricle. *J Thorac Cardiovasc Surg* 1995;109:1116–26.

64. Sanjay OP, Srikrishna SV, Prashanth P, Kajrekar P, Vincent V. Antegrade versus antegrade with retrograde delivery of cardioplegia solution in myocardial revascularisation. A clinical study in patients with triple vessel coronary artery disease. *Ann Card Anaesth* 2003;6:143–8.

65. Radmehr H, Soleimani A, Tatari H, Salehi M. Does combined antegrade-retrograde cardioplegia have any superiority over antegrade cardioplegia? *Heart Lung Circ* 2008;17:475–7.

66. Louagie YA, Jamart J, Gonzalez M, et al. Continuous cold blood cardioplegia improves myocardial protection: a prospective randomized study. *Ann Thorac Surg* 2004;77:664–71.

67. Li G, Tian W, Wang J, et al. The effects of simultaneous antegrade/retrograde cardioplegia on cellular volumes and energy metabolism. *J Card Surg* 2008;23:437–43.

68. Mentzer RM, Bartels C, Bolli R, et al. Sodium–hydrogen exchange inhibition by cariporide to reduce the risk of ischemic cardiac events in patients undergoing coronary artery bypass grafting: results of the EXPEDITION study. *Ann Thorac Surg* 2008;85:1261–70.

69. Carrier M, Pellerin M, Perrault LP, et al. Cardioplegic arrest with L-arginine improves myocardial protection: results of a prospective randomized clinical trial. *Ann Thorac Surg* 2002;73:837–42.

70. Rao V, Borger MA, Weisel RD, et al. Insulin cardioplegia for elective coronary bypass surgery. *J Thorac Cardiovasc Surg* 2000;119:1176–84.

71. Vinten-Johansen J, Zhao ZQ, Corvera JS, et al. Adenosine in myocardial protection in on-pump and off-pump cardiac surgery. *Ann Thorac Surg* 2003;75:S691–9.

72. Ji B, Liu J, Liu M, et al. Effect of cold blood cardioplegia enriched with potassium-magnesium aspartate during coronary artery bypass grafting. *J Cardiovasc Surg (Torino)* 2006;47:671–5.

73. Yeatman M, Caputo M, Narayan P, et al. Magnesium-supplemented warm blood cardioplegia in patients undergoing coronary artery revascularization. *Ann Thorac Surg* 2002;73:112–8.

74. Albacker TB, Carvalho G, Schricker T, Lachapelle K. Myocardial protection during elective coronary artery bypass grafting using high-dose insulin therapy. *Ann Thorac Surg* 2007;84:1920–7.

75. Koramaz I, Pulathan Z, Usta S, et al. Cardioprotective effect of cold-blood cardioplegia enriched with N-acetylcysteine during coronary artery bypass grafting. *Ann Thorac Surg* 2006;81:613–8.

76. El-Hamamsy I, Stevens LM, Carrier M, et al. Effect of intravenous N-acetylcysteine on outcomes after coronary artery bypass surgery: a randomized, double-blind, placebo-controlled clinical trial. *J Thorac Cardiovasc Surg* 2007;133:7–12.

77. Smith PK, Carrier M, Chen JC, et al. Effect of pexelizumab in coronary artery bypass graft surgery with extended aortic cross-clamp time. *Ann Thorac Surg* 2006;82:781–8.

78. Carrier M, Ménasché P, Levy JH, et al. Inhibition of complement activation by pexelizumab reduces death in patients undergoing combined aortic valve replacement and coronary artery bypass surgery. *J Thorac Cardiovasc Surg* 2006;131:352–6.

79. Fannelop T, Dahle GO, Matre K, et al. Esmolol before 80 min of cardiac arrest with oxygenated cold blood cardioplegia alleviates systolic dysfunction. An experimental study in pigs. *Eur J Cardiothorac Surg* 2008;33:9–17.

80. Luo WJ, Qian JF, Jiang HH. Pretreatment with aminophylline reduces release of Troponin I and neutrophil activation in the myocardium of patients undergoing cardioplegic arrest. *Eur J Cardiothorac Surg* 2007;31:360–5.

81. Edwards R, Treasure T, Hossein-Nia M, Murday A, Kantidakis GH, Holt DW. A controlled trial of substrate-enhanced, warm reperfusion ("hot shot") versus simple reperfusion. *Ann Thorac Surg* 2000;69:551–5.

82. Buckberg GD. Substrate enriched warm blood cardioplegia reperfusion: an alternate view. *Ann Thorac Surg* 2000;69:334–5.

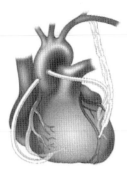

CHAPTER 7

Admission to the ICU and Monitoring Techniques

7 Admission to the ICU and Monitoring Techniques

I. Admission to the ICU

A. The first critical phase of postoperative care starts at the completion of the surgical procedure. During transfer from the operating room table to an intensive care unit (ICU) bed, from one monitoring system to another, and from the operating room to the ICU, the potential exists for airway and ventilation problems, sudden hypotension or hypertension, arrhythmias, inadvertent medication changes, and unidentified problems with invasive catheters, monitoring, and bleeding. The electrocardiogram (ECG) and pressure tracings (arterial, central venous, and/or pulmonary artery) are transferred one at a time from the operating room monitor to the transport module to ensure that the patient is monitored at all times. Ventilation is provided by an Ambu bag connected to a portable oxygen tank. Drug infusions should be placed on battery-powered infusion pumps to ensure accurate infusion rates. A selection of cardiac medications should always be available in the event of an emergency during transport.

B. Upon arrival in the ICU, the endotracheal tube is connected to a mechanical ventilator, and the ECG and pressure lines are transduced on a bedside monitor. A pulse oximeter is attached to one of the patient's fingertips. Medication drip rates are confirmed or readjusted on controlled infusion pumps, preferably using the same pumps that were used in the operating room to avoid temporary disconnection from the patient. The thoracic drainage system is connected to suction.

C. During this transition phase, much attention is directed to getting the patient connected to the monitors and attached to the ventilator. To ensure that the patient remains stable while getting settled in, it is critical that the accompanying anesthesia and/or surgical personnel as well as the accepting nurses and respiratory therapists make sure that:

    1. The patient is being well-ventilated by observing chest movement and auscultating bilateral breath sounds.

    2. The ECG tracing demonstrates satisfactory rate and rhythm on the transport and then the bedside monitor.

    3. The blood pressure is adequate on the portable monitor and remains so after the arterial line is transduced and calibrated on the bedside monitor.

D. Immediate assessment and response to any abnormalities suspected to be present at the time of admission to the ICU, whether real or spurious, is imperative. The two most common problems encountered are a low blood pressure and an indecipherable ECG.

Manual of Perioperative Care in Adult Cardiac Surgery, 5th Edition. By Robert M. Bojar.
Published 2011 by Blackwell Publishing Ltd.

E. **Low blood pressure** (systolic BP <90 mm Hg or mean BP <60 mm Hg) is caused most commonly by hypovolemia or sudden termination of a drug infusion. However, the possibility of a more critical problem, such as acute blood loss, myocardial ischemia, severe myocardial dysfunction, arrhythmias, or ventilatory problems, should always be kept in mind. Low blood pressure may also result from inadequate zeroing of the transducer, or kinking or transient occlusion of the line, producing a dampened tracing. If the transduced blood pressure is low, do the following:

1. Resume manual ventilation and listen for bilateral breath sounds.

2. Palpate the brachial or femoral artery to confirm a pulse and a satisfactory blood pressure. Attach the blood pressure cuff above the radial arterial line site and take an auscultatory or occlusion blood pressure. The latter is done by inflating the cuff until the arterial tracing is obliterated; when the pressure tracing reappears, the systolic pressure can be read from the sphygmomanometer. **Never assume that a low blood pressure recording is caused by dampening of the arterial line unless a higher pressure can be confirmed by another method**. Insertion of an additional arterial monitoring line (usually in the femoral artery) may be indicated.

3. Make sure that all medication bottles are appropriately labeled and are connected to the patient and infusing at the designated rate through patent intravenous lines. **Note:** If hypotension is present, quickly ascertain whether the patient is receiving nitroglycerin or nitroprusside (in the silver wrapper), because they can lower the blood pressure precipitously. Unless you know how to change the drip rate on the particular drug infusion pump, let someone else who is familiar with it take care of it!

4. Quickly examine the chest tubes for massive mediastinal bleeding. Exsanguinating hemorrhage may require emergency sternotomy.

5. Evaluate the cardiac filling pressures on the transport monitor or the ICU monitor. Confirm that the transducers are at the appropriate levels relative to the patient's position in the bed and that the monitors are calibrated. Not uncommonly, during the very early stages of admission to the ICU, the observed filling pressures will not be accurate and this can confound an assessment of the patient's volume status. The anesthesiologist should be aware of the filling pressures during transport and can assist in assessing whether the patient has low filling pressures, indicating hypovolemia, or very high filling pressures, perhaps suggesting myocardial dysfunction.

6. The initial **treatment** of hypotension should include volume infusion, and, if there is no immediate response, administration of calcium chloride 500 mg IV. Vasoactive medications may be started or the rate of medications already being used can be adjusted. **If there is no response to these measures, and the ECG is abnormal, assume the worst and prepare to treat the patient as an imminent cardiac arrest until the problem is sorted out. If the patient cannot be immediately resuscitated, call for help and prepare for an emergency sternotomy.**

F. An indeterminate or undecipherable **ECG** is usually caused by artifact with jostling or detachment of the ECG leads. If the arterial waveform is normal or the pulse oximeter sounds normal, this is usually the case. However, if the arterial pressure is low or not transduced, the pulse is irregular or slow, or the monitor is difficult to interpret, palpate for a pulse and take the steps mentioned above. **If the blood pressure is undetectable and an ECG reading is not available, assume the worst and treat the patient as a cardiac arrest**. Readjust the ECG leads on the patient and monitor. If interpretation remains difficult, attach a standard ECG machine to limb leads to ascertain the rhythm.

Table 7.1 • Initial Evaluation of the Patient in the Intensive Care Unit

1. The patient should be examined thoroughly (heart, lungs, peripheral perfusion)

2. Obtain hemodynamic measurements including the CVP, PA pressures, PCW pressure, obtain a cardiac output and calculate the systemic vascular resistance (SVR) (see Table 11.1, page 441)

3. A portable supine chest x-ray should be obtained either in the operating room or soon after arrival in the ICU. Specific attention should be paid to the position of the endotracheal tube and Swan-Ganz catheter, the width of the mediastinum, and the presence of a pneumothorax, fluid overload, atelectasis, or pleural effusion (hemothorax)

4. A 12-lead ECG should be reviewed for ischemic changes or arrhythmias

5. Laboratory tests should be drawn (see Table 7.2 for sample admission order sheet)

---

1. If ventricular fibrillation or tachycardia is present, immediate defibrillation and a cardiac arrest protocol are indicated (see page 506).

2. If a pacemaker is being used, examine the connections and settings and confirm capture on the bedside monitor or an ECG. Make sure that the pacemaker is appropriately sensing the patient's rhythm, since inappropriate sensing may trigger malignant ventricular arrhythmias.

3. Attach a pacemaker and initiate pacing if bradycardia or heart block is present. The initial default setting on most external pacemakers is the VVI setting, which should produce a ventricular contraction. One should then attempt to pace the atrium (AOO) or initiate AV pacing (DDD or DVI) if atrial pacing wires are present and heart block is present. If there is no response to atrial pacing, ventricular pacing (VVI) should be used. If the patient has a rhythm, but the ventricle fails to pace, consider placing a skin wire as a ground in case one of the wires has been dislodged from the heart.

4. Look for the undetected development of atrial fibrillation that can develop during AV pacing. This may account for a fall in cardiac output and blood pressure despite an adequate ventricular pacing rate.

5. Obtain a 12-lead ECG, looking for evidence of arrhythmias or ischemia that may require treatment.

G. Once the patient's heart rate, rhythm, and blood pressure are found to be satisfactory and adequate ventilation from the ventilator is confirmed, a full report should be given to the ICU staff by the accompanying anesthesiologist and/or surgical house staff/PA/NP. This should include the patient's cardiac disease, comorbidities, operative procedure, intraoperative course, medications being administered, and special instructions for postoperative care. Further assessment as delineated in Table 7.1 can then be carried out to address the subtleties of patient care. A standardized set of preprinted orders that can be adapted to each patient is invaluable in ensuring that no essential elements of the early postoperative care are overlooked (Table 7.2 and Appendix 3).

H. It is very important to review the immediate postoperative chest x-ray to assess the position of the endotracheal tube and make sure that a pneumothorax is not missed. Obtaining this chest x-ray prior to departure from the operating room is beneficial. In addition, review of an ECG obtained soon after arrival in the ICU is essential to identify any ischemic changes that might require urgent attention.

Table 7.2 • Typical Orders for Admission to the ICU

1. Admit to ICU on _____ MD service
2. Procedure:_____
3. Vital signs q15 minutes until stable, then q30 min or per protocol
4. Continuous ECG, arterial, PA tracings, SaO_2 on bedside monitor
5. Cardiac output q15 min × 1 hour, then q1h × 4 hours, then q2–4h when stable
6. IABP 1:1; check distal pulses manually or with Doppler q1h
7. Chest tubes to chest drainage system with −20 cm H_2O suction; record hourly until <30 mL/h, then q8h
8. Bair Hugger warming system if core temperature <35 °C
9. Urinary catheter to gravity drainage and record hourly
10. Elevate head of bed 30°
11. Hourly I & O
12. Daily weights
13. Advance activity after extubation (dangle, OOB to chair)
14. VTE prophylaxis
    - ☐ T.E.D. elastic stockings (apply on POD #1)
    - ☐ Sequential compression devices
    - ☐ Heparin 5000 units SC bid starting on POD #_____
    - ☐ Low-molecular-weight heparin (Lovenox) 40 mg SC daily starting on POD #_____
15. GI/Nutrition: ☐ NPO while intubated
    - ☐ Nasogastric tube to low suction
    - ☐ Clear liquids as tolerated 1h after extubation and removal of NG tube
16. Ventilator settings

    FiO_2:_____in SIMV mode

    IMV rate: _____breaths/min

    Tidal volume: _____ mL

    PEEP: _____cm H_2O

    Pressure support: _____ cm H_2O
17. Respiratory care
    - ☐ Endotracheal suction q4h, then prn
    - ☐ Wean ventilator to extubate per protocol (see Tables 10.3–10.5, pages 400–402)
    - ☐ O_2 via face mask with FiO_2 0.6–1.0 per protocol
    - ☐ O_2 via nasal prongs @ 2–6 liters/min to keep SaO_2 >95%
    - ☐ Incentive spirometer q1h when awake
    - ☐ Cough pillow at bedside
    - ☐ Albuterol 0.5 mL of 0.5% solution (2.5 mg) in 3 mL normal saline q6h via nebulizer or metered dose inhaler 6 puffs via endotracheal tube (90 μg/inhalation)

Table 7.2 • (Continued)

18. Laboratory tests

  ☐ On arrival: STAT ABGs, CBC, electrolytes, glucose

  STAT PT, PTT, platelet count if chest tube output >100/h
  (thromboelastogram if available)

  STAT chest x-ray (if not done in operating room)

  STAT ECG

  ☐ 4 and 8 hours after arrival and prn: potassium, hematocrit, ABGs (respiratory distress)

  ☐ ABGs per protocol (prior to weaning and prior to extubation)

  ☐ 3 AM on POD #1: CBC, lytes, BUN, creatinine, blood glucose, ECG, CXR, INR
  (if patient to receive warfarin after valve procedure)

19. Pacemaker settings: Mode: ☐ Atrial   ☐ VVI   ☐ DVI   ☐ DDD

  Atrial output:_____ mA Ventricular output _____mA

  Rate: _____/min   AV interval:_____ msec

  Sensitivity: ☐ Asynchronous   ☐ Demand

  ☐ Pacer off but attached

20. Cardiac Rehab consult

21. Notify MD/PA for:

  a. Systolic blood pressure <90 or >140 mm Hg

  b. Cardiac index <2.0 L/min/m^2

  c. Urine output <30 mL/h for 2 hours

  d. Chest tube drainage >100 mL/h

  e. Temperature >38.5 °C

22. IV Drips/Medications (with suggested ranges)

  Allergies_____

  a. IV drips:

  ☐ Dextrose 5% in 0.45 NS 250 mL via Cordis/triple lumen to KVO

  ☐ Arterial line and distal Swan-Ganz port: NS flushes at 3 mL/h

  ☐ Epinephrine 1 mg/250 mL D5W: _____ µg/min to maintain cardiac index >2.0
  (0.01–0.06 µg/kg/min or 1–4 µg/min)

  ☐ Milrinone 20 mg/100mL D5W: _____ µg/kg/min (0.375–0.625 µg/kg/min)

  ☐ Dopamine 400 mg/250 D5W: _____ µg/kg/min (2–20 µg/kg/min)

  ☐ Dobutamine 250 mg/250 D5W: _____ µg/kg/min (5–20 µg/kg/min)

  ☐ Norepinephrine 4–8 mg/250 mL D5W: _____ µg/min to keep systolic BP >100
  (0.01–1.0 µg/kg/min)

  ☐ Phenylephrine 20 mg/250 mL NS: _____ µg/min to keep systolic BP >100
  (0.1–3.0 µg/kg/min)

(continued)

Table 7.2 • (Continued)

☐ Vasopressin 15 units/150 mL D5W: _____ units/min (0.01–0.07 units/min)

☐ Nitroprusside 50 mg/250 mL D5W: _____μg/kg/min to keep systolic BP <130 (0.1–5 μg/kg/min)

☐ Clevidipine 50mg/100 mL D5W: _____ mg/h to keep systolic BP <130 (2–5 mg/h)

☐ Nicardipine 25 mg/250 mL D5W: _____ mg/h to keep BP <130 (5–15 mg/h)

☐ Nitroglycerin 50 mg/250 mL D5W: _____ μg/kg/min (0.1–2.0 μg/kg/min)

☐ Diltiazem: 100 mg/100 mL D5W: _____ mg/h (for radial artery prophylaxis)

☐ Esmolol 2.5 g/250 NS: _____ μg/kg/min (25–100 μg/kg/min)

☐ Amiodarone: after initial IV load in OR, 900 mg/500 D5W: 1 mg/min × 6 hours, then decrease to 0.5 mg/min × 18 hours

☐ Lidocaine 2 g/250 mL D5W: _____ mg/min IV; wean off at 06:00 POD #1

☐ Nesiritide: 1.5 mg/100 mL DSW:_____μg/kg/min (0.01–0.03 μg/kg/min)

☐ Fenoldopam: 10 mg/250 D5W: 0.1 μg/kg/min

b. Antibiotics

☐ Cefazolin 1 g IV q8h for 6 doses

☐ Vancomycin 1 g IV q12h for 4 doses

c. Sedatives/analgesics

☐ Propofol infusion 10 mg/mL: 25–50 μg/kg/min; wean to off per protocol

☐ Dexmedetomidine: 400 μg (2 vials of 2 mL of 100 μg/mL solution)/100 mL NS: bolus dose of _____ (1 μg/kg) over 10 minutes, then maintenance infusion of _____ (0.2–0.7 μg/kg/h)

☐ Midazolam 2 mg IV q2h prn agitation; stop after extubation

☐ Morphine sulfate _____ mg IV q2h prn for pain (while intubated)

☐ Meperidine 25–50 mg IV prn shivering

☐ Ketorolac 30–60 mg IV q6h prn for moderate-to-severe pain (4–10 on pain scale); stop after 72 hours

☐ Percocet 5/325 mg 1–2 tablets PO q4h prn for pain after extubation; start with 1 tablet for mild pain (1–3 on pain scale); give additional tablet 60 minutes later if no change in pain. Give 2 tablets for moderate-to-severe pain (4–10 on pain scale)

d. Other medications

☐ β-blocker starting at 08:00 on POD #1, then q12 h; hold for HR <60 or SBP <100

  ☐ Metoprolol 25 mg PO/per NG tube bid

  ☐ Carvedilol 3.125 mg PO/per NG tube bid

☐ Amiodarone 400 mg PO bid to start after amiodarone infusion discontinued

☐ Magnesium sulfate 2 g in 50 mL NS IV over 2 hours on POD #1 in AM

☐ Sucralfate 1 g per NG tube q6h until NG tube removed

Table 7.2 • (Continued)

☐ Pantoprazole (Protonix) 40 mg IV/PO qd

☐ Aspirin ☐ 81 mg ☐ 325 mg PO qd (starting 8 hours after arrival); hold for platelet count <75,000 or chest tube drainage >50 mL/h

☐ Warfarin _____ mg starting _____; check with HO for daily dose (use warfarin protocol) – see Appendix 8

☐ Nitroglycerin 100 mg/250 mL D5W at 10–15 μg/min until taking PO (radial artery prophylaxis); then convert to:

    ☐ Amlodipine 5 mg PO qd

    ☐ Amlodipine 10 mg PO qd

    ☐ Isosorbide mononitrate sustained release (Imdur) 20 mg PO qd

☐ Simvastatin _____ mg qd hs (no more than 20 mg if on amiodarone)

☐ Mupirocin 2% (Bactroban ointment) via Q-tip nasal swab the evening after surgery and bid × 3 days

☐ Chlorhexidine 0.12% oral wash (Peridex) 15 mL with brushing q12 hr (at 0900 and 2100 while intubated)

e. PRN medications

    ☐ Acetaminophen 650 mg PO/PR q4h prn temp >38.5 °C

    ☐ Metoclopramide 10 mg IV/PO q6h prn nausea

    ☐ Ondansetron 4 mg IV q4h prn nausea

    ☐ KCl 80mEq/250 mL D5W via central line to keep K^+ >4.5 mEq/L:

        ☐ K^+ 4.0–4.5 KCl 10 mEq over 30 min

        ☐ K^+ 3.5–3.9 KCl 20 mEq over 60 min

        ☐ K^+ <3.5   KCl 40 mEq over 90 min

    ☐ Initiate hyperglycemia protocol if blood glucose >150 mg/dL on admission or any time within the first 48 hours (see Appendix 6)

    ☐ Other

II. Monitoring in the ICU: Techniques and Problems

Careful monitoring is required in the early postoperative period to optimize patient management and outcome. A continuous display of the ECG is provided, and pressures derived from invasive catheters, including arterial and Swan-Ganz catheters placed in the operating room, are transduced on bedside monitors (Figure 7.1). The endotracheal tube is securely connected to the mechanical ventilator and appropriate ventilator settings are selected. A continuous readout of the arterial oxygen saturation (SaO_2) determined by pulse oximetry should be displayed. The drainage outputs of chest tubes and the Foley catheter are measured and recorded. A comprehensive flowsheet, whether handwritten or entered into a computerized system, is

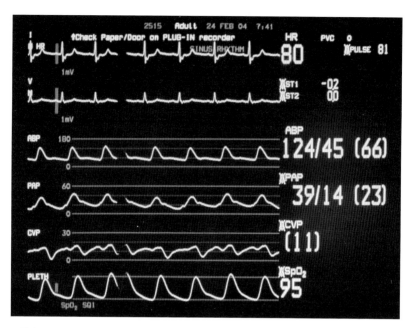

Figure 7.1 • Monitoring in the ICU. From top to bottom: ECG leads, arterial blood pressure (ABP), pulmonary artery systolic/diastolic waveforms (PAP), central venous pressure (CVP), and pulse oximetry (SpO$_2$).

essential (Appendix 5). Each invasive technique is used to provide an essential function or obtain special information about the patient's postoperative course, but each has potential complications. Each should be used only as long as necessary to maximize benefit while minimizing morbidity.

    A. **ECG display** on a bedside monitor is critical to allow for rapid interpretation of rhythm changes. The use of cartridge modules allows for the simultaneous display and recording of standard limb leads and atrial electrograms for an analysis of complex rhythms (see Chapter 11, pages 529–554). Most bedside monitors have a memory, and abnormal rhythms will activate a printout. This is helpful in detecting the mechanism of arrhythmia development (such as an R-on-T phenomenon leading to ventricular tachycardia or fibrillation). ST segment analysis is provided by most monitoring systems, but abnormalities must be thoroughly analyzed from a 12-lead ECG.

    B. Mechanical ventilation via an endotracheal tube is used for all patients except those who are extubated in the operating room. The initial settings are determined by the anesthesiologist and respiratory therapist and generally provide a tidal volume of 8–10 mL/kg at a rate of 8–10/min with the initial FiO$_2$ set at 1.0. Confirmation of bilateral breath sounds and chest movement, intermittent re-checking of ventilator settings, and assessment of the adequacy of gas exchange are essential.

1. **Pulse oximetry** is routinely used to continuously assess the status of peripheral perfusion and arterial oxygen saturation (SaO_2).[1] It can draw attention to major problems with oxygenation during the period of intubation and following extubation. If the patient is severely vasoconstricted, the recordings from the patient's fingers may be inadequate and a better signal may be derived from the earlobe. Use of pulse oximetry obviates the need to draw arterial blood gases more than a few times during the period of intubation.[2] Nonetheless, it should be kept in mind that pulse oximetry only provides a measurement of SaO_2 (and heart rate), but does not provide the same information as an arterial blood gas (ABG), which measures the PCO_2 and pH. These values may be important in assessing the patient's respiratory drive during the weaning process and can identify whether the patient has a metabolic or respiratory acidosis/alkalosis. This is particularly valuable in identifying when a metabolic acidosis reflects borderline hemodynamic function that requires further pharmacologic intervention.

2. Suctioning should be performed gently every few hours or as necessary to maintain a tube free of secretions but not so frequently as to induce endobronchial trauma or bronchospasm.[3] The endotracheal tube bypasses the protective mechanism of the upper airway and predisposes the patient to pulmonary infection. It should be removed as soon as the patient can maintain satisfactory ventilation and oxygenation and is able to protect his/her airway. This is generally accomplished within 12 hours of surgery. A standard protocol for weaning and extubation is essential in any cardiac surgical ICU (see Tables 10.3–10.5, pages 400–402).

C. **Arterial lines** are placed in either the radial or femoral artery and are transduced on the bedside monitor.[4] Occasionally, a brachial arterial line may be necessary when a radial line cannot be placed and there are issues that preclude placement of a femoral arterial line. These may include extensive iliofemoral disease, vascular reconstructive grafts in the groin, or limited availability of the femoral vessels because of an intra-aortic balloon pump (IABP) or femoral cannulation for cardiopulmonary bypass. Accurate pressure recording depends on proper calibration and elimination of air from the transducer. Although radial arterial pressure measurements may not reflect the central aortic pressure immediately after bypass, this problem usually abates by the time the patient reaches the ICU. If a discrepancy persists, a femoral arterial line may need to be placed in the ICU. This usually produces comparable mean pressures to radial lines, although it frequently demonstrates systolic overshoot that can be eliminated by resonance overshoot filters.

1. There is often a discrepancy noted between the auscultatory or occlusion blood pressure and that recorded digitally on the bedside monitor. This may be ascribed to the dynamic response characteristics of catheter-transducer systems.[5] The overdampening of signals usually results from gas bubbles within the fluid-filled system. Underdampening of signals is related to excessive compliance, length, or diameter of the tubing connecting the arterial line to the transducer. If the intra-arterial pressure appears to be dampened or exhibits overshoot, the analog display of the mean pressure is most reliable. The occlusion pressure is probably the most accurate measurement of the systolic pressure.

2. Arterial lines should be connected to continuous saline flushes to improve patency rates and minimize thrombus formation. Heparin flushes do not provide any advantage in maintaining line patency and may potentially increase the risk of

developing heparin-induced thrombocytopenia, although this problem has not been documented in studies of cardiac surgical ICU patients.[6,7]

3. The incidence of complications associated with radial arterial lines, such as digital ischemia or infection, is extremely low, and empiric changing of arterial lines is not mandatory. However, attention must always be directed to perfusion of the hand when a radial arterial line is present so that prompt therapy can be initiated if problems develop. Digital ischemia can occur within a few days and usually is caused by thrombosis at the insertion site with distal embolization.[8] This is a serious problem that mandates immediate removal of the arterial line. It usually does not respond to radial revascularization but can be treated with vasodilators to minimize tissue loss. Infections usually respond to line removal and antibiotics. An infected pseudoaneurysm usually requires surgery.[9]

4. Arterial lines are invaluable for sampling arterial blood gas specimens and obtaining blood for other laboratory tests, but they are often retained when invasive pressure monitoring is no longer essential but intravenous access for blood sampling is limited. Arterial lines should generally be removed when there is no longer a requirement for pharmacologic support and when satisfactory post-extubation arterial blood gases have been achieved. A room-air blood gas before removal may give a baseline assessment of the patient's oxygenation. However, as long as the PaO_2 and oxygen saturation obtained from an ABG are consistent with the oxygen saturation measured by pulse oximetry, the latter may then be used to follow the patient's oxygenation. After removal of a femoral arterial catheter, adequate manual pressure should be maintained over the femoral artery to produce adequate hemostasis. A falling hematocrit of unclear etiology could result from bleeding into the groin or retroperitoneum from iliofemoral arterial wall puncture.

D. **Central venous pressure (CVP)** monitoring may provide adequate information about filling pressures in patients with preserved ventricular function undergoing coronary surgery. Several studies have shown comparable outcomes in patients undergoing on- or off-pump surgery managed with CVP lines or pulmonary artery (PA) catheters.[10–12] In most patients, the CVP and PA diastolic pressures correlate reasonably well and can guide appropriate fluid management.

1. However, studies have suggested that there is an imprecise correlation of CVP with circulatory blood volume, and PA catheter monitoring provides a better assessment of intracardiac volumes in patients undergoing valve surgery.[13,14] Thus, although avoidance of a PA catheter should not compromise postoperative care of a routine coronary patient, it does provide more objective and accurate data upon which therapeutic decisions can be based. However, patients with PA catheters tend to receive more volume than those managed with only CVP lines, with a tendency towards delayed extubation.[10]

2. Venous oxygen saturation reflects the balance between oxygen delivery and consumption by the tissues.[15] The mixed venous oxygen saturation (SvO_2) obtained from the distal PA port of a Swan-Ganz catheter has been considered the best means of assessing this balance and, although subject to many variables, it is generally reflective of the cardiac output. An inexpensive alternative to the SvO_2 is the central venous oxygen saturation (CvO_2) obtained from a CVP line. However, there is often a significant discrepancy between these two values which reflects variation in regional blood flow, and it is most marked when the SaO_2, hemoglobin, or cardiac

index is low.[16-18] There is also a discrepancy noted between co-oximetric readings and those obtained from continuous monitoring devices, such as the CeVOX device (Pulsion Medical Systems).[19] Thus, the SvO_2 may have some value in assessing the cardiac output, but the lack of correlation with the CvO_2 suggests that the latter should only be used as a relative means of detecting trends in oxygen extraction.

3. One study of goal-directed therapy in moderate-to-high-risk patients asssessed whether use of the Vigileo/FloTrac device (see pages 293–294) to measure cardiac outputs along with continuous CvO_2 measurements influenced results compared with standard monitoring including a CVP line. This approach increased volume infusions and adjustment of inotropic medications but did decrease the duration of ventilation. Otherwise, there were few clinical benefits.[20]

E. **Swan-Ganz pulmonary artery catheters** are commonly placed in patients undergoing open-heart surgery to assist with intraoperative and postoperative hemodynamic management. They are valuable in making evidence-based, scientific decisions about fluid, inotropic, or vasopressor support, although their impact on clinical outcome may only be evident in high-risk patients. They are generally placed either prior to or after the induction of anesthesia, but may need to be placed preoperatively in the cardiac cath lab or the ICU in hemodynamically unstable patients.

1. These catheters measure the CVP, pulmonary artery (PA) and pulmonary capillary wedge (PCW) pressures indicative of left-sided filling, and allow for the determination of a thermodilution cardiac output. Sampling blood from the PA port allows for measurement of a mixed venous oxygen saturation (SvO_2). Although the correlation of SvO_2 and cardiac output is subject to many variables (see pages 442–443), the SVO_2 is helpful when the thermodilution output seems inconsistent with the patient's clinical course.[21] It is also useful in patients with tricuspid regurgitation, in whom the thermodilution cardiac output is inaccurate and tends to underestimate the cardiac output.[22,23]

2. The interpretation of hemodynamic parameters derived from the PA catheter requires an understanding of the patient's underlying disease process, baseline values, the nature and extent of the operative procedure, the effects of surgery on ventricular compliance, and an integration with intraoperative echocardiographic assessments of ventricular volumes and function. It can provide information on volume status, systolic dysfunction, diastolic dysfunction, suspicion of ischemia, regurgitant heart lesions, and intracardiac shunting.[24,25] Thus, when utilized appropriately, a Swan-Ganz catheter provides invaluable information for patient management.

3. Some Swan-Ganz catheters have the capability of providing continuous cardiac output measurements and in-line SvO_2. They are particularly useful in patients undergoing off-pump surgery. Other catheters calculate right ventricular volumes and ejection fraction, while others have additional ports for volume infusions or pacing wires.

4. The introducer sheath for a PA catheter (the "Cordis") is an 8.5 Fr cannula with a side port for volume infusions. In patients with limited access, a 9 Fr advanced venous access (AVA) catheter with multiple ports can be used.

5. The proximal port of the Swan-Ganz catheter (30 cm from the tip) is used for CVP measurements from the right atrium and for fluid injections to determine the cardiac output. Care must be exercised when injecting sterile fluid for cardiac outputs to

prevent bolusing of vasoactive medications that might be running through the CVP port. **Note:** One must *never* infuse anything through this port if the catheter has been pulled back so that the tip of the catheter lies in the right atrium and the CVP port is not within the bloodstream!

6. The distal port should always be transduced and displayed on the bedside monitor to allow for detection of catheter advancement into the permanent wedge position, which could result in pulmonary artery injury. This will be detected by loss of the phasic PA trace on the monitor and is suggested by the position of the catheter on a chest x-ray. Balloon inflation ("wedging" of the catheter) need not be performed more than once every few hours, and the balloon should not be inflated for more than two respiratory cycles to prevent PA injury. Balloon inflation should be performed cautiously with minimal inflation volume or should be avoided entirely in patients with pulmonary hypertension. Medications should never be given through the distal PA port.

7. Although there is a significant incidence of minor complications associated with the insertion and use of the Swan-Ganz catheter, serious life-threatening complications are very uncommon. The catheter is more commonly placed through the internal jugular vein than the subclavian vein for cardiac surgery, as the catheter may become displaced during sternal retraction with the latter approach.[26] Identification of the location of the internal jugular vein using an echo probe is helpful in avoiding arterial puncture (Figure 4.2, page 178).

   a. Complications associated with insertion include:
   - Arrhythmias and heart block (especially in patients with a LBBB)
   - Arterial puncture
   - Pneumothorax
   - Air embolism
   - Perforation of the right atrium or ventricle
   - Catheter knotting

   b. Complications of indwelling PA catheters include:
   - Arrhythmias and heart block
   - Heparin-induced thrombocytopenia (from heparin-coated catheters)
   - Infection
   - Pulmonary artery rupture and hemorrhage; pulmonary pseudoaneurysms
   - Endocardial and valvular damage
   - Pulmonary infarction
   - Pulmonary infiltrates
   - Venous thrombosis

8. **Pulmonary artery perforation** is a very serious complication that may occur during insertion of the catheter, during surgery, or at any time in the ICU.[27–29] The position of the catheter should always be inspected on an immediate postoperative or any post-insertion chest x-ray. Migration of the catheter into the wedge position should be noted on the bedside monitor and the catheter should be pulled back immediately. Perforation may lead to hemoptysis, bleeding into the endotracheal tube, or intrapleural hemorrhage. The chest x-ray may demonstrate a hematoma surrounding the tip of the catheter. If perforation is suspected, the catheter should be

withdrawn and positive end-expiratory pressure (PEEP) added to the ventilator circuit. If bleeding persists, bronchoscopy can be performed with placement of a bronchial blocker to isolate the lung. Use of a double-lumen endotracheal tube or even a thoracotomy with pulmonary resection may be indicated for ongoing pulmonary hemorrhage. Rarely, a false aneurysm of the pulmonary artery branches may develop. This has been treated by transcatheter embolization.[30] The management of pulmonary artery perforation occurring during surgery is discussed on page 180.

9. The PA catheter should be removed when the patient no longer requires vasoactive drug support. If the catheter is removed but the introducer sheath is left in place for fluid or medication administration, the port must be covered with a small adhesive drape to minimize the risk of infection. A one-way valve present on most introducer sheaths eliminates the possibility of air embolism. The introducer should be removed as soon as possible because of its size to minimize the risk of infection and venous thrombosis (let alone patient discomfort). If less intensive central venous monitoring is required or there is limited venous access, a smaller double- or triple-lumen catheter should replace the large-bore introducer.

F. **Alternative means of assessing cardiac output.** Although the Swan-Ganz catheter is the gold standard for measuring cardiac outputs, it is an invasive catheter associated with a number of potential complications. Alternative less invasive means of determining the cardiac output have been developed that can provide comparable cardiac output measurements.

1. There are a number of arterial pressure-based technologies that can be used to assess cardiac output.[31] Of particular value in cardiac surgery is the Edwards Vigileo/FloTrac device, which performs an analysis of the pressure wave signal from the arterial line, correlates the standard deviation of the pulse pressure with the stroke volume using patient demographic data, adjusts for vascular compliance, and then provides continuous cardiac output calculations (Figure 7.2).[32,33] This is very valuable when a Swan-Ganz catheter has not been placed, is not functioning well, or provides cardiac output values that appear inconsistent with the patient's clinical picture (e.g., the patient with tricuspid regurgitation). During off-pump surgery, it is extremely helpful in assessing cardiac function when the heart is displaced for posterior anastomoses or when significant ischemia occurs. The correlation with thermodilution cardiac outputs is reasonably accurate.[34,35]

2. Esophageal Doppler is rarely used in cardiac surgery patients, but can also provide comparable cardiac output measurements to thermodilution technology. It provides Doppler flow velocity waveforms that include flow time and peak velocity. These waveforms allow for assessment of left ventricular contractility, filling, and systemic vascular resistance (Figure 7.3).[36,37]

G. **Left atrial (LA) lines** can be used in special circumstances to give the most accurate assessment of left-sided filling pressures. They are placed through the right superior pulmonary vein and passed into the left atrium during surgery.

1. LA lines are particularly helpful in patients with a high transpulmonary gradient, in whom the pulmonary artery diastolic pressure is significantly greater than true left-sided filling pressures. They may be used in patients with severe left ventricular dysfunction, severe pulmonary hypertension secondary to mitral valve disease, during use of circulatory assist devices, or following heart transplantation.

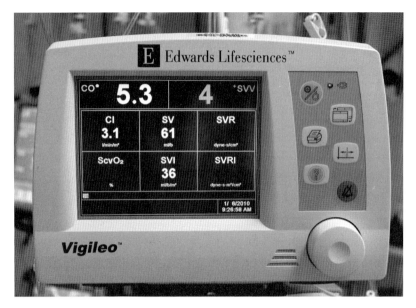

Figure 7.2 • The Edwards Vigileo FloTrac continuous cardiac output monitor which is connected to the arterial line.

2. Although LA lines may provide important hemodynamic information, they are associated with rare but potentially significant complications.[38,39] An LA line should always be considered dangerous because of the risk of air embolism. It must always be aspirated before being flushed to make sure there is no air or thrombus present within the system. It is then connected to a constant infusion flush line that includes an air filter to reduce the risk of systemic air embolism. The line should be removed when the chest tubes are still in place in the event that bleeding from the insertion site occurs.

H. **Chest tubes** are placed in the mediastinum and into the pleural spaces if they are entered during surgery. Drainage should be recorded hourly or more frequently if there is evidence of significant bleeding.

1. The chest tubes are connected to a drainage system to which -20 cm of H_2O suction is applied. The tubes should be gently milked or stripped to prevent blood from clotting within them. There is no particular advantage of any of the common practices (milking, stripping, fanfolding, or tapping) in maintaining chest tube patency.[40–42] Aggressive stripping creates a negative pressure of up to -300 cm H_2O in the mediastinum. This may actually increase bleeding and is quite painful to the patient who has regained consciousness and is not adequately sedated. Suctioning of clotted chest tubes with endotracheal suction catheters is discouraged because of the risk of introducing infection.

2. Bloody drainage through chest tubes can be best observed if the tubes are not completely covered with tape. Plastic connectors must be tightly and securely attached to both the chest tubes and the drainage tubing to maintain sterility and prevent air leaks within the system. Although an air leak should always raise the

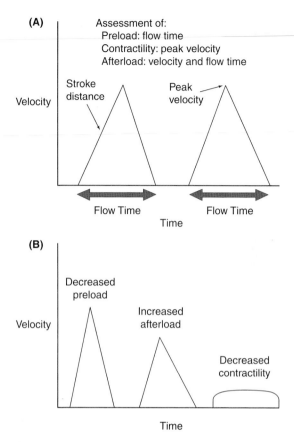

Figure 7.3 • Doppler flow waveforms obtained with the esophageal Doppler. (A) A normal waveform. Preload is estimated by the flow time, contractility by the peak velocity, and afterload (systemic resistance) assessed by both velocity and flow time. (B) Waveforms associated with decreased preload, increased afterload, or decreased contractility. These conditions can be improved by volume infusions, vasodilators, and inotropes, respectively.

possibility of a pulmonary parenchymal leak, the connections should be checked first since a loose connection or disconnection is an easily remediable problem. The development of subcutaneous emphysema may reflect an active air leak with clotted chest tubes, but more frequently is the result of kinking of the tubes.

3. Excessive mediastinal bleeding requires immediate attention because it often leads to hemodynamic instability, metabolic acidosis, the requirement for multiple blood products, and the potential for cardiac tamponade (see Chapter 9).

4. Autotransfusion of shed mediastinal blood can be used as a component of a blood conservation strategy, but its benefits are controversial. It provides volume expansion with the potential for reducing transfusion requirements. However, shed blood also has a low level of platelets, fibrinogen, and factor VIII and a high level of fibrin split products.[43] Although reinfusion in moderate amounts (less than 1 liter) does not significantly alter coagulation parameters, larger amounts may.[44] If the patient has

bled that much, reexploration is probably indicated. Autotransfusion can be accomplished either from soft plastic collection bags or directly from the plastic shell via a pump through a 20–40 μm filter.

I. The **urinary Foley catheter** is attached to gravity drainage and the urine output is recorded hourly. Urine output is subject to many variables, but in a patient with normal renal function, it generally reflects the level of renal perfusion, which may be compromised in a low cardiac output state.

1. Foley catheters incorporating temperature probes are commonly used during surgery and can be used in the ICU to record the patient's core temperature.

2. The Foley catheter is usually removed at midnight entering the second postoperative day.[45] It may be left in place if the patient is undergoing a significant diuresis or has a history of prostatic hypertrophy or urinary retention and has not been mobilized. The risk of urinary infection increases with a longer duration of indwelling catheter time, and early removal should be considered in patients with prosthetic valves and grafts when its use is no longer essential.

3. Suprapubic tubes should be left in place and clamped after several days to see if the patient can void per urethra.

J. **Nasogastric tubes** or orogastric tubes may be inserted in the operating room or after the patient's arrival in the ICU to aid with gastric decompression. Insertion may cause hypertension, bradycardia, tachycardia, or arrhythmias if the patient is not well sedated. Insertion may also cause nasopharyngeal bleeding if the patient is still heparinized (during surgery) or has a coagulopathy. Instillation of a medication to reduce stress ulceration, such as sucralfate, should be considered for all patients during the first 12–24 hours. This is equally as efficacious as the H_2 blockers and proton pump inhibitors, both of which raise gastric pH. One could consider the supplemental use of a proton pump inhibitor if the patient is at extremely high risk for stress ulcer-related bleeding.[46–48]

K. **Pacing wires**. Most surgeons place two atrial and two ventricular temporary epicardial pacing wire electrodes at the conclusion of open-heart surgery. If the pacing wires are being used, they must be securely attached to the patient and to the cable connector, and the cable must be securely attached to the pacing box. The pacemaker box itself should be easily accessible. **Everyone caring for the patient should understand how the particular pacemaker generator works and what the current pacemaker settings are**. Pacing wires that are not being used should be placed in insulating needle caps to isolate them from stray electrical currents that could potentially trigger arrhythmias. Particular issues of concern are pacing thresholds in patients with complete heart block and no escape mechanism, and inappropriate sensing and pacing that could trigger malignant arrhythmias.

III. Summary of Guidelines for Removal of Lines and Tubes in the ICU

A. The Swan-Ganz catheter should be removed when inotropic support and vasodilators are no longer necessary. If central venous access is required after several days but hemodynamic monitoring is no longer essential, the Swan-Ganz catheter should be replaced by a double- or triple-lumen catheter.

B. Any central line should be removed when no longer necessary to reduce the risk of infection. The catheter need only be replaced for a clinical indication, such as a fever of unknown origin or suspected bacteremia. If the catheter site is infected or bacteremia is confirmed, the catheter should be withdrawn and another inserted in a different site. If neither of these indications is present, the catheter can be changed over a guidewire to reduce the risk of mechanical complications associated with a new insertion site. The catheter tip is cultured. If this returns positive, the catheter should be changed to a new site.[49,50]

C. The arterial line should be removed after a stable post-extubation blood gas has been obtained. An additional ABG obtained on room air is frequently worthwhile because it provides a relative indication of the patient's baseline postoperative oxygenation and it can be correlated with the oxygen saturation measured by pulse oximetry. Subsequently, the latter may be used to follow the patient's oxygenation. The arterial line should not be left in place as a convenience for blood sampling. Adequate pressure should be maintained over the groin upon removal of a femoral arterial catheter.

D. LA lines must be removed in the ICU while the chest tubes remain in place in the event that intrapericardial bleeding occurs.

E. The urinary catheter can be left in place if the patient is undergoing a vigorous diuresis or has an increased risk of urinary retention. It should otherwise be removed once the patient is mobilized out of bed, usually at midnight entering the second postoperative day.

F. Chest tubes should be removed when the total drainage is less than 100 mL for 8 hours. Prolonging the duration of drainage may increase total chest-tube output without any effect on the incidence of postoperative pericardial effusions.[51] One study showed that there was no difference in the incidence of pericardial effusions if tubes were withdrawn when drainage was less than 50 mL over 5 hours or when the fluid became serosanguineous (either upon visual inspection or when the drain/blood hematocrit ratio was <0.3).[52]

1. Straight and right-angled 32 Fr PVC or silicone-coated tubes are usually placed in the mediastinum, with either two anterior tubes or one anterior and one posterior tube. The latter must be tacked by the surgeon away from inferior wall grafts, as compression could precipitate inferior wall ischemia, which should be noted on a postoperative ECG. Pleural tubes can be placed either through the upper abdominal wall lateral to the mediastinal tubes or through the lateral chest wall. Tubes placed laterally can produce more chest wall pain, but are theoretically less prone to contribute to mediastinal infection if left in place for a prolonged period of time.

2. Alternatively, silastic fluted (Blake) drains may be placed in the mediastinum or into the pleural space. These drains usually provide comparable drainage efficiency and are more comfortable for the patient.[53] One study showed that use of an infracardiac Blake drain rather than a semirigid drain resulted in more drainage, less residual effusion, and a lower risk of atrial fibrillation.[54] Leaving a supplemental drain in the pleural space for 3–5 days is useful in reducing the incidence of symptomatic pleural effusions, and this should preferably be placed through the lateral chest wall, rather than through the mediastinum.[55]

3. Mediastinal tubes should always be removed off suction, because graft avulsion might theoretically occur if suction is maintained. A chest x-ray is not essential after mediastinal tube removal, but should be performed after removal of pleural chest tubes to rule out a pneumothorax.

References

1. Bierman MI, Stein KL, Snyder JV. Pulse oximetry in the postoperative care of cardiac surgical patients. A randomized controlled trial. *Chest* 1992;102:1367–70.

2. Durbin CG Jr, Rostow SK. More reliable oximetry reduces the frequency of arterial blood gas analyses and hastens oxygen weaning after cardiac surgery: a prospective randomized trial of the clinical impact of a new technology. *Crit Care Med* 2002;30:1735–40.

3. Guglielminotti J, Desmonts JM, Dureuil B. Effects of tracheal suctioning on respiratory resistances in mechanically ventilated patients. *Chest* 1999;113:1135–8.

4. Haddad F, Zeeni C, El Rassi I, et al. Can femoral artery pressure monitoring be used routinely in cardiac surgery? *J Cardiothorac Vasc Anesth* 2008;22:418–22.

5. Gibbs NC, Gardner RM. Dynamics of invasive pressure monitoring systems: clinical and laboratory evaluation. *Heart Lung* 1988;17:43–51.

6. Whitta RK, Hall KF, Bennetts TM, Welman L, Rawlins P. Comparison of normal or heparinised saline flushing on function of arterial lines. *Crit Care Resusc* 2006;8:205–8.

7. Hall KF, Bennetts TM, Whitta RK, Welman L, Rawlins P. Effect of heparin in arterial line flushing solutions on platelet count: a randomised double-blind study. *Crit Care Resusc* 2006;8:294–6.

8. Valentine RJ, Modrall JG, Clagett GP. Hand ischemia after radial artery cannulation. *J Am Coll Surg* 2005;201:18–22.

9. El-Hamamsy I, Dürrleman N, Stevens LM, et al. Incidence and outcome of radial artery infections following cardiac surgery. *Ann Thorac Surg* 2003;76:801–4.

10. Stewart RD, Psyhojos T, Lahey SJ, Levitsky S, Campos CT. Central venous catheter use in low-risk coronary artery bypass grafting. *Ann Thorac Surg* 1998;66:1306–11.

11. Schwann TA, Zacharias A, Riordan CJ, Durham SJ, Engoren M, Habib RH. Safe, highly selective use of pulmonary artery catheters in coronary artery bypass grafting: an objective patient selection method. *Ann Thorac Surg* 2002;73:1394–402.

12. Resano FG, Kapetanakis EI, Hill PC, Haile E, Corso PJ. Clinical outcomes of low-risk patients undergoing beating-heart surgery with and without pulmonary artery catheterization. *J Cardiothorac Vasc Anesth* 2006;20:300–6.

13. Yamauchi H, Biuk-Aghai EN, Yu M, et al. Circulating blood volume measurements correlate poorly with pulmonary artery catheter measurements. *Hawaii Med J* 2008;67:8–11.

14. Breukers RM, Trof RJ, de Wilde R.B. et al. Relative value of pressures and volumes in assessing fluid responsiveness after valvular and coronary artery surgery. *Eur J Cardiothorac Surg* 2009;35:62–8.

15. Shepherd SJ, Pearse RM. Role of central and mixed venous oxygen saturation measurement in perioperative care. *Anesthesiology* 2009;111:649–56.

16. Yazigi A, El Khoury C, Jebara S, Haddad F, Hayeck G, Sleilaty G. Comparison of central venous to mixed venous oxygen saturation in patients with low cardiac index and filling pressures after coronary artery surgery. *J Cardiothorac Vasc Anesth* 2008;22:77–83.

17. Lorentzen AG, Lindskov C, Sloth E, Jakobsen CJ. Central venous oxygen saturation cannot replace mixed venous saturation in patients undergoing cardiac surgery. *J Cardiothorac Vasc Anesth* 2008;22:853–7.

18. Sander M, Spies CD, Foer A, et al. Agreement of central venous saturation and mixed venous saturation in cardiac surgery patients. *Intensive Care Med* 2007;33:1719–25.

19. Baulig W, Dullenkopf A, Kobler A, Baulig B, Roth HR, Schmid ER. Accuracy of continuous central venous oxygen saturation monitoring in patients undergoing cardiac surgery. *J Clin Monit Comput* 2008;22:183–8.

20. Kapoor PM, Kakani M, Chowdhury U, Choudhury M, Lakshmy R, Kiran U. Early goal-directed therapy in moderate to high-risk cardiac surgery patients. *Ann Card Anaesth* 2008;11:27–34.

21. Sommers MS, Stevenson JS, Hamlin RL, Ivey TD, Russell AC. Mixed venous oxygen saturation and oxygen partial pressure as predictors of cardiac index after coronary artery bypass grafting. *Heart Lung* 1993;22:112–20.

22. Balik M, Pachl J, Hendl J. Effect of the degree of tricuspid regurgitation on cardiac output measurements by thermodilution. *Intensive Care Med* 2002;28:1117–21.

23. Heerdt PM, Blessios GA, Beach ML, Hogue CW. Flow dependency of error in thermodilution measurement of cardiac output during acute tricuspid regurgitation. *J Cardiothorac Vasc Anesth* 2001;15:183–7.

24. Ranucci M. Which cardiac surgical patients can benefit from placement of a pulmonary artery catheter? *Crit Care* 2006;10 Suppl 3:S6.

25. Mark JB. Multimodal detection of perioperative myocardial ischemia. *Tex Heart Inst J* 2005;32:461–6.

26. Ruesch S, Walder B, Tramèr MR. Complications of central venous catheters: internal jugular versus subclavian access – a systematic review. *Crit Care Med* 2002;30:454–60.

27. Mullerworth MH, Angelopoulos P, Couyant MA, et al. Recognition and management of catheter-induced pulmonary artery rupture. *Ann Thorac Surg* 1998;66:1242–5.

28. Bossert T, Gummert JF, Bittner HB, et al. Swan-Ganz catheter-induced severe complications in cardiac surgery: right ventricular perforation, knotting, and rupture of the pulmonary artery. *J Card Surg* 2006;21:292–5.

29. Abreu AR, Campos MA, Krieger BP. Pulmonary artery rupture induced by a pulmonary artery catheter: a case report and review of the literature. *J Intensive Care Med* 2004;19:291–6.

30. Karak P, Dimick R, Hamrick KM, Schwartzberg M, Saddekni S. Immediate transcatheter embolization of Swan-Ganz catheter-induced pulmonary artery pseudoaneurysm. *Chest* 1997;111:1450–2.

31. Maus TM, Lee DE. Arterial pressure-based cardiac output assessment. *J Cardiothorac Vasc Anesth* 2008;22:468–73.

32. Manecke GR. Edwards FloTrac sensor and Vigileo monitor: easy, accurate, reliable cardiac output assessment using the arterial pulse wave. *Expert Rev Med Devices* 2005;2:523–7.

33. Zimmermann A, Kufner C, Hofbauer S, et al. The accuracy of the Vigileo/FloTrac continuous cardiac output monitor. *J Cardiothorac Vasc Anesth* 2008;22:388–93.

34. Mehta Y, Chand RK, Sawhney R, Bhise M, Singh A, Trehan N. Cardiac output monitoring: comparison of a new arterial pressure waveform analysis to the bolus thermodilution technique in patients undergoing off-pump coronary artery bypass surgery. *J Cardiothorac Vasc Anesth* 2008;22:394–9.

35. Breukers RMBGE, Sepehrkhouy S, Speigelenberg SR, Groeneveld ABJ. Cardiac output measured by a new arterial pressure waveform analysis method without calibration compared with thermodilution after cardiac surgery. *J Cardiothorac Vasc Anesth* 2007;21:632–5.

36. DiCorte CJ, Latham P, Greilich PE, Cooley MV, Grayburn PA, Jessen ME. Esophageal Doppler monitor determinations of cardiac output and preload during cardiac operations. *Ann Thorac Surg* 2000;69:1782–6.

37. Bein B, Worthmann F, Tonner PH, et al. Comparison of esophageal Doppler, pulse contour analysis, and real-time pulmonary artery thermodilution for the continuous measurement of cardiac output. *J Cardiothorac Vasc Anesth* 2004;18:185–9.

38. Santini F, Gatti G, Borghetti V, Oppido G, Mazzucco A. Routine left atrial catheterization for the post-operative management of cardiac surgical patients: is the risk justified? *Eur J Cardiothorac Surg* 1999;16:218–21.

39. Feerick AE, Church JA, Zwischenberger J, Conti V, Johnston WE. Systemic gaseous microembolism during left atrial catheterization: a common occurrence? *J Cardiothorac Vasc Anesth* 1995;9:395–8.

40. Wallen M, Morrison A, Gillies D, O'Riordan E, Bridge C, Stoddart F. Mediastinal chest drain clearance for cardiac surgery. *Cochrane Database Syst Rev* 2004;4:CD003042.

41. Day TG, Perring RR, Gofton K. Is manipulation of mediastinal chest drains useful or harmful after cardiac surgery? *Interact Cardiovasc Thorac Surg* 2008;7:888–90.

42. Charnock Y, Evans D. Nursing management of chest drains: a systematic review. *Aust Crit Care* 2001;14:156–60.

43. Hartz RS, Smith JA, Green D. Autotransfusion after cardiac operation. Assessment of hemostatic factors. *J Thorac Cardiovasc Surg* 1988;96:178–82.

44. Axford TC, Dearani JA, Ragno G, et al. Safety and therapeutic effectiveness of reinfused shed blood after open heart surgery. *Ann Thorac Surg* 1994;57:615–22.

45. Griffiths R, Fernandez R. Strategies for the removal of short-term indwelling urethral catheters in adults. *Cochrane Database Syst Rev* 2007;2:CD004011.

46. van der Voort PH, Zandstra DF. Pathogenesis, risk factors, and incidence of upper gastrointestinal bleeding after cardiac surgery: is specific prophylaxis in routine bypass procedures needed? *J Cardiothorac Vasc Anesth* 2000;14:293–9.

47. Hata M, Shiono M, Sekino H, et al. Prospective randomized trial for optimal prophylactic treatment of the upper gastrointestinal complications after open heart surgery. *Circ J* 2005;69:331–4.

48. Jung R, MacLaren R. Proton-pump inhibitors for stress ulcer prophylaxis in critically ill patients. *Ann Pharmacother* 2002;36:1929–37.

49. Cobb DK, High KP, Sawyer RG, et al. A controlled trial of scheduled replacement of central venous and pulmonary-artery catheters. *N Engl J Med* 1992;327:1062–8.

50. Hagley MT, Martin B, Gast P, Traeger SM. Infectious and mechanical complications of central venous catheters placed by percutaneous venipuncture and over guidewires. *Crit Care Med* 1992;20:1426–30.

51. Smulders YM, Wiepking ME, Moulijn AC, Koolen JJ, van Wezel HB, Visser CA. How soon should drainage tubes be removed after cardiac operations? *Ann Thorac Surg* 1989;48:540–3.

52. Gercekoglu H, Aydin NB, Dagdeviren B, et al. Effect of timing of chest tube removal on development of pericardial effusion following cardiac surgery. *J Card Surg* 2003;18:217–24.

53. Sakopoulos AG, Hurwitz AS, Suda RW, Goodwin JN. Efficacy of Blake drains for mediastinal and pleural drainage following cardiac operations. *J Card Surg* 2005;20:574–7.

54. Ege T, Tatli E, Canbaz S, et al. The importance of intrapericardial drain selection in cardiac surgery. *Chest* 2004;126:1559–62.

55. Payne M, Magovern GJ Jr, Benckart DH, et al. Left pleural effusion after coronary artery bypass decreases with a supplemental pleural drain. *Ann Thorac Surg* 2002;73:149–52.

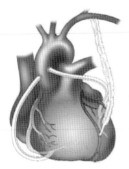

CHAPTER 8

Early Postoperative Care

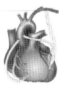

8 Early Postoperative Care

The early postoperative course for most patients undergoing cardiac surgery with use of cardiopulmonary bypass (CPB) is characterized by a typical pattern of pathophysiologic derangements that benefits from standardized management. Intraoperative monitoring with Swan-Ganz catheter measurements and transesophageal echocardiography (TEE) are routinely used to direct hemodynamic management and fluid administration. Anesthetic techniques and early extubation protocols should be designed to achieve "fast-track" recovery of most patients (Table 8.1).[1,2] The pathophysiology noted after off-pump surgery is slightly different in that patients are not subjected to the insults of CPB and cardioplegia, two factors that contribute to a systemic inflammatory response and transient myocardial depression. This chapter will summarize the basic clinical features of the post-CPB patient and will then present scenarios commonly seen in the early postoperative period. It will then discuss aspects of postoperative care unique to various types of cardiac surgical procedures. The subsequent chapters will describe in greater detail the assessment and management of the major concerns of the postoperative period: mediastinal bleeding, respiratory, cardiovascular, renal, and metabolic problems.

I. Basic Features of the Early Postoperative Period

A. Overview

1. Following most cardiac procedures, patients arrive in the intensive care unit (ICU) fully anesthetized and sedated, requiring mechanical ventilation for several hours. Adequate pharmacologic sedation and pain control is essential at this time and during the weaning process from the ventilator, which generally should be started once standard criteria are met (Table 10.3, page 400). Early extubation is usually defined as withdrawal of mechanical ventilation within 8 hours of surgery, although many protocols are designed to achieve "ultra-fast" extubation within a few hours.[3]

2. Extubation can be accomplished at the conclusion of surgery following both on- and off-pump surgery. The blood pressure may be better maintained with increased sympathetic tone and less requirement for vasodilating medications such as propofol and narcotics. Right ventricular function may be improved when positive-pressure ventilation is not required. However, it is important to provide adequate analgesia to these patients without producing respiratory depression, generally using nonsteroidal anti-inflammatory drugs or low doses of narcotics.

Manual of Perioperative Care in Adult Cardiac Surgery, 5th Edition. By Robert M. Bojar.
Published 2011 by Blackwell Publishing Ltd.

Table 8.1 • Options for a Fast-Track Protocol

Operating Room	
Anesthetic agents	Sufentanil 0.5 μg/kg for induction, then 0.25 μg/kg/h Fentanyl 5–10 μg/kg, then 0.3–5 μg/kg/h or inhalational agents + propofol Remifentanil 1 μg/kg for induction, then 0.05–2 μg/kg/min
Sedatives	Midazolam 2.5–5 mg before bypass Propofol 50–75 μg/kg/min (2–10 mg/kg/h) after bypass
Cardiopulmonary bypass	Withdrawal of autologous blood before starting bypass Consider retrograde autologous priming to maintain higher hematocrit Echo imaging for aortic atherosclerosis Maintain blood glucose <180 mg/dL Consider nesiritide/fenoldopam if renal dysfunction Warm to 37 °C before terminating bypass
Myocardial protection	Antegrade/retrograde blood cardioplegia with terminal "hot shot"
Antifibrinolytic agents	ε-aminocaproic acid 5 g at skin incision and in pump prime, and 1 g/h infusion Tranexamic acid 10 mg/kg, then 1 mg/kg/h
Fluids	Minimize fluid administration
Other medications	Amiodarone 150 mg IV over 30 minutes, then continue as an infusion in the ICU for 24 hours Methylprednisolone 1 g before bypass, then dexamethasone 4 mg q6h × 4 doses
Intensive Care Unit	
Analgesia	Morphine as small boluses or an infusion of 0.01–0.02 mg/kg/h depending on age Ketorolac 15–30 mg IV after extubation × 72 hours PCA pump with morphine on POD #1
Anxiolysis	Propofol 25 μg/kg/min Dexmedetomidine 1 μg/kg over 10 minutes followed by a continuous infusion of 0.2–0.7 μg/kg/h
Shivering	Meperidine 25–50 mg IV
Hypertension	Sodium nitroprusside/clevidipine/nicardipine/esmolol (avoid sedatives)
Anemia	Tolerate hematocrit of 22% if stable
Other medications	Metoprolol by POD #1 (AF prophylaxis) Magnesium sulfate 2 g on POD #1 (AF prophylaxis) Consider amiodarone for AF prophylaxis

3. Ventricular function is commonly compromised for several hours following operations on CPB with cardioplegic arrest. Inotropic medications may be required for postcardiotomy hemodynamic support during this time as the heart recovers from the insult imposed by ischemia and reperfusion. Furthermore, diastolic function is impaired with reduced compliance. Therefore, volume administration to achieve satisfactory preload will require higher filling pressures than noted preoperatively.

4. Urine output may be copious because of hemodilution during surgery. However, even though the patient is total body fluid overloaded, fluid administration is usually necessary to maintain intravascular volume to optimize hemodynamic status. Hypokalemia associated with excellent urine output must be monitored and treated. Renal function is generally a good marker of hemodynamic function, although it is subject to numerous variables. Consequently, an initial good urine output may be noted despite poor cardiac function, but a low urine output is of more concern.

5. Patients may have mediastinal bleeding as a result of technical factors or a coagulopathy, and careful monitoring of chest tube drainage is essential. Blood or blood product transfusions may be indicated for profound anemia or ongoing bleeding.

6. Postoperative care requires an integration of a myriad of hemodynamic measurements and laboratory tests to ensure a swift and uneventful recovery from surgery. Use of a comprehensive hand-written or computerized flowsheet is essential in evaluating the patient's course in the ICU (see Appendix 5).

B. **Warming from hypothermia to 37 °C**

1. Hypothermia ($< 36 °C$) upon admission to the ICU has been associated with adverse outcomes.[4,5] Therefore, it is imperative that adequate rewarming be performed during surgery and that hypothermia be actively treated in the ICU since it may:

   a. Predispose to atrial and ventricular arrhythmias and lower the ventricular fibrillation threshold.

   b. Produce peripheral vasoconstriction, increasing the systemic vascular resistance (SVR). This will elevate filling pressures and mask hypovolemia, increase afterload, raising myocardial oxygen demand, and often cause hypertension, potentially increasing mediastinal bleeding.

   c. Precipitate shivering, which increases peripheral O_2 consumption and CO_2 production.

   d. Produce platelet dysfunction and a generalized impairment of the coagulation cascade.

   e. Prolong the duration of action of anesthetic drugs and prolong the time to extubation.

   f. Increase the risk of wound infection, possibly related to immunosuppression.

2. CPB is usually accompanied by moderate systemic hypothermia to $32-34 °C$ and is terminated after the patient has been rewarmed to a core body temperature of at least $36 °C$. Although it is common practice to warm patients to $37 °C$ before terminating bypass, this may require higher arterial inflow temperatures and may be associated with impairment in neurocognitive function.[6] In fact, studies have shown that the

brain temperature is several degrees warmer than the nasopharyngeal temperature during rewarming, suggesting that temperatures measured at other sites may underestimate the degree of cerebral hyperthermia.[7] Even the rectum or bladder, two commonly monitored sites considered to represent the core temperature, are in an "intermediate compartment" where the temperature is close, but not identical, to core temperature. Thus, although hypothermia has potential adverse effects, aggressive "overwarming" during CPB may also prove detrimental.

3. Despite adequate core rewarming on pump, progressive hypothermia may ensue in the post-pump period when the chest is still open and hemostasis is being achieved (so-called "temperature afterdrop"). This results from insufficient rewarming of peripheral tissues that leaves a significant temperature gradient between the core temperature and the periphery. Thus, heat is subsequently redistributed to the periphery, resulting in a gradual reduction in core temperature. Heat loss is further exacerbated by continued intraoperative heat loss from exposure to cool ambient temperatures, poor peripheral perfusion, and anesthetic-induced inhibition of normal thermoregulatory control.[6,7] Even with normothermic bypass, active warming is usually required to maintain patients at temperatures greater than 35 °C on CPB, and even these patients may cool down several degrees.

4. Prevention of afterdrop can be achieved by prolonging the warming phase on CPB, warming the periphery, or using pharmacologic vasodilation. Heat loss during surgery occurs by convection from the anterior surface of the body and may be minimized by increasing the ambient air temperature, especially in patients undergoing off-pump surgery. In these patients, maintaining a higher room temperature and using either the Kimberly-Clark (formerly Arctic Sun) temperature-controlling system or a cutaneous forced-air warming device, such as the Bair Hugger (Arizant) are helpful in avoiding hypothermia (Figure 8.1).[8,9] These devices are also very helpful in preventing temperature afterdrop when deep hypothermic circulatory arrest (DHCA) is used, but they cannot actively warm the patient or reduce redistribution of heat.[8–13] Sodium nitroprusside has been successful in reducing postbypass afterdrop because it produces peripheral vasodilation and improves peripheral perfusion. However, this benefit is usually noticed only in patients cooled to less than 32 °C.[14]

5. In the ICU, most patients are peripherally vasoconstricted as a compensatory mechanism to provide core warming. Pharmacologic vasodilation with medications such as nitroprusside or propofol may facilitate the redistribution of core heat to peripheral tissues and improve tissue perfusion, but at the same time they may delay central warming because peripheral vasodilation augments heat loss. Forced-air warming systems (such as the Bair Hugger) are superior to radiant heaters or warming blankets in increasing the rate of rewarming.[8,10–13]

6. Other measures, such as heating intravenous fluids or using heated humidifiers in the ventilator circuit, are of some benefit in preventing progressive hypothermia, but generally do not contribute to warming.

7. Shivering is associated with hypothermia and increases oxygen consumption and patient discomfort. Control of shivering is important in the postoperative period and is best controlled with meperidine (25 mg), which has specific anti-shivering properties related to several possible mechanisms.[15] Dexmedetomidine is also effective in controlling shivering.[16]

(A)

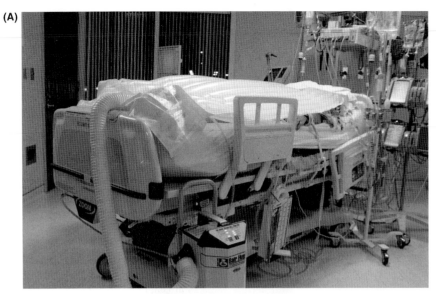

(B)

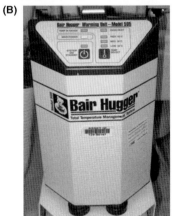

Figure 8.1 • The Bair Hugger warming system, used to warm patients arriving in the ICU at temperatures <36 °C.

8. Occasionally a patient may rapidly rewarm to 37 °C and then "overwarm" to higher temperatures due to resetting of the central thermoregulating system. Narcotics tend to increase the core temperature required for sweating and may contribute to this problem.[17] Since warming may lead to profound peripheral vasodilation and hypotension, gradual vasodilation with nitroprusside and concomitant volume infusion can minimize this problem (see postoperative scenarios II.A and II.B, pages 312–315).

C. **Control of mediastinal bleeding** (see Chapter 9)

1. Numerous factors may predispose to mediastinal bleeding following CPB. These include residual heparin effect, thrombocytopenia and platelet dysfunction, clotting factor depletion, fibrinolysis, technical issues during surgery, hypothermia, and postoperative hypertension.[18]

2. Antifibrinolytic medications, including ε-aminocaproic acid and tranexamic acid, are recommended for all cardiac surgical procedures to reduce intraoperative bleeding.[19,20] These medications not only inhibit fibrinolysis, but, to varying degrees, also preserve platelet function. Aprotinin was generally felt to be the most effective medication to reduce bleeding, but was withdrawn from the market in 2007.

3. Careful monitoring of the extent of postoperative bleeding dictates the aggressiveness with which bleeding should be treated. Many patients with "nonsurgical" causes will drain about 100 mL/h for several hours before bleeding eventually tapers. A faster rate of bleeding without evidence of diminution requires systematic evaluation and treatment, often prompting reexploration, as described in Chapter 9. Coagulation studies tend to be abnormal in patients with coagulopathic bleeding, but may also be abnormal in patients with ongoing surgical bleeding. Nonetheless, abnormal coagulation studies should not delay exploration for significant bleeding. Persistent bleeding with normal coagulation studies tends to be more surgical in nature.

4. Recognition of the early signs of cardiac tamponade and the importance of prompt mediastinal exploration for severe bleeding or tamponade are critical to improving patient outcomes.[21]

D. **Ventilatory support, emergence from anesthesia, weaning and extubation** (see Chapter 10)

1. Following off-pump or uneventful on-pump surgery, some groups prefer to extubate patients in the operating room or upon arrival in the ICU.[22] This can be accomplished using short-acting narcotics, such as remifentanil, low doses of other narcotics, or primarily inhalational agents. Careful monitoring of the patient's mental status and respiratory drive is imperative during recovery from anesthesia, especially since some analgesia needs to be provided. High thoracic epidural analgesia or spinal (intrathecal) analgesia, with bupivacaine, fentanyl, or morphine with clonidine, have been successfully utilized.[23–26]

2. Early extubation (within 8 hours) is feasible in most patients, conditional upon their mental status, gas exchange, and hemodynamic performance. As long as certain criteria are met, there is no reason to exclude a patient from a protocol of early extubation based upon age, comorbidities, cardiac disease, or the extent of surgery. Even if it takes a few hours longer to extubate a patient, the benefits of earlier extubation usually translate into a quicker recovery from surgery.[27–32] Propofol is commonly used for sedation, neuromuscular blocking agents are allowed to wear off, low-dose narcotics may be used for analgesia, and hypertension is controlled with non-sedating antihypertensive medications. Once standard criteria for weaning are met (Table 10.3, page 400), the propofol is weaned off, and the patient is extubated once extubation criteria are satisfied. Some groups use dexmedotomidine instead of propofol because it is less of a sedative but can "take the edge off" because of its anxiolytic properties.

3. Residual sedation from anesthestic agents and hypoxemia are the two primary reasons for prolonged ventilation.[32]

   a. Selection of anesthetic agents often influences the ability to extubate patients early. For example, use of remifentanil rather than sufentanil or fentanyl (the most commonly used agents) and use of sevoflurane rather than isoflurane as an inhalational agent generally allow for very early awakening and extubation, often soon after arrival in the ICU.[26,33–35] Neuromuscular blockers that have a short duration of action and do not require renal or hepatic elimination, such as cisatracurium or rocuronium, are best in this regard.[36]

   b. With use of sufentanil or fentanyl, most patients arrive in the ICU requiring mechanical ventilation for a short period of time. Supplemental propofol is added to provide adequate sedation as the narcotic effects dissipate. The initial fraction of inspired oxygen (FiO_2) of 1.0 is gradually weaned to below 0.5 as long as the PaO_2 remains above 80 torr or the arterial oxygen saturation (SaO_2) exceeds 95%. The respiratory rate or tidal volume of the mechanical ventilator is adjusted to accommodate the increased CO_2 production that occurs with warming, awakening, and shivering.

   c. Oxygenation is influenced by the patient's baseline pulmonary status (COPD, CHF), hemodynamic performance, the use and duration of CPB, and the amount of fluid administered during surgery. CPB produces a systemic inflammatory response with a "capillary leak" that increases interstitial lung water. Various measures can be used in the operating room to optimize postoperative pulmonary function. Minimizing the positive fluid balance during surgery (as well as in the ICU), using a centrifugal pump, membrane oxygenator, heparin-coated circuit, steroids, and/or leukocyte filter during CPB may reduce the systemic inflammatory response and contribute to a faster convalesence.

4. Despite the desirability of early extubation, there are patients in whom it is ill-advised to "rush to extubate" (Table 10.2, page 397).

   a. **Preoperative** factors predictive of prolonged postoperative ventilation include cardiogenic shock, pulmonary edema, and severe COPD. Additional risk factors include marked obesity, peripheral vascular disease, renal dysfunction, left ventricular (LV) dysfunction, emergency surgery, and need for an intra-aortic balloon pump (IABP) for hemodynamic support.[27,30,31,37] In these cases, use of sufentanil or fentanyl is advisable, rather than shorter-acting medications. It is reasonable to use narcotics for control of hypertension.

   b. **Postoperative** clinical issues that may necessitate prolonged ventilation include hemodynamic instability requiring multiple inotropes and/or IABP dependence, low cardiac output syndrome, altered mental status, bleeding, oliguria from renal failure, and especially poor oxygenation or poor respiratory mechanics.[31] In these patients, propofol can provide adequate sedation for several days and may be converted to other sedatives, such as fentanyl, if prolonged intubation is required.[38] Careful review of the patient's chest x-ray, ECG, arterial blood gases, hemodynamic parameters, and renal function should allow for identification of problems that need to be addressed. Issues related to the management of hypoxia and acute respiratory failure are discussed in detail in Chapter 10.

E. Analgesia and sedation

1. An essential element of postoperative care is the provision of adequate analgesia and sedation.[39-42]

   a. Parasternal intercostal blocks or subcutaneous local anesthetic infusions (On-Q pain relief system, I-Flow Corporation) initiated at the time of surgery can ameliorate chest wall pain and decrease opioid requirements.[43,44] This is especially beneficial in patients extubated in the operating room.

   b. Patients still intubated upon arrival in the ICU are commonly anesthetized from the residual effects of anesthetic agents which also provide some element of analgesia. When early extubation is anticipated, a short-acting sedative such as propofol can be used to provide sedation, but additional analgesia is usually required within a few hours. Dexmedetomidine can be used instead of propofol, because it provides both sedative and analgesic properties. Midazolam is also a short-acting sedative, but its effects tends to last longer and it is a less desirable option when early extubation is planned.

   c. Adequate analgesia can be provided by a variety of medications and via different routes. Epidural narcotics are beneficial in providing adequate analgesia.[23-25] Small bolus doses of IV narcotics or a continuous infusion of narcotics (such as morphine sulfate 0.02 mg/kg/h for patients under age 65 and 0.01 mg/kg/h for patients over age 65) may also be given to provide analgesia while minimizing respiratory depression. Alternatively, just before the propofol is discontinued, a nonsteroidal anti-inflammatory medication, such as ketorolac 30 mg IV, indomethacin 50 mg PR or diclofenac 75 mg PR, can be given to provide analgesia.[45] One advantage of ketorolac is that it is primarily a COX-1 inhibitor that inhibits platelet aggregation; this may prove beneficial in CABG patients.[46]

2. If the patient does not tolerate the weaning process, often becoming agitated with the weaning of propofol, substitution of dexmedetomidine can provide anxiolysis, analgesia, sympatholysis, and mild sedation to expedite a more tolerable weaning process from the ventilator.[47] It can be continued after the patient is extubated. If delayed extubation is anticipated, propofol remains an excellent choice for several days and may be converted to fentanyl for longer-term sedation. It should be noted that the offset of action of propofol depends on the duration of use, the depth of sedation, and body habitus. One study showed that with light sedation for up to 24 hours, emergence occurs in only 13 minutes, but in heavily sedated patients it may take up to 25 hours![48] Although use of dexmedetomidine has only been recommended for 24 hours, several studies have found it to be comparable to or better than propofol or midazolam for long-term sedation.[49,50]

3. Breakthrough pain may be treated with small additional doses of IV morphine or IV ketorolac (15–30 mg) for 72 hours, which is quite effective in bridging the patient to oral analgesics. An alternative approach, especially in patients with more prominent postoperative pain, is use of a patient-controlled analgesia (PCA) pump starting on the first postoperative day. Studies suggest that morphine (1 g bolus and 0.3 mg/h infusion), fentanyl (10 μg bolus and 1 μg/kg/h infusion), and remifentanil (0.25–0.5 mg/kg bolus and a 0.05 μg/kg/min infusion) administered via a PCA pump provide comparable analgesia.[51,52]

F. Hemodynamic support during a period of transient myocardial depression (see Chapter 11)[53,54]

1. Myocardial function following a period of cardioplegic arrest may be temporarily depressed from ischemia/reperfusion injury and will often benefit from low-dose inotropic support for several hours. The reduction in ejection fraction is about 10–15% in patients with relatively normal ventricles, and it may be even greater in those with preexisting LV dysfunction.[54] Additionally, hypothermia and elevated levels of catecholamines lead to an increase in SVR and systemic hypertension, which increase afterload and can further depress myocardial performance. Factors influencing the need for inotropic support include the extent of preoperative left ventricular dysfunction, a recent infarction or ongoing ischemia at the time of surgery, and the duration of aortic cross-clamping. In patients sustaining a perioperative infarction, the period of myocardial depression tends to last somewhat longer, and may require more prolonged support.

2. Serial assessments of filling pressures, cardiac output, and SVR allow for the appropriate selection of fluids, inotropes, and/or vasodilators to optimize preload, afterload, and contractility to provide hemodynamic support during this period of temporary myocardial depression. The objective is to maintain a cardiac index above 2.2 L/min/m^2 with a stable blood pressure (systolic 100–130 mm Hg) or a mean pressure above 70–80 mm Hg. Adequate tissue oxygenation is the primary goal of hemodynamic management and can be assessed by measuring the mixed venous O_2 saturation (SvO_2) from the pulmonary artery port of the Swan-Ganz catheter (normal > 65%).

3. The initial intervention to augment cardiac output is fluid administration. The filling pressures tend to underestimate volume status because of impaired ventricular compliance. Furthermore, the response to volume may differ depending on whether the heart is hypertrophied with a "pressure overload" condition, as noted with hypertension or aortic stenosis, or somewhat dilated from a "volume overload" condition, as noted with long-standing mitral regurgitation.[54]

4. Atrial or atrioventricular pacing at a rate of 90–100 beats/min is commonly required at the conclusion of surgery to achieve optimal hemodynamics, especially in hypertrophied hearts. Pacing is generally required in patients taking β-blockers before surgery. A slow heart rate may reduce myocardial oxygen demand but will compromise cardiac output. In a well-revascularized heart, raising the heart rate to augment cardiac output is indicated and generally well tolerated.

5. Inotropes should be selected based on an understanding of their hemodynamic benefits and potential complications (see pages 457–472). If a marginal cardiac output is present after adequate fluid status has been achieved, inotropic support is initiated and should improve the cardiac output to acceptable levels. If a satisfactory cardiac output still cannot be achieved or begins to deteriorate, additional inotropes, an IABP, or rarely an assist device may be necessary. However, in most patients, cardiac function improves to baseline within a few hours and inotropes can be usually weaned off within 12 hours of surgery. In patients with preexisting severe ventricular dysfunction or acute perioperative cardiac insults (ischemia, prolonged cross-clamp time), it may take somewhat longer.

6. Monitoring of serial hematocrits is important to ensure the adequacy of tissue oxygen delivery. The hematocrit may be influenced by hemodilution or mediastinal bleeding and should generally be maintained at a level greater than 22–24%. In elderly or

critically ill patients, especially those with a low cardiac output state, hypotension, tachycardia, low mixed venous oxygen saturation, evidence of ischemia, metabolic acidosis, or hypoxemia, transfusion to a higher level should be considered, weighing the potential benefits and risks of transfusion.[55]

G. **Fluid administration** to maintain filling pressures in the presence of a capillary leak and vasodilation (see Chapter 12)

1. Following CPB, the patient will be total body salt and water overloaded and should theoretically be diuresed. However, the use of CPB results in a "systemic inflammatory response" which produces a capillary leak. Furthermore, peripheral vasoconstriction masks intravascular hypovolemia despite adequate left-heart filling pressures.

2. Fluid resuscitation is therefore necessary to offset the capillary leak and the vasodilation caused by numerous medications and warming to normothermia. Crystalloid and colloid infusions are used to maintain intravascular volume, although this usually occurs at the expense of expansion of the interstitial space. After the capillary leak has ceased and hemodynamics have stabilized, the patient may be aggressively diuresed to eliminate the excessive salt and water administered during surgery and the early postoperative period.

H. Monitoring of serum **potassium** is essential in the early postoperative period. Potassium levels may be elevated from cardioplegia solutions delivered for myocardial protection, but most patients with normal renal function and preserved myocardial function will make large quantities of urine during the first few hours after CPB, often resulting in hypokalemia. To minimize the risk of developing arrhythmias, potassium levels should be checked every 4 hours and replaced as necessary.

I. Strict management of **hyperglycemia** has been shown to reduce the incidence of sternal wound infection and surgical mortality.[56,57] Factors that contribute to hyperglycemia are insulin resistance, endogenous catecholamine release on pump, and use of epinephrine post-pump for hemodynamic support. A hyperglycemia protocol should be utilized to determine the appropriate amount of insulin to be given to maintain blood glucose less than 180 mg/dL (see Appendix 6).

II. Management of Common Postoperative Scenarios

There are several typical hemodynamic scenarios that are noted during the early phase of recovery from open-heart surgery. An understanding of these patterns allows for therapeutic maneuvers to be undertaken in anticipation of hemodynamic changes, rather than as reactions to problems once they have occurred.

A. **Vasoconstriction from hypothermia with hypertension and borderline cardiac output**

1. The patient arriving in the ICU with a temperature below 35–36 °C will vasoconstrict in an attempt to increase core body temperature. The elevation in SVR may produce hypertension at a time when cardiac function is still somewhat depressed from surgery. These patients should be managed by a combination of fluid replacement to reach a pulmonary artery diastolic (PAD) pressure or pulmonary capillary wedge pressure (PCWP) around 15–20 mm Hg, pharmacologic vasodilation to maintain a systolic pressure of 100–120 mm Hg (mean pressure 70–80 mm Hg), and inotropic support if the cardiac index remains less than 2.0 L/min/m². Warming methods noted above should also be employed. Among the commonly used vasodilators,

nitroprusside is preferable to nitroglycerin, which tends to lower preload and reduce cardiac output to a greater degree while producing less systemic vasodilation. Nicardipine and clevidipine are both excellent vasodilators, but the latter may be preferable since it is a short-acting calcium channel blocker.[58]

2. The use of arterial vasodilators is beneficial in the vasoconstricted patient in that they:

   a. Reduce afterload, improving myocardial metabolism and LV function
   b. Improve peripheral tissue perfusion and redistribute heat to the periphery
   c. Facilitate gentle and adequate fluid administration

3. Vasodilators will reduce the SVR and blood pressure, and left-sided filling pressures will fall modestly, requiring the simultaneous infusion of fluids to maintain cardiac output. The optimal left-sided filling pressures depend on the state of myocardial contractility and compliance. Preload should generally not be raised above 20 mm Hg because of the deleterious effects of elevated wall tension on myocardial metabolism and function. However, if preload is allowed to fall too low, the patient may become hypovolemic and hypotensive when normothermia is achieved. The general principle is to "optimize preload → reduce afterload → restore preload".

4. If the patient has a marginal cardiac index (less than $2.0\,L/min/m^2$), has adequate filling pressures, yet is somewhat hypertensive, a low dose of a vasodilator can be initiated. If the patient is already on inotropic support, it is imperative to assess the cardiac index before modifying the therapeutic approach. Despite the temptation to do so, **stopping an inotropic medication in a hypertensive patient without first ensuring that a satisfactory cardiac output is present can be very dangerous**. Some patients with very marginal cardiac function maintain a satisfactory blood pressure by intense vasoconstriction from enhanced sympathetic tone. Loss of this compensatory mechanism may result in rapid deterioration from loss of perfusion pressure.

B. Vasodilation and hypotension during the rewarming phase

1. Vasodilation reduces filling pressures and, in the hypovolemic patient, may produce hypotension and often a decrease in cardiac output despite good cardiac function. There are several reasons why a patient may vasodilate during the early postoperative period.

   a. Medications used for analgesia and anxiolysis are vasodilators (narcotics, propofol, midazolam). Recent use of angiotensin-converting enzyme (ACE) inhibitors or angiotensin receptor blockers (ARBs) tends to cause hypotension during and after bypass.

   b. Nitroglycerin (NTG) used in the operating room or in the ICU to control blood pressure, minimize ischemia, or prevent radial artery spasm will lower preload and cardiac output as well as the blood pressure. To counteract these problems, significant fluid administration is frequently required. Unless active ischemia is present, IV NTG is best avoided during the rewarming phase to reduce fluid requirements.

   c. Resolution of hypothermia leads to peripheral vasodilation, which is accentuated in patients who warm to higher than 37 °C.

   d. Improvement in cardiac output often leads to relaxation of peripheral vasoconstriction.

e. A vasoplegic state of refractory hypotension may develop despite the presence of an adequate cardiac output. This may be a consequence of a systemic inflammatory response (although it has been noted after off-pump surgery as well) and may be related to nitric oxide-induced vasodilation.

2. To avoid hypotension, fluids must be given to maintain filling pressures. The quandary is whether crystalloid or colloid should be selected and how much should be given. If the basic reason for hypovolemia is a capillary leak syndrome, the use of colloid could be detrimental, because its oncotic elements may pass into the interstitial tissues, exacerbating tissue edema and compromising organ function. However, if vasodilation of the peripheral and splanchnic beds is the major problem, then colloids should be preferable, because they will augment the intravascular volume to a greater extent than crystalloids. Generally, if filling pressures are not elevated, the amount of extravascular lung water will not be influenced significantly by whether colloid or crystalloid is infused.[59] Volume resuscitation is usually required during the initial 6 hours after arrival in the ICU, following which most mechanisms for vasodilation are no longer present and the capillary leak begins to abate.

3. It is generally best to start with a 500 mL bolus of lactated Ringer's or normal saline. If there is minimal increase in filling pressures, a colloid such as 5% albumin may be chosen. Hetastarch compounds increase the intravascular volume more effectively than crystalloid and for longer than 5% albumin and can be safely given in the absence of significant mediastinal bleeding or renal dysfunction. Nonetheless, the total infusion volume should be limited to 1500–1750 mL (20 mL/kg) per 24 hours.[60] If the patient's hematocrit is low, a packed red cell transfusion is the most appropriate means of increasing intravascular volume. If the patient is bleeding, use of blood component transfusions may be indicated as well. It must always be remembered that these colloid solutions will also lower the hematocrit from hemodilution.

4. There is often a tendency to administer a tremendous amount of fluid during the period of vasodilation in order to maintain filling pressures and systemic blood pressure. Furthermore, most patients with satisfactory cardiac function are simultaneously producing a copious amount of urine. One should resist the temptation to "flood" the patient with fluid. Excessive fluid administration (>2 liters within 6 hours) may exacerbate interstitial edema and delay extubation. It also produces significant hemodilution, often necessitating blood transfusions for anemia, and reduces the levels of clotting factors, possibly increasing mediastinal bleeding and necessitating plasma or platelet administration. **Preload should be increased only as necessary to maintain satisfactory cardiac output and tissue perfusion.**

5. The response to fluid administration is not always predictable and depends on the compliance of the left atrium and ventricle, the degree of "capillary leak", and the intensity of peripheral vasoconstriction.

   a. An increase in preload with repeated fluid challenges will generally raise the cardiac output and blood pressure to satisfactory levels. Peripheral vasoconstriction tends to relax as the cardiac output improves and the patient warms. As this occurs, filling pressures tend to fall and some additional volume may be necessary. If cardiac function and filling pressures are adequate, yet the blood pressure remains marginal, use of an α-agent (phenylephrine or norepinephrine) to support the blood pressure can limit the amount of fluid that needs to be given. If these drugs cannot maintain a satisfactory BP with adequate filling pressures, yet the cardiac output is satisfactory, a "vasoplegic syndrome" may be present. This generally responds to vasopressin 0.01–0.07 units/min.[61] This syndrome may be attributable to leukocyte activation and release of proinflammatory mediators caused by the systemic inflammatory response to CPB, although it has been described after off-pump surgery as well.[62]

b. Failure of filling pressures to rise with volume infusions may be noted in patients with highly compliant, volume-overloaded hearts (such as mitral regurgitation), in whom the cardiac output improves before the filling pressures are noted to increase. Thus, further fluid therapy can be guided by the cardiac output. However, in other patients, filling pressures may not rise due to persistent vasodilation and the capillary leak of fluid into the interstitial space rather than retention in the intravascular space. This is particularly common in very sick patients with a long duration of CPB. Sometimes it seems virtually impossible to maintain filling pressures and cardiac output despite a tremendous amount of fluid administration, yet, on occasion, this may be necessary. One often has to accept the adverse consequences of excessive total body water to improve hemodynamics. Use of drugs to provide inotropic support and some increase in systemic resistance may reduce the amount of fluid that is administered.

c. If filling pressures do rise with fluid administration, but the blood pressure and cardiac output remain marginal, right and left ventricular distention may ensue, increasing myocardial oxygen demand and decreasing coronary blood flow. Further fluid administration is contraindicated, and inotropic support must be initiated.

6. The following is a general guideline to hemodynamic management during the rewarming phase.

a. If the blood pressure is marginal, push the PAD pressure or PCWP to 18–20 mm Hg (often up to 25 mm Hg in hypertrophied hearts) using crystalloid and then colloid. Once this level is reached, if the patient remains hypotensive, if the urine volume begins to match the infused volume, or if more than 2000 mL of fluid has been administered and filling pressures are not rising, consider the following:

i. If CI >2.2 L/min/m², use phenylephrine (pure α), or if unsuccessful, vasopressin for a potential "vasoplegic" state

ii. If CI is 1.8–2.2 L/min/m², use norepinephrine (α and β)

iii. If CI <1.8 L/min/m², use an inotrope, then norepinephrine prn

b. **Note:** Use of an α agent may not be able to minimize a capillary leak, but it does counteract vasodilation. This may decrease the volume requirement and improve SVR and blood pressure with little effect on myocardial function.

C. **Copious urine output and falling filling pressures**. Some patients will make large quantities of urine, resulting in a reduction in filling pressures, blood pressure, and cardiac output. Several factors should be considered when determining why this might be occurring.

1. Is the patient on a vasoactive drug that may produce copious urine output out of proportion to its hemodynamic effects? This may occur with use of nesiritide,

fenoldopam, or "renal dose" dopamine that may be used during surgery to optimize renal function. If this impairs the ability to maintain adequate filling pressures and cardiac output, consider changing to another drug, such as low-dose epinephrine, dobutamine, or milrinone, or stopping the "renoprotective" drug.

2. Did the patient receive mannitol or furosemide in the operating room because of a low urine output or hyperkalemia? Urine output is no longer a direct reflection of myocardial function when a diuretic has been administered. Excessive urine output often necessitates a significant amount of fluid administration to maintain filling pressures and confounds the selection of the appropriate fluid to administer (crystalloid vs. colloid).

3. Is the patient hyperglycemic and developing an osmotic diuresis? A hyperglycemia protocol should be used routinely to maintain the blood glucose below 180 mg/dL (see Appendix 6).[57]

4. Does the patient have normal left ventricular function and the kidneys are simply mobilizing excessive interstitial fluid from hemodilution on pump? This beneficial effect is often seen in healthy patients with a short CPB run, and reflects excellent cardiac output and renal function that should lead to a rapid postoperative recovery. However, copious urine output can be problematic when it lowers filling pressures, blood pressure, and cardiac output.

   a. Any contributing factors or medications causing the diuresis should be addressed.

   b. Crystalloid and colloid should be administered to keep the fluid balance modestly negative during this phase of spontaneous diuresis. The temptation to administer too much colloid should be resisted, because this can produce hemodilution and progressive anemia despite the negative fluid balance and can dilute clotting factors, potentially contributing to mediastinal bleeding. Use of an α-agent may maintain filling pressures and decrease the volume requirement in some of these patients.

D. **Low cardiac output syndrome with impaired left ventricular function**

1. Isolated left ventricular dysfunction requiring postcardiotomy inotropic support may be noted in patients with preexisting LV dysfunction from a remote or recent myocardial infarction or advanced valvular heart disease, or in patients with active ischemia going into the operating room. It may also result from intraoperative problems, such as a prolonged period of cardioplegic arrest, inadequate myocardial protection, incomplete revascularization or compromised graft flow. Poor LV function often reflects reversible myocardial stunning rather than perioperative ischemia and infarction. Both are managed in similar fashion, but the suspicion of ongoing ischemia by ECG may require reevaluation in the cardiac cath lab.

2. Appropriate measures should be taken at the conclusion of surgery to assess and optimize a patient's hemodynamic status before arrival in the ICU, including pacing, optimal preload, inotropic support, and use of an IABP, if indicated. It is critical that the surgeon, along with the anesthesiologist, establish a "game plan" for how the patient should be managed in the ICU. Assessment of cardiac function by direct visualization and TEE allows for correlation with hemodynamic parameters obtained with the Swan-Ganz catheter to establish an individualized therapeutic approach. Decisions on desired filling pressures, inotropic selection, plans for maintaining or weaning inotropes, ventilatory requirements, and drugs for renal

support, must be communicated to those caring for the patient in the ICU on a minute-by-minute basis. Careful monitoring and continuous reevaluation in the ICU are essential to identify whether the patient is recovering as desired or requires further evaluation and intervention.

3. In addition to careful examination and standard monitoring of critically ill patients, **echocardiography** in the ICU is very beneficial in clarifying potential problems. A typical scenario that may benefit from echo evaluation is the patient with a low cardiac output on substantial doses of inotropes, borderline and labile blood pressure, elevated filling pressures (often ascribed to volume infusions), worsening oxygenation, and bleeding that has tapered. In such a situation, an echo is indicated to assess whether there are factors other than LV dysfunction that may be causing the low cardiac output syndrome. Conditions such as circumferential or regional cardiac tamponade, severe diastolic dysfunction, RV dysfunction, regurgitant valvular lesions or septal shunting may be identified. The most likely alternative cause of the scenario noted is cardiac tamponade, which, fortunately, is the most remediable. If a transthoracic echo does not provide adequate acoustic windows, a transesophageal study can easily be performed, especially in the intubated patient.[63]

4. A comprehensive discussion of the management of the low cardiac output syndrome is provided starting on page 444 of Chapter 11.

E. **Normal left ventricular function but low cardiac output (diastolic dysfunction and right ventricular failure)**

1. A disturbing postoperative scenario is that of a low cardiac output syndrome associated with normal or elevated left-heart filling pressures yet preserved left ventricular function. This scenario is noted most commonly in small women with systemic hypertension who have small, hypertrophied left ventricles. A variant of this problem is seen in patients with aortic stenosis and hyperdynamic hearts that manifest near cavity obliteration.[64]

2. The problem of severe diastolic dysfunction is characterized by reduced ventricular compliance exacerbated by myocardial edema from ischemia/reperfusion injury. Contributing factors to the low cardiac output are lack of atrioventricular (AV) synchrony with impaired ventricular filling, occasionally impaired right ventricular function, and perhaps excessive use of inotropic agents.

3. The hemodynamic data derived from the Swan-Ganz catheter typically show elevated filling pressures and a low cardiac output, suggestive of left ventricular dysfunction. Thus, a typical therapeutic response would be to ensure AV conduction, administer some volume, and initiate inotropic support. However, this may lead to little improvement in cardiac output, even higher filling pressures leading to pulmonary congestion, a reduction in renal blood flow (often exacerbated by systemic venous hypertension), and progressive oliguria. The use of inotropes may also produce a significant sinus tachycardia that is detrimental to myocardial metabolism and recovery.

4. Transesophageal echocardiography (TEE) has been invaluable in the assessment and management of this problem. TEE will usually confirm a hypertrophic, stiff left ventricle with hyperdynamic systolic function and signs of diastolic dysfunction. Fluid should be administered to raise the pulmonary artery diastolic (PAD) pressure to about 20–25 mm Hg. This will increase the left ventricular end-diastolic volume,

which tends to be smaller than would be suggested by pressure measurements because of poor LV compliance. Lusitropic drugs that relax the left ventricle should be substituted for catecholamines that have β-adrenergic inotropic and chronotropic properties. Milrinone may be beneficial in this regard and can support RV function as well. Nesiritide exerts lusitropic properties that may be the mechanism of its pulmonary vasodilatory effects. Anecdotally, it has been noted to benefit patients with severe diastolic dysfunction.

5. Other considerations include use of low-dose calcium channel blockers or β-blockers to improve diastolic relaxation, although it is conceptually difficult to start these when the cardiac output is compromised. Aggressive diuresis to reduce interstitial edema while providing colloid (salt-poor albumin) to maintain intravascular volume may also improve diastolic relaxation. If the patient can survive the first few days of low output syndrome without end-organ dysfunction, a gradual improvement in cardiac output generally results.

6. The problem of a marginal cardiac output and blood pressure with preserved LV function may also be noted in patients with markedly impaired RV function. This may result from right ventricular infarction or poor intraoperative protection of a hypertrophied right ventricle in patients with pulmonary hypertension. This problem is not uncommon in cardiac transplant recipients with preexisting pulmonary hypertension and may be noted in patients with advanced mitral valve disease. The use of blood products also increases pulmonary vascular resistance (PVR) and can exacerbate RV dysfunction. Right ventricular distention can then cause septal shift, compromising left ventricular filling. Fluid administration, inotropic support with medications such as milrinone, use of nesiritide, inhaled nitric oxide, a pure pulmonary vasodilator, or prostacyclin analogs may be beneficial.[65] If not, a circulatory assist device might be necessary. The management of RV dysfunction is discussed in more detail on pages 327–328 and 452–457.

III. Postoperative Considerations Following Commonly Performed Procedures

A. On-pump coronary artery bypass grafting (CABG)

1. Even with relatively normal preoperative left ventricular function, most centers use low-dose inotropes to support myocardial function at the termination of bypass and for several hours in the ICU. Although propofol tends to mitigate the extent of hypertension, blood pressure tends to creep upwards as the level of sedation is weaned. At this point, if the patient is otherwise hemodynamically stable, it is advisable to start a vasodilator rather than give additional sedation or narcotics to control hypertension, in order to minimize respiratory depression.

2. Although patients who are β-blocked preoperatively frequently require pacing at the conclusion of bypass, tachycardia may be present in those who are not β-blocked, especially in young anxious patients. Although the potential causes of a tachycardia always need to be assessed, the combination of hypertension and tachycardia with a supranormal cardiac output can be managed by β-blockers (esmolol or intermittent doses of IV metoprolol). Patients with a **hyperdynamic left ventricle** may develop progressive tachycardia when vasodilators are used to control hypertension. This should be managed by allowing the blood pressure to

drift up to 140 mm Hg systolic and then using β-blockers to control both the tachycardia and the hypertension.

3. Atrial and ventricular pacing wires should be placed in all patients undergoing CABG. If the patient has sinus bradycardia or a junctional rhythm, atrial pacing at 90 beats/min should be used to ensure optimal LV filling and improve the cardiac output. If there is normal AV conduction, it is always preferable to use atrial pacing rather than AV sequential pacing, since the latter involves pacing of the right atrium (RA) and right ventricle (RV), which will produce ventricular dyssynchrony. If second- or third-degree heart block is present, pacing in the DVI or DDD mode is appropriate. In patients with moderate-to-severe LV dysfunction, biventricular pacing (RA-BiV) using an extra sets of leads will provide a superior cardiac output to standard RA-RV pacing.[66] If the patient has a slow ventricular response to atrial fibrillation, VVI pacing should be initiated.

4. Use of nitroglycerin to control hypertension will reduce preload and cardiac output because of its venodilatory effects. Sodium nitroprusside is the preferable medication because it primarily lowers the SVR with less effect on preload and thus requires less volume infusion. However, nitroglycerin should be used if there is any evidence of ischemia. Clevidipine is another satisfactory alternative to control hypertension.[58] Nicardipine is also an effective antihypertensive, but has a longer duration of action. Its use could be problematic if the patient becomes hemodynamically unstable.

5. **Inotropic support** is usually initiated at the termination of bypass and may be required for several hours in the ICU to support cardiac output during the early phase of transient myocardial dysfunction. The initial first-line drug may be epinephrine, dobutamine, or dopamine. Epinephrine (1–2 μg/min) is the preferred inotrope and usually produces less tachycardia than the other drugs. If there is an inadequate response to one of these catecholamines, milrinone is of great benefit in improving cardiac output. It is a positive inotrope that produces systemic vasodilation that frequently requires the addition of norepinephrine to support systemic resistance. When hemodynamic performance remains very marginal, placement of an IABP should be considered. In contrast to the catecholamines, the IABP can reduce myocardial oxygen demand and improve coronary perfusion. Inotropic support beyond 6–12 hours may be necessary if the patient has sustained a perioperative infarction or has a severely "stunned" myocardium that exhibits a prolonged period of dysfunction in the absence of infarction. A persistent low output state despite optimal pharmacologic therapy and an IABP may require placement of an assist device.

6. A common practice is to initiate antiarrhythmic therapy with lidocaine in the operating room to suppress ventricular arrhythmias, although there is little documented evidence of benefit.[67] It is given at the time of removal of the aortic cross-clamp and then continued on a prophylactic basis until the following morning. Prophylactic amiodarone has been found to reduce the incidence of postoperative atrial fibrillation (AF), especially in elderly patients, and can also provide benefits in controlling ventricular ectopy. A common approach is to give the initial load intravenously during surgery, although protocols of preoperative oral loading or a postoperative IV load may be just as effective in reducing the incidence of postoperative AF.[68,69]

7. The development of ventricular arrhythmias later during the postoperative course raises the specter of ischemia, but reentrant ventricular tachycardias are usually related to prior heart damage. Nonsustained VT in patients with an ejection fraction >35% is best managed with β-blockers. In patients with a low ejection fraction, an electrophysiologic study may be indicated, and placement of an implantable cardioverter-defibrillator (ICD) may be considered (see pages 58–59). The timing of placement may depend on the frequency and severity of VT, since randomized studies have generally suggested waiting 3 months after revascularization, during which time improvement in LV function may occur.

8. **Atrial fibrillation (AF)** is noted in about 25% of patients following CABG. It may be related to poor atrial preservation during surgery or to withdrawal of β-blockers. Most centers initiate β-blockers by the first postoperative morning (usually metoprolol 25–50 mg bid) because of the overwhelming evidence that β-blockers reduce the incidence of AF.[70–72] Magnesium sulfate has been shown in some, but not all, studies to reduce the incidence of AF as well as the occurrence of ventricular arrhythmias.[73] Administration of 2 g at the termination of CPB and on the first postoperative morning can be recommended. Amiodarone should be considered for AF prophylaxis in patients at higher risk.[68,74] A detailed discussion of the prevention and management of atrial fibrillation is presented on pages 538–547.

9. Close attention must be paid to the postoperative **ECG**. Evidence of ischemia may represent incomplete revascularization, poor myocardial protection, or impaired myocardial perfusion due to anastomotic stenosis, acute graft occlusion, or coronary spasm (Figure 8.2). Regardless of the etiology, intravenous nitroglycerin (starting at 0.25 µg/kg/min) is usually indicated. Calcium channel blockers (nifedipine 30 mg SL or diltiazem 0.25 mg/kg IV over 2 minutes, then 5–15 mg/h IV) are useful if coronary spasm is suspected. These medications may resolve ischemic changes or minimize infarct size if necrosis is already under way. Placement of an IABP should also be considered. If a problem with a bypass graft is suspected as the cause of the ischemia, emergency angiography followed by percutaneous coronary intervention or reexploration may be indicated. ST elevation noted in multiple leads is often consistent with acute pericarditis, although computerized interpretation of these ECGs often indicates "acute infarct" (Figure 8.3). The ECG must be interpreted carefully, taking into consideration the heart's hemodynamic performance and an accurate perception by the surgeon of the quality of revascularization. An echocardiogram should be considered to assess for regional wall motion abnormalities.

10. The diagnosis of a perioperative **myocardial infarction** (PMI) can be difficult to make, but is usually confirmed by persistent ECG changes and new regional wall motion abnormalities on echocardiography (see page 513). The use of cardiac biomarkers to define a PMI is controversial, since they are elevated in all patients. Troponin levels are very sensitive to myocardial injury, but their significance needs to be defined.[75] Average values following CABG range from 6 to 18 ng/mL in the absence of infarction,[76] yet one study found that levels exceeding 8.5 ng/mL did correlate with worse short- and long-term outcomes.[77] Definitions of PMI therefore are based on the premise that higher levels of biomarkers result from more myocardial necrosis and correlate with adverse outcomes.[78]

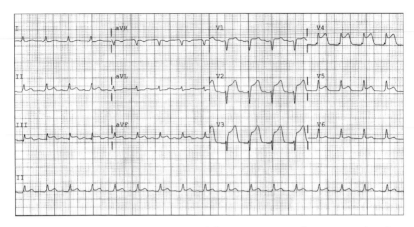

Figure 8.2 • An ECG obtained from a patient following a coronary bypass operation that required an endarterectomy of a diffusely diseased LAD. Note the profound ST elevations in precordial leads consistent with a current of injury. The patient was returned to the cath lab and found to have an obstruction distal to the anastomosis from elevated plaque, and a stent was satisfactorily placed.

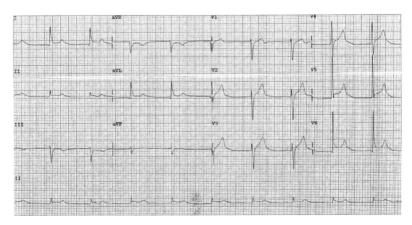

Figure 8.3 • An ECG obtained several hours after an uneventful valve operation. Note the diffuse elevation in ST segments with PR depression, which is consistent with acute pericarditis.

    a. The 2008 Society of Thoracic Surgeons data specifications defined a perioperative MI based upon creatine kinase myocardial band (CK-MB) levels and ECG changes. Within the first 24 hours of surgery, a CK-MB level $>5 \times$ the upper limit of normal was selected as the criterion, independent of the presence of Q waves. Numerous publications have addressed the correlation of troponin levels with perioperative MI, and a joint task force of 4 major cardiology societies published a consensus statement in 2007 that provided a universal definition of myocardial infarction, including that occurring in the postoperative CABG patient.[79] The 2011 STS data specifications have been updated to correspond with that definition.

    b. The widely-accepted definition of a perioperative MI is an elevation of biomarkers (either CK or troponin) to > 5 × the 99th percentile of the normal reference range during the first 72h after a CABG *plus*:

       i. New pathological Q waves or LBBB *or*

       ii. Angiographically documented new graft or native coronary artery occlusion *or*

       iii. Imaging evidence of new loss of viable myocardium

    c. Management of a PMI consists of hemodynamic support and other standard measures. A common finding in the patient sustaining a small PMI is a low SVR that requires a vasopressor for several days to support blood pressure. A more extensive infarction may require pharmacologic support or an IABP for longer periods of time and is associated with increased operative mortality and a decrease in long-term survival.

11. For patients receiving **radial artery grafts**, a vasodilator is used to prevent graft spasm. A variety of "cocktails" including nitroglycerin with verapamil or nicardipine are used during preparation of the conduit, and diltiazem 10 mg/h IV or nitroglycerin 10−15 μg/min (0.1−0.2 μg/kg/min) is given intraoperatively and continued for 18−24 hours postoperatively.[80,81] These intravenous medications are then converted to amlodipine 5 mg qd, long-acting diltiazem 120−180 mg PO qd, or Imdur (sustained release) 20 mg PO qd, and arbitrarily continued for 6 months.[82]

12. **Antiplatelet therapy** has been shown to inhibit platelet deposition on vein grafts and may delay or attenuate the development of fibrointimal hyperplasia and atherosclerosis. The immediate postoperative period is a time of increased platelet reactivity, and thus enteric-coated aspirin should be started within 6−24 hours after surgery. Although the generally recommended dose is 75−100 mg,[83] there are concerns that platelet aggregation may not be sufficiently inhibited at these doses.[84] In fact, both the 2005 STS and 2008 European guidelines suggest use of 325 mg/day, although higher and lower doses may have equal efficacy.[85,86] Aspirin can be recommended for 1 year to improve graft patency and indefinitely for secondary prevention of coronary disease. Thus it should also be given to patients receiving all arterial grafts. In patients unable to take aspirin, a 300 mg clopidogrel load followed by 75 mg daily is recommended, since failure to give a load will cause inadequate platelet inhibition for several days.[87] Both aspirin and clopidogrel are recommended for patients undergoing surgery for NSTEMI.[88]

B. **Off-pump coronary artery bypass grafting (OPCAB)** is performed through a sternotomy incision and should achieve complete revascularization comparable to traditional on-pump surgery. Numerous studies have documented that OPCAB is associated with reduced blood loss, reduced transfusion requirements, less renal dysfunction, and arguably less atrial fibrillation, less neurocognitive decline, and a lower risk of stroke.[89,90] Patients are intensively monitored during OPCAB using continuous cardiac output measurements, in-line mixed venous oxygen saturations, and TEE to ensure stability during the procedure. Aspects of this operation which can impact postoperative care include temperature regulation, the influence of intraoperative ischemia on cardiac performance, potential anastomotic problems or incomplete revascularization causing perioperative ischemia or infarction, fluid administration to maintain hemodynamics during cardiac positioning, and bleeding due to use of heparin or transfusion of scavenged blood.

1. Patient temperature tends to drift during surgery and must be maintained by having a higher temperature in the operating room, warming all intravenous fluids and using a topical warming device, such as the Bair Hugger or Kimberly-Clark temperature-controlling system.[9,91] The Thermogard endovascular heating system (Alsius Corporation) which lies within the inferior vena cava has also been found to be very effective in maintaining normothermia.[92] If the patient arrives in the unit hypothermic, the standard measures noted on pages 305–307 should be taken.

2. Hemodynamic performance is generally stable after arrival in the ICU, although ischemia occurring during construction of anastomoses may lead to transient diminution in cardiac performance. Generally, the initial deterioration in cardiac output noted in CPB patients does not occur. However, low doses of inotropes are commonly used during surgery, especially in patients with impaired ventricular function, and should be continued until a satisfactory output can be maintained.

3. The immediate postoperative ECG must be evaluated. Intraoperative assessment of graft patency by Doppler flow analysis should be considered. The likelihood of an anastomotic problem is greater during OPCAB due to suboptimal visualization from bleeding or movement. This may be evident by ECG changes or regional wall motion abnormalities on TEE, but this is not always the case. Occasionally, an abnormal ECG reflects incomplete revascularization when small coronary arteries are not bypassed. There should be a low threshold for postoperative coronary angiography if there is any question about graft flow and patency.

4. Pacing wires should be placed on all patients, because patients well-managed preoperatively on β-blockers will have slower heart rates that will persist into the postoperative period. Although heart rates of 60–70 bpm are acceptable, cardiac output can be optimized by achieving a heart rate of at least 80 bpm in the early postoperative period.

5. The benefits of OPCAB in reducing the incidence of atrial fibrillation are controversial, with benefits most likely seen in elderly patients.[93–95] Thus, the early initiation of β-blockers remains essential. Magnesium is usually given in the operating room to raise the arrhythmia threshold during construction of anastomoses, and may also be given on the first postoperative day to reduce the risk of AF.

6. Many centers extubate patients in the operating room or soon after arrival in the ICU. Standard criteria for weaning and extubation should be used. These include the achievement of normothermia, hemodynamic stability, absence of bleeding, an adequate level of alertness without significant pain, and satisfactory gas exchange. Use of short-acting anesthetic agents and propofol should allow for the safe early extubation of most patients once these criteria are met. Although OPCAB is performed without CPB, there is little evidence that avoidance of CPB preserves respiratory function any better when evaluating postoperative pulmonary function tests, arterial blood gases, or the duration of intubation.[96,97]

7. Although the hemodilution of CPB has been avoided, there is a tendency for anesthesiologists to administer a significant amount of fluid during surgery to

maintain preload and offset the adverse effects of cardiac manipulation and positioning on hemodynamic performance. Thus, patients tend to be somewhat fluid overloaded and need to be diuresed once hemodynamic stability has been achieved. Although the incidence of renal dysfunction may be less with OPCAB, there is an obligatory period of relative hypotension during the construction of proximal anastomoses with an aortic side-clamp that can adversely affect kidney function in patients with preexisting renal dysfunction. This is less of a problem when proximal anastomoses are constructed using devices such as the HEART-STRING proximal seal system (Maquet Cardiovascular).

8. Anemia is less common after OPCAB than on-pump surgery because hemodilution and other adverse effects of CPB on the coagulation system are avoided.[98] Thus, significant mediastinal bleeding should be extremely uncommon in the absence of a surgical bleeding site. However, the potential for a coagulopathy may still exist.

   a. Heparinization is necessary during the procedure, and some degree of fibrinolysis is also probably present. The antifibrinolytic drugs have been shown to be beneficial in reducing bleeding in OPCAB, and thus should be utilized.[99]

   b. Insidious blood loss occurring during the construction of distal anastomoses is scavenged into a cell-saving device. Centrifugation and washing eliminates clotting factors and platelets from reinfused blood.

   c. Both pleural spaces are entered during OPCAB, and failure to place a chest tube in a pleural cavity (or poor drainage through a pleural tube that is placed) may result in the undetected collection of blood that spills over from the mediastinum. Vigilance remains necessary in assessing and managing significant mediastinal bleeding, with a high level of suspicion that it might be occurring if the patient is hemodynamically unstable.

9. Following OPCAB, there is arguably a hypercoagulable state in part related to enhanced platelet reactivity and less platelet dysfunction than noted with use of CPB.[100,101] Early institution of aspirin plus clopidogrel has been shown to reduce postoperative cardiac events without an increased risk of bleeding.[101] One study showed no additional benefit of giving clopidogrel for longer than 1 month after surgery.[102]

C. **Minimally invasive direct coronary artery surgery (MIDCAB)** entails performance of an anastomosis of the left internal thoracic artery (LITA) to the left anterior descending artery (LAD). This is performed through a left thoracotomy incision using one-lung anesthesia. The LITA may be taken down with direct vision, thoracoscopically or robotically.

   1. Patients are generally extubated in the operating room or soon after arrival in the ICU. Epidural or intrathecal morphine analgesia (Duramorph) is helpful in reducing splinting and improving respiratory efforts in patients who might otherwise have significant chest wall pain from rib retraction, resection, or fracture.[103] A local infusion of bupivacaine into the wound is also helpful and may provide superior pain relief than PCA alone.[104]

   2. No pacing wires are placed, so a heart rate in the 60–70 bpm range is acceptable. Ventricular pacing wires placed through the Swan-Ganz catheter can be used for bradycardia, but generally do not provide optimal hemodynamics. External pacing may be used, if necessary.

3. A postoperative ECG must be obtained and carefully reviewed for any evidence of ischemia because anastomotic problems are more common when surgery is performed on a beating, rather than an arrested, heart.

4. Intrapericardial or intrapleural bleeding may originate from the chest wall, the anastomotic site, or side branches of the ITA. Blood will more readily accumulate in the pleural space during spontaneous ventilation. The possibility of bleeding should be monitored by observing chest tube drainage and a postoperative chest x-ray.

D. Aortic valve surgery

1. Aortic stenosis

a. Aortic stenosis (AS) leads to the development of a hypertrophied, noncompliant left ventricle that depends on synchronized atrial and ventricular contractions for nearly 30% of its stroke volume. Postoperatively, it is imperative that sinus rhythm be present or that atrial or AV pacing be used. The optimal heart rate is probably around 90–100 bpm for patients with LVH. There should be a low threshold for cardioversion of atrial fibrillation because profound hemodynamic deterioration may occur, especially during the first 24 hours after surgery.

b. Adequate **preload** must be maintained (PCWP often > 20 mm Hg) to ensure adequate left ventricular filling. Filling pressures may rise rapidly with minimal volume infusion because of the noncompliant hypertrophied ventricle.

c. Although the left ventricular pressure is often very high in patients with high transvalvular gradients, significant **systolic hypertension** is usually not seen at the conclusion of bypass despite elimination of most of the gradient by valve replacement. However, hypertension tends to develop after several hours in the ICU and must be controlled to reduce myocardial oxygen demand and protect the aortic suture line. Use of vasodilators for a hyperdynamic heart may reduce diastolic perfusion pressure and produce a tachycardia. A β-blocker, such as esmolol, is beneficial in this situation.

d. The patient with a hypertrophied, hyperdynamic left ventricle may demonstrate midcavity obliteration and intracavitary flow acceleration, a problem associated with increased perioperative risk.[64] The left ventricle demonstrates diastolic dysfunction, being stiff and unable to fill well. This results in elevated filling pressures, low stroke volumes, and a low cardiac output. TEE in the operating room can define the nature of the pathophysiology and direct management appropriately. Volume infusions to improve left ventricular filling are beneficial despite the high filling pressures, but initiation of inotropic support with catecholamines for a low cardiac output state is counterproductive. Milrinone or nesiritide might be beneficial because of their lusitropic effects that promote ventricular relaxation. β-blockers can be used cautiously.

2. Aortic regurgitation

a. Aortic regurgitation (AR) produces both volume and pressure overload of the left ventricle, resulting in a dilated and frequently hypertrophied chamber. Maintenance of a supraventricular rhythm is important. Filling pressures often rise minimally despite large fluid challenges because of the enlarged, compliant left ventricle, although the cardiac output will usually improve.

b. Despite the placement of a competent aortic valvular prosthesis, most patients with AR remain vasodilated after surgery and require the use of an α-agent, such as phenylephrine or norepinephrine, to maintain a satisfactory blood pressure. Systolic hypertension is often better controlled with β-blockers than with vasodilators.

3. **Heart block** may complicate an aortic valve replacement (AVR) because of edema, hemorrhage, suturing, or debridement near the conduction system, which lies adjacent to the base of the right coronary cusp near the commissure with the noncoronary cusp. It is more likely to occur in patients with preoperative conduction system disease, aortic regurgitation, or following operations for endocarditis or reoperations, which require more manipulation in the region of the conduction system. Epicardial AV pacing may be necessary for several days. The presence of a bundle branch block following AVR is of adverse prognostic significance.[105] If complete heart block persists for more than a few days, during which time edema or hemorrhage should subside, placement of a permanent DDD pacemaker should be considered. The overall incidence of pacemaker placement following AVR is about 5%.[106]

4. **Anticoagulation.** The following recommendations are from the American College of Chest Physicians (ACCP) and the American College of Cardiology/ American Heart Association (ACC/AHA) guidelines, published every few years or updated online (ACC/AHA guidelines at www.cardiosource.com).[107,108]

   a. Tissue aortic valves: antiplatelet therapy with aspirin 81 mg (50–100 mg) once daily is considered as effective as warfarin in the prevention of thromboembolism from tissue aortic valves.[109] Warfarin with a target INR of 2.0–3.0 is recommended if specific risk factors are present, such as prior thromboembolism, atrial fibrillation, a hypercoagulable state, or LV dysfunction (ejection fraction < 35%).

   b. Mechanical aortic valves: all patients with current-generation single tilting-disc or bileaflet valves should receive warfarin indefinitely to achieve a target INR of 2.5 (range 2.0–3.0). Aspirin 81 mg should also be taken. The ACC guidelines recommend a higher target INR of 2.5–3.5 during the first 3 months.[107] This level of INR is also recommended if the above risk factors are present (ACC), or if there is left atrial enlargement or an anteroapical ST-elevation infarction (ACCP).

   c. In patients receiving mechanical valves, there is a potential increased risk of thromboembolism when the patient is not therapeutically anticoagulated. Therefore use of heparin is recommended until the INR becomes therapeutic. However, the timing of initiation of heparin as a bridge is not well defined. Early postoperative use of either unfractionated heparin (UFH) or low-molecular-weight heparin (LMWH) increases the risk of cardiac tamponade.[110,111] Since patients are generally hypocoagulable for several days after surgery, a safe approach would be to start unfractionated heparin (UFH) on the 4th–5th postoperative day if the INR is less than 1.8.

   d. The ACCP 2008 guidelines recommend that either IV UFH or LMWH be given until the INR is > 2.0 for 2 consecutive days.[108] Several studies have documented the safety and efficacy of LMWH as a bridge until the INR is in the therapeutic range, with the total duration of therapy averaging about 1 week. Thus, the patient can be discharged home at any level of INR on LMWH. One study used enoxaparin 1 mg/kg bid and another used a weight-unadjusted dose of 40 mg bid with comparable safety and efficacy.[112,113] A bridge is important if the INR is <2.0 in patients with a mechanical valve, atrial fibrillation, or a hypercoagulable disorder. Fondaparinux may be a reasonable alternative to LMWH, but data on its efficacy are lacking.

E. **Mitral valve surgery**

1. **Mitral stenosis (MS).** Most patients with MS have a small left ventricular cavity with preserved function. They are prone to a low cardiac output syndrome following surgery because of small LV end-diastolic and end-systolic volumes. Maintenance of adequate filling pressures is essential to ensure a satisfactory stroke volume. The "ideal" filling pressure varies for each patient, depending on the level of preexisting pulmonary hypertension and the degree of its reversibility. Generally, there is a substantial reduction in PA pressures postoperatively, even in patients with severe preoperative pulmonary hypertension, using low-dose vasodilators such as nitroglycerin and inducing mild hypocarbia during postoperative mechanical ventilation for more than 12 hours.[114] Hemodynamic support may be required more commonly for RV than LV dysfunction.

   a. Postoperative ventilatory failure is not uncommon in patients with chronic MS as a result of pulmonary hypertension, fluid overload, and chronic cachexia with poor ventilatory reserve. Aggressive diuresis, nutritional support, and a plan for ventilatory support and weaning are essential.

   b. Most patients with MS are diuretic-dependent. Despite correction of their valvular abnormality, they often require substantial doses of diuretics during the hospital stay to achieve their preoperative weight. They should be maintained on diuretics for several months after discharge.

2. **Mitral regurgitation (MR)** reduces left ventricular wall stress by systolic unloading through the regurgitant valve. When mitral valve competence has been restored, there may be unmasking of left ventricular dysfunction because of the greater systolic wall stress required to achieve forward ejection. This may be attenuated to some degree by a reduction in volume overload. This so-called "afterload mismatch" may result in LV failure and require inotropic support and systemic unloading with vasodilators.

3. **Right ventricular dysfunction** is not uncommon following mitral valve surgery, especially in patients with preexisting pulmonary hypertension. RV failure may be precipitated by poor myocardial protection or factors that increase RV afterload. These include positive-pressure ventilation, increased extravascular lung water, blood and blood component transfusions, blood gas and acid–base abnormalities, and reversible pulmonary vascular spasm associated with perfusion-related phenomena and the systemic inflammatory response.

   a. Isolated RV dysfunction is manifested by a high CVP, variable PA pressures, a hypovolemic left ventricle, and a low cardiac output. The use of volumetric Swan-Ganz catheters can better define the degree of RV dysfunction by calculating the RV ejection fraction, but the presence of functional tricuspid regurgitation may render thermodilution cardiac outputs unreliable. In this situation, an alternative means of measuring cardiac output may be necessary, such as the FloTrac system.[115]

b. The initial management of RV dysfunction is fluid administration to optimize preload. However, if the CVP rises above 20 mm Hg without achieving a satisfactory cardiac output, further volume should not be given. This may cause further deterioration of RV function and also impair LV filling by producing a septal shift.

c. Inotropic drugs should be given to support both RV and LV performance. Preferably, those that can also reduce the PVR, such as milrinone, should be chosen. Low-dose epinephrine or dobutamine may be helpful. Probably the strongest drug to improve RV performance is isoproterenol, which is commonly used following heart transplantation, but its utility may be limited by a significant tachycardia.

d. Nesiritide is very effective in reducing PA pressures with minimal effect on the systemic circulation.[116] Its benefits are more related to a lusitropic effect on the ventricles that improves loading conditions than to any direct pulmonary vasodilatory effect. It is more beneficial in patients with pulmonary hypertension from mitral regurgitation rather than mitral stenosis. It also produces a strong diuretic effect.

e. In patients with severe RV dysfunction, selective pulmonary vasodilators may improve RV function by lowering RV afterload. Nitroglycerin is effective in reducing preload, although it also produces systemic vasodilation at higher doses. Selective pulmonary vasodilators include inhaled nitric oxide (20–40 ppm through the ventilator), inhaled epoprostenol (Flolan) (up to 50 ng/kg/min), or inhaled iloprost (Ventavis) (25 μg of a 20 μg/mL mixture via nebulizer).[117–119]

f. Additional comments on the management of RV failure are noted on pages 452–457.

4. Left ventricular dysfunction may occur after surgery for mitral regurgitation because a newly competent mitral valve reduces low pressure unloading of the left ventricle and may unmask LV dysfunction. Deterioration of LV function is minimized by mitral valve reparative techniques or preservation of the subchordal apparatus during mitral valve replacement (MVR). However, an early decline in ejection fraction may be noted after both repair or replacement, especially in symptomatic patients with enlarged left ventricular dimensions. In these patients, the end-diastolic dimensions decrease due to reduced volume overload, but the end-systolic volume remains the same, resulting in a reduction in ejection fraction.[120] Recovery of a normal ejection fraction at later follow-up is more common when surgery is performed when LV dimensions are smaller (LV end-systolic dimension < 36 mm) and after mitral valve repair.[121] On rare occasions, LV dysfunction may be attributable to inadvertent circumferential entrapment of the circumflex coronary artery during suture placement, either for valve repair or replacement (usually in left dominant circulations) or during a left atrial reduction procedure.[122] This should be identified by significant regional wall motion abnormalities on TEE and by ECG changes in the distribution of the artery.

a. To optimize the systemic output, the LV volume status usually has to be maintained at fairly high levels. Administering a large quantity of fluid is frequently required because of increased left atrial and ventricular chamber size and compliance. In the presence of severe RV dysfunction, this can be problematic, because attempts to achieve adequate left-sided filling may lead to progressive RV dilatation and failure, with subsequent impairment in LV filling. Careful monitoring of CVP and RV end-diastolic volumes may indicate when fluid challenges are detrimental rather than beneficial.

b. Assessment of LV end-diastolic volumes is difficult using Swan-Ganz catheter measurements. The extent of reversibility of preexisting pulmonary hypertension is unpredictable and PAD pressures may not correlate well with volume status. The PCWP is more accurate than PAD pressures, especially in patients with a high transpulmonary gradient (PA mean pressure minus PCWP), but "wedging of the balloon" is ill-advised in patients with pulmonary hypertension. Left atrial pressures measured through a left atrial line provide the most accurate assessment of LV filling. They are safe as long as certain precautions regarding air embolism and observation after their removal are taken.[123] They also permit the selective infusion of α-agents to counteract the systemic vasodilation of some vasodilators, although this is rarely necessary.

c. It is generally best to correlate the PAD pressure with direct observation of LV volumes by TEE at the conclusion of surgery. This can establish a baseline from which trends can be identified in the ICU.

5. Left ventricular outflow tract obstruction (LVOTO) has been described following mitral valve replacement due to strut malposition in the outflow tract, in patients with small LV cavities or septal thickening, and most commonly with retention of the anterior mitral leaflet. In many patients, the obstruction requires reoperation, but in some it is dynamic and can be minimized by avoiding hypovolemia and catecholamines, increasing afterload, and using β-blockers.[124,125] Systolic anterior motion (SAM) producing LVOTO is most commonly noted following mitral valve repair when there is excess posterior leaflet height. If it does not respond to the above measures, it may require revision of the repair with a "sliding plasty" technique.[126] SAM is commonly noted preoperatively in patients with hypertrophic obstructive cardiomyopathy due to mitral–septal apposition with a hypertrophied basal septum. This produces not only outflow tract obstruction but also mitral regurgitation from incomplete leaflet apposition. With an adequate extended septal myectomy, SAM and mitral regurgitation should be eliminated, but, if present, similar steps may be taken before considering surgical revision.

6. Maintenance of **sinus rhythm** is beneficial to optimize cardiac output after mitral valve surgery, although it is not as critical as in hypertrophied hearts. Faster heart rates are preferable in volume-overloaded hearts to reduce diastolic filling, which, by reducing wall stress, may improve systolic emptying.[54] It is controversial whether exposure to the mitral valve through the dome of the left atrium (superior approach), the superior transseptal approach which divides the sinus node artery, or a biatrial transseptal approach with or without connecting the atrial incisions ("minitransseptal" approach) is associated with more junctional rhythms or increased need for pacemakers than the standard posterior left atriotomy approach.[127–129] Nonetheless, it is not uncommon to have some difficulty with atrial pacing despite preoperative sinus rhythm. In patients with long-standing persistent atrial fibrillation, it is frequently possible to atrially or AV pace the heart for several hours or days after surgery. Maintenance of sinus rhythm beyond the early

postoperative period is highly unlikely, however, when AF has been present for more than 1 year or the left atrial dimension exceeds 50 mm. β-blockers or calcium channel blockers may be used for rate control, but medications to maintain sinus rhythm, such as amiodarone, are generally not indicated in patients with long-standing persistent AF.

7. The Maze procedure (Figures 1.25 and 1.26, pages 56 and 57) can be used to treat paroxysmal or persistent atrial fibrillation and is most commonly performed as an adjunct to mitral valve surgery.[130] Bilateral pulmonary vein isolation with resection and oversewing of the left atrial appendage is an acceptable operation for paroxysmal AF, but additional ablation lines within the left atrium are essential for persistent AF. The added benefit of right atrial ablation lines is not clear. Although ablative technologies including radiofrequency and cryoablation are successful in restoring sinus rhythm, their results remain inferior to the elaborate "cut and sew" Cox-Maze III operation. Notably, about 10–15% of patients required pacemakers after this procedure, although some patients will require a pacemaker using other ablative technologies. Amiodarone and warfarin are generally recommended for 3–6 months after a successful ablation. If AF persists, elective cardioversion may be considered after 3 months. If the cardioversion is unsuccessful, only warfarin is continued.

8. The acute onset of exsanguinating bleeding through the chest tubes or the development of tamponade soon after mitral valve replacement suggests the possibility of **left ventricular rupture**. This may occur at the atrioventricular groove, at the base of the papillary muscles, or in between. This problem can be avoided by meticulous surgical technique, chordal preservation during MVR, and avoiding tissue valves in patients with very small left ventricles (usually in elderly women with mitral stenosis). Tissue valves have three protruding struts, although the profiles of newer tissue valves are much lower than in the past. Left ventricular rupture may be precipitated by LV distention or excessive afterload after bypass. Once identified, emergency surgical intervention on bypass is required and carries a significant mortality rate.[131]

9. **Anticoagulation**

   a. **Mitral annuloplasty rings.** There are insufficient studies to determine whether warfarin or aspirin is preferable following prosthetic annuloplasty rings for patients who are in sinus rhythm. The European Society of Cardiology recommends 3 months of warfarin, but smaller studies suggest that aspirin alone may be sufficient.[132,133]

   b. **Tissue mitral valves.** Warfarin or aspirin may be recommended for the first 3 months following tissue MVR.
      i. The 2008 ACCP recommendation is for use of warfarin to achieve a target INR of 2.5 (range 2.0–3.0) with conversion to aspirin after 3 months, based upon evidence that the risk of thromboembolism is higher during the first 3 postoperative months. This is the approach most commonly recommended and utilized.[108,109] Low-dose aspirin should be added if the patient has evidence of peripheral vascular disease. One might consider initiating heparin before the INR becomes therapeutic, usually starting it on the 4th–5th postoperative day and continuing it until the INR exceeds 1.8 if the patient is in sinus rhythm. After 3 months, aspirin may be substituted if the patient remains in sinus rhythm.

  ii. The 2008 ACC/AHA recommendation is for use of aspirin 75–100 mg daily in patients with no risk factors, considering it "reasonable" (Class IIa indication) to use warfarin instead with a target INR of 2.0–3.0. Both are recommended if risk factors are present (prior thromboembolism, atrial fibrillation, hypercoagulable state, ejection fraction <35%, or an enlarged left atrium).[107] In patients with these risk factors, the warfarin should be given indefinitely.

 c. Mechanical mitral valves. Warfarin is started on the first postoperative day to achieve a target INR of 3.0 (range 2.5–3.5) and is given indefinitely along with aspirin 75–100 mg to further reduce the thromboembolic risk. Heparin should be started around the fourth postoperative day if the INR is <2.0. As noted on page 326, the ACCP guidelines recommend that either IV UFH or LMWH be given until the INR is >2.0 for 2 consecutive days, and this can easily be accomplished using LMWH as an outpatient. Again, it should be reemphasized that early postoperative initiation of either UFH or LMWH may increase the risk of tamponade.[110,111]

F. Minimally invasive/robotic surgery

1. Procedures performed through small incisions limit surgical exposure to the heart. Since all minimally invasive valve procedures and some totally endoscopic/robotic coronary bypass grafting are performed on-pump, problems related to use of CPB, whether pulmonary, cardiac, or renal, are similar to those noted above for specific valve pathology. However, there are a few specific issues that may arise in these patients.

2. Pain control is essential following ministernotomy and rib-spreading procedures. Similar to MIDCABs, use of epidural analgesia or intercostal blocks can optimize patient comfort and pulmonary status.

3. Access to the right ventricle is limited, making placement of pacemaker wires somewhat difficult. The ability to pace the heart using pacing pads (which are fairly uncomfortable) or using a ventricular pacing wire placed through specially designed PA catheters is useful.

4. Placement of chest tubes may not be ideal because of exposure limitations. Usually one pleural and one anterior mediastinal tube are placed, but may not provide ideal drainage. It is essential to be alert to the potential for undetected accumulation of blood in the pleural space or for the development of tamponade when the patient is hemodynamically unstable.

5. Although some minimally invasive incisions allow for central aortic and venous cannulation, all robotic cases and other minimally invasive cases with limited exposure require alternative cannulation sites – usually the femoral artery and/or vein. The presence of aortoiliac disease, very small femoral arteries, or thoracic or abdominal aneurysmal disease contraindicates this approach, such that axillary or central cannulation must be used. Insertion of a femoral cannula is accomplished by direct cutdown or percutaneous cannula placement. Following decannulation, the artery is usually repaired under direct vision unless placed percutaneously. The potential for hemorrhage, femoral artery injury, focal thrombosis, or distal ather-oembolism may exist. It is absolutely essential that distal perfusion be assessed at the conclusion of surgery by pulse examination.

6. Because these operations can be tedious, especially in the early part of the learning curve, the bypass run may be quite long, often over 4 hours. This leads to the potential for development of a lower-extremity compartment syndrome. Since the anesthetized patient cannot complain of pain or sensory changes or exhibit motor function, assessment of calf size and tenseness at the conclusion of surgery and in the ICU on a frequent basis is essential to recognize the very early stages of a compartment syndrome. Early fasciotomy can salvage muscle and limb function; delayed fasciotomy may be the first step towards an amputation.

G. **Aortic dissections**

1. Virtually all patients with dissections that involve the ascending aorta (type A dissections) undergo surgical repair (Figure 1.19, page 47). The reestablishment of vascular continuity involves suturing of a Dacron graft to very fragile tissues, and suture-line bleeding is commonly noted. In addition, surgical repair is predicated on stabilization of the entry site of the dissection, but does not completely eliminate the distal false channel. Thus surgery is palliative and leaves the patient predisposed to distal aneurysm formation in the future.

2. Aggressive management of hypertension following surgery is just as important as preoperative control. Similar antihypertensive medications should be used to reduce systolic blood pressure and the force of cardiac contraction (dp/dt). The most common regimens are a β-blocker (intravenous esmolol, metoprolol, or labetalol) alone or in combination with nitroprusside. The patient is then converted to oral metoprolol or labetalol with use of additional antihypertensives, such as calcium channel blockers or ACE inhibitors, as necessary. The risk of subsequent aneurysmal disease in the descending aorta is reduced with use of β-blockers, reinforcing that heart rate control is an important component of postoperative long-term care.[134] This is also true for patients with type B dissections (not involving the ascending aorta), in whom control of both blood pressure and heart rate reduces the frequency of aortic events, including distal ischemia, recurrent dissection, aortic rupture, and expansion.[135]

3. The repair of a type A dissection usually involves a period of DHCA while the distal anastomosis is performed. The extensive period of profound cooling and rewarming may be associated with a significant coagulopathy, but bleeding can be minimized by use of felt reinforcement at the suture lines and use of the tissue adhesive BioGlue. Early and aggressive use of blood products is indicated if a coagulopathy is suspected to be the cause of significant bleeding.

4. Careful preoperative and postoperative neurologic assessments are important to distinguish a preoperative neurologic deficit from a stroke related to DHCA or cerebral malperfusion.

5. For type B dissections, surgery is usually reserved for patients with "complicated" dissections, yet even in the most experienced centers the mortality rate for this operation is 20–35%.[136,137] The most common postoperative complications are respiratory failure and those related to aortic cross-clamping or malperfusion (renal failure and paraplegia). The latter complications may be lessened but not eliminated with endovascular repair.[138,139] Careful preoperative assessment of branch artery flow is essential, and additional fenestration or branch artery stenting/ grafting may be necessary if there is mesenteric ischemia. A careful preoperative and

postoperative neurologic examination of the lower extremities, and measures to support renal function in the perioperative period are important. Other comments on descending thoracic aortic surgery are noted below.

H. Ascending aortic and arch aneurysms

1. Ascending aortic aneurysms commonly develop in patients with bicuspid aortic valves due to a congenital abnormality of the aortic wall with a deficient extracellular matrix that predisposes to aortic enlargement. These patients tend to have few other significant comorbid problems, and complications are more related to surgical technique than to other medical issues.

2. In contrast, degenerative aneurysms tend to develop in elderly patients with hypertension, chronic lung disease, and diffuse atherosclerosis, including cerebrovascular, coronary, and renovascular disease. Thus, recognition and management of problems involving these organ systems are essential to optimize surgical recovery.

3. An ascending aortic aneurysm that tapers before the aortic arch can often be repaired with the aortic cross-clamp in place using mildly hypothermic CPB. Although the mid-arch can be cannulated for bypass, use of the femoral artery (in the absence of significant distal atherosclerosis) or the axillary artery is preferable. It is important to confirm satisfactory distal flow into the limb beyond the cannulation site after decannulation. The risk of stroke is low unless there is atherosclerotic disease at the level of the aortic cross-clamp, in which case clamping should be avoided. With careful suturing of the aortic anastomoses, often with felt reinforcement, surgical bleeding should be readily controlled, but still may require use of multiple blood products. Furthermore, control of hypertension is essential in the ICU to minimize suture-line bleeding.

4. Ascending aortic aneurysms that extend into the arch may require a hemiarch or total arch repair. Neuroprotection by provision of cerebral blood flow may extend the tolerable period of DHCA during construction of the arch and reduce the neurologic risk. The most significant postoperative complications of this type of surgery are those of stroke or neurocognitive dysfunction and bleeding.

   a. Although DHCA alone may suffice for short periods of circulatory arrest (< 30−40 minutes), a means of providing cerebral perfusion during DHCA will extend the safe period of arrest.[140,141] Selective antegrade cerebral perfusion (SACP) (either directly or via axillary artery cannulation) reduces the mortality and stroke rate of open arch replacements more than use of retrograde cerebral perfusion (RCP) via the superior vena cava.[142] Although some surgeons use cold SACP with moderate (25 °C) systemic perfusion to eliminate some of the issues related to deep hypothermia, this may not be safe in older patients with long DHCA times and multiple comorbidities.[143] An alternative approach in aortic arch surgery is a "debranching" operation, which restores cerebral flow to individual arch vessels before the distal aortic anastomosis is sewn. This may limit the duration of DHCA and optimize cerebral protection.[144]

   b. Following operations using DHCA, neurologic recovery may take up to 24 hours in some patients, and the anesthetic agents and postoperative protocols for sedation and control of hypertension should be selected anticipating a slightly prolonged duration of ventilation. It is enticing to promptly awaken the patient to assess a response to verbal commands and motor function of all extremities, but this could result in a period of inadequate analgesia and hypertension that is best avoided.

c. Use of DHCA to 18 °C requires a substantial time to rewarm to normothermia because it is important to maintain a perfusion gradient of <10 °C. Despite active rewarming to 37 °C on bypass, significant temperature afterdrop is common, and a temperature-controlling device during surgery (Bair Hugger or Kimberly-Clark) and a forced-air system in the ICU (Bair Hugger) should be used. Coagulopathies are commonly present and require aggressive management to minimize mediastinal bleeding.

I. **Descending thoracic and thoracoabdominal aneurysms**

1. Repair of descending thoracic and thoracoabdominal aneurysms involves a thoracotomy incision and often takedown of the diaphragm. Furthermore, extensive blood loss requiring massive transfusions of blood is not uncommon and usually produces a coagulopathy requiring multiple blood components and often a reexploration. Prolonged ventilation should be anticipated and medications selected accordingly. The extensive incisions required for these operations can produce significant pain that requires adequate analgesia. More than 10% of patients undergoing these repairs may require a postoperative tracheostomy for prolonged ventilatory support.[145,146]

2. Cross-clamping of the descending aorta can result in paraplegia or renal failure, even if distal perfusion is provided during the cross-clamp period. Because hypoperfusion is considered to be the mechanism producing spinal cord ischemia, intraoperative blood pressure management (avoidance of hypotension) and cerebrospinal fluid (CSF) drainage initiated before surgery are important to improve spinal cord perfusion pressure.[147] The drain is left in place for up 3 days after surgery to keep the CSF pressure less than 10 mm Hg. A mean arterial pressure of at least 90 mm Hg should be maintained with an understanding that this could worsen bleeding.[148] Particular attention to a pre- and postoperative neurologic evaluation on a daily basis is essential. **Delayed onset of paraplegia** occurring in the ICU may develop after several days and is actually more common than immediate postoperative paraplegia when protective steps, including distal perfusion, CSF drainage, or circulatory arrest, are used.[148–150] It is usually, but not always, triggered by an episode of hypotension. If recognized immediately, it is usually reversible with elevation of the systemic blood pressure, high-dose steroids, and reinsertion of the CSF drain if it has been removed.

3. Cross-clamping of the aorta impairs renal perfusion and can produce acute kidney injury. Measures should be taken during surgery to optimize renal perfusion, which may include use of mannitol, furosemide, or an infusion of fenoldopam or nesiritide.[151] The incidence of renal failure after thoracoabdominal surgery is about 10–15%.[145]

4. The use of endovascular stent repair for descending thoracic aneurysms has improved results compared with open repair.[152] However, spinal cord ischemia still occurs in 3–12% of patients. Use of somatosensory evoked potentials, CSF drainage, and maintaining a mean arterial pressure >90 mm Hg may be beneficial in improving neurologic outcomes.[153,154]

J. Left ventricular aneurysms and ventricular arrhythmia surgery

1. Patients undergoing resection of a left ventricular aneurysm usually have markedly depressed LV function. Although ventricular size and geometry are better preserved using the endoaneurysmorrhaphy or endoventricular circular patch plasty techniques than with a linear closure, the stroke volume of the left ventricle after left ventricular aneurysm repair is usually lower after surgery. Achieving adequate filling pressures (usually a PCWP around 20–25 mm Hg) is essential to optimize stroke volume. Filling pressures may rise precipitiously with minimal volume infusion because of the small noncompliant LV chamber. Many patients generate a satisfactory cardiac output by virtue of a faster heart rate, which should not be reduced pharmacologically unless the stroke volume is satisfactory. Hemodynamic support and an IABP are frequently necessary to allow weaning from CPB.

2. Surgery for ventricular tachycardia is relatively uncommon and usually involves blind endocardial resection with cryoablation. To minimize the risk of postoperative ventricular arrhythmias, lidocaine should be used prophylactically for 24 hours. Most of these patients will be candidates for postoperative ICD placement with or without electrophysiologic testing.

3. ICDs are usually placed in the electrophysiology lab in patients with sustained ventricular tachycardia, other suspected life-threatening arrhythmias, or prophylactically in patients with poor LV function. If the patient has had heart surgery and had a preoperative indication for the device, it is placed several days after surgery. Similarly, if the patient has poor ventricular function and develops nonsustained or sustained VT after surgery, an ICD may be considered before hospital discharge. The device is tested and usually left in the active mode. There should be a card posted above the head of the patient's bed indicating the status of the ICD so that anyone who responds to an emergency knows whether the device is activated or not. Generally, patients are placed on either β-blockers or amiodarone if they have malignant ventricular arrhythmias.

References

1. Svircevic V, Nierich AP, Moons KG, Brandon Bravo Bruinsma GJ, Kalkman CJ, van Dijk D. Fast-track anesthesia and cardiac surgery: a retrospective cohort study of 7989 patients. *Anesth Analg* 2009;108:727–33.

2. Hawkes CA, Dhileepan S, Foxcroft D. Early extubation for adult cardiac surgical patients. *Cochrane Database Syst Rev* 2003;4:CD003587.

3. Hemmerling TM, Preito I, Choinière JL, Basile F, Fortier JD. Ultra-fast-track anesthesia in off-pump coronary artery bypass grafting: a prospective audit comparing opioid-based anesthesia vs thoracic epidural-based anesthesia. *Can J Anaesth* 2004;51:163–8.

4. Insler SR, Sessler DI. Perioperative thermoregulation and temperature monitoring. *Anesthesiol Clin* 2006;24:823–37.

5. Reynolds L, Beckmann J, Kurz A. Perioperative complications of hypothermia. *Best Pract Res Clin Anaesthesiol* 2008;22:645–57.

6. Mora CT, Henson MB, Weintraub WS, et al. The effect of temperature management during cardiopulmonary bypass on neurologic and neuropsychologic outcomes in patients undergoing coronary revascularization. *J Thorac Cardiovasc Surg* 1996;112:514–22.

7. Jones T, Roy RC. Should patients be normothermic in the immediate postoperative period? *Ann Thorac Surg* 1999;68:1454–5.

8. Forbes SS, Eskicioglu C, Nathens AB, et al. Evidence-based guidelines for prevention of perioperative hypothermia. *J Am Coll Surg* 2009;209:492–503.

9. Grocott HP, Mathew JP, Carver EH, et al. A randomized controlled trial of the Arctic Sun Temperature Management System versus conventional methods for preventing hypothermia during off-pump cardiac surgery. *Anesth Analg* 2004;98:298–302.

10. Rajek A, Lenhardt R, Sessler DI, et al. Efficacy of two methods for reducing postbypass afterdrop. *Anesthesiology* 2000;92:447–56.

11. Pathi V, Berg GA, Morrison J, Cramp G, McLaren D, Faichney A. The benefits of active rewarming after cardiac operations: a randomized prospective trial. *J Thorac Cardiovasc Surg* 1996;111:637–41.

12. Bräuer A, English MJ, Steinmetz N, et al. Efficacy of forced-air warming systems with full body blankets. *Can J Anaesth* 2007;54:34–41.

13. Bräuer A, Weyland W, Kazmaier S, et al. Efficacy of postoperative rewarming after cardiac surgery. *Ann Thorac Cardiovasc Surg* 2004;10:171–7.

14. Noback CR, Tinker JH. Hypothermia after cardiopulmonary bypass in man: amelioration by nitroprusside-induced vasodilatation during rewarming. *Anesthesiology* 1980;53:277–80.

15. De Witte J, Sessler DI. Perioperative shivering. Physiology and pharmacology. *Anesthesiology* 2002;96:467–84.

16. Bicer C, Esmaoglu A, Akin A, Boyaci A. Dexmedetomidine and meperidine prevent postanaesthetic shivering. *Eur J Anaesthesiol* 2006;23:149–53.

17. Kurz A, Go JC, Sessler DI, Kaer K, Larson MD, Bjorksten AR. Alfentanil slightly increases the sweating threshold and markedly reduces the vasoconstriction and shivering thresholds. *Anesthesiology* 1995;83:293–9.

18. Despotis GJ, Hogue CW Jr. Pathophysiology, prevention, and treatment of bleeding after cardiac surgery: a primer for cardiologists and an update for the cardiothoracic team. *Am J Cardiol* 1999;83:15B–30B.

19. Despotis GJ, Avidan MS. Hogue CW Jr. Mechanisms and attenuation of hemostatic activation during extracorporeal circulation. *Ann Thorac Surg* 2001;72:S1821–31.

20. McIlroy DR, Myles PS, Phillips LE, Smith JA. Antifibrinolytics in cardiac surgical patients receiving aspirin: a systematic review and meta-analysis. *Br J Anaesth* 2009;102:168–78.

21. Karthik S, Grayson AD, McCarron EE, Pullan DM, Desmond MJ. Reexploration for bleeding after coronary artery bypass surgery: risk factors, outcomes, and effect of time delay. *Ann Thorac Surg* 2004;78:527–34.

22. Reis J, Mota JC, Ponce P, Costa-Pereira A, Guerreiro M. Early extubation does not increase complication rates after coronary artery bypass surgery with cardiopulmonary bypass. *Eur J Cardiothorac Surg* 2002;21:1026–30.

23. Hemmerling TM, Lê N, Olivier JF, Choinière JL, Basile F, Prieto I. Immediate extubation after aortic valve surgery using high thoracic epidural analgesia or opioid-based analgesia. *J Cardiothorac Vasc Anesth* 2005;19:176–81.

24. Turker G, Goren S, Sahin S, Korfali G, Sayan E. Combination of intrathecal morphine and remifentanil infusion for fast-track anesthesia in off-pump coronary artery bypass surgery. *J Cardiothorac Vasc Anesth* 2005;19:708–13.

25. Parlow JL, Steele RG, O'Reilly D. Low dose intrathecal morphine facilitates early extubation after cardiac surgery: results of a retrospective continuous quality improvement audit. *Can J Anaesth* 2005;52:94–9.

26. Lena P, Balarac N, Lena D, et al. Fast-track anesthesia with remifentanil and spinal analgesia for cardiac surgery: the effect on pain control and quality of recovery. *J Cardiothorac Vasc Anesth* 2008;22:536–42.

27. Toraman F, Evrenkaya S, Yuce M, Göksel O, Karabulut H, Alhan C. Fast-track recovery in noncoronary cardiac surgery patients. *Heart Surg Forum* 2005;8:E61–4.

28. Alhan C, Toraman F, Karabulut EH, et al. Fast track recovery of high risk coronary bypass surgery patients. *Eur J Cardiothorac Surg* 2003;23:678–83.

29. Kogan A, Ghosh P, Preisman S, et al. Risk factors for failed "fast-tracking" after cardiac surgery in patients older than 70 years. *J Cardiothorac Vasc Anesth* 2008;22:530–5.

30. Parlow JL, Ahn R, Milne B. Obesity is a risk factor for failure of "fast track" extubation following coronary artery bypass surgery. *Can J Anaesth* 2006;53:288–94.

31. Wong DT, Cheng DC, Kustra R, et al. Risk factors of delayed extubation, prolonged length of stay in the intensive care unit, and mortality in patients undergoing coronary artery bypass graft with fast-track cardiac anesthesia: a new cardiac risk score. *Anesthesiology* 1999;91:936–44.

32. Yende S, Wunderlink R. Causes of prolonged mechanical ventilation after coronary artery bypass surgery. *Chest* 2002;122:245–52.

33. Lison S, Schill M, Conzen P. Fast-tract cardiac anesthesia: efficacy and safety of remifentail versus sufentanil. *J Cardiothorac Vasc Anesth* 2007;21:35–40.

34. Delphin E, Jackson D, Gubenko Y, et al. Sevoflurane provides earlier tracheal extubation and assessment of cognitive recovery than isoflurane in patients undergoing off-pump coronary artery bypass surgery. *J Cardiothorac Vasc Anesth* 2007;21:690–5.

35. Hemmerling T, Olivier JR, Le N, Prieto I, Bracco D. Myocardial protection by isoflurane vs. sevoflurane in ultra-fast-track anaesthesia for off-pump aortocoronary bypass grafting. *Eur J Anaesthesiol* 2008;25:230–6.

36. Hemmerling TM, Russo G, Bracco D. Neuromuscular blockade in cardiac surgery: an update for clinicians. *Ann Card Anaesth* 2008;11:80–90.

37. Constantinides VA, Tekkis PP, Fazil A, et al. Fast-track failure after cardiac surgery: development of a prediction model. *Crit Care Med* 2006;34:2875–82.

38. Ho KM, Ng JY. The use of propofol for medium and long-term sedation in critically ill adult patients: a meta-analysis. *Intensive Care Med* 2008;34:1969–79.

39. Roediger L, Larbuisson R, Lamy M. New approaches and old controversies to postoperative pain control following cardiac surgery. *Eur J Anaesthesiol* 2006;23:539–50.

40. Erstad BL, Puntillo K, Gilbert HC, et al. Pain management principles in the critically ill. *Chest* 2009;135:1075–86.

41. Sessler CN, Varney K. Patient-focused sedation and analgesia in the ICU. *Chest* 2008;133:552–65.

42. Gommers D, Bakker J. Medications for analgesia and sedation in the intensive care unit: an overview. *Crit Care* 2008;12(suppl 3):S4. (available at ccforum.com/content/12/S3/S4)

43. Barr AM, Tutungi E, Almeida AA. Parasternal intercostal block with ropivacaine for pain management after cardiac surgery: a double-blind, randomized controlled trial. *J Cardiothorac Vasc Anesth* 2007;21:547–53.

44. White PF, Rawal S, Lathan P, et al. Use of a continuous local anesthetic infusion for pain management after median sternotomy. *Anesthesiology* 2003;99:918–23.

45. Ralley FE, Day FJ, Cheng DCH. Pro: Nonsteroidal anti-inflammatory drugs should be routinely administered for postoperative analgesia after cardiac surgery. *J Cardiothorac Vasc Anesth* 2000;14:731–4.

46. Engoren MC, Habib RH, Zacharias A, et al. Postoperative analgesia with ketorolac is associated with decreased mortality after isolated coronary artery bypass graft surgery in patients already receiving aspirin: a propensity-matched study. *J Cardiothorac Vasc Anesth* 2007;21:820–6.

47. Herr DL, Sum-Ping ST, England M. ICU sedation after coronary artery bypass graft surgery: dexmedetomidine-based versus propofol-based sedation regimens. *J Cardiothorac Vasc Anesth* 2003;17:576–84.

48. Barr J, Egan TD, Sandoval NF, et al. Propofol dosing regimens for ICU sedation based upon an integrated pharmacokinetic-pharmacodynamic model. *Anesthesiology* 2001;95:324–33.

49. Ruokonen E, Parviainen I, Jakob SM, et al. Dexmedetomidine versus propofol/midazolam for long-term sedation during mechanical ventilation. *Intensive Care Med* 2009;35:282–90.

50. Riker RR, Shehabi Y, Bokesch PM, et al. Dexmedetomidine vs midazolam for sedation of critically ill patients: a randomized trial. *JAMA* 2009;301:489–99.

51. Gurbet A, Goren S, Sahin S, Uckunkaya N, Korfali G. Comparison of analgesic effects of morphine, fentanyl, and remifentanil with intravenous patient-controlled analgesic after cardiac surgery. *J Cardiothorac Vasc Anesth* 2004;18:755–8.

52. Baltali S, Turkoz A, Bozdogan N, et al. The efficacy of intravenous patient-controlled remifentanil versus morphine anesthesia after coronary artery surgery. *J Cardiothorac Vasc Anesth* 2009;23:170–4.

53. Griffin MJ, Hines RL. Management of perioperative ventricular dysfunction. *J Cardiothorac Vasc Anesth* 2001;15:90–106.

54. St. André AC, DelRossi A. Hemodynamic management of patients in the first 24 hours after cardiac surgery. *Crit Care Med* 2005;33:2082–93.

55. Murphy GJ, Reeves BC, Rogers CA, Rizvi SIA, Culliford L, Angelini GD. Increased mortality, postoperative morbidity, and cost after red blood cell transfusions in patients having cardiac surgery. *Circulation* 2007;116:2544–52.

56. Jones KW, Cain AS, Mitchell JH, et al. Hyperglycemia predicts mortality after CABG: postoperative hyperglycemia predicts dramatic increases in mortality after coronary artery bypass graft surgery. *J Diabetes Complications* 2008;22:365–70.

57. Lazar HL, McDonnell M, Chipkin SR, et al. The Society of Thoracic Surgeons practice guidelines series: blood glucose management during adult cardiac surgery. *Ann Thorac Surg* 2009;87:663–9.

58. Singla N, Warltier DC, Gandhi SD, et al. Treatment of acute postoperative hypertension in cardiac surgery patients: an efficacy study of clevidipine assessing its postoperative antihypertensive effect in cardiac surgery-2 (ESCAPE-2), a randomized, double-blind, placebo controlled trial. *Anesth Analg* 2008;107:59–67.

59. Gallagher JD, Moore RA, Kerns D, et al. Effects of colloid or crystalloid administration on pulmonary extravascular water in the postoperative period after coronary artery bypass grafting. *Anesth Analg* 1985;64:753–8.

60. Boldt J. Pro: use of colloids in cardiac surgery. *J Cardiothorac Vasc Anesth* 2007;21:453–6.

61. Tayama E, Ueda T, Shojima T, et al. Arginine vasopressin is an ideal drug after cardiac surgery for the management of low systemic vascular resistant hypotension concomitant with pulmonary hypertension. *Interact Cardiovasc Thorac Surg* 2007;6:715–9.

62. Gomes WJ, Erlichman MR, Batista-Filho ML, et al. Vasoplegic syndrome after off-pump coronary artery bypass surgery. *Eur J Cardiothorac Surg* 2003;23:165–9.

63. Imren Y, Tasoglu I, Oktar GL, et al. The importance of transesophageal echocardiography in diagnosis of pericardial tamponade after cardiac surgery. *J Card Surg* 2008;23:450–3.

64. Bartunek J, Sys SU, Rodrigues AC, Schuerbeeck E, Mortier L, de Bruyne B. Abnormal systolic intracavity flow velocities after valve replacement for aortic stenosis. Mechanisms, predictive factors, and prognostic significance. *Circulation* 1996;93:712–9.

65. Winterhalter M, Simon A, Fischer S, et al. Comparison of inhaled iloprost and nitric oxide in patients with pulmonary hypertension during weaning from cardiopulmonary bypass in cardiac surgery: a prospective randomized trial. *J Cardiothorac Vasc Anesth* 2008;22:406–13.

66. Cannesson M, Farhat F, Scarlata M, Cassar E, Lehot JJ. The impact of atrio-biventricular pacing on hemodynamics and left ventricular dyssynchrony compared with atrio-right ventricular pacing alone in the postoperative period after cardiac surgery. *J Cardiothorac Vasc Anesth* 2009;23:306–11.

67. Johnson RG, Goldberger AL, Thurer RL, Schwartz M, Sirois S, Weintraub RM. Lidocaine prophylaxis in coronary revascularization patients: a randomized, prospective trial. *Ann Thorac Surg* 1993;55:1180–4.

68. Mitchell LB, Exner DV, Wyse DG, et al. Prophylactic oral amiodarone for the prevention of arrhythmias that begin early after revascularization, valve replacement or repair: PAPABEAR: a randomized controlled trial. *JAMA* 2005;294:3093–100.

69. Zebis LR, Christensen TD, Thomsen HF, et al. Practical regimen for amiodarone use in preventing postoperative atrial fibrillation. *Ann Thorac Surg* 2007;83:1326–31.

70. Bradley D, Creswell LL, Hogue CW Jr, et al. Pharmacologic prophylaxis: American College of Chest Physicians guidelines for the prevention and management of postoperative atrial fibrillation after cardiac surgery. *Chest* 2005;128(2 Suppl):39S–47S.

71. Echahidi N, Pibarot P, O'Hara G, Mathieu P. Mechanisms, prevention, and treatment of atrial fibrillation after cardiac surgery. *J Am Coll Cardiol* 2008;51:793–801.

72. Budeus M, Feindt P, Gams E, et al. β-blocker prophylaxis for atrial fibrillation after coronary artery bypass grafting in patients with sympathovagal imbalance. *Ann Thorac Surg* 2007;84:61–6.

73. Henyan NN, Gillespie EL, White CM, Kluger J, Coleman CI. Impact of intravenous magnesium on post-cardiothoracic surgery atrial fibrillation and length of hospital stay: a meta-analysis. *Ann Thorac Surg* 2005;80:2402–6.

74. Magee MJ, Herbert MA, Dewey TM, et al. Atrial fibrillation after coronary artery bypass grafting: development of a predictive risk algorithm. *Ann Thorac Surg* 2007;83:1707–12.

75. Tzimas PG, Milionis HJ, Arnaoutoglou HM, et al. Cardiac troponin I versus creatine kinase-MB in the detection of postoperative cardiac events after coronary artery bypass grafting surgery. *J Cardiovasc Sug (Torino)* 2008;49:95–101.

76. Adabag AS, Rector T, Mithani S, et al. Prognostic significance of elevated cardiac troponin I after heart surgery. *Ann Thorac Surg* 2007;83:1744–50.

77. Croal BL, Hillis GS, Gibson PH, et al. Relationship between postoperative cardiac troponin I levels and outcome of cardiac surgery. *Circulation* 2006;114:1468–75.

78. Bignami E, Landoni G, Crescenzi G, et al. Role of cardiac biomarkers (troponin I and CK-MB) as predictors of quality of life and long-term outcome after cardiac surgery. *Ann Card Anaesth* 2009;12:22–6.

79. Thygesen K, Alpert JS, White HD on behalf of the Joint ESC/ACCF/AHA/AHF task force for the redefinition of myocardial infarction. Universal definition of myocardial infarction. *Circulation* 2007;116:2634–53. and *J Am Coll Cardiol* 2007;50:2173–95.

80. He GW, Fan L, Furnary A, Yang Q. A new antispastic solution for arterial grafting: nicardipine and nitroglycerin cocktail in preparation of internal thoracic and radial arteries for coronary surgery. *J Thorac Cardiovasc Surg* 2008;136:673–80.

81. Attaran S, John L, El-Gamel A. Clinical and potential use of pharmacological agents to reduce radial artery spasm in coronary artery surgery. *Ann Thorac Surg* 2008;85:1483–9.

82. Bond BR, Zellner JL, Dorman BH, et al. Differential effects of calcium channel antagonists in the amelioration of radial artery vasospasm. *Ann Thorac Surg* 2000;69:1035–40.

83. Becker RC, Meade TW, Berger PB, et al. The primary and secondary prevention of coronary artery disease. American College of Chest Physicians evidence-based clinical practice guidelines (8th edition). *Chest* 2008;133:776S–814S.

84. Bednar F, Osmancik P, Hlavicka J, Jedlickova V, Paluch Z, Vanek T. Aspirin is insufficient in inhibition of platelet aggregation and thromboxane formation early after coronary artery bypass surgery. *J Thromb Thrombolysis* 2009;27:394–9.

85. Ferraris VA, Ferraris SP, Moliterno DJ, et al. The Society of Thoracic Surgeons practice guideline series: aspirin and other antiplatelet agents during operative coronary revascularization (executive summary). *Ann Thorac Surg* 2005;79:1454–61.

86. Dunning J, Versteegh M, Fabbri A, et al. Guidelines on antiplatelet and anticoagulation management in cardiac surgery. *Eur J Cardiothorac Surg* 2008;34:73–92.

87. Lim E, Coirnelissen J, Routledge T, et al. Clopidogrel did not inhibit platelet function early after coronary artery bypass surgery: a prospective randomized trial. *J Thorac Cardiovasc Surg* 2004;128:432–5.

88. Kunadian B, Thornely AR, Babu TN, Dunning J. Should high risk patients receive clopidogrel as well as aspirin post coronary artery bypass grafting? *Interact Cardiovasc Thorac Surg* 2006;5:755–60.

89. Møller CH, Penninga L, Wettersley J, Steinbrüchel DA, Gluud C. Clinical outcomes in randomized trials of off- vs. on-pump coronary artery bypass surgery: systematic review with meta-analyses and trial sequential analyses. *Eur Heart J* 2008;29:2601–16.

90. Sellke FW, DiMaio JM, Caplan LR, et al. Comparing on-pump and off-pump coronary artery bypass grafting: numerous studies but few conclusions: a scientific statement from the American Heart Association council on cardiovascular surgery and anesthesia in collaboration with the interdisciplinary working group on quality of care and outcomes research. *Circulation* 2005;111:2858–64.

91. Jeong SM, Hahm KD, Jeong YB, Yang HS, Choi IC. Warming of intravenous fluids prevents hypothermia during off-pump coronary artery bypass graft surgery. *J Cardiothorac Vasc Anesth* 2008;22:67–70.

92. Allen GS. Intraoperative temperature control using the Thermogard system during off-pump coronary artery bypass grafting. *Ann Thorac Surg* 2009;87:284–8.

93. Athanasiou T, Aziz O, Mangoush O, et al. Do off-pump techniques reduce the incidence of postoperative atrial fibrillation in elderly patients undergoing coronary artery bypass grafting? *Ann Thorac Surg* 2004;77:1567–74.

94. Athanasiou T, Aziz O, Mangoush O, et al. Does off-pump coronary artery bypass reduce the incidence of postoperative atrial fibrillation? A question revisited. *Eur J Cardiothorac Surg* 2004;26:701–10.

95. Salamon T, Michler RE, Knott KM, Brown DA. Off-pump coronary artery bypass grafting does not decrease the incidence of atrial fibrillation. *Ann Thorac Surg* 2003;75:505–7.

96. Staton GW, Williams WH, Mahoney EM, et al. Pulmonary outcomes of off-pump vs on-pump coronary artery bypass surgery in a randomized trial. *Chest* 2005;127:892–901.

97. Cimen S, Ozkul V, Ketenci B, et al. Daily comparison of respiratory functions between on-pump and off-pump patients undergoing CABG. *Eur J Cardiothorac Surg* 2003;23:589–94.

98. Puskas JD, Williams WH, Duke PG, et al. Off-pump coronary artery bypass grafting provides complete revascularization with reduced myocardial injury, transfusion requirements, and length of stay: a prospective randomized comparison of two hundred unselected patients undergoing off-pump versus conventional coronary artery bypass grafting. *J Thorac Cardiovasc Surg* 2003;125:797–808.

99. Murphy GJ, Mango E, Lucchetti V, et al. A randomized trial of tranexamic acid in combination with cell salvage plus a meta-analysis of randomized trials evaluating tranexamic acid in off-pump coronary artery bypass grafting. *J Thorac Cardiovasc Surg* 2006;132:475–80.

100. Bednar F, Osmancik P, Vanek T, et al. Platelet activity and aspirin efficacy after off-pump compared with on-pump coronary artery bypass surgery: results from the prospective randomized PRAGUE-11-Coronary Artery Bypass and REactivity of Thrombocytes (CABARET). *J Thorac Cardiovasc Surg* 2008;136:1054–60.

101. Halkos ME, Cooper WA, Petersen R, et al. Early administration of clopidogrel is safe after off-pump coronary artery bypass surgery. *Ann Thorac Surg* 2006;81:815–9.

102. Gurbuz AT, Zia AA, Vuran AC, Cui H, Aytac A. Postoperative clopidogrel improves mid-term outcome after off-pump coronary artery bypass graft surgery: a prospective study. *Eur J Cardiothorac Surg* 2006;29:190–5.

103. Zisman E, Shenderey A, Ammar R, Eden A, Pizov R. The effects of intrathecal morphine on patients undergoing minimally invasive direct coronary artery bypass surgery. *J Cardiothorac Vasc Anesth* 2005;19:40–3.

104. Chiu KM, Wu CC, Wang MJ, et al. Local infusion of bupivacaine combined with intravenous patient-controlled analgesia provides better pain relief than intravenous patient-controlled analgesia alone in patients undergoing minimally invasive cardiac surgery. *J Thorac Cardiovasc Surg* 2008;135:1348–52.

105. Thomas JL, Dickstein RA, Parker FB Jr, et al. Prognostic significance of the development of left bundle conduction defects following aortic valve replacement. *J Thorac Cardiovasc Surg* 1982;84:382–6.

106. Dawkins S, Hobson AR, Kalra PR, Tang ATM, Monro JL, Dawkins KD. Permanent pacemaker implantation after isolated aortic valve replacement: incidence, implications, and predictors. *Ann Thorac Surg* 2008;85:108–12.

107. Bonow RO, Carabello BA, Chatterjee K, et al. 2008 focused update incorporated into the ACC/AHA 2006 guidelines for the management of patients with valvular heart disease. A report of the American College of Cardiology/American Heart Association task force on practice guidelines (Writing committee to revise the 1998 guidelines for the management of patients with valvular heart disease). Endorsed by the Society of Cardiovascular Anesthesiologists, Society for Cardiovascular Angiography and Interventions, and Society of Thoracic Surgeons. *J Am Coll Cardiol* 2008;52:e1–142. (available at acc.org).

108. Salem DN, O'Gara PT, Madias C, Pauker SG; American College of Chest Physicians. Valvular and structural heart disease. American College of Chest Physicians evidence-based practice guidelines (8th edition). *Chest* 2008;133(6 Suppl):593S–629S.

109. El Bardissi AW, DiBardino DJ, Chen FY, Yamashita MH, Cohn LH. Is early antithrombotic therapy necessary with bioprosthetic aortic valves in normal sinus rhythm? *J Thorac Cardiovasc Surg* 2010;139:1137–45.

110. Jones HU, Mulestein JB, Jones KW, et al. Early postoperative use of unfractionated heparin or enoxaparin is associated with increased surgical re-exploration for bleeding. *Ann Thorac Surg* 2005;80:519–22.

111. Kulik A, Rubens FD, Wells PS, et al. Early postoperative anticoagulation after mechanical valve replacement: a systematic review. *Ann Thorac Surg* 2006;81:770–81.

112. Meurin P, Tabet JY, Weber H, Renaud N, Ben Driss A. Low-molecular-weight heparin as a bridging anticoagulant early after mechanical valve replacement. *Circulation* 2006;113:564–9.

113. Steger V, Bail DH, Graf D, Walker T, Rittig K, Ziemer G. A practical approach for bridging anticoagulation after mechanical heart valve replacement. *J Heart Valve Dis* 2008;17:335–42.

114. Tempe DK, Hasija S, Datt V, et al. Evaluation and comparison of early hemodynamic changes after elective mitral valve replacement in patients with severe and mild pulmonary arterial hypertension. *J Cardiothorac Vasc Anesth* 2009;23:298–305.

115. Zimmermann A, Kufner C, Hofbauer S, et al. The accuracy of the Vigileo/FloTrac continuous cardiac output monitor. *J Cardiothorac Vasc Anesth* 2008;22:388–93.

116. Salzberg SP, Filsoufi F, Anyanwu A, et al. High-risk mitral valve surgery: perioperative hemodynamic optimization with nesiritide (BNP). *Ann Thorac Surg* 2005;80:502–6.

117. Rex S, Schaelte G, Metzelder S, et al. Inhaled iloprost to control pulmonary artery hypertension in patients undergoing mitral valve surgery: a prospective, randomized-controlled trial. *Acta Anaethesiol Scand* 2008;52:65–72.

118. Santini F, Casali G, Franchi G, et al. Hemodynamic effects of inhaled nitric oxide and phosphodiesterase inhibitor (dipyridamole) on secondary pulmonary hypertension following heart valve surgery in adults. *Int J Cardiol* 2005;103:156–63.

119. Yurtseven N, Karaca P, Uysal G, et al. A comparison of the acute hemodynamic effects of inhaled nitroglycerin and iloprost in patients with pulmonary hypertension undergoing mitral valve surgery. *Ann Thorac Cardiovasc Surg* 2006;12:319–23.

120. Suri RM, Schaff HV, Dearani JA, et al. Determinants of early decline in ejection fraction after surgical correction of mitral regurgitation. *J Thorac Cardiovasc Surg* 2008;136:442–7.

121. Suri RM, Schaff HV, Dearani JA, et al. Recovery of left ventricular function after surgical correction of mitral regurgitation caused by leaflet prolapse. *J Thorac Cardiovasc Surg* 2009;137:1071–6.

122. Grande AM, Fiore A, Massetti M, Viganò M. Iatrogenic circumflex coronary lesion in mitral valve surgery: case report and review of the literature. *Tex Heart Inst J* 2008;35:179–83.

123. Santini F, Gatti G, Borghetti V, Oppido G, Mazzucco A. Routine left atrial catheterization for the post-operative management of cardiac surgical patients: is the risk justified? *Eur J Cardiothorac Surg* 1999;16:218–21.

124. Wu Q, Zhang L, Zhu R. Obstruction of left ventricular outflow tract after mechanical mitral valve replacement. *Ann Thorac Surg* 2008;85:1789–91.

125. Okamoto K, Kiso I, Inoue Y, Matayoshi H, Takahashi R, Umezu Y. Left ventricular outflow obstruction after mitral valve replacement preserving native anterior leaflet. *Ann Thorac Surg* 2006;82:735–7.

126. Crescenzi G, Landoni G, Zangrillo A, et al. Management and decision-making strategy for systolic anterior motion after mitral valve repair. *J Thorac Cardiovasc Surg* 2009;137:320–5.

127. Tambuer L, Meyns B, Flameng W, Daenen W. Rhythm disturbances after mitral valve surgery: comparison between left atrial and extended transseptal approach. *Cardiovasc Surg* 1996;4:820–4.

128. Little S, Flynn M, Pettersson GB, Gillinov AM, Blackstone EH. Revisiting the dome approach to partial sternotomy/minimally invasive mitral valve surgery. *Ann Thorac Surg* 2009;87:694–7.

129. Nienaber JJ, Glower DD. Minitransseptal versus left atrial approach to the mitral valve: a comparison of outcomes. *Ann Thorac Surg* 2006;82:834–9.

130. vonOppell UO, O'Callaghan P, Eheler R, Dimitrakakis G, Schiffelers S. Mitral valve surgery plus concomitant atrial fibrillation ablation is superior to mitral valve surgery alone with intensive rhythm control strategy. *Eur J Cardiothorac Surg* 2009;35:641–50.

131. Karlson KH, Ashraf MM, Berger RL. Rupture of the left ventricle following mitral valve replacement. *Ann Thorac Surg* 1988;46:590–7.

132. Asopa S, Patel A, Dunning J. Is short-term anticoagulation necessary after mitral valve repair? *Interact Cardiovasc Thorac Surg* 2006;5:761–5.

133. Oprea D, Memet R, Jovin A, et al. Anticoagulation at discharge after mitral valve repair and long-term mortality. *Circulation* 2006;114:II–734.

134. Zierer A, Voeller RK, Hill KE, Kouchoukos NT, Damiano RJ Jr, Moon MR. Aortic enlargement and late reoperation after repair of type A aortic dissection. *Ann Thorac Surg* 2007;84:479–86.

135. Kodama K, Nishigami K, Sakamoto T, et al. Tight heart rate control reduces secondary adverse events in patients with type B aortic dissection. *Circulation* 2008;118(14 Suppl):S167–70.

136. Bozinovski J, Coselli JS. Outcomes and survival in surgical treatment of descending thoracic aorta with acute dissection. *Ann Thorac Surg* 2008;85:965–71.

137. Fattori R, Tsai TT, Myrmel T, et al. Complicated acute type B dissection: is surgery still the best option? A report from the International Registry of Acute Aortic Dissection. *J Am Coll Cardiol Interv* 2008;1:395–402.

138. Parker JD, Golledge J. Outcome of endovascular treatment of acute type B aortic dissection. *Ann Thorac Surg* 2008;86:1707–12.

139. Szeto WY, McGarvey M, Pochettino A, et al. Results of a new surgical paradigm: endovascular repair for acute complicated type B aortic dissection. *Ann Thorac Surg* 2008;86:87–94.

140. Harrington DK, Fragomeni F, Bonser RS. Cerebral perfusion. *Ann Thorac Surg* 2007;83:S799–804.

141. Percy A, Widman S, Rizzo JA, Tranquilli M, Elefteriades JA. Deep hypothermic circulatory arrest in patients with high cognitive needs: full preservation of cognitive abilities. *Ann Thorac Surg* 2009;87:117–23.

142. Sundt TM III, Orzulak TA, Cook DJ, Schaff HV. Improving results of open arch replacement. *Ann Thorac Surg* 2008;86:787–96.

143. Khaladj N, Shrestha M, Meck S, et al. Hypothermic circulatory arrest with selective antegrade cerebral perfusion in ascending aortic and aortic arch surgery: a risk factor analysis for adverse outcome in 501 patients. *J Thorac Cardiovasc Surg* 2008;135:908–14.

144. Spielvogel D, Etz CD, Silovitz D, Lansman SL, Griepp RB. Aortic arch replacement with a trifurcated graft. *Ann Thorac Surg* 2007;83:S791–5.

145. Cambria RP, Clouse WD, Davison JK, Dunn PF, Corey M, Dorer D. Thoracoabdominal aneurysm repair: results with 337 operations performed over a 15-year interval. *Ann Surg* 2002;236:471–9.

146. Gloviczki P. Surgical repair of thoracoabdominal aneurysms: patient selection, techniques and results. *Cardiovasc Surg* 2002;10:434–41.

147. Estrera AL, Sheinbaum R, Miller CC, et al. Cerebrospinal fluid drainage during thoracic aortic repair: safety and current management. *Ann Thorac Surg* 2009;88:9–15.

148. Maniar HS, Sundt T.M. III, Prasad SM, et al. Delayed paraplegia after thoracic and thoracoabdominal aneurysm repair: a continuing risk. *Ann Thorac Surg* 2003;75:113–20.

149. Hunt I, Deshpande RP, Aps C, Young CP. Delayed paraplegia after thoracic and thoracoabdominal aneurysm repair: timing of reinsertion of spinal drain. *Ann Thorac Surg* 2004;78:2213.

150. Cheung AT, Weiss SJ, McGarvey ML, et al. Interventions for reversing delayed-onset postoperative paraplegia after thoracic aortic reconstruction. *Ann Thorac Surg* 2002;74:413–21.

151. Sheinbaum R, Ignacio C, Safi HJ, Estrera A. Contemporary strategies to preserve renal function during cardiac and vascular surgery. *Rev Cardiovasc Med* 2003;4(suppl 1):S21–8.

152. Svensson LG, Kochoukos NT, Miller DC, et al. Expert consensus document on the treatment of descending thoracic aortic disease using endovascular stent grafts: report from the Society of Thoracic Surgeons endovascular surgery task force. *Ann Thorac Surg* 2008;85(1 suppl):S1–41.

153. Weigang E, Hartert M, Siegenthaler MP, et al. Perioperative management to improve neurologic outcome in thoracic and thoracoabdominal aortic stent-grafting. *Ann Thorac Surg* 2006;82:1679–87.

154. Cheung AT, Pochettino A, McGarvey ML, et al. Strategies to manage paraplegia risk after endovascular stent repair of descending thoracic aortic aneurysms. *Ann Thorac Surg* 2005;80:1280–8.

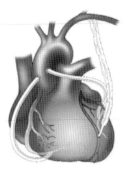

CHAPTER 9

Mediastinal Bleeding

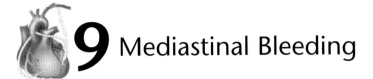

9 Mediastinal Bleeding

I. Overview

    A. The use of cardiopulmonary bypass (CPB) during cardiac surgical procedures causes a significant disruption of the coagulation system that may contribute to a coagulopathy of varying degrees.[1] In addition to hemodilution from a crystalloid prime, which reduces levels of clotting factors and platelets, contact of blood with the extracorporeal circuit activates platelets and the extrinsic and intrinsic coagulation systems, and triggers fibrinolysis. In fact, systemic heparinization alone causes platelet dysfunction and induces fibrinolysis.[2] In addition, cell-saving devices that are routinely used for red cell salvage eliminate platelets and coagulation factors from the blood.

    B. Off-pump coronary artery bypass surgery (OPCAB) avoids hemodilution and minimizes platelet activation, and is associated with reduced usage of blood products.[3] The ability of the antifibrinolytic agents to reduce bleeding suggests that low-grade fibrinolysis is still present.[4] Although a coagulopathy after OPCAB is very unusual, it may occur in patients who have sustained substantial blood loss with blood scavenged in and returned from the cell-saving device. This will result in depletion of coagulation factors and platelets. The occurrence of substantial bleeding after an OPCAB procedure generally indicates a surgical source.

    C. Either 28–32 Fr PVC or silicone malleable chest tubes or 24 Fr silastic fluted (Blake) drains are placed in the mediastinum and opened pleural cavities. They are connected to a drainage system and placed to −20 cm of H_2O suction. They are gently milked or stripped to maintain patency after surgery. Both are equally effective in evacuating blood, although the Blake drains may be more comfortable for the patient.[5,6]

        1. Some surgeons do not obligatorily place chest tubes into widely opened pleural spaces, especially after off-pump surgery. However, any bleeding that occurs in the pleural space will tend to accumulate and not be drained by the mediastinal tubes. This can produce a deceptive picture with insidious bleeding that can only be detected by chest x-ray.

        2. Following minimally invasive surgery, the number and location of tubes may vary. After MIDCABs, only one pleural chest tube is placed, so blood could potentially accumulate around the heart and not be drained through the pericardial opening. Following ministernotomy incisions, one mediastinal tube is placed unless the pleural cavity is entered. With right thoracotomy approaches to the aortic or mitral valve, one mediastinal and one pleural tube are placed. Chest-tube positioning is difficult and

Manual of Perioperative Care in Adult Cardiac Surgery, 5th Edition. By Robert M. Bojar.
Published 2011 by Blackwell Publishing Ltd.

not ideal after these procedures, so the potential for undetected blood accumulation around the heart or in the pleural spaces is enhanced. Thus, extra vigilance for undrained blood in the unstable patient is imperative.

D. Postoperative bleeding gradually tapers over the course of several hours in the majority of patients, but about 1–3% of patients will require reexploration in the operating room for persistent mediastinal bleeding. Prompt assessment and aggressive treatment in the intensive care unit (ICU) may frequently arrest "medical bleeding", but evidence of persistent or increasing amounts of bleeding should prompt early exploration (see section VIII, pages 373–374).

E. Bleeding invariably requires use of various blood products to maintain normovolemia and adequate hemodynamic parameters, correct anemia to ensure adequate tissue oxygen delivery, and correct a coagulopathy to help arrest the bleeding. Transfused blood is not benign and can cause a variety of complications that may increase operative mortality.[7–9] The safe lower limit for hematocrit (HCT) is not precisely defined, but in the bleeding patient in the early postoperative period, hemodynamic considerations and potential impairment of tissue oxygen delivery mandate transfusions to maintain a safe HCT, which is probably at least 25%. Blood component therapy ideally should be selected based upon identification of specific coagulation abnormalities by point-of-care testing and treatment algorithms, although clinical judgment remains essential in making prompt therapeutic decisions.

F. Mediastinal bleeding can be a highly morbid and lethal problem. Although hypovolemia can be corrected by volume infusions, the bleeding patient tends to be hemodynamically unstable out of proportion to the degree of bleeding and fluid replacement. Most importantly in the immediate postoperative period is the potential for blood to accumulate around the heart, causing **cardiac tamponade**. The restriction to cardiac filling may produce severe hemodynamic compromise that can precipitously cause cardiac arrest. Constant attention to the degree of bleeding and to trends in hemodynamic parameters should allow steps to be taken to avert this problem. If profound hypotension or a cardiac arrest develop, emergency sternotomy in the ICU is indicated.

II. Etiology of Mediastinal Bleeding (Table 9.1)

Mediastinal bleeding is somewhat arbitrarily categorized as "surgical" or "medical" in nature. Significant bleeding after uneventful surgery is usually "surgical", especially when initial coagulation studies are fairly normal. However, persistent bleeding depletes coagulation factors and platelets, causing a coagulopathy that is self-perpetuating. Bleeding that is noted after complex operations with long durations of CPB is frequently associated with abnormal coagulation studies and is considered "medical". However, even after correction of coagulation abnormalities, discrete bleeding sites may be present that will not stop without reexploration. Thus, the initial approach to bleeding is to try to identify any contributing factors that might account for the degree of bleeding and then take the appropriate steps to correct them.[1]

A. A number of risk factors have been identified that increase perioperative bleeding and/or the requirement for transfusions (Table 9.2).[7] Aside from stopping antiplatelet or anticoagulant medications preoperatively, most of these factors cannot be modified. However, they should alert the healthcare team to the increased risk of a coagulopathy, the necessity of utilizing blood conservation measures, and the importance of early aggressive treatment of bleeding to minimize or prevent hemodynamic compromise and organ system dysfunction.

Table 9.1 • Etiology of Mediastinal Bleeding

1. Surgical bleeding sites
2. Heparin effect – residual or rebound
3. Excessive protamine administration
4. Platelet dysfunction
5. Thrombocytopenia
6. Clotting factor deficiency
7. Fibrinolysis

Table 9.2 • Patients at Increased Risk for Mediastinal Bleeding

Patient-related Variables

1. Older patients
2. Females or smaller body surface area
3. Preoperative anemia
4. Advanced cardiac disease (shock, poor LV function)
5. Comorbidities (renal or hepatic dysfunction, diabetes, peripheral vascular disease)
6. Known coagulopathies (von Willebrand's disease, uremia)

Preoperative Medications

1. High-dose aspirin
2. Clopidogrel/prasugrel
3. Low-molecular-weight heparin within 18 hours
4. Fondaparinux within 48 hours
5. Incomplete reversal of INR off warfarin
6. Emergency surgery after IIb/IIIa inhibitors or thrombolytic therapy

Procedure-related Variables

1. Complex operations (valve-CABG, thoracic aortic surgery, especially requiring deep hypothermic circulatory arrest)
2. Urgent/emergent operations
3. Reoperations
4. Use of bilateral ITA grafting

B. Surgical bleeding is usually related to:
1. Anastomotic sites (suture lines)
2. Side branches of arterial or venous conduits
3. Substernal soft tissues, sternal suture sites, bone marrow, periosteum
4. Raw surfaces caused by previous surgery, pericarditis, or radiation therapy

C. Anticoagulant effect related to heparin or excessive protamine
1. Preoperative use of low-molecular-weight heparin (enoxaparin) within 12–18 hours of surgery or of fondaparinux, a factor Xa inhibitor, within 48 hours of surgery are associated with increased perioperative bleeding since neither can be completely reversed with protamine.[10–12]
2. Residual heparin effect may result from inadequate neutralization with protamine at the conclusion of CPB. Administering fully heparinized "pump" blood towards the end of the protamine infusion will reintroduce unneutralized heparin into the blood. Blood washed in cell-saving devices is usually given after protamine administration, but has been shown to contain insignificant amounts of heparin.[13]
3. Heparin rebound may occur when heparin reappears from tissue stores after protamine administration. This is more common in patients receiving large amounts of heparin, especially obese patients.
4. Excessive protamine may cause a coagulopathy.

D. Quantitative platelet defects
1. Preoperative thrombocytopenia may result from use of heparin, drug reactions (especially antibiotics and IIb/IIIa inhibitors), infection, hypersplenism in patients with liver disease, and other chronic conditions (idiopathic thrombocytopenic purpura [ITP]). If a patient developing thrombocytopenia has recently been given heparin, it is essential to rule out heparin-induced thrombocytopenia (HIT).
2. Hemodilution on CPB and consumption in the extracorporeal circuit reduce the platelet count by about 30–50%, and thrombocytopenia will be progressive as the duration of CPB lengthens.
3. Protamine administration transiently reduces the platelet count by about 30%.

E. Qualitative platelet defects are a major concern with the liberal use of antiplatelet agents in patients with acute coronary syndromes.
1. Preoperative platelet dysfunction may result from antiplatelet medications (aspirin, clopidogrel, prasugrel), glycoprotein IIb/IIIa inhibitors (tirofiban, eptifibatide, abciximab), herbal medications and vitamins (fish oils, ginkgo products, vitamin E), or uremia.
2. Exposure of platelets to the CPB circuit with α-granule release and alteration of platelet membrane receptors impairs platelet function. The degree of platelet dysfunction correlates with the duration of CPB and the degree of hypothermia after bypass.
3. Inadequate heparinization is a potent trigger for thrombin release, which activates platelets.

F. Depletion of coagulation factors
1. Preoperative hepatic dysfunction, residual warfarin effect, vitamin K-dependent clotting factor deficiencies, von Willebrand's disease, and thrombolytic therapy reduce the level of clotting factors.

2. Hemodilution on CPB reduces most factors by 50%, including fibrinogen. This is most pronounced in patients with a small blood volume.

3. Loss of clotting factors results from use of intraoperative cell-saving devices.

G. Fibrinolysis results in clotting factor degradation and platelet dysfunction.

1. Preoperative use of thrombolytic agents causes fibrinolysis.

2. Use of CPB causes plasminogen activation.

3. Heparinization itself induces a fibrinolytic state.

III. Prevention of Perioperative Blood Loss: Blood Conservation Measures (Table 9.3)[7]

A. Preoperative assessment of the patient's coagulation system should entail measurement of a prothrombin time (INR), partial thromboplastin time (PTT), and platelet count. Any abnormality should be investigated and corrected, if possible, prior to surgery. Although additional screening with bleeding times is not indicated for patients on aspirin, platelet function testing to assess platelet responsiveness to clopidogrel is helpful in determining when the bleeding risk is low enough to proceed with nonurgent surgery.

B. **Heparin-induced thrombocytopenia (HIT)** may develop in patients receiving intravenous heparin for several days before surgery. Thus, it is very important to recheck the platelet count on a daily basis in these patients. If the patient develops thrombocytopenia, with documented heparin antibodies by ELISA testing and a positive functional assay (serotonin release assay or heparin-induced platelet aggregation test), an alternative means of anticoagulation will be necessary during surgery (see pages 202–204).[14]

C. **Cessation of medications** with antiplatelet or anticoagulant effects is essential to allow their effects to dissipate to minimize blood loss. A more detailed discussion of these medications is presented in Chapter 3 (pages 133–139). Specific recommendations are as follows:[7,15,16]

1. **Warfarin** should be stopped 4 days before surgery to allow for resynthesis of vitamin K-dependent clotting factors and normalization of the INR. If interim anticoagulation is required for patients at high thromboembolic risk, heparin is substituted, either as unfractionated heparin or as low-molecular-weight heparin. If the patient requires urgent surgery, vitamin K should be given to normalize the INR. A slow IV infusion of 5 mg over 30 minutes is effective in promptly correcting the INR, but it is preferable to give 5 mg of oral Vitamin K if surgery can be delayed a day or two to avoid the risk of anaphylaxis. If emergency surgery is indicated, fresh frozen plasma (FFP) may be necessary.

2. **Unfractionated heparin** (UFH) is used for patients with acute coronary syndromes, during catheterization, for critical coronary disease, or during use of an intra-aortic balloon pump (IABP). It is reversible with protamine and can be continued up to the time of surgery without increasing morbidity during line placement or increasing the risk of perioperative bleeding.

3. **Low-molecular-weight heparin** (LMWH) is given in a dose of 1 mg/kg SC q12h for acute coronary syndromes or as a bridge to surgery once warfarin has been stopped. The last dose should be given 18–24 hours prior to surgery to minimize the perioperative bleeding risk, since only 60–80% of LMWH is reversible with

---

Table 9.3 • Methods of Minimizing Operative Blood Loss and Transfusion Requirements

1. Stop all anticoagulant and antiplatelet medications preoperatively (except low-dose ASA for CABG patients)
2. Consider erythropoietin with iron for anemic patients prior to elective surgery
3. Identify preoperative hematologic abnormalities (HIT, antiphospholipid syndrome)
4. Transfuse patients requiring urgent surgery to a HCT >28% preoperatively
5. Use antifibrinolytic therapy (ε-aminocaproic acid or tranexamic acid)
6. Consider off-pump coronary bypass grafting, if feasible
7. Perfusion considerations
   a. Autologous blood withdrawal prior to CPB if HCT >30%
   b. Use heparin-coated circuit, if available
   c. Use miniaturized CPB circuit, if available
   d. Use heparin-protamine titration test to optimize anticoagulation and heparin reversal
   e. Consider retrograde autologous priming of the bypass circuit
   f. Avoid use of cardiotomy suction
   g. Salvage pump blood via either hemofiltration or cell saver
8. Employ meticulous surgical technique with careful inspection of anastomotic sites and all artery and vein side branches before coming off bypass
9. Complete neutralization of heparin with protamine to return ACT to baseline
10. Administer appropriate blood component therapy based upon suspicion of the hemostatic defect (especially platelet dysfunction) or use point-of-care testing to direct blood component therapy
11. Use recombinant factor VIIa for intractable coagulopathic bleeding
12. Exercise patience

---

protamine.[10–12] Fondaparinux must be stopped at least 48 hours prior to surgery because it has a half-life of nearly 20 hours.

4. **Aspirin** (ASA) should be continued up to the time of surgery in patients with acute coronary syndromes or critical anatomy.[7,15,16] A dose of 81 mg has not been associated with an increased risk of bleeding.[17] Aspirin can probably be stopped 3 days prior to elective CABG or valve surgery to minimize the risk of bleeding. However, one can consider continuing aspirin in all CABG patients since some studies indicate that the risk of infarction and mortality may be lower when aspirin is continued up to the time of surgery.[18,19] Antifibrinolytic drugs are useful in reducing bleeding associated with preoperative use of aspirin.[20]

5. **Clopidogrel** has antiplatelet effects that last for the life span of the platelet, and it should therefore be stopped 5–7 days prior to elective surgery.[7,15,16] However, it is commonly given as a 300–600 mg load in patients with an acute coronary syndrome in anticipation of a stenting procedure, which will achieve significant platelet inhibition within a few hours. If surgery is required on an urgent basis, significant bleeding may be encountered. Exogenously administered platelets may be ineffective if given within 6 hours of a loading dose or 4 hours of a

maintenance dose because the active metabolite may still be present in the bloodstream. In patients with drug-eluting stents placed within the previous year, the risk of stent thrombosis is increased if clopidogrel is stopped. In these patients, the options are to:

   a. Continue the clopidogrel and accept the potential for more bleeding.

   b. Stop the clopidogrel for 3 days to restore some platelet function while maintaining a lesser degree of platelet inhibition.

   c. Stop the clopidogrel and use a short-acting glycoprotein IIb/IIIa inhibitor as a bridge to surgery.

6. **Prasugrel** is a strong antiplatelet agent that may supplant use of clopidogrel in patients with acute coronary syndromes undergoing a percutaneous coronary intervention (PCI).[21] It is associated with more periprocedural bleeding and may pose significant bleeding problems in patients requiring emergency surgery. Surgery should be delayed 7 days after the last dose is taken.

7. **Tirofiban** (Aggrastat) and **eptifibatide** (Integrilin) are short-acting IIb/IIIa inhibitors which allow for recovery of 80% of platelet function within 4–6 hours of being discontinued. They should be stopped about 4 hours prior to surgery.[7] Some studies have shown that continuing these medications up to the time of surgery may preserve platelet function on pump, leading to increased platelet number and function after bypass with no adverse effects on bleeding.[22]

8. **Abciximab** (ReoPro) is a long-acting IIb/IIIa inhibitor used for high-risk PCI that has a half-life of 12 hours. If surgery needs to be performed on an emergency basis, platelets are effective in producing hemostasis since there is very little circulating unbound drug. Ideally, surgery should be delayed at least 12 hours and preferably 24 hours. Although platelet function remains abnormal for up to 48 hours, there is little hemostatic compromise at receptor blockade levels less than 50%.

9. **Direct thrombin inhibitors** are primarily used in patients with HIT, but bivalirudin has been used as an alternative to UFH in patients undergoing PCI. It has a short half-life of 25 minutes and should not pose a significant issue if emergency surgery is required. Its use as an alternative to heparin during surgery in patients with HIT has been associated with comparable outcomes, although bleeding tends to be more problematic.[23]

10. **Thrombolytic therapy** is an alternative to primary PCI in patients presenting with ST-elevation myocardial infarctions (STEMIs). Although currently used agents have short half-lives measured in minutes, the systemic hemostatic defects persist much longer. These effects include depletion of fibrinogen, reduction in factors II, V, and VIII, impairment of platelet aggregation, and the appearance of fibrin split products. If surgery is required for persistent ischemia after failed thrombolytic therapy, it should be delayed at least 12–24 hours. If it is required emergently, fresh frozen plasma and cryoprecipitate will probably be necessary to correct the anticipated coagulopathy.

D. **Antifibrinolytic therapy** should be used to reduce intraoperative blood loss in all on- and off-pump surgical cases (see doses on page 199).[24–27]

   1. **ε-aminocaproic acid** (Amicar) is an antifibrinolytic agent that preserves platelet function by inhibiting the conversion of plasminogen to plasmin. It is effective in

reducing blood loss and the amount of transfusions, although it has not been shown to reduce the rate of reexploration for bleeding.[7] Because of its low cost, it is usually the drug of choice for most cardiac surgical procedures.

2. **Tranexamic acid** (Cyclokapron) has similar properties and benefits to ε-amino-caproic acid. It has been shown to reduce perioperative blood loss in both on- and off-pump surgery.[4]

3. **Aprotinin** is a serine protease inhibitor that was the most effective drug available to reduce blood loss, transfusion requirements, and reexploration for bleeding. It preserves adhesive platelet receptors during the early period of CPB, exhibits antifibrinolytic properties by inhibiting plasmin, and also inhibits kallikrein, blocking the contact phase of coagulation and inhibiting the intrinsic coagulation cascade. Because of concerns that it increased the risks of mortality, renal dysfunction, myocardial infarction, and stroke (most of which have not been confirmed in numerous studies), aprotinin was no longer available in the USA as of late 2007.[28]

E. **Heparin and protamine dosing**

1. Ideal anticoagulation for CPB should minimize activation of the coagulation cascade, be fully reversible, and minimize perioperative bleeding. The most commonly used drug is heparin, which binds to antithrombin III to inhibit thrombin and factor Xa. Empiric dosing of heparin (3–4 mg/kg) to achieve an activated clotting time (ACT) >480 seconds is routine, although patients with antithrombin III deficiency may be heparin-resistant and require fresh frozen plasma or Thrombate to achieve a satisfactory ACT.[29] Inadequate heparin dosing increases thrombin generation which in turn activates platelets and can trigger clotting within the CPB circuit. Lower doses of heparin may be used in biocompatible circuits (see section F.3, below).

2. Systems that provide heparin–protamine titration tests measure circulating heparin concentrations and determine dose–response curves to achieve the desired ACT. These systems provide the optimal level of heparin and allow for calculation of the precise amount of protamine sulfate needed to reverse heparin effect. The end result is generally a reduction in perioperative bleeding. Some studies with the Medtronic Hepcon system have found that it is necessary to use higher doses of heparin, yet this is associated with less thrombin and platelet activation, preservation of higher levels of clotting factors, and a reduction in fibrinolysis, and subsequently less bleeding.[7,30] In contrast, another study using dose–response curves with the Hemochron RxDx system (International Technidyne) found that lower doses of heparin are sufficient and associated with less blood loss.[31]

3. One of heparin's advantages is that its anticoagulant effect can be reversed with protamine. In contrast, other effective anticoagulants that can be used for CPB, such as the direct thrombin inhibitors (bivalirudin or argatroban used in HIT patients), are not reversible.

4. Protamine is usually given in a 1:1 ratio or a 0.5:1 ratio to the dose of heparin. Using point-of-care hemostasis systems with dose–response curves, lower doses of protamine are usually used to adequately reverse heparin, which may result in less bleeding. Excessive protamine (varying from 1.5:1 up to 2.6:1 in three studies) serves as an anticoagulant that directly impairs platelet function and elevates the ACT.[32–34]

F. **Perfusion considerations** that may be considered to optimize blood conservation include the following (see also Chapter 5):

1. **Autologous blood withdrawal** before instituting bypass (acute normovolemic hemodilution) protects platelets from the damaging effects of CPB. This has been demonstrated to preserve red cell mass and reduce transfusion requirements. However, its efficacy in reducing perioperative bleeding is controversial.[7,35] It can be considered when the calculated on-pump hematocrit after withdrawal remains satisfactory (greater than 20–22%). This can be calculated using the following equation:

$$\text{amount withdrawn} = \text{EBV} - \frac{0.22\ (\text{EBV} + \text{PV} + \text{CV})}{\text{HCT}}$$

where:
   EBV = estimated blood volume (70 × kg)
   PV = priming volume
   CV = estimated cardioplegia volume
   HCT = prewithdrawal hematocrit

2. **Platelet-rich plasmapheresis** entails the withdrawal of platelet-rich plasma using a plasma separator at the beginning of the operation with its readministration after protamine infusion. This improves hemostasis and reduces blood loss. Although it might be beneficial in reoperations, it is expensive, time-consuming, and probably of little benefit when prophylactic antifibrinolytic medications are used, and probably is of no greater benefit than fresh whole blood withdrawn before CPB.[7,36]

3. The use of **biocompatible circuits** (usually heparin-bonded) may reduce activation of platelets and the coagulation cascade with a subsequent reduction in blood loss. These systems may allow for use of lower doses of heparin in uncomplicated cases (ACT of 350 seconds). However, one study suggested that reduction of heparin dosing reduced platelet loss, but did not suppress the platelet release reaction, and thus was not beneficial to platelet function.[37] The potential remains that inadequate heparinization may increase thrombin generation, causing more platelet activation on CPB that may in fact increase perioperative bleeding. Furthermore, use of low-dose heparin combined with antifibrinolytic medications might theoretically raise the risk for thrombotic events.[7] Thus, biocompatible circuits may improve hemostasis, but the lower limit of heparinization has not been well defined. Additional considerations, such as avoiding cardiotomy suction, are important in realizing clinical advantages with these circuits.

4. **Avoidance of cardiotomy suction** may reduce perioperative bleeding. Blood aspirated from the pericardial space has been in contact with tissue factor and contains high levels of factor VIIa, procoagulant particles, fat particles, and activated complement proteins, and exhibits fibrinolytic activity.[7,38] Blood aspirated with cardiotomy suckers drains into a reservoir and mixes directly with the pump blood that is reinfused in the CPB circuit. Most groups use cardiotomy suction routinely and do not find that it has a significant effect on bleeding.

5. **Miniaturized CPB circuits** require low priming volumes (500–800 mL) that limit the degree of hemodilution, thus maintaining a higher HCT on pump. Studies

have arguably demonstrated that these systems reduce activation of coagulation and fibrinolysis, and minimize blood loss. However, the lack of a cardiotomy reservoir increases the risk of air embolism.[7,39]

6. **Retrograde autologous priming** of the extracorporeal circuit entails initial withdrawal of crystalloid prime to minimize hemodilution, thus maintaining a higher HCT and colloid oncotic pressure on pump. This also reduces extravascular lung water. In some studies, this has been shown to reduce the rate of transfusion.[7,40,41]

7. **Intraoperative autotransfusion** of blood that is aspirated from the field into a cell-saving device is recommended as a routine means of salvaging red blood cells if cardiotomy suction is not utilized. It is most helpful in salvaging red cells from dilute fluids (e.g., after cold saline is poured on the heart during cardioplegic arrest). Cell salvage of pump contents at the conclusion of CPB is routinely performed as well. The cells are washed to remove heparin and cytokines, and the red cells are concentrated, but the washing results in loss of coagulation factors and platelets from the blood. Although most studies suggest that intraoperative cell salvage does not influence bleeding or reduce transfusion requirements,[7,42–45] one study found that it increased both.[46] The routine use of ultrafiltration to remove the pump prime is not recommended.[7]

G. **Meticulous surgical technique** is the mainstay of hemostasis. Warming the patient to normothermia before terminating bypass improves the function of the coagulation system.

IV. Assessment of Bleeding in the ICU (Table 9.4)[47]

A. The appropriate assessment of bleeding in the ICU requires the following steps:

1. Frequent documentation of the amount of blood draining into the collection system and attention to tube patency.

2. Determination of the color (arterial or venous) and pattern of drainage (sudden dump when turned or continuous drainage).

3. Monitoring of hemodynamic parameters with ongoing awareness of the possibility of cardiac tamponade.

4. Identification of potential causative factors by review of coagulation studies.

5. Suspicion of undrained blood in the mediastinum or pleural spaces by review of a chest x-ray (looking for a widened mediastinum or haziness in the pleural cavity as blood layers posteriorly), auscultating decreased breath sounds on examination, or noting elevation of peak inspiratory pressures on the ventilator.

6. Obtaining an echocardiogram if tamponade is suspected based upon the pattern of bleeding, hemodynamic derangements, or abnormalities on chest x-ray.

B. **Quantitate the amount of chest tube drainage**. Make sure that the chest tubes are patent because the extent of ongoing hemorrhage may be masked when the tubes have clotted or blood has drained into an open pleural space. **Note:** When patients are turned or moved, they will occasionally drain a significant volume of blood that has been accumulating in the chest for several hours. This may suggest the acute onset of bleeding and the need for surgical exploration. The presence of dark

---

Table 9.4 • *Assessment of Postoperative Mediastinal Bleeding*

1. Obtain immediate postoperative chest x-ray as baseline evaluation of mediastinum and pleural spaces
2. Quantify the degree of bleeding into drainage unit frequently
3. Optimize hemodynamic status while addressing bleeding issues
4. Obtain coagulation studies
   a. PT/INR, PTT, platelet count, fibrinogen level
   b. Platelet function testing
   c. Thromboelastogram, if available
5. Repeat coagulation studies after blood products administered if still bleeding
6. Repeat chest x-ray if concerned about tamponade or undrained blood
7. Obtain TEE if concerned about tamponade

---

blood and minimal additional drainage are clues that this does not represent active bleeding. Serial chest x-rays may be helpful in identifying residual blood in the pleural space.

C. **Assess hemodynamics** with the Swan-Ganz catheter. Maintenance of adequate filling pressures and cardiac output is essential and is generally accomplished using crystalloid or colloid solutions. However, in the bleeding patient, these will produce hemodilution and progressive anemia, and may potentiate a coagulopathy. It should be noted that unstable hemodynamics are frequently seen in the bleeding patient even if filling pressures are maintained.

1. If filling pressures are decreasing and nonheme fluid is administered, one needs to anticipate a decrease in the HCT from hemodilution, but more so with ongoing bleeding. Five percent albumin will have a dilutional effect on clotting factors and the HCT and is the preferable colloid (other than fresh frozen plasma). High-molecular-weight hetastarch-based compounds have additional adverse effects on fibrin formation and platelet function (perhaps slightly less with Hextend than Hespan).[48–51] Although the low-molecular-weight hetastarch compounds such as pentastarch and tetrastarch appear to have minimal effect on coagulation, they may still be associated with postoperative bleeding.[52,53]

2. The administration of volume in the form of clotting factors and platelets promotes hemostasis but must be accompanied by red cell transfusions to maintain a safe hematocrit. Anemia not only reduces oxygen-carrying capacity of the blood, but also results in a reduction in blood oncotic pressure and viscosity which contributes to hypotension.

3. Evidence of rising filling pressures and decreasing cardiac outputs may suggest the development of cardiac tamponade. Equilibration of intracardiac pressures may be noted with postoperative tamponade, but, more commonly, accumulation of clot adjacent to the right or left atrium will produce variable elevation in intracardiac pressures that is also consistent with right or left ventricular failure, respectively.

4. If hemodynamic measurements suggest borderline cardiac function and tamponade cannot be ruled out, **transesophageal echocardiography** is invaluable in

making the correct diagnosis. Tamponade should be suspected when hemodynamic compromise is associated with excessive bleeding, bleeding that has abruptly stopped, or even minimal chest tube drainage caused by clotted tubes or spillage into the pleural space. A transesophageal echocardiogram is more accurate than a transthoracic study in detecting clot behind the heart, because the latter is often compromised by inability to obtain the acoustic windows to adequately identify an effusion.[54]

D. Obtain **coagulation studies** upon arrival in the ICU and serial **hematocrits** if the patient is bleeding. Coagulation studies do not need to be ordered if the patient has minimal mediastinal bleeding. Furthermore, if they are obtained and are abnormal, but the patient has insignificant bleeding, use of blood component therapy is **not** indicated.

1. If hemostasis was difficult to achieve in the operating room or hemorrhage persists in the ICU (generally greater than 100 mL/h), lab tests may be helpful in assessing whether a coagulopathy is contributing to mediastinal bleeding. Tests for some of the more common nonsurgical causes of bleeding (residual heparin effect, thrombocytopenia, and clotting factor deficiency) are readily available, but documentation of platelet dysfunction requires additional technology.[55] Athough no individual test correlates that well with the amount of bleeding, together they can usually direct interventions in a somewhat scientific manner.[56]

2. No matter what the results of coagulation testing are, clinical judgment remains paramount in trying to ascertain whether the bleeding is more likely to be of a surgical nature (which tends to persist) or due to a coagulopathy (which might improve). If normal coagulation studies are present upon arrival in the ICU, significant bleeding usually requires surgical reexploration (see pages 371–373). If markedly abnormal coagulation studies are present, yet bleeding persists despite their correction, surgical exploration is also indicated.

3. **Prothrombin time (PT)** measured as the international normalized ratio (INR) assesses the extrinsic coagulation cascade. The INR may be slightly increased after a standard pump run, but clotting factor levels exceeding 30% of normal should allow for satisfactory hemostasis. An abnormal INR can be corrected with fresh frozen plasma.

4. **Partial thromboplastin time (PTT)** assesses the intrinsic coagulation cascade and can also detect residual or recurrent heparin effect ("heparin rebound"). When an elevated PTT occurs as an isolated abnormality, or with slight elevation of the INR, protamine is beneficial in correcting the PTT and controlling bleeding. One study found that heparin rebound documented by elevated Xa levels and an abnormal clotting time was present in virtually all patients after surgery and could be abolished by a continuous infusion of 25 mg/h of protamine.[57] However, another study found little correlation of elevated anti-Xa levels and elevated PTTs, even though both were noted in about 40% of patients.[58] This study concluded that an elevated PTT is not necessarily related to excessive heparin – it may be due to clotting factor deficiency or even excessive protamine, which acts as a coagulation inhibitor. If available, it is sometimes worthwhile obtaining an ACT, yet it also may be elevated in conditions other than residual heparin.

5. **Platelet count.** Although CPB reduces platelet count by about 30–50% and also produces platelet dysfunction, platelet function is usually adequate to produce

hemostasis. Platelet transfusions may be justified in the bleeding patient with thrombocytopenia (generally <100,000/μL) or for suspicion of platelet dysfunction (usually for patients on aspirin or clopidogrel) even in the absence of thrombocytopenia.

6. **Platelet function** can be assessed by a variety of available technologies, including those that measure platelet aggregometry and other sophisticated tests of clot formation and retraction.[55,59,60] Although the correlation of these tests with the occurrence of bleeding is not specific, qualitative platelet abnormalites in the bleeding patient do suggest that platelet transfusions are indicated. In most centers, suspicion of platelet dysfunction is based upon preoperative use of antiplatelet agents and prompts platelet transfusions without point-of-care testing.

7. **Fibrinogen** (factor I) is essential to proper platelet function by promoting platelet–platelet interaction leading to platelet aggregation. It is also a cell adhesion molecule that enhances platelet adhesion to endothelial cells. If the patient has significant bleeding and a fibrinogen level <100 mg/dL, transfusion of cryoprecipitate, which is rich in factors I, VIII, and XIII, is helpful.

8. **Fibrinolysis** is invariably present in all patients having heart surgery, although it may be attenuated by use of lysine analogs which exhibit antifibrinolytic properties. Test results consistent with fibrinolysis are nonspecific and include elevations in the INR and PTT, decreased level of factors I and VIII, and elevated fibrin split products (such as D-dimer). Additional dosing of Amicar may be considered if fibrinolysis is confirmed, but is of undefined value.[61] The best means of identifying fibrinolysis are thromboelastography/thromboelastometry and a Sonoclot analysis.

9. The **thromboelastogram** (TEG) and **ROTEM thromboelastometry** (Pentapharm) give a qualitative measurement of clot strength.[62–67] These tests evaluate the interaction of platelets with the coagulation cascade from the onset of clot formation through clot lysis and have a distinct contour for a variety of coagulation abnormalities, including fibrinolysis (Figure 9.1). Although these tests are very helpful in guiding therapy in patients with coagulopathic bleeding, they do not necessarily identify patients who are going to bleed, and treatment is not indicated for abnormalities noted in the absence of bleeding. However, in the bleeding patient, they provide more rapid assessment of hemostatic abnormalities than standard blood coagulation testing, thus allowing for more prompt and effective therapy.[64] ROTEM has been used to identify platelet dysfunction and also exclude residual heparin in patients with elevated ACTs.[67] One comparative study of TEG and platelet aggregometry found that both were effective in determining impaired hemostasis, but neither was superior to the other in minimizing blood loss.[59]

10. **Sonoclot analysis** (Figure 9.2) is another viscoelastic method of evaluating clot formation and retraction that allows for assessment of coagulation factors, fibrinogen, and platelet activity. The device measures the changing impedance to movement imposed by the developing clot on a small probe that vibrates at an ultrasonic frequency within a blood sample. Studies have suggested that both a TEG and Sonoclot are more predictive of bleeding than routine coagulation studies. This device has seen limited use, but can direct appropriate therapy in patients with persistent bleeding.[68]

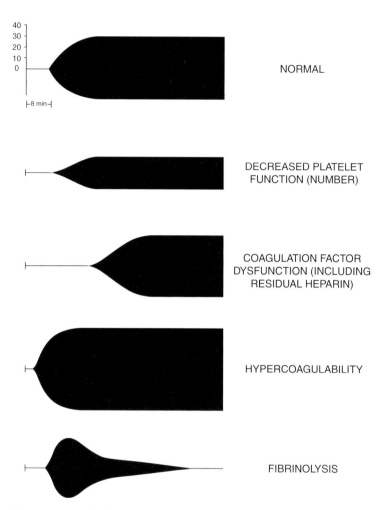

Figure 9.1 • Representative thromboelastogram tracings.

E. Repeat a chest x-ray

1. Note the overall width of the mediastinum. A widened mediastinum may suggest undrained clotted blood accumulating within the pericardial cavity that could cause cardiac tamponade. Comparison with preoperative films can be misleading because of differences in technique, but any difference noted between the immediate postoperative supine film and a repeat film should be noted (Figure 9.3). A widened superior mediastinum is noted when there is significant clot accumulation around the great vessels.

2. Note the distance between the edge of the Swan-Ganz catheter in the right atrium or the location of the right atrial pacing wires (if placed on the right atrial free wall) and the edge of the mediastinal silhouette. If this distance widens, suspect clot accumulation adjacent to the right atrium.

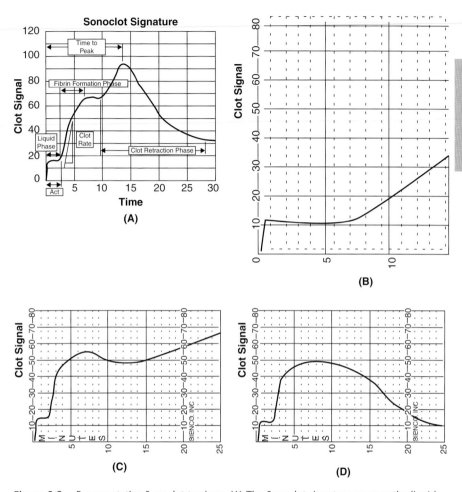

Figure 9.2 • Representative Sonoclot tracings. (A) The Sonoclot signature assesses the liquid phase of initial clot formation, the rate of fibrin and clot formation, further fibrinogenesis and platelet–fibrin interaction, a peak impedance after completion of fibrin formation, and a downward slope as platelets induce contraction of the completed clot. (B) Heparinization. (C) Poor platelet function (slow clot retraction). (D) Hyperfibrinolysis (no tightening associated with clot retraction). (Courtesy of Sienco, Inc.)

3. Note any accumulation of blood within the pleural space that has not drained through the pleural chest tubes. This can be difficult to assess since fluid will layer out on a supine film, so a discrepancy in the haziness of the two pleural spaces should be sought.

F. Consider obtaining an **echocardiogram** if any of the above suggest the presence of cardiac tamponade. If the transthoracic study is inconclusive, obtain a transesophageal study.

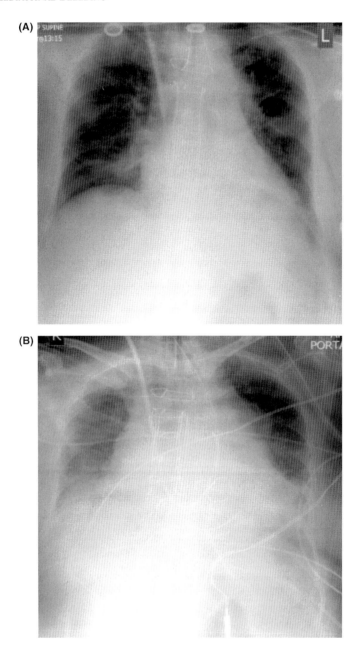

Figure 9.3 • (A) Supine chest x-ray obtained at the conclusion of surgery. (B) Supine chest x-ray obtained 6 hours later in the same patient with minimal mediastinal bleeding but hemodynamic compromise. Since neither pleural space was entered, blood accumulated primarily around the heart, producing a wide mediastinum consistent with cardiac tamponade.

V. Management of Mediastinal Bleeding (Table 9.5)[47,69-71]

Although there is no role for prophylactic blood product transfusions in the prevention of bleeding following open-heart surgery, persistent bleeding must be treated immediately and aggressively based on the suspected etiology of hemorrhage. It is a truism that the longer a patient bleeds, the worse the coagulopathy becomes. In general, the most benign and least invasive treatments should be considered first. If a patient was "dry" at the time of closure and suddenly starts to bleed, the source is usually surgical in nature and requires reexploration. In contrast, the patient with persistent bleeding may have a surgical or medical cause for the bleeding.

A. Ensure chest tube patency. Ongoing bleeding without drainage leads to cardiac tamponade. Gently milk the tubes to remove clot. Aggressive stripping is not necessary.

B. Warm the patient to 37 °C. Hypothermia produces a generalized suppression of the coagulation mechanism and also impairs platelet function.[72] The use of a heated humidifier in the ventilator circuit and a forced-air warming blanket are beneficial and will reduce the tendency to shiver. All blood products should be delivered through blood-warming devices.

C. Control hypertension with vasodilators (nitroprusside, clevidipine, nicardipine) or β-blockers (esmolol for the hyperdynamic heart). Higher doses of propofol or morphine can also be used since extubation should not be contemplated in the bleeding patient.

Table 9.5 • *Management of Postoperative Mediastinal Bleeding*

1. Explore early for significant ongoing bleeding or tamponade
2. Ensure that chest tubes are patent
3. Warm patient to normothermia
4. Control hypertension, agitation, and shivering
5. Check results of coagulation studies (INR, PTT, platelet count or TEG)
6. Protamine 25 mg IV for two doses if elevated PTT
7. Consider use of 10 cm PEEP with caution
8. Packed cells if hematocrit <26%
9. Platelets, 1–2 "six packs"
10. Fresh frozen plasma, 2–4 units
11. Cryoprecipitate, 6 units
12. Desmopressin (DDAVP) 0.3 µg/kg IV over 20 minutes (if suspect platelet dysfunction from uremia or aspirin)
13. Recombinant factor VIIa 60 µg/kg if severe coagulopathy
14. **Transesophageal echocardiography** if concerned about tamponade
15. **Urgent exploration** for significant ongoing bleeding or tamponade
16. **Emergency exploration** for exsanguinating hemorrhage or near cardiac arrest from tamponade

D. Control agitation in the awake patient with short-acting sedatives:
   1. Propofol 25–50 μg/kg/min
   2. Dexmedetomidine 1 μg/kg load over 10 minutes followed by a continuous infusion of 0.2–0.7 μg/kg/h
   3. Midazolam 2.5–5.0 mg IV q1–2h
   4. Morphine 2.5–5 mg IV q1–2h

E. Control shivering with:
   1. Meperidine 25–50 mg IV
   2. Pancuronium 0.1 mg/kg IV over 5–10 minutes, then 0.01 mg/kg q1h or a continuous infusion of 2–4 mg/h (always with sedation)

F. Use of increasing level of positive end-expiratory pressure (PEEP) to augment mediastinal pressure has been shown to reduce microvascular bleeding.[7] However, prophylactic PEEP at levels of either 5 or 10 cm H_2O has not been found to be effective in reducing bleeding or transfusion requirements.[73] If it is elected to increase PEEP to control bleeding, careful attention to its effects on hemodynamics is essential.

G. Use of blood components to treat early significant bleeding should be based on suspicion of the hemostatic defect. This is often necessary before the results of coagulation studies are available. For example, the patient who has received aspirin, clopidogrel, or IIb/IIIa inhibitors, or is uremic, is likely to have platelet dysfunction and will benefit primarily from platelet transfusions, even if the platelet count is normal. In contrast, the patient who has recently been on warfarin or has hepatic dysfunction is more likely to have clotting factor deficiencies and may benefit more from an initial transfusion of fresh frozen plasma. Platelets, FFP, and cryoprecipitate may be necessary in patients who have had a long duration of CPB (>3 hours) or who have received multiple blood products during surgery. Aggressive treatment with blood components should be provided promptly for significant bleeding from a suspected coagulopathy, because persistent bleeding causes progressive depletion of clotting factors and platelets ("coagulopathy begets coagulopathy").

H. Once the results of coagulation studies become available, there is more objective information upon which to base therapy. Point-of-care testing in the operating room is the most expeditious way of assessing the hemostatic profile (Figure 9.4). Some groups preferentially use the thromboelastogram to identify the exact nature of the hemostatic defect, allowing for more prompt initiation of appropriate therapy. This may result in lower transfusion requirements.[64] The results of routine coagulation studies drawn after bypass is terminated are usually available in the operating room or soon after arrival in the ICU. If bleeding persists despite corrective measures, clotting studies can be repeated to reassess the status of the coagulation system.
   1. An elevated PT implies the need for clotting factors provided by FFP and/or cryoprecipitate.
   2. An elevated PTT or ACT suggests a problem with the intrinsic coagulation cascade or persistent heparin effect. Additional protamine should be given first, with an understanding that an elevated PTT may not be related to heparin, and protamine could exacerbate a coagulopathy.[57] FFP and/or cryoprecipitate may also be indicated.

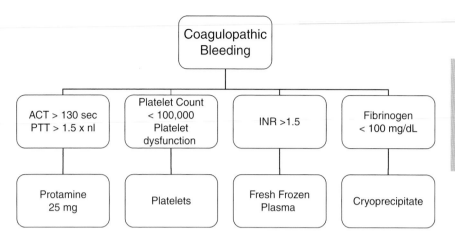

Figure 9.4 • Point-of-care testing of routine coagulation studies to treat postoperative bleeding.

3. Fibrinogen levels <100 mg/dL warrant administration of cryoprecipitate when bleeding is persistent.

4. A platelet count below 100,000/μL suggests the need for platelet transfusions. Because CPB induces platelet dysfunction, suspicion of a qualitative defect in the actively bleeding patient should be treated with platelets even if the platelet count is adequate.

5. **Note:** Abnormal results do not need to be treated if the patient has minimal bleeding. Blood samples are frequently drawn from heparinized lines, so they should be repeated if results are markedly abnormal or inconsistent with the amount of bleeding. Platelet transfusions are not indicated in the nonbleeding patient until the platelet count approaches 20,000–30,000/μL, although most patients in the immediate postoperative period will tend to bleed at platelet counts less than about 60,000/μL.

I. Blood transfusions are often neglected in the bleeding patient when anemia may be progressive and exacerbated by hemodilution from the administration of fresh frozen plasma and platelet transfusions. Although a low transfusion trigger (hematocrit of 21%) might be acceptable in a nonbleeding, stable young patient with no comorbidities, this is **not** safe in the bleeding patient. The patient with ongoing mediastinal bleeding should be transfused to maintain a hematocrit at a reasonable level (>25%) as a safety margin to maintain satisfactory tissue oxygenation. Furthermore, there are a number of clinical indications for transfusion to a higher hematocrit, especially those suggestive of an impairment in tissue oxygen supply (see section VI.D, page 367). Notably, platelet function is impaired in the profoundly anemic patient.[74] Red cells increase platelet-to-platelet interaction and facilitate the interaction of platelets with the subendothelium to improve hemostasis.

J. Protamine may be given in a dose of 25–50 mg (5 mg/min) if the PTT is elevated. Generally ACTs correlate with the PTT but are usually not drawn once the patient leaves the operating room. Although the ACT should return to baseline after protamine administration, reinfusion of cell-saver blood may reintroduce a small amount of heparin, and release of heparin from tissue stores can introduce residual unneutralized heparin that contributes to bleeding. This may occur because the half-life of protamine is only about 5 minutes, with virtual elimination from the bloodstream in about 20–30 minutes.[75] Thus, a continuous infusion of low-dose protamine or additional doses for potential heparin rebound is a feasible approach.[57] Notably, it has been shown that prolonged ACTs (and inferentially PTTs) may be noted in the absence of free heparin, as confirmed by use of the Hepcon system.[76] Thus, if additional protamine is given and the PTT remains elevated, unneutralized heparin may not be the problem. In fact, excessive use of protamine will elevate the ACT and cause bleeding. Excess protamine causes platelet dysfunction, enhances fibrinolysis, and decreases clot strength, emphasizing that indiscriminate use of excessive protamine should be avoided.[32–34,77]

K. Desmopressin (DDAVP) has no role in the prophylaxis of postoperative bleeding but might be considered in patients with documented von Willebrand's disease, uremia, and possibly drug-induced platelet dysfunction, although the latter has not been studied.[7,78]

1. Bleeding following cardiac surgery is often secondary to an acquired defect in the formation of the platelet plug caused by a deficiency in von Willebrand's factor. DDAVP increases the level of factor VIII precursors, von Willebrand's factor (by approximately 50%) and tissue-type plasminogen activator by releasing them from vascular endothelium. These factors are responsible for promoting platelet adhesion to the subendothelium.

2. DDAVP is given in a dose of 0.3–0.4 μg/kg IV over 20 minutes. A slow infusion may attenuate the peripheral vasodilation and hypotension that often follows DDAVP infusion.[79] Peak effects are seen in 30–60 minutes.

L. Recombinant factor VIIa (rFVIIa) has been used successfully in arresting bleeding in patients with a severe uncontrollable coagulopathy after various types of open-heart surgery.[80–85] It combines with tissue factor at the site of vessel injury and to the surface of activated platelets, activating factor X. This results in thrombin generation, platelet activation, and an explosive "thrombin burst" that promotes localized hemostasis at the site of tissue injury. It produces a prompt improvement in the INR. Because tissue factor and activated platelets are present systemically after CPB, systemic thrombosis may occur, being noted in 5–10% of patients.[81,82,86,87] The usual dose is 60 μg/kg with a second dose given after 2 hours, if necessary. The half-life of rFVIIa is 2.9 hours.

M. Calcium chloride 1 g IV (10 mL of 10% solution) over 15 minutes may be administered if the patient has received multiple transfusions of CPD preserved blood during a short period of time (e.g., more than 10 units within 1–2 hours). The citrate used as a preservative in CPD blood binds calcium, but hypocalcemia is unusual because of the rapid metabolism of citrate by the liver. However, calcium administration is not necessary when adenine-saline (AS-1) is used as the preservative. If hypocalcemia is present, as it often is following CPB, calcium chloride is preferable to calcium gluconate because it provides three times more ionized calcium.

VI. Blood Transfusions: Red Cells

A. **Red cell transfusions** are indicated primarily to increase the oxygen-carrying capacity of blood to avoid end-organ ischemia and dysfunction. Tissue oxygen delivery depends on the cardiac output, the hemoglobin level, and the oxygen extraction ratio in tissues. Because the early postoperative period is associated with delayed myocardial metabolic recovery, reduced cardiac output, and significant anemia, oxygen delivery is commonly reduced by at least 25% postoperatively. There is evidence that tissue oxygenation may be maintained in healthy patients with hemoglobins as low as 6–7 g/dL (hematocrit around 18–21%), and studies suggest that the safe lower limit for the hematocrit in the **stable** postoperative patient is probably around 22–24%.[7,88–90] In fact, one study showed that a hematocrit <24% was associated with a lower incidence of Q-wave infarctions.[91]

B. Nonetheless, the approach to the bleeding patient requires extra vigilance and a margin of safety to ensure adequate tissue oxygenation, minimize myocardial ischemia, and prevent hemodynamic compromise. It is therefore safest in the bleeding patient to administer blood when the hematocrit is less than 26%, especially when there is ongoing blood loss and predictable hemodilution from administration of blood components and platelets. There is no indication for transfusing to a hematocrit greater than 30%.

C. Blood transfusions contain cytokines and proinflammatory mediators and are immunomodulatory.[7,92,93] They are associated with numerous potential complications, including viral infections, such as HIV, hepatitis B, hepatitis C (all of which are currently very rare), and cytomegalovirus (CMV) (in up to 50% of units); bacterial infections, especially pneumonia;[94,95] immunologic reactions, including transfusion-related acute lung injury (TRALI); and multisystem organ failure. Pulmonary morbidity is especially common, whether related to TRALI or not.[96] Transfusions also increase short- and long-term mortality after open-heart surgery.[7,8,97–99] Leukocyte depletion by the blood bank can reduce the risk of infection (especially CMV) and lower mortality rates as well.[100]

D. Transfusion triggers should be determined by clinical criteria, including hypotension, tachycardia, low cardiac output states with low mixed venous oxygen saturation, metabolic acidosis, evidence of neurologic impairment, respiratory insufficiency, or renal dysfunction. Even in these situations, it must be recognized that transfusions may provide minimal improvement in oxygen-carrying capacity immediately after transfusion, may reduce microcirculatory flow, and in fact could prove more detrimental than beneficial. This is because the 2,3-diphosphoglycerate (2,3-DPG) level in blood is very low, especially with longer durations of storage, resulting in a leftward shift of the oxyhemoglobin dissociation curve with more avid binding of oxygen to hemoglobin and less release to tissues. Fortunately, 2,3-DPG levels return to 50% of normal within 24 hours after transfusion.[92]

E. Use of blood filters is beneficial in removing microaggregates of blood. Blood filters of at least 170 μm pore size must be used for all blood transfusions. Filters of 20–40 μm pore size are more effective in removing microaggregates of fibrin, platelet debris, and leukocytes that accumulate in stored blood. These filters have been shown to decrease the incidence of nonhemolytic febrile transfusion reactions and may reduce the adverse effects of multiple transfusions on pulmonary function. Blood lines should be primed with isotonic solutions (preferably normal saline), avoiding lactated Ringer's, which contains calcium, and D5W, which is hypotonic and will produce significant red cell hemolysis.

F. **Note:** Care should be taken to avoid transfusing cold blood products. Blood warmers should generally be used if the patient receives rapid transfusions. If one unit is to be transfused, it should be allowed to sit at ambient room temperature or under a heating hood for several minutes to warm.

G. **Packed red blood cells** (RBCs) contain approximately 200 mL of red cells, 100 mL of Optisol AS, and about 30 mL of plasma per unit. Each unit has an average hematocrit of 70% and one unit will raise the hematocrit of a 70 kg man by 3%. At least 70% of transfused cells survive 24 hours, and these cells have a normal life span. Since packed cells contain no clotting factors, administration of fresh frozen plasma should be considered to replace clotting factors if a large number of units (generally more than five) is given over a short period of time.

1. Although the shelf-life of packed RBCs stored at 1−6 °C in Optisol AS solutions is 42 days, significant changes occur in the red cells with storage. These include increased levels of cytokines, which produce more systemic inflammation, loss of deformability, which increases capillary transit time, and depletion of 2,3-DPG, which reduces oxygen unloading from hemoglobin.

2. Several studies suggest that transfusion of blood with prolonged storage results in an increased risk of bacterial infections, especially pneumonia, with a longer duration of intubation, more acute renal dysfunction, and a longer ICU stay,[101,102] but other studies have confirmed this only in blood stored for over 28 days.[103,104]

3. Leukoreduction of red cells is beneficial in reducing some of the febrile and nonhemolytic transfusion reactions. In some hospitals, this is done routinely.

H. **Fresh whole blood** (less than 6 hours old) has a hematocrit of about 35% and contains clotting factors and platelets. One unit has been shown to provide equivalent, if not superior, hemostasis to that of 10 units of platelets.[105] It is probably the best replacement product, but most blood banks fractionate blood into components and fresh whole blood is usually not available for use.

I. **Cell-saver blood** (shed and washed in the operating room) is rinsed with heparinized saline and is devoid of clotting factors and platelets. A small amount of heparin may be present after centrifugation, but is not considered to be clinically significant.[13] The survival, function, and hemolysis of washed red blood cells is equivalent to that of nonprocessed blood.[106]

J. **Hemofiltration blood** is obtained by placing a hemofilter in the extracorporeal circuit. This provides concentrated red cells and also preserves platelets and clotting factors. Studies have shown superior blood salvage and hemostasis with use of a hemofilter than with cell-saving devices, but ultrafiltration of pump blood is generally not recommended.[7]

K. **Autotransfusion** of shed mediastinal blood is a controversial means of blood salvage. It has arguably been shown to reduce the need for transfusions, and most systems have been designed for reinfusion through 20−40 μm blood filters without washing. Blood filters do not completely remove lipid particles and blood micro-aggregates, and the reinfused blood contains low levels of factor I and VIII, a low level of platelets which are dysfunctional, elevated levels of fibrinolytics (fibrin split products), inflammatory cytokines, endotoxin, tissue factor, and free hemoglo-bin.[7,107] Washing is able to remove some of these factors but will also eliminate all clotting factors and platelets. If unwashed blood is returned in moderate amounts (>500 mL), an apparent coagulopathy will be present with an elevation in INR, PTT, and D-dimers, and a reduction in fibrinogen.[108] Several studies have noted an increased risk of wound infections with reinfusion of unwashed shed mediastinal blood.[109,110] Thus, it is recommended that if autotransfusion is to be used as part of a blood conservation program, blood should be washed in a cell-saving device prior to reinfusion.[7]

VII. Blood Components, Colloids, and Blood Substitutes

A. **Platelets** should be given to the bleeding patient if the platelet count is less than 100,000/μL. Furthermore, since platelets are dysfunctional in patients receiving antiplatelet medications and IIb/IIIa inhibitors and after CPB, one should not hesitate to administer platelets for ongoing bleeding even if the platelet count exceeds 100,000/μL. Platelets are not indicated in the nonbleeding patient unless the count is perilously low (<20–30,000/μL).

1. Platelets are provided as a pooled preparation from one or several donors, usually as a 6-unit bag, which is the usual amount given to an average-sized adult. Each unit contains approximately 8×10^{10} platelets and should increase the platelet count by about 7000–10,000/μL in a 75 kg adult. One unit of platelets contains 70% of the platelets in a unit of fresh blood, but platelets lose some of their functional capacity during storage. Platelets stored at room temperature can be used for up to 5 days and have a life span of 8 days. Those stored at 4 °C are useful for only 24 hours (only 50–70% of total platelet activity is present at 6 hours) and have a life span of only 2–3 days.[93]

2. **Note:** Platelet function is impaired in patients with hypofibrinogenemia and when the hematocrit is less than 30%.[74] Thus, use of cryoprecipitate and red cell transfusion to raise the hematocrit towards 30% can be considered to improve platelet function.

3. Transfused platelets will be less effective when given within 6 hours of a loading dose or 4 hours of a maintenance dose of clopidogrel or prasugrel, because the active compound may still be present in the bloodstream.

4. ABO compatibility should be observed for platelets, but is not essential. For each donor used, there is a similar risk of transmitting hepatitis and HIV as for one unit of blood.

5. Platelets should be administered through a 170 μm filter. Several filters are available (such as the Pall LRF 10 filter) that can be used to remove leukocytes from platelet transfusions. Use of these filters may be beneficial in reducing the risk of allergic reactions caused by red and white cells present in platelet packs. Pretreatment with diphenhydramine (50 mg IV), ranitidine (150 mg IV) (H_1 and H_2 blockers), and steroids (hydrocortisone 100 mg IV) might also attenuate these reactions, but is usually not necessary.

6. Despite some claims that platelet transfusions are associated with higher risks of infection, respiratory complications, stroke, and death, it is more likely that the need for platelets is simply a surrogate marker for sicker patients.[111] A study of

nearly 33,000 patients from the Cleveland Clinic confirmed increased postoperative morbidity in patients receiving platelets, but after risk adjustment, there was no increase in morbidity or mortality from transfused platelets.[112]

B. **Fresh frozen plasma** (FFP) contains all clotting factors at normal concentrations with a slight reduction in factor V (66% of normal) and factor VIII (41% of normal). It is devoid of red cells, white cells, and platelets. However, levels of factor VIII, von Willebrand's factor, factor I (fibrinogen), fibronectin, and factor XIII will be reduced to 30% if cryoprecipitate is also obtained from the same unit of blood.[93] Only 30% of the normal level of most clotting factors is essential to provide hemostasis, and the INR generally has to exceed 1.5 before a clinically significant factor deficiency exists. However, due to the hemodilutional effects of CPB and the progressive loss of clotting factors during ongoing bleeding, one should not hesitate to administer FFP to improve hemostasis even if the INR is minimally abnormal. Because of the importance of factors I and VIII in promoting platelet aggregation and adhesion to the endothelium, transfusion of cryoprecipitate may be helpful as well.

1. One unit of FFP contains about 250 mL of volume. The amount given is usually **2–4 units for the average adult**. Four units will increase the level of clotting factors by 10%, which is considered to be the amount necessary to improve coagulation status.[113]

2. FFP should be ABO compatible and given through a 170 μm filter. Since each unit is derived from one unit of whole blood from one donor, FFP has a similar risk of transmitting hepatitis or HIV as one unit of blood.

3. FFP may be given to patients with antithrombin III (AT III) deficiency, which may only be recognized when significant heparin resistance is noted in the operating room. To minimize the amount of volume infused, a concentrated source of AT III is commercially available (Thrombate III).[29] The amount required is based on an estimate of the level of AT III present (see calculation on page 201).

4. **Note:** The administration of plasma and platelets not only provides clotting factors, but also raises filling pressures. These blood products will therefore lower the hematocrit and can precipitate fluid overload. If the hematocrit is less than 26% or not yet available and the patient is bleeding, anticipate the need for blood if other volume is being administered. Remember that the hematocrit does not change with acute blood loss until replacement fluids are administered.

C. **Cryoprecipitate**

1. Cryoprecipitate represents the cold insoluble portion of plasma that precipitates when FFP is thawed at 1–6 °C. It is then refrozen at −18 °C within 1 hour. Approximately 15 mL is derived from 1 unit which is then suspended in 15 mL of plasma and pooled into a concentrate of 6 units, containing about 200 mL.[93]

2. Each unit provides concentrated levels of several coagulation factors, including 150–250 mg of fibrinogen, 80–100 units of factor VIII:C, 40–50% of the original plasma content of von Willebrand's factor, factor XIII (fibrin-stabilizing factor), and fibronectin (a tissue integrin involved in wound healing). Both factors I and VIII are essential for proper platelet aggregation and adherence to endothelium.

3. The amount given is usually 1 unit/7–10 kg of body weight (e.g., 7 units to a 70 kg patient). Ten individual units will raise the fibrinogen level of a 70 kg man by 70 mg/dL. One can also calculate the number of units that will be required from the following equations:

$$\text{Blood volume (BV)} = 70 \text{ mL/kg} \times \text{weight in kg}$$

$$\text{Plasma volume (PV)} = \text{BV} \times (1 - \text{hematocrit})$$

$$\text{Fibrinogen required (mg)} = 0.01 \times \text{PV} \times (\text{desired level} - \text{current level})$$

$$\text{Bags of cryo required} = \text{mg fibrinogen required}/250 \text{ mg per bag}$$

For example, to raise the fibrinogen to 200 mg/dL for a 75 kg man with a hematocrit of 25% and a fibrinogen level of 100 mg/dL, one would give $70 \times 75 \times (1 - 0.25) \times 0.01 \times (200 - 100) = $ about 4000 mg/250 = 15 units.

4. Cryoprecipitate is especially beneficial for patients with von Willebrand's disease or documented hypofibrinogenemia. It may also benefit patients requiring surgery soon after thrombolytic therapy, which significantly reduces fibrinogen levels.

5. Cryoprecipitate should be given through a 170 μm filter within 4–6 hours of thawing. ABO compatibility should be observed, but is not essential.

D. **Hetastarch** 6% in saline (Hespan), hetastarch in balanced electrolyte solution (Hextend), and 5% **albumin** are colloid solutions that are used as volume expanders. Albumin can be given if the patient is hypovolemic and blood components are not available as it has primarily a dilutional effect on clotting factors. In contrast, all of the high-molecular-weight hetastarch compounds are best avoided in the bleeding patient because they can produce a coagulopathy by reducing levels of factor VIII, von Willebrand's factor and fibrinogen, impairing fibrin polymerization and clot strength. These issues, as well as reduced availability of the platelet glycoprotein IIb/IIIa receptor, contribute to the antiplatelet effects.[48–53] If the patient is not bleeding, they can be safely used by limiting infusion volume to 1500 mL per day (about 20–25 mL/kg).

E. **Blood substitutes**. Extensive research has been carried out into the development of red blood cell substitutes that consist of hemoglobin-based oxygen carriers (HBOC). A study of one such compound, HBOC-201, a polymerized bovine hemoglobin solution (Hemopure, Biopure Corporation) found that it preserved oxygen transport and eliminated the need for transfusions in 34% of patients after cardiac surgery, although substantial doses of this short-acting product were required.[114] Polymerized hemoglobin preparations appear to be the best blood substitutes undergoing evaluation.[115]

VIII. Mediastinal Reexploration for Bleeding or Tamponade

A. The presence of untapering mediastinal bleeding or suspected cardiac tamponade is an indication for urgent mediastinal reexploration. Emergency reexploration in the intensive care unit is indicated for exsanguinating hemorrhage or tamponade with incipient cardiac arrest.[116] Surgical exploration should be considered when there is the acute onset of rapid bleeding (>300 mL/h) after minimal blood loss, or persistent bleeding above arbitrary threshold levels at various times after surgery.

These must take into consideration the extent of coagulopathy that may be in the process of being treated and the hemodynamic effects of ongoing bleeding. General guidelines for reexploration include hourly bleeding rates of approximately:

1. More than 400 mL/h for 1 hour (>200 mL/m^2)
2. More than 300 mL/h for 2–3 hours (>150 mL/m^2/h × 2–3 hours)
3. More than 200 mL/h for 4 hours (>100 mL/m^2/h × 4 hours)

B. Reexploration for **bleeding** is associated with increased operative morbidity and mortality, primarily because of a delay in returning the patient to the operating room and occasionally because of the necessity for open-chest resuscitation in the intensive care unit.[116–118] There should be a low threshold for returning a patient to the operating room early for bleeding using the guidelines noted above. The benefits of doing so greatly outweigh any risks. Early exploration (<12 hours in several studies)[118,119] reduces the risk of adverse outcomes because it can mitigate factors that contribute to increased morbidity and mortality. Early exploration can:

1. Minimize the use of multiple transfusions, which are associated with a higher risk of respiratory and renal failure, sepsis, and death.[96,117]
2. Avert periods of hemodynamic instability and low cardiac output syndrome, which can lead to multisystem organ failure.
3. Reduce the risk of tamponade and cardiac arrest – events that frequently occur in the middle of the night due to reluctance to explore a patient earlier.
4. Lower the risk of wound complications.[120]

C. The diagnosis of **cardiac tamponade** is suggested by hemodynamic compromise with elevated filling pressures, usually in a patient with significant mediastinal bleeding or significant bleeding that has stopped. In the early postoperative period, the following findings alone, but often in combination, should heighten the suspicion of cardiac tamponade:

1. Sudden cessation of significant mediastinal bleeding.
2. A persistent low cardiac output state with respiratory variation (either spontaneously or with mechanical ventilation) and narrowing of the pulse pressure noted on the arterial tracing. An increasing requirement for inotropic or vasopressor medications is commonly necessary in response to increasing filling pressures, low blood pressure, and a dwindling cardiac ouput.
3. Equilibration of intracardiac pressures with RA = PCW = LA pressure resulting from increased intrapericardial pressure. **Note:** It is not unusual for clot to accumulate next to the right or left atrium and cause unequal elevations of RA and LA pressures.
4. Radiographic findings of an enlarged cardiac silhouette or widened mediastinum compared with an earlier postoperative chest x-ray (Figure 9.3). However, this finding is helpful only if present since it is absent in 80% of patients with tamponade.[121] Displacement of the right heart border from the cardiac silhouette, indicated by an increased distance from right atrial free wall pacing wires to the edge of the cardiac silhouette, suggests accumulation of clot adjacent to the right atrium. A very large pleural effusion can also cause tamponade.
5. ECG changes, including decreased voltage, a compensatory tachycardia, dysrhythmias, and, terminally, electromechanical dissociation.

D. The diagnosis of tamponade may be obvious on a clinical basis when the typical abnormalities just noted are present. However, occasionally, tamponade may be suspected when in fact ventricular dysfunction is the primary problem. The scenario of hypotension, tachycardia, and elevated filling pressures with moderate mediastinal bleeding is not an uncommon scenario in a patient with marginal myocardial function. If hemodynamics do not improve after volume infusion and inotropic support, tamponade should be suspected and ruled out. If the diagnosis is not clear, and if time allows, an **echocardiogram** should be performed to differentiate ventricular failure from tamponade. Transthoracic echocardiography usually can detect blood compressing the atria and ventricles, but will fail to provide adequate visualization due to unsatisfactory acoustic windows in up to 60% of patients.[122] Thus, in equivocal situations, a **transesophageal echocardiogram** should be performed to make the diagnosis.[54] Even then, an occasional finding is a small, localized effusion producing selective chamber compression without the classic features of tamponade, such as right atrial and right ventricular diastolic collapse. Left ventricular diastolic collapse is a reliable sign of tamponade in the postoperative patient.[123]

E. Once tamponade is diagnosed clinically or by echocardiography, or when suspicion remains high despite echocardiographic findings, emergency mediastinal exploration should be performed. CT scanning is also very sensitive in detecting a large hemopericardium, but it cannot provide an assessment of tamponade physiology; furthermore, it requires moving an unstable patient out of the monitoring environment of the ICU.

   1. If the patient can be temporarily stabilized, plans should be made for exploration in the operating room as soon as possible.

   2. If the patient is markedly hypotensive and cardiac arrest is imminent or has occurred, emergency exploration in the ICU is indicated. With appropriate technique, this is associated with low infection rates and excellent survival.[124]

IX. Technique of Emergency Resternotomy

A. Emergency reexploration is indicated for exsanguinating hemorrhage or tamponade with incipient cardiac arrest. Every member of the house staff must be thoroughly familiar with the location and use of emergency thoracotomy equipment as he/she may be the only individual available to perform an emergency sternotomy and save a patient's life. A small subxiphoid incision may initially relieve some of the pressure around the heart, but in dire circumstances, it is easier and more expeditious to open the entire sternotomy wound.

B. An emergency resternotomy pack must be available and readily accessible in all cardiac surgical ICUs. This must include all the essential equipment to perform the procedure, including gowns, gloves, and masks, antiseptic solutions and drapes to prep and drape the patient expeditiously, and a preselected assortment of essential instruments. Having a separate small kit with instruments required to open the chest (knife, heavy needle holder and wire cutter, sponges, one-piece retractor) is helpful while the larger pack of instruments is being opened.

C. Technique of emergency resternotomy

1. Remove the dressing.

2. Pour antiseptic on skin and then place four towels around the sternotomy incision and other drapes over the rest of the patient. Alternatively, some have recommended use of a one-piece sterile thoracic drape that covers the entire field and may immobilize bacteria.[116] This allows for external compressions to be immediately restarted after the drape is applied. When antiseptic solutions are placed, the wound can be emergently opened, but external compressions have to be applied over a towel since the skin has not dried.

3. Open the wound down to the sternum with a knife. If skin staples are present, make the incision adjacent to the staples.

4. If sternal wires were used, cut with a wire cutter; if a wire cutter is not available, untwist the wires with a heavy needle holder until they fatigue and break. If the sternum was not closed with wire, simply cut the sutures with the knife. If other means of sternal reinforcement were used, additional devices should be available at the bedside (e.g., a sterile screwdriver for sternal talons (KLA Martin), or heavy metal cutters for Biomet or Synthes plates).

5. Place the sternal retractor to expose the heart (a one-piece retractor is essential).

6. Place a finger over the bleeding site if it can be identified and suction the remainder of the chest to improve exposure.

7. Resuscitate with volume through central or peripheral lines.

8. Initiate internal massage if the chest is opened for cardiac arrest or marginal blood pressure. Commonly, improvement in cardiac activity and blood pressure will be noted upon relief of tamponade (and often from the bolus of epinephrine given as the patient is deteriorating). Performing internal massage mandates attention to the location of bypass grafts, especially the left internal thoracic artery (LITA) graft to the left anterior descending artery (LAD), which can easily be avulsed. An experienced individual can achieve satisfactory compression using one-hand massage (usually the left hand), placing the fingers behind the heart and compressing the ventricles against the thenar eminence. Use of the right hand may result in perforation of the right ventricular outflow tract and is more difficult to perform. Therefore, it is generally recommended that two hands be used, compressing the heart between the right hand, placed around the left ventricular apex and behind the heart, and the palm and flattened fingers of the left hand anteriorly.

9. Control major and then minor bleeding sites. Manual control of a bleeding site should be obtained while the chest is suctioned and the patient receives volume resuscitation. Only then should specific attention be paid to placing sutures or ties to control bleeding. Manual control can usually minimize bleeding and "buys time" until a more experienced person arrives or the operating room can be made available. If the patient remains hemodynamically unstable, it is preferable to resuscitate the patient in the ICU rather than rush the patient to the operating room. Invariably the bleeding site can be controlled and the patient stabilized.

10. If the patient has arrested, but tamponade is not present, an IABP usually should be placed, and the patient brought back to the operating room as soon as possible.

11. Irrigate the mediastinum extensively with warm saline or antibiotic solution and consider leaving drainage catheters for postoperative antibiotic irrigation.

12. Note that patients who have had cardiac surgery via a right thoracotomy incision or a short left anterior thoracotomy incision cannot be resuscitated with internal massage, although opening of the incision may allow for drainage of tamponade. Either equipment for a full sternotomy must be available in the ICU or the patient will need to be returned to the operating room for further resuscitation.

References

1. Despotis GJ, Hogue CW Jr. Pathophysiology, prevention, and treatment of bleeding after cardiac surgery: a primer for cardiologists and an update for the cardiothoracic team. *Am J Cardiol* 1999;83:15B–30B.

2. Khuri SF, Valeri CR, Loscalzo J, et al. Heparin causes platelet dysfunction and induces fibrinolysis before cardiopulmonary bypass. *Ann Thorac Surg* 1995;60:1008–14.

3. Puskas JD, Williams WH, Duke PG, et al. Off-pump coronary artery bypass grafting provides complete revascularization with reduced myocardial injury, transfusion requirements, and length of stay: a prospective randomized comparison of two hundred unselected patients undergoing off-pump versus conventional coronary artery bypass grafting. *J Thorac Cardiovasc Surg* 2003;125:797–808.

4. Murphy GJ, Mango E, Lucchetti V, et al. A randomized trial of tranexamic acid in combination with cell salvage plus a meta-analysis of randomized trials evaluating tranexamic acid in off-pump coronary artery bypass grafting. *J Thorac Cardiovasc Surg* 2006;132:475–80.

5. Bjessmo S, Hylander S, Vedin J, Mohlkert D, Ivert T. Comparison of three different chest drainages after coronary artery bypass surgery – a randomised trial in 150 patients. *Eur J Cardiothorac Surg* 2007;31:372–5.

6. Sakopoulos AG, Hurwitz AS, Suda RW, Goodwin JN. Efficacy of Blake drains for mediastinal and pleural drainage following cardiac operations. *J Card Surg* 2005;20:574–7.

7. Society of Thoracic Surgeons Blood Conservation Guidelines Task Force, Ferraris VA, Ferraris SP, Saha SP, et al. Perioperative blood transfusion and blood conservation in cardiac surgery: the Society of Thoracic Surgeons and the Society of Cardiovascular Anesthesiologists clinical practice guideline. *Ann Thorac Surg* 2007;83(5 suppl):S27–86.

8. Kuduvalli M, Oo AY, Newall N, et al. Effect of peri-operative red blood cell transfusion on 30-day and 1-year mortality following coronary artery bypass surgery. *Eur J Cardiothorac Surg* 2005;27:592–8.

9. Engoren MC, Habib RH, Zacharias A, Schwann TA, Riordan CJ, Durham SJ. Effect of blood transfusion on long-term survival after cardiac operation. *Ann Thorac Surg* 2002;74:1180–6.

10. Kincaid EH, Monroe ML, Saliba DL, Kon ND, Byerly WG, Reichert MG. Effects of preoperative enoxaparin versus unfractionated heparin on bleeding indices in patients undergoing coronary artery bypass grafting. *Ann Thorac Surg* 2003;76:124–8.

11. Jones HU, Muhlestein JB, Jones KW, et al. Preoperative use of enoxaparin compared with unfractionated heparin increases the incidence of re-exploration for postoperative bleeding after open-heart surgery in patients who present with an acute coronary syndrome: clinical investigation and reports. *Circulation* 2002;106(supp I):I-19–22.

12. Renda G, Di Pillo R, D'Alleva A, et al. Surgical bleeding after pre-operative unfractionated heparin and low molecular weight heparin for coronary bypass surgery. *Haematologica* 2007;92:366–73.

13. Gravlee GP, Hopkins MB, Yetter CR, Buss DH. Heparin content of washed red blood cells from the cardiopulmonary bypass circuit. *J Cardiothorac Vasc Anesth* 1992;6:140–2.

14. Warkentin TE, Greinacher A, Koster A, Lincoff AM. Treatment and prevention of heparin-induced thrombocytopenia. American College of Chest Physicians evidence-based clinical practice guidelines (8th edition). *Chest* 2009;133:340S–80S.

15. Ferraris VA, Ferraris SP, Moliterno DJ, et al. The Society of Thoracic Surgeons practice guidelines series: aspirin and other antiplatelet agents during operative coronary revascularization (executive summary). *Ann Thorac Surg* 2005;79:1454–61.

16. Dunning J, Versteegh M, Fabbri A, et al. Guideline on antiplatelet and anticoagulation management in cardiac surgery. *Eur J Cardiothorac Surg* 2008;34:73–92.

17. Sun JC, Whitlock R, Cheng J, et al. The effect of pre-operative aspirin on bleeding, transfusion, myocardial infarction, and mortality in coronary artery bypass surgery: a systematic review of randomized and observational studies. *Eur Heart J* 2008;29:1057–71.

18. Dacey LJ, Munoz JJ, Johnson ER, et al. Effects of preoperative aspirin use on mortality in coronary artery bypass grafting patients. *Ann Thorac Surg* 2000;70:1986–90.

19. Bybee KA, Powell BD, Valeti U, et al. Preoperative aspirin therapy is associated with improved postoperative outcomes in patients undergoing coronary artery bypass grafting. *Circulation* 2005;112(9 Suppl):I-296–92.

20. McIlroy DR, Myles PS, Phillips LE, Smith JA. Antifibrinolytics in cardiac surgical patients receiving aspirin: a systematic review and meta-analysis. *Br J Anaesth* 2009;102:168–78.

21. Brandt JT, Payne CD, Wiviott SD, et al. A comparison of prasugrel and clopidogrel loading doses on platelet function: magnitude of platelet inhibition is related to active metabolite formation. *Am Heart J* 2007;153:66.

22. Bizzari F, Scolletta S, Tucci E, et al. Perioperative use of tirofiban hydrochloride (Aggrastat) does not increase surgical bleeding after emergency or urgent coronary artery bypass grafting. *J Thorac Cardiovasc Surg* 2001;122:1181–5.

23. Dyke CM, Smedira NG, Koster A.M. et al. A comparison of bivalirudin to heparin with protamine reversal in patients undergoing cardiac surgery with cardiopulmonary bypass: The EVOLUTION-ON study. *J Thorac Cardiovasc Surg* 2006;131:533–9.

24. Chauhan S, Gharde P, Bisoi A, Kale S, Kiran U. A comparison of aminocaproic acid and tranexamic acid in adult cardiac surgery. *Ann Card Anaesth* 2004;7:40–3.

25. Henry DA, Carless PA, Moxey AJ, et al. Anti-fibrinolytic use for minimising perioperative allogenic blood transfusions. *Cochrane Database Syst Rev* 2007;4:CD001886.

26. Mengistu AM, Röhm KD, Boldt J, Mayer J, Suttner SW, Piper SN. The influence of aprotinin and tranexamic acid on platelet function and postoperative blood loss in cardiac surgery. *Anesth Analg* 2008;107:391–7.

27. Henry D, Carless P, Fergusson D, Laupacis A. The safety of aprotinin and lysine-derived antifibrinolytic drugs in cardiac surgery: a meta-analysis. *CMAJ* 2009;180:183–93.

28. Mangano DT, Tudor IC, Dietzel L: Multicenter Study of Perioperative Ischemia Research Group; Ischemia Research and Education Foundation. The risk associated with aprotinin in cardiac surgery. *N Engl J Med* 2006;354:353–65.

29. Spiess BD. Treating heparin resistance with antithrombin or fresh frozen plasma. *Ann Thorac Surg* 2008;85:2153–60.

30. Despotis GJ, Joist JH, Hogue GW Jr, et al. The impact of heparin concentration and activated clotting time monitoring on blood conservation. A prospective, randomized evaluation in patients undergoing cardiac operation. *J Thorac Cardiovasc Surg* 1995;110:46–54.

31. Runge M, Møller CH, Steinbrüchel DA. Increased accuracy in heparin and protamine administration decreases bleeding: a pilot study, *J Extra Corpor Technol* 2009;41:10–4.

32. Mochizuki T, Olson PJ. Szlam F, Ramsay JG, Levy JH. Protamine reversal of heparin affects platelet aggregation and activated clotting time after cardiopulmonary bypass. *Anesth Analg* 1998;87:781–5.

33. McLaughlin KE, Dunning J. In patients post cardiac surgery do high doses of protamine cause increased bleeding? *Interact Cardiovasc Thorac Surg* 2003;2:424–6.

34. Griffin MJ, Rinder HM, Smith BR, et al. The effect of heparin, protamine, and heparin/protamine reversal on platelet function under conditions of arterial shear stress. *Anesth Analg* 2001;93:20–7.

35. Ramnath AN, Naber HR, de Boer A, Leusink JA. No benefit of intraoperative whole blood sequestration and autotransfusion during coronary artery bypass grafting: results of a randomized clinical trial. *J Thorac Cardiovasc Surg* 2003;125:1432–7.

36. Carless PA, Rubens FD, Anthony DM, O'Connell D, Henry DA. Platelet-rich plasmapheresis for minimising peri-operative allogeneic blood transfusion. *Cochrane Database Syst Rev* 2003;2: CD004172.

37. Nakajima T, Kawazoe K, Ishibashi K, et al. Reduction of heparin dose is not beneficial to platelet function. *Ann Thorac Surg* 2000;70:186–90.

38. Chung JH, Gikakis N, Rao AK, Drake TA, Colman RW, Edmunds LH Jr. Pericardial blood activates the extrinsic coagulation pathway during clinical cardiopulmonary bypass. *Circulation* 1996;93:2014–8.

39. Nollert G, Schwabenland I, Maktav D, et al, Miniaturized cardiopulmonary bypass in coronary artery bypass surgery: marginal impact on inflammation and coagulation but loss of safety margins. *Ann Thorac Surg* 2005;80:2326–32.

40. Balachandran S, Cross MH, Karthikeyan S, Mulpur A, Hansbro SD, Hobson P. Retrograde autologous priming of the cardiopulmonary bypass circuit reduces blood transfusion after coronary artery surgery. *Ann Thorac Surg* 2002;73:1912–8.

41. Murphy GS, Szokol JW, Nitsun M, et al. The failure of retrograde autologous priming of the cardiopulmonary bypass circuit to reduce blood use after cardiac surgical procedures. *Anesth Analg* 2004;98:1201–7.

42. Niranjan G, Asimakopoulos G, Karagounis A, Cockerill G, Thompson M, Chandrasekaran V. Effects of cell saver autologous blood transfusion on blood loss and homologous blood transfusion requirements in patients undergoing cardiac surgery on- versus off-cardiopulmonary bypass: a randomised trial. *Eur J Cardiothorac Surg* 2006;30:271–7.

43. Carless PA Henry DA, Moxey AJ, O'Connell DL, Brown T, Fergusson DA. Cell salvage for minimising perioperative allogeneic blood transfusions. *Cochrane Database Syst Review* 2006;4: CD001888.

44. Klein AA, Nashef SA, Sharples L, et al. A randomized controlled trial of cell salvage in routine cardiac surgery. *Anesth Analg* 2008;107:1487–95.

45. Sirvinskas E, Veikutiene A, Benetis R, et al. Influence of early re-infusion of autologous shed mediastinal blood on clinical outcome after cardiac surgery. *Perfusion* 2007;22:345–52.

46. Rubens FD, Boodhwani M, Mesana T, et al. The cardiotomy trial. A randomized, double-blind study to assess the effect of processing of shed blood during cardiopulmonary bypass on transfusion and neurocognitive function. *Circulation* 2007;116(suppl I):I-89–97.

47. Levy JH, Tanaka KA, Steiner ME. Evaluation and management of bleeding during cardiac surgery. *Curr Hematol Rep* 2005;4:368–72.

48. Schramko AA, Suojaranta-Ylinen RT, Kuitunen AH, Kukkonen SI, Niemi TT. Rapidly degradable hydroxyethyl starch solutions impair blood coagulation after cardiac surgery: a prospective randomized trial. *Anesth Analg* 2009;108:30–6.

49. Dailey SE, Dysart CB, Langan DR, et al. An *in vitro* study comparing the effects of Hextend, Hespan, normal saline, and lactated Ringer's solution on thromboelastography and the activated partial thromboplastin time. *J Cardiothorac Vasc Anesth* 2005;19:358–61.

50. Deusch E, Thaler U, Kozek-Langenecker SA. The effects of high molecular weight starch solutions on platelets. *Anesth Analg* 2004;99:665–8.

51. Moskowitz DM, Shander A, Javidroozi M, et al. Postoperative blood loss and transfusion associated with use of Hextend in cardiac surgery patients at a blood conservation center. *Transfusion* 2008;48:768–75.

52. Franz A, Bräunlich P, Gamsjäger T, Felfernig M, Gustorff B, Kozek-Langenecker SA. The effects of hydroxyethyl starchs of varying molecular weights on platelet function. *Anesth Analg* 2001;92:1402–7.

53. Haynes GR. Fluid management in cardiac surgery: is one hydroxyethyl starch solution safer than another? *J Cardiothorac Vasc Anesth* 2006;20:916–7.

54. Imren Y, Tasoglu I, Oktar GL, et al. The importance of transesophageal echocardiography in diagnosis of pericardial tamponade after cardiac surgery. *J Card Surg* 2008;23:450–3.

55. Shore-Lesserson L. Point-of-care coagulation monitoring for cardiovascular patients: past and present. *J Cardiothorac Vasc Anesth* 2002;16:99–106.

56. Gelb AB, Roth RI, Levin J, et al. Changes in blood coagulation during and following cardiopulmonary bypass. Lack of correlation with clinical bleeding. *Am J Clin Pathol* 1996;106:87–99.

57. Teoh KH, Young E, Blackall MH, Roberts RS, Hirsh J. Can extra protamine eliminate heparin rebound following cardiopulmonary bypass surgery? *J Thorac Cardiovasc Surg* 2004;128:211–9.

58. Taneja R, Marwaha G, Sinha P, et al. Elevated activated partial thromboplastin time does not correlate with heparin rebound following cardiac surgery. *Can J Anaesth* 2009;56:489–96.

59. Mengistu AM, Wolf MW, Boldt J, Röhm KD, Lang J, Piper SN. Evaluation of a new platelet function analyzer in cardiac surgery: a comparison of modified thromboelastography and whole-blood aggregometry. *J Cardiothorac Vasc Anesth* 2008;22:40–6.

60. Rahe-Meyer N, Winterhalter M, Boden A, et al. Platelet concentrates transfusion in cardiac surgery and platelet function assessment by multiple electrode aggregometry. *Acta Anesthesiol Scand* 2009;53:168–75.

61. Ray MJ, Hales MM, Brown L, O'Brien MF, Stafford EG. Postoperatively administered aprotinin or epsilon aminocaproic acid after cardiopulmonary bypass has limited benefit. *Ann Thorac Surg* 2001;72:521–6.

62. Tuman KJ, Spiess BD, McCarthy RJ, Ivankovich AD. Comparison of viscoelastic measures of coagulation after cardiopulmonary bypass. *Anesth Analg* 1989;69:69–75.

63. Ronald A, Dunning J. Can thromboelastography predict and decrease bleeding and blood and blood product requirements in adult patients undergoing cardiac surgery? *Interact Cardiovasc Thorac Surg* 2005;1:456–63.

64. Shore-Lesserson L, Manspeizer HE, DePerio M, Francis S, Vela-Cantos F, Ergin MA. Thromboelastography-guided transfusion algorithm reduces transfusions in complex cardiac surgery. *Anesth Analg* 1999;88:312–9.

65. Davidson SJ, McGrowder D, Roughton M, Kelleher AA. Can ROTEM thromboelastometry predict postoperative bleeding after cardiac surgery? *J Cardiothorac Vasc Anesth* 2008;22:655–61.

66. Swallow RA, Agarwala RA, Dawkins KD, Curzen NP. Thromboelastography: potential bedside tool to assess the effects of antiplatelet therapy? *Platelets* 2006;17:385–92.

67. Mittermayr M, Velik-Salchner C, Stalzer B, et al. Detection of protamine and heparin after termination of cardiopulmonary bypass by thromboelastometry (ROTEM): results of a pilot study. *Anesth Analg* 2009;108:743–50.

68. Hett DA, Walker D, Pilkington SN, Smith DC. Sonoclot analysis. *Br J Anaesth* 1995;75:771–6.

69. Despotis G, Eby C, Lublin DM. A review of transfusion risks and optimal management of perioperative bleeding with cardiac surgery. *Transfusion* 2008;48(1 Suppl):2S–30S.

70. Brevig J, McDonald J, Zelinka ES, Gallagher T, Jin R, Grunkemeier GL. Blood transfusion reduction in cardiac surgery: multidisciplinary approach at a community hospital. *Ann Thorac Surg* 2009;87:532–9.

71. Levy JH. Pharmacologic methods to reduce perioperative bleeding. *Transfusion* 2008;48(1 Suppl): 31S–8S.

72. Valeri CR, Khabbaz K, Khuri SF, et al. Effect of skin temperature on platelet function in patients undergoing extracorporeal bypass. *J Thorac Cardiovasc Surg* 1992;104:108–16.

73. Collier B, Kolff J, Devineni R, Gonzalez LS III. Prophylactic positive end-expiratory pressure and reduction of postoperative blood loss in open-heart surgery. *Ann Thorac Surg* 2002;74:1191–4.

74. Fernandez F. Goudable C, Sie P, et al. Low haematocrit and prolonged bleeding time in uremic patients: effect of red cell transfusions. *Br J Haematol* 1985;59:139–48.

75. Butterworth J, Lin YA, Prielipp RC, Bennett J, Hammon JW, James RL. Rapid disappearance of protamine in adults undergoing cardiac operation with cardiopulmonary bypass. *Ann Thorac Surg* 2002;74:1589–95.

76. Gundry SR, Drongowski RA, Klein MD, Coran AG. Postoperative bleeding in cardiovascular surgery. Does heparin rebound really exist? *Am Surg* 1989;55:162–5.

77. Nielsen VG. Protamine enhances fibrinolysis by decreasing clot strength: role of tissue-factor-initiated thrombin generation. *Ann Thorac Surg* 2006;81:1720–7.

78. Cattaneo M. The use of desmopressin in open-heart surgery. *Haemophilia* 2008;14 (Suppl 1):40–7.

79. Frankville DD, Harper GB, Lake CL, Johns RA. Hemodynamic consequences of desmopressin administration after cardiopulmonary bypass. *Anesthesiology* 1991;74:988–96.

80. Gelsomino S, Lorusso R, Romagnoli S. et al. Treatment of refractory bleeding after cardiac operations with low-dose recombinant activated factor VII (NovoSeven): a propensity score analysis. *Eur J Cardiothorac Surg* 2008;33:64–71.

81. Warren O, Mandal K, Hadjianastassiou V, et al. Recombinant activated factor VII in cardiac surgery: a systematic review. *Ann Thorac Surg* 2007;83:707–14.

82. Bowman LJ, Uber WE, Stroud MR, et al. Use of recombinant activated factor VII concentrate to control postoperative hemorrhage in complex cardiovascular surgery. *Ann Thorac Surg* 2008;85:1669–77.

83. Hardy JF, Belisle S, Van der Linden P. Efficacy and safety of recombinant activated factor VII to control bleeding in nonhemophiliac patients: a review of 17 randomized controlled trials. *Ann Thorac Surg* 2008;86:1038–48.

84. Karkouti K, Beattie WS. Pro: the role of recombinant factor VIIa in cardiac surgery. *J Cardiothorac Vasc Anesth* 2008;22:779–82.

85. Al-Ruzzeh S, Ibrahim K, Navia JL. Con: the role of recombinant factor VIIa in the control of bleeding after cardiac surgery. *J Cardiothorac Vasc Anesth* 2008;22:783–5.

86. Lichtman AD, Carullo V, Minhaj M, Karkouti K. Massive intraoperative thrombosis and death after recombinant activated factor VII administration. *J Cardiothorac Vasc Anesth* 2007;21:897–902.

87. Tanos M, Dunning J. Is recombinant factor VII useful for intractable bleeding after cardiac surgery? *Interact Cardiovasc Thorac Surg* 2006;5:493–8.

88. Johnson RG, Thurer RL, Kruskall MS, et al. Comparison of two transfusion strategies after elective operations for myocardial revascularization. *J Thorac Cardiovasc Surg* 1992;104:307–14.

89. Doak GJ, Hall RI. Does hemoglobin concentration affect perioperative myocardial lactate flux in patients undergoing coronary artery bypass surgery? *Anesth Analg* 1995;80:910–6.

90. Murphy GJ, Angelini GD. Indications for blood transfusion in cardiac surgery. *Ann Thorac Surg* 2006;82:2323–34.

91. Spiess BD, Ley C, Body SC, et al. Hematocrit value on intensive care unit entry influences the frequency of Q-wave myocardial infarction after coronary artery bypass grafting. *J Thorac Cardiovasc Surg* 1998;116:460–7.

92. Spiess BD. Choose one: damned if you do/damned if you don't! *Crit Care Med* 2005;33:1871–3.

93. American Red Cross. American Red Cross. Practice Guidelines for Blood Transfusion. A compilation from recent peer-reviewed literature. 2nd edition, 2007 (available at www.redcross.org)

94. Chelemer SB, Prato BS, Cox PM Jr, O'Connor GT, Morton JR. Association of bacterial infection and red blood cell transfusion after coronary artery bypass surgery. *Ann Thorac Surg* 2002;73:138–42.

95. Ali ZA, Lim E, Motalleb-Zadeh R, et al. Allogeneic blood transfusion does not predispose to infection after cardiac surgery. *Ann Thorac Surg* 2004;78:1542–6.

96. Koch C, Li L, Figueroa P, Mihaljevic T, Svensson L, Blackstone EH. Transfusion and pulmonary morbidity after cardiac surgery. *Ann Thorac Surg* 2009;88:1410–8.

97. Scott BH, Seifert FC, Grimson R. Blood transfusion is associated with increased resource utilisation, morbidity and mortality in cardiac surgery. *Ann Card Anaesth* 2008;11:15–9.

98. Whitson BA, Huddleston SJ, Savik K, Shumway SJ. Bloodless cardiac surgery is associated with decreased morbidity and mortality. *J Card Surg* 2007;22:373–8.

99. Reeves BC, Murphy GJ. Increased mortality, morbidity, and cost associated with red blood cell transfusion after cardiac surgery. *Curr Opin Anaesthesiol* 2008;21:669–73.

100. van de Watering LMG, Hermans J, Houbiers JGA, et al. Beneficial effects of leukocyte depletion of transfused blood on postoperative complications in patients undergoing heart surgery. A randomized clinical trial. *Circulation* 1998;97:562–8.

101. Basran S, Frumento RJ, Cohen A, et al. The association between duration of storage of transfused red blood cells and morbidity and mortality after reoperative cardiac surgery. *Anesth Analg* 2006;103:15–20.

102. Koch CG, Li L, Sessler DI, et al. Duration of red cell storage and complications after cardiac surgery. *N Engl J Med* 2008;358:1229–39.

103. Leal-Noval SR, Jara-López I, Garcia-Garmendia JL, et al. Influence of erythrocyte concentrate storage time on postsurgical morbidity in cardiac surgery patients. *Anesthesiology* 2003;98:815–22.

104. Yap CH, Lau L, Krishnaswamy M, Gaskell M, Yii M. Age of transfused red cells and early outcomes after cardiac surgery. *Ann Thorac Surg* 2008;86:554–9.

105. Mohr R, Martinowitz U, Lavee J, Amroch D, Ramot B, Goor DA. The hemostatic effects of transfusing fresh whole blood versus platelet concentrates after cardiac operations. *J Thorac Cardiovasc Surg* 1988;96:530–4.

106. Valeri CR, Dennis RC, Ragno G, Pivacek LE, Hechtman HB, Khuri SF. Survival, function, and hemolysis of shed red blood cells processed as nonwashed and washed blood cells. *Ann Thorac Surg* 2001;72:1598–602.

107. Hartz R, Smith JA, Green D. Autotransfusion after cardiac operation. Assessment of hemostatic factors. *J Thorac Cardiovasc Surg* 1988;96:178–82.

108. Griffith LD, Billman GF, Daily PO, Lane TA. Apparent coagulopathy caused by infusion of shed mediastinal blood and its prevention by washing of the infusate. *Ann Thorac Surg* 1989;47:400–6.

109. Body SC, Birmingham J, Parks R, et al. Safety and efficacy of shed mediastinal blood transfusion after cardiac surgery: a multicenter observational study. Multicenter Study of Perioperative Ischemia Research Group. *J Cardiothorac Vasc Anesth* 1999;13:410–6.

110. Dial S, Nguyen D, Menzies D. Autotransfusion of shed mediastinal blood. A risk factor for mediastinitis after cardiac surgery? Results of a cluster investigation. *Chest* 2003;124:1847–51.

111. Spiess BD, Royston D, Levy JH, et al. Platelet transfusions during coronary artery bypass graft surgery are associated with serious adverse outcomes. *Transfusion* 2004;44:1143–8.

112. McGrath T, Koch CG, Xu M, et al. Platelet transfusion in cardiac surgery does not confer increased risk for adverse morbid outcomes. *Ann Thorac Surg* 2008;86:543–53.

113. Puget Sound Blood Center. Puget Sound Blood Center. Blood component therapy. psbc.org/therapy/ffp.htm.

114. Levy JH, Goodnough LT, Greilich PE, et al. Polymerized bovine hemoglobin solution as a replacement for allogeneic red blood cell transfusions after cardiac surgery: results of a randomized, double-blind trial. *J Thorac Cardiovasc Surg* 2002;124:35–42.

115. Napolitano LM. Hemoglobin-based oxygen carriers: first, second, or third generation? Human or bovine? Where are we now? *Crit Care Clin* 2009;25:279–301.

116. Dunning J, Fabbri A, Kolh PH, et al. Guideline for resuscitation in cardiac arrest after cardiac surgery. *Eur J Cardiothorac Surg* 2009;36:3–28.

117. Ranucci M, Bozzetti G, Ditta A, Cotza M, Carboni G, Ballotta A. Surgical reexploration after cardiac operations: why a worse outcome? *Ann Thorac Surg* 2008;86:1557–62.

118. Karthik S, Grayson AD, McCarron EE, Pullan DM, Desmond MJ. Reexploration for bleeding after coronary artery bypass surgery: risk factors, outcomes, and the effect of time delay. *Ann Thorac Surg* 2004;78:527–34.

119. Choong CK, Gerrard C, Goldsmith KA, Dunningham H, Vuylsteke A. Delayed re-exploration for bleeding after coronary artery bypass surgery results in adverse outcomes. *Eur J Cardiothorac Surg* 2007;31:834–8.

120. Talamonti MS, LoCicero J. III, Hoyne WP, Sanders JH, Michaelis LL. Early reexploration for excessive postoperative bleeding lowers wound complication rates in open heart surgery. *Am Surgeon* 1987;53:102–4.

121. Hamid M, Khan MU, Bashour AC. Diagnostic value of chest x-ray and echocardiography for cardiac tamponade in post cardiac surgery patients. *J Pak Med Assoc* 2006;56:104–7.

122. Price S, Prout J, Jaggar SI, Gibson DG, Pepper JR. "Tamponade" following cardiac surgery: terminology and echocardiography may both mislead. *Eur J Cardiothorac Surg* 2004;26:1156–60.

123. Chuttani K, Pandian NG, Mohanty PK, et al. Left ventricular diastolic collapse. An echocardiographic sign of regional cardiac tamponade. *Circulation* 1991;83:1999–2006.

124. Charalambous CP, Zipitis CS, Keenan DJ. Chest reexploration in the intensive care unit: a safe alternative to returning to the operating theater. *Ann Thorac Surg* 2006;81:191–4.

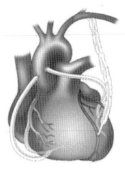

CHAPTER 10

Respiratory Management

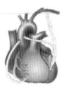 **10** Respiratory Management

I. General Comments

A. Virtually all patients undergoing open-heart surgery will have some element of postoperative pulmonary dysfunction. However, in the vast majority of patients, it is well tolerated with minimal impairment in oxygenation and ventilation. Thus, it is possible and desirable in most patients to achieve early endotracheal extubation within the first 8–12 hours after surgery. This reduces pulmonary complications, encourages earlier mobilization, and reduces costs and the hospital length of stay.[1-3]

B. The use of general anesthesia and a median sternotomy incision for most open-heart operations and the use of the internal thoracic artery (ITA) for virtually all coronary bypass operations have significant adverse effects on pulmonary function and chest wall mechanics.[4-6] Although the use of cardiopulmonary bypass (CPB) is associated with a systemic inflammatory response that has been incriminated as the major cause of postoperative pulmonary dysfunction, studies comparing postoperative pulmonary function in patients undergoing on- and off-pump surgery have not demonstrated a significant difference, except perhaps in patients with advanced pulmonary disease.[7-9] Thus, anesthetic management and intensive care unit (ICU) protocols to achieve early extubation should be the goal after both types of operations.

C. Minimally invasive incisions preserve a more stable chest wall and have less impact on chest wall mechanics. Ministernotomies for aortic valve replacement, for example, are associated with less atelectasis than a full sternotomy incision.[10] Although a thoracotomy incision does produce moderate pain with splinting, this can be minimized using epidural or intercostal analgesia or a continuous infusion pump (On-Q, I-Flow Corporation).[11,12] Generally, pulmonary function is better preserved with limited incisions. However, the potential adverse influence of CPB on gas exchange will still be noted following minimally invasive valve operations that require CPB.

D. Postoperative respiratory impairment and the likelihood of "delayed extubation" or the need for prolonged ventilatory support can be predicted fairly reliably based on clinical variables.[13-20] Careful preoperative evaluation for obstructive or restrictive pulmonary disease with review of baseline arterial blood gases (ABGs) should identify patients at high risk for pulmonary complications after surgery. However, most patients without severe preoperative respiratory compromise have adequate pulmonary reserve to tolerate the insults imposed by cardiac surgery. Standard protocols for ventilatory management and early extubation can be applied to all but the very highest-risk patients with excellent results. In approximately 5–10% of patients, mechanical ventilatory support beyond 48 hours is necessary because of marked hemodynamic compromise, poor oxygenation, or inadequate ventilation.

Manual of Perioperative Care in Adult Cardiac Surgery, 5th Edition. By Robert M. Bojar.
Published 2011 by Blackwell Publishing Ltd.

E. An understanding of the postoperative changes in pulmonary function, basic concepts in oxygenation and ventilation, routine pulmonary management, and contributing factors to respiratory dysfunction allows for the early identification and treatment of problems to optimize the recovery of pulmonary function.

II. Postoperative Changes in Pulmonary Function

During the early postoperative period, the principal mechanisms underlying poor gas exchange with borderline oxygenation are ventilation/perfusion (V/Q) mismatch and intrapulmonary shunting.[6,21] Contributing factors include the following:

A. General anesthetics, neuromuscular relaxants, and narcotics that decrease the central respiratory drive and contribute to decreased respiratory muscle function.

B. The median sternotomy incision that produces chest wall splinting and reduces most pulmonary function testing variables; the presence of chest tubes for mediastinal or pleural drainage also impairs respiratory function.[22]

C. Harvesting of the internal thoracic artery (ITA) with pleural entry is associated with a decrease in chest wall compliance and deterioration of pulmonary function testing to a greater degree than when no ITA is harvested.[8,23–25]

1. A significant reduction in the peak expiratory flow rate (PEFR) and forced expiratory volume in 1 second (FEV_1), as well as in the forced vital capacity (FVC), functional residual capacity (FRC), and expiratory reserve volume, has been documented postoperatively and may be exacerbated by the presence of pleural chest tubes.[26,27]

2. ITA harvesting is associated with a higher incidence of pleural effusions and atelectasis, but these may be minimized if ITA harvesting can be accomplished without pleural entry.[28]

3. There is the potential for phrenic nerve injury and devascularization during ITA harvesting, the latter arguably being more frequent in diabetic patients.[29,30]

4. Interestingly, one study showed that the incidence of respiratory complications and the degree of respiratory impairment were no greater if bilateral, rather than just unilateral, ITA harvesting was performed.[31]

D. Effects of cardiopulmonary bypass[6,32]

1. Cardiogenic pulmonary edema may result from hemodilution, fluid overload, and reduction in oncotic pressure. Postcardiotomy left ventricular (LV) dysfunction with elevated pulmonary artery (PA) pressures may contribute to pulmonary edema and lead to impairment of right ventricular (RV) function.

2. Noncardiogenic interstitial pulmonary edema is a manifestation of the "systemic inflammatory response" which produces an increase in endothelial permeability and accumulation of extravascular lung water; this also decreases lung surfactant, contributing to atelectasis. Contributory factors to this syndrome include:

a. Complement activation

b. Release of cytokines and other inflammatory mediators

c. Pulmonary sequestration of neutrophils activated by blood contact with the extracorporeal circuit, resulting in release of proteolytic enzymes, such as neutrophil elastase, that may damage tissue and increase alveolar-endothelial permeability.

3. Hyperoxia may increase oxygen free-radical damage.

4. Hypothermia, pulmonary ischemia, or failure to ventilate the lungs may impair pulmonary function.[33,34]

E. Blood transfusions introduce microemboli and proinflammatory mediators that may elevate the pulmonary vascular resistance and PA pressures, increase inspiratory pressures, impair oxygenation, and reduce RV function. Transfusions are associated with an increased risk of pulmonary morbidity that may be associated with or independent of the development of transfusion-related acute lung injury (TRALI), which is considered to be an immune-mediated phenomenon.[35-37] Transfusions also increase the risk of wound infection.[38]

F. Preexisting comorbidities may impair postoperative pulmonary function, such as preexisting lung disease, especially chronic obstructive pulmonary disease (COPD) with any active bronchitic component, and obesity, which produces V/Q imbalance and impairs oxygenation.[39]

G. Diaphragmatic dysfunction from phrenic nerve injury may result from the use of iced saline slush in the pericardial well or from direct injury or devascularization from harvesting of the ITA.[40]

H. Studies have shown that impairment of pulmonary function persists for several months after surgery. One study showed that the values for FEV_1, forced expiratory flow at 50% of vital capacity (FEF_{50}), and maximum voluntary ventilation remained more than 25% less than preoperative values at 3.5 months after surgery.[27]

III. Routine Ventilator, Sedation, and Analgesia Management (Table 10.1)

A. For open-heart surgery, patients generally receive a balanced anesthestic regimen consisting of a narcotic (fentanyl, sufentanil, or remifentanil), an inhalational anesthetic, a neuromuscular blocker, and a sedative, such as midazolam or propofol.[41-43] In addition to their selection based on the patient's underlying cardiac disease, the use and dosing of these medications should be modified based upon the plans for postoperative extubation. Generally, remifentanil is used only in patients for whom very early extubation is planned because of its rapid offset of action. This allows for very early awakening and is associated with less respiratory depression and less atelectasis after extubation.[44]

B. If not extubated in the operating room, the patient should be placed on a volume-cycled respirator for full ventilator support upon arrival in the ICU, using either the synchronized intermittent mandatory ventilation (SIMV) or assist/control (A/C) mode. The patient remains anesthetized from the residual effects of narcotics, anxiolytic medications, and muscle relaxants given during surgery.

1. Before the patient can initiate and achieve adequate spontaneous ventilation, controlled ventilation will provide efficient gas exchange and decrease oxygen consumption by reducing the work of breathing. This may be very important during the first few postoperative hours when hypothermia, acid-base and electrolyte disturbances, and hemodynamic instability are most pronounced.

Table 10.1 • Initial Respiratory Orders

1. Initial ventilator settings
    a. Tidal volume 8–10 mL/kg
    b. Respiratory rate (usually in the IMV mode): 8–10/min
    c. FiO_2: 1.0
    d. PEEP: 5 cm H_2O
    e. Pressure support: 5–8 cm H_2O

2. Display pulse oximetry on bedside monitor

3. Chest x-ray after arrival in ICU (or in OR)

4. Check ABGs 15–30 minutes after arrival

5. Reduce FiO_2 to 0.4 as long as PaO_2 >100 torr or O_2 sat >95%

6. Adjust ventilator settings to maintain PCO_2 >30 torr with pH 7.30–7.50

7. Propofol 25–50 µg/kg/min; gradually decrease dose once standard weaning criteria are present and then initiate weaning when patient is mentally alert with reversal of neuromuscular blockade

8. Utilize dexmedetomidine if propofol weaning is not tolerated

2. Several studies have evaluated the effects of assist/control ventilation, SIMV, and biphasic intermittent positive airway pressure (BiPAP) in the early postoperative period. All three modes of ventilation were found to have comparable effects on hemodynamics and gas exchange, but BiPAP reduced the use of analgesics and sedatives and the duration of ventilation. BiPAP allows for unrestricted spontaneous breathing during all phases of respiration and may be more comfortable for the patient during the early return of spontaneous ventilation.[45,46]

C. Initial ventilator settings are as follows:
Tidal volume: 8–10 mL/kg
Intermittent mandatory ventilation (IMV) rate: 8–10 breaths/min
Fraction of inspired oxygen (FiO_2): 1.0
Positive end-expiratory pressure (PEEP): 5 cm H_2O
Pressure support of 5–8 cm H_2O
Inspiratory:expiratory (I:E) ratio of 1:2–1:3

D. The tidal volume and respiratory rate are selected to achieve a minute ventilation of approximately 100 mL/kg/min. Patients with COPD often benefit from lower respiratory rates and higher tidal volumes with increased inspiratory flow rates. The latter allows more time for the expiratory phase and can reduce the potential for developing high levels of "auto-PEEP" and air-trapping that may adversely affect hemodynamics. Lower tidal volumes with higher respiratory rates are often beneficial for patients with restrictive lung disease.

E. A low level (5 cm H_2O) of PEEP is routinely added to the respiratory circuit to prevent atelectasis. Despite this common practice, studies suggest that this level of PEEP does not reopen atelectactic lung and produces no significant improvement in oxygenation over zero PEEP.[47] A PEEP level of 10 cm H_2O or higher is usually necessary to improve lung recruitment, but it must be used judiciously because it may reduce venous return and impair right and left ventricular function. Caution is required when the patient is hypovolemic from peripheral vasodilation or when impaired RV function is already present.

F. Continuous pulse oximetry is used during mechanical ventilation with display of the arterial oxygen saturation (SaO_2) on the bedside monitor. This can bring attention to abrupt changes in oxygenation and should obviate the need to obtain ABGs on a frequent basis in the stable patient. Concern should be raised when the SaO_2 is <95%.

G. Although not commonly used in the ICU, capnography (end-tidal CO_2) can be used to provide a relative assessment of the level of PCO_2, although it is inaccurate when V/Q mismatch is present. For example, the end-tidal CO_2 will be much lower than the PCO_2 when there is an increase in physiologic dead space (increased V/Q). It is also affected by the degree of CO_2 production, the minute ventilation, and the cardiac output. Nonetheless, an abrupt change in the contour of the capnogram signifies an acute problem with the patient's ventilatory status, hemodynamics, or metabolic state.

H. A chest x-ray should be checked after arrival in the ICU. The position of the endotracheal tube, Swan-Ganz catheter or any central line, and intra-aortic balloon pump (IABP) should be identified. The lung fields should be evaluated for lung expansion/atelectasis, pneumothorax, undrained pleural effusion, pulmonary edema, or infiltrates. Attention should be paid to the width of the mediastinum, primarily for later comparison in the event of postoperative hemorrhage.

I. An initial ABG should be checked about 15–20 minutes after arrival in the ICU. The FIO_2 is gradually reduced to 0.40 and the tidal volume and respiratory rate are adjusted to maintain the ABGs within a normal range. The extent of hypothermia should be taken into consideration when making these adjustments, anticipating that the PCO_2 will rise as the patient warms. The metabolic demand and CO_2 production are decreased 10% for every degree less than 37 °C. Acceptable ABGs include:

PaO_2 >80 torr (SaO_2 >95%)

PCO_2 32–48 torr

pH 7.32–7.48

J. Adequate sedation and analgesia must be provided in the early postoperative period to minimize anxiety, pain, and hemodynamic stress that may contribute to myocardial ischemia and hypertension. This often seems difficult when the goal is to have a stable and comfortable patient who is awakening from anesthesia with an indwelling endotracheal tube.

1. For patients extubated in the operating room, adequate analgesia must be provided while minimizing sedation. Thoracic epidural analgesia or a continuous suprasternal infusion of bupivacaine using the On-Q system are beneficial in reducing pain.[11,41,42] Nonsteroidal anti-inflammatory drugs are useful non-sedating analgesics that may supplement the use of low-dose narcotics.

2. Most patients will arrive in the ICU sedated from narcotics and short-acting medications, such as propofol (usually at a dose of 25 µg/kg/min), started at the conclusion of surgery. Once standard criteria for weaning are met, the propofol infusion is weaned off over a short period of time. Most patients will awaken within 20 minutes of termination of a propofol infusion, although it may take several more

hours before they can be extubated. The offset of propofol is related to its dose, the duration of use, and the patient's body habitus. For example, with light sedation for up to 24 hours, emergence occurs in only 13 minutes, but in heavily sedated patients, it may take up to 25 hours![48]

3. Dexmedetomidine is an α-2 adrenergic agonist that may be used as an alternative medication to propofol when very early extubation is planned or when weaning of propofol is poorly tolerated. It may be started in the operating room or later with a loading dose of 1 μg/kg over 10 minutes followed by a continuous infusion of 0.2−0.7 μg/kg/h. It provides analgesia, anxiolysis, and sympatholysis, but only mild sedation and no amnesia. It allows for use of lower doses of other medications and can be continued after extubation.[49]

4. If early extubation is contemplated, midazolam is best avoided after cardiopulmonary bypass is terminated, because it has a half-life of over 10 hours after surgery.

5. If delayed extubation is anticipated, propofol remains an excellent choice for several days and may be converted to fentanyl for longer-term sedation. Although use of dexmedetomidine has only been recommended for 24 hours, several studies been found it to be comparable to or better than propofol or midazolam for long-term sedation.[50,51] Figure 10.3 on page 411 presents an algorithm for sedation in mechanically ventilated patients for whom drug selection is dictated by the patient's clinical condition.

6. Numerous options can be used to optimize perioperative analgesia.

   a. Most commonly, initial analgesia consists of intravenous narcotics, which are then transitioned to oral medications. With plans for early extubation, lower doses of narcotics should be selected to minimize respiratory depression. Small doses of IV narcotics or a continuous infusion of narcotics (such as morphine sulfate 0.02 mg/kg/h for patients under age 65 and 0.01 mg/kg/h for patients over age 65) may be given to provide analgesia and blunt the sympathetic response while minimizing respiratory depression associated with the peaks and valleys of bolus doses of narcotics. It may also be given safely after the patient is extubated. Alternatively, just before the propofol is discontinued, ketorolac (Toradol) 30 mg IV can be used to decrease narcotic requirements. Its use should be limited to 72 hours, and it should be avoided in patients with renal dysfunction. Other nonsteroidal anti-inflammatory medications, such as indomethacin 50 mg PR, may be administered safely without concerns about renal dysfunction.

   b. Epidural narcotics are beneficial in providing analgesia, but there may be reluctance to place these catheters because of concerns about heparinization.

   c. Patient-controlled analgesia (PCA) using narcotics (morphine, fentanyl, or remifentanil) provides adequate analgesia in patients with a low pain threshold with few side effects.[52,53]

K. Arterial blood gases should be checked if there is a significant change in the patient's clinical picture or if noninvasive monitoring (pulse oximetry or end-tidal CO_2) suggests a problem. A cautious approach is to check the ABGs after 4−6 hours, before initiating weaning, and just before extubation. Once criteria for weaning have been met, the IMV rate is gradually decreased or the patient may be directly given a spontaneous breathing trial on continuous positive airway pressure (CPAP) with 5 cm of PEEP. If satisfactory mechanics and ABGs are present, the patient is extubated.

IV. Basic Concepts of Oxygenation

   A. The first of the two primary goals of mechanical ventilation is the achievement of satisfactory arterial oxygenation. Although this is usually assessed by the arterial PO_2 (PaO_2), it should be remembered that the PaO_2 is a measurement of the partial pressure of oxygen dissolved in the bloodstream – it indirectly reflects oxygen saturation of hemoglobin (Hb) in the blood and does not measure the oxygen content of the blood.

   B. Blood oxygen content is determined primarily by the Hb level and the amount of oxygen bound to Hb (the arterial oxygen saturation or SaO_2) and to a minimal extent by that dissolved in solution (the PaO_2). Each gram of Hb can transport 1.39 mL of oxygen per 100 mL of blood (vol%), whereas each 100 torr of PaO_2 transports 0.031 vol%. Thus, correction of anemia does significantly more to improve blood oxygen content than does raising the level of dissolved oxygen (PaO_2) by increasing the FiO_2.

   1. The oxygen–hemoglobin dissociation curve demonstrates the relationship between PaO_2 and O_2 saturation (Figure 10.1). The amount of oxygen delivered to tissues depends on a number of factors that can affect this relationship. A shift to the left, as noted with hypothermia and alkalosis, indicates more avid binding of oxygen and less release to the tissues, whereas a shift to the right, noted with acidosis, improves tissue oxygen delivery. Blood transfusions have very low levels of

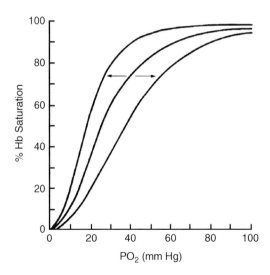

Figure 10.1 • Oxygen–hemoglobin dissociation curve. The sigmoid curve delineates the saturation of hemoglobin at increasing levels of PO_2. Note that a PO_2 of 65 mm Hg (torr) corresponds to a saturation of 90%. Higher levels of O_2 produce only small increments in blood oxygen content, but a PO_2 below this level results in a precipitous fall in O_2 saturation. A shift of the curve to the left, as is noted with alkalosis and hypothermia, increases the affinity of hemoglobin for oxygen and decreases tissue oxygen delivery. A shift to the right occurs with acidosis and improves tissue oxygen delivery.

2,3-DPG, which will also result in a leftward shift of the curve, resulting in less tissue oxygen delivery.

2. Note that a PaO_2 of 65 torr corresponds to an O_2 saturation of 90%, but this lies at the shoulder of the sigmoid curve. Below this level, a small decrease in PaO_2 causes a precipitous fall in O_2 saturation. Therefore, although a PaO_2 of 60–70 torr is certainly acceptable, there is little margin of safety in the event of a sudden change in hematocrit, cardiac output, or ventilator function.

3. The correlation of PaO_2 and oxygen saturation dissociates when methemoglobinemia is present. This occurs when more than 1% of available Hb is in an oxidized form (methemoglobin, metHb) and unable to bind oxygen. It has been noted in patients receiving high-dose IV nitroglycerin (over 10 μg/kg/min for several days), especially when hepatic or renal dysfunction is present.[54] When methemoglobinemia is present, the PaO_2 may be high, but the O_2 saturation measured by oximetry is lower than expected because the O_2 saturation of metHb is only 85%. Because some of the hemoglobin is not carrying oxygen, ischemia may be exacerbated by a reduced oxygen-carrying capacity despite the high PaO_2. It should be remembered that the O_2 saturation reported back from the blood gas laboratory is usually calculated from a nomogram based on the PaO_2, pH, and temperature – it is not measured directly.

4. Pulse oximetry is beneficial in measuring O_2 saturations continuously when the PaO_2 is low, but, because it measures several forms of hemoglobin, it will overestimate the oxyhemoglobin content when methemoglobinemia is present.

5. The amount of oxygen available to tissues depends not only on the SaO_2, pH, and the blood Hb content, but also on the cardiac output. An attempt to improve oxygen saturation at the expense of a decrease in cardiac output is counterproductive. This may be noted when increasing levels of PEEP are applied in the hypovolemic patient.

C. The PaO_2 is generally used to assess the adequacy of oxygenation, but its relationship to the FIO_2 should be examined. The PaO_2/FIO_2 ratio is a reliable predictor of pulmonary dysfunction and can also be used to assess whether weaning is feasible.[49] The calculation of the alveolar–arterial oxygen difference $(D(A − a)O_2)$ also takes the FIO_2 into consideration and is a very sensitive index of the efficiency of gas exchange. This is calculated according to the following equation:

$$D(A − a)O_2 = (FIO_2)(713) − PaO_2 − PCO_2/0.8$$

D. In patients with normal pulmonary function, the PaO_2 should usually be greater than 350 torr on 100% oxygen immediately after surgery. The FIO_2 should be gradually decreased to 0.40 as tolerated to prevent adsorption atelectasis and oxygen toxicity. However, it should not be lowered any further even if the PaO_2 seems high in order to maintain a safety margin for oxygenation in the event that hypotension, dysrhythmias, bleeding, or a pneumothorax should suddenly develop.

E. The definitions of adult respiratory distress syndrome (ARDS) and TRALI include poor oxygenation with a PaO_2/FIO_2 ratio less than 200 and 300, respectively. However, such ratios are not that uncommon following open-heart surgery, especially in patients with significant COPD or in hypertensive smokers with low preoperative

PaO$_2$ levels.[55] Impaired oxygenation may be both cardiogenic and noncardiogenic in etiology, caused by fluid overload and/or a transient capillary leak from CPB. Acute pulmonary dysfunction is of concern when the PaO$_2$/FiO$_2$ ratio is <150 torr. This would correspond, for example, to a PaO$_2$ of only 150 torr on an FiO$_2$ of 1.0 or only 75 torr on an FiO$_2$ of 0.5. This is more likely to occur in patients with advanced age, obesity, pulmonary hypertension, low cardiac output syndromes, surgery requiring very long pump runs, and postoperative renal dysfunction.[17]

F. Some patients with chronic pulmonary disease have a relatively "fixed shunt" with a PaO$_2$ of 60–70 torr despite a high FiO$_2$ and moderate levels of PEEP. It is best to avoid an FiO$_2$ greater than 0.5 for more than a few days, if possible, to avoid complications associated with oxygen toxicity. Keep in mind that a PaO$_2$ of 65 torr corresponds to an O$_2$ saturation of 90% and is acceptable in these patients.

V. Basic Concepts of Alveolar Ventilation

A. The second goal of mechanical ventilation is that of alveolar ventilation, which regulates the level of PCO$_2$. This is controlled by setting the tidal volume and the respiratory rate on the ventilator and should provide a minute ventilation of approximately 8–10 L/min. The level of PCO$_2$ is determined most reliably by the arterial blood gases. Noninvasive monitoring with end-tidal CO$_2$ gives a reasonably accurate assessment of PCO$_2$, although the correlation depends on the amount of physiologic dead space.

B. **Hypocarbia**

1. Mild hypocarbia (PCO$_2$ of 30–35 torr) is quite acceptable in the immediate postoperative period, especially when the patient is hypothermic. It produces a mild respiratory alkalosis that:

   a. Decreases the patient's respiratory drive.

   b. Allows for increased CO$_2$ production to occur from the increased metabolic rate associated with warming and shivering without producing respiratory acidosis. Remember that the metabolic rate is decreased 10% for every degree below 37 °C and most patients return to the ICU from the operating room with a core temperature around 35–36 °C.

   c. Compensates for the mild metabolic acidosis that frequently develops from hypoperfusion and peripheral vasoconstriction when the patient is still hypothermic.

2. A more profound respiratory alkalosis has potential detrimental effects and must be avoided.

   a. It leads to hypokalemia and may predispose to ventricular arrhythmias.

   b. It shifts the oxygen–hemoglobin dissociation curve to the left, decreasing oxygen release to the tissues.

   c. It induces cerebral vasoconstriction, reducing cerebral blood flow.

   d. **Note:** Hypocarbia with a normal pH is masking a metabolic acidosis that may need to be evaluated and addressed.

3. **Management** of hypocarbia is best accomplished by lowering the IMV rate. The amount of dead space in the tubing can also be increased. Adding 10% of the tidal volume in mL/kg to the tubing will raise the PCO$_2$ approximately 5 torr.

    a. Although the addition of PEEP to the ventilator circuit usually prevents alveolar collapse by maintaining volume in the lungs above the critical closing volume, alveolar hypoventilation and atelectasis are best prevented by maintaining an adequate tidal volume of 8–10 mL/kg. The tidal volume can be lowered, but usually should be decreased only if peak inspiratory pressures are excessively high (over 35–40 cm H_2O).

    b. Occasionally, hypocarbia may develop in a patient who is "fighting the ventilator" with repeated triggering. These patients seem to be unable to breathe in synchrony with delivered breaths, such that the phases of respiration vary between the patient and the ventilator. This may be noted in patients with hypoxia, mental confusion or delirium, anxiety, or inadequate sedation. Some patients also become very agitated when spontaneous breaths are initiated against high levels of PEEP. Patient-ventilator dyssynchrony usually occurs in the assist mode when the patient's breath does not trigger the demand valve due to too insensitive a trigger. It may also occur when the tidal volume is set too high with a low inspiratory flow rate, resulting in an increase in the inspiratory time. Thus the patient becomes short of breath and has an increased work of breathing.

       i. It is important to assess the adequacy of ventilation and oxygenation first and ensure there are no major pleuropulmonary issues (mucus plugs, bronchospasm, tension pneumothorax) or mechanical issues with the ventilator.

      ii. The ventilator settings can be readjusted to increase the inspiratory flow rate or increase the time between the end of inspiration and the beginning of expiration with an end-inspiratory pause.

     iii. If no specific issues can be identified, additional sedation or selection of a different medication (propofol, fentanyl, or dexmedetomidine) and/or paralysis may be necessary to minimize the patient's respiratory drive.

     iv. Full ventilation is then resumed in the controlled mandatory ventilation (CMV) mode. PEEP levels should be decreased to 5 cm H_2O or less if PaO_2 permits.

      v. Pressure support ventilation (PSV) (see page 424) increases the comfort of the spontaneously breathing patient and may reduce the work of breathing.

C. Hypercarbia

  1. Hypercarbia indicates that the minute ventilation provided by the ventilator is inadequate to meet ventilatory demands. Adjustment of ventilator settings must accommodate the progressive increase in PCO_2 that occurs during the early postoperative period as the metabolic rate increases from warming and post-anesthetic shivering. During the weaning process, a slightly elevated PCO_2 in the range of 48–50 torr is usually acceptable, since the patient is still somewhat sedated. Higher levels of PCO_2 usually mean that the patient is not awake enough to maintain adequate ventilation.

  2. A lower tidal volume may be requested by the surgeon to minimize tension on a short ITA pedicle. In these patients, it is preferable to increase the IMV rate rather than the tidal volume to compensate for an elevated PCO_2.

3. During weaning from mechanical ventilation, hypercarbia may represent compensatory hypoventilation in response to a metabolic alkalosis. This frequently results from aggressive diuresis in the early postoperative period. Use of acetazolamide (Diamox) 250–500 mg IV q8–12h in conjunction with other diuretics is beneficial in correcting a primary metabolic alkalosis. However, the metabolic component should only be partially corrected in patients with chronic CO_2 retention.

4. **Manifestations** of significant hypercarbia and respiratory acidosis include tachycardia, increasing PA pressures, hypertension, and arrhythmias.

5. **Treatment**

   a. Moderate hypercarbia in the fully ventilated patient is corrected by increasing either the respiratory rate or tidal volume, as long as the peak inspiratory pressure is less than 40 cm H_2O.

   b. Significant hypercarbia usually indicates a mechanical problem such as ventilator malfunction, endotracheal tube malposition, or a pneumothorax. The latter may still be present even when bilateral breath sounds seem to be heard above all the other extraneous noises of the ICU setting. Temporary hand bag ventilation, adjustment of ventilator settings, repositioning of the endotracheal tube, or insertion of a chest tube will usually resolve the problem.

   c. Sedation can be obtained with short-acting narcotics or other sedatives. These include:

      i. Propofol 25–75 µg/kg/min

      ii. Morphine sulfate 2.5–5 mg IV q1–2 h

      iii. Dexmedetomidine 1 µg/kg over 10 minutes followed by a continuous infusion of 0.2–0.7 µg/kg/h. The loading dose provides sedation within 10–15 minutes after the infusion is started with offset of action of over 2 hours. The mix is 2 mL/50 mL normal saline, which gives a final concentration of 4 µg/mL.

      iv. Midazolam 2–4 mg IV q1h or 2–10 mg/h as a continuous infusion. This can reduce the total narcotic requirement but will delay extubation.

      v. Fentanyl drip can be used when a more prolonged period of sedation is indicated. The usual dose is a 50–100 µg IV bolus over 5 minutes with subsequent doses every 2 hours prn or an infusion of 50–200 µg/h of a 2.5 mg/250 mL mix.

   d. Shivering is best controlled using meperidine 25–50 mg IV. More persistent and refractory shivering that is deleterious to hemodynamics may need to be controlled with pharmacologic paralysis. **It is important never to paralyze an awake patient without also administering sedation.** Paralytic agents, including pancuronium, vecuronium, or atracurium can be used if meperidine fails to control the shivering (see Appendix 11 for doses).

6. If the patient becomes hypercarbic because of "fighting the ventilator" and is receiving inadequate tidal volumes, the steps noted above (change in ventilator settings, sedation, and conversion to PSV) will allow for improved ventilation.

7. The persistence of hypercarbia despite standard therapeutic measures usually indicates significant ventilatory failure. This will be discussed in the sections on acute and chronic respiratory insufficiency later in this chapter.

VI. Considerations To Achieve Early Extubation

A. An initial period of sedation is usually beneficial to allow for warming to normothermia, the achievement of hemodynamic stability, and evaluation of bleeding, following which "early extubation" can be achieved. This approach improves hemodynamic performance, decreases pulmonary complications, requires less medication, and allows for more rapid mobilization and a faster recovery. Virtually all studies have demonstrated the safety and efficacy of early extubation, with documentation of decreased length of stay and hospital costs.[1-3] Early extubation is feasible with most narcotics, although ultrafast extubation (within 1–3 hours) may be best with remifentanil because of its short half-life.[44] Although some centers try to extubate in the operating room or within 1 hour of arrival in the ICU, there is little difference in pulmonary function if one waits a few hours longer, and in high likelihood, ultrafast extubation does not reduce the length of stay in the ICU or the overall hospital stay.[2,56,57] In contrast, there is a potential benefit in being able to observe the patient for a short time to ensure stability. The important concept is that **extubation**, no matter when it is accomplished, **requires that standard criteria be met**. It should never represent "premature" extubation, when discontinuation of mechanical ventilation may prove deleterious to the patient's recovery.

B. The potential disadvantages of early extubation must always be taken into consideration. These include:

1. Increased sympathetic tone causing tachycardia and hypertension that can adversely affect myocardial recovery and can contribute to myocardial ischemia during the first 4–6 hours in the ICU.

2. Increased risk of bleeding if hypertension develops.

3. More chest pain and splinting if less analgesia is given. This may result in hypoventilation and atelectasis, potentially contributing to oxygen desaturation and the need for reintubation. Ineffective lung expansion is less capable of tamponading chest wall bleeding than positive-pressure ventilation (PPV).

4. Compromise of ventilatory status if there is significant fluid overload.

C. The selection of patients for early extubation should not be overly restrictive, yet it does depend on an understanding of potential risk factors for pulmonary dysfunction and delayed extubation. Some of these factors can be modified or influenced by therapeutic measures, whereas others cannot. The Society of Thoracic Surgeons (STS) risk model for operative mortality also provides a risk calculator for numerous complications, including prolonged ventilation beyond 48 hours. This can be accessed at the www.sts.org website. In addition, several studies have identified risk factors for acute pulmonary dysfunction upon arrival in the ICU and for increased respiratory morbidity and prolonged ventilation (Figure 10.2).[13,17-20,58-61] All of these factors must be taken into consideration when deciding whether early extubation is feasible or whether more prolonged support will be in the patient's best interest. Generally, about 5–10% of patients require ventilation for over 48 hours.[18,19] Evaluating these risk factors, one can define some exclusion criteria for early extubation (Table 10.2). Factors that delay extubation include:

1. Preoperative factors: older patient age, females, lower body surface area, preexisting impairment of cardiac (NYHA class IV/CHF, poor LV function, shock), respiratory (smoking, COPD, preoperative ventilation), and renal subsystems

Risk Factor	Score
Age 66-75	2
Age 76-80	5
Age > 80	5.5
$FEV_1 < 70\%$	1.5
Current smoker	1.5
Scr > 125-175 µmol/L (1.4-2 mg/dL)	2
Scr > 175 µmol/L (> 2 mg/dL)	4
PVD	2
EF < 30%	2
MI < 90 days	2
Preop ventilation	4
Reoperation	2.5
Urgent surgery	1.5
Emergent surgery	2
MV surgery	2
Aortic surgery	5.5
CPB	1.5

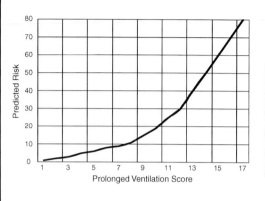

Figure 10.2 • Logistic model to predict risk of postoperative respiratory failure following cardiac surgery. A score ≥18 had a greater than 80% risk of requiring prolonged ventilation >48 hours (Adapted with permission from Reddy et al., *Ann Thorac Surg* 2007;84:528–36.)[19]

(elevated creatinine), obesity, diabetes,[62] urgent or emergent surgery with hemodynamic instability, and active endocarditis.

2. **Intraoperative factors:** reoperations, long duration of CPB (often for combined valve-CABGs or double valve operations), requirement for multiple blood

Table 10.2 • Exclusion Criteria for Early Extubation

Preoperative Criteria	Intraoperative Criteria	Postoperative Criteria
Pulmonary edema	Deep hypothermic circulatory arrest	Mediastinal bleeding
Intubated	Coagulopathy	Hemodynamic instability or need for an IABP
Cardiogenic shock	Severe myocardial dysfunction	Respiratory failure or hypoxia
Sepsis	Long pump run >4–6 hours	Stroke

products, significant fluid administration, elevated blood glucose on CPB, poor hemodynamic performance requiring inotropes or IABP support, perioperative MI.

3. **Postoperative factors:** excessive mediastinal bleeding, reexploration for bleeding or use of multiple blood products; low cardiac output syndromes, sepsis, pneumonia, renal dysfunction, stroke or depressed level of consciousness, GI bleeding.

D. The pharmacologic protocol for postoperative sedation should be similar for most patients, since propofol can be used for several days if prolonged support is not anticipated. Otherwise, more liberal use of a longer-acting medication (such as fentanyl) can be considered. Lorazepam has been used successfully as well, but is associated with a higher incidence of delirium and is not recommended.[63] Use of standard protocols and criteria for weaning should allow for extubation when clinically indicated, even if it takes a little longer than desired. The duration of intubation should not be based on risk factors alone or dictated by a rigid time schedule. Of interest, although smoking is a significant risk factor for postoperative morbidity, one study showed that it is advantageous to extubate smokers earlier rather than later to reduce the risk of respiratory complications.[64]

VII. Therapeutic Interventions to Optimize Postoperative Respiratory Performance and Early Extubation

A. Recognition of risk factors for pulmonary dysfunction can direct attention to potential therapeutic steps that can be taken to optimize postoperative respiratory performance. The treatment of modifiable factors, performance of a proficient operation, and aggressive postoperative management of all subsystems are essential to achieve early extubation and minimize the risk of postoperative respiratory failure.

B. **Preoperative considerations**

1. Attempt to convince the patient to stop cigarette smoking at least 1 month prior to surgery. Recommend use of nicotine patches or start the patient on varenicline (Chantix) or bupropion HCL (Wellbutrin, Zyban).

2. Treat all active cardiopulmonary disease processes, such as pneumonia, bronchospasm, or CHF, to optimize oxygenation and ventilatory status.

3. Consider intensive inspiratory muscle training in patients at high risk for pulmonary complications.[65,66]

4. Transfuse patients to a hematocrit of at least 28% prior to surgery to minimize the degree of hemodilution during surgery and the requirement for blood and blood components.

5. Optimize hemodynamic performance and renal function as best possible prior to surgery.

C. **Intraoperative considerations**

1. Modify the CPB circuit to minimize the inflammatory response, hemodilution and bleeding: use membrane oxygenators, centrifugal pumps, biocompatible circuits, or miniaturized circuits, if available; avoid cardiotomy suction; consider retrograde autologous priming and perhaps use of leukocyte-depleting filters.[67,68]

2. Process shed mediastinal blood at the conclusion of CPB through a cell-saving device to eliminate fat, particulate matter, and vasoactive mediators. This has

been shown to improve cardiopulmonary hemodynamics and may reduce ventilatory requirements after surgery.[69]

3. Minimize fluid administration during CPB or off-pump surgery.

4. Use antifibrinolytic therapy to minimize perioperative bleeding.

5. Perform an expeditious, technically proficient operation with excellent myocardial protection to achieve complete revascularization or satisfactory valve function.

6. Use inotropic support or an IABP as necessary to achieve satisfactory hemodynamic performance (cardiac index >2 L/min/m^2) and avoid excessively high filling pressures.

7. Pay fastidious attention to hemostasis.

8. Minimize use of blood and blood components.

9. Consider use of steroids (methylprednisolone or dexamethasone) to decrease the inflammatory response, although this has not conclusively been shown to produce much clinical benefit on pulmonary function.[70,71]

10. Control blood glucose on CPB with intravenous insulin (keep glucose <180 mg/dL).[72]

11. Consider ventilating the lungs during bypass (shown to improve post-pump oxygenation).[34]

12. Use pharmacologic intervention with either fenoldopam, nesiritide, or a bicarbonate infusion in patients with renal dysfunction (creatinine >1.4 mg/dL) to optimize renal function during CPB (see Chapter 12, pages 598–600).[73–76]

13. Consider hemofiltration to remove fluid in patients with preoperative CHF or renal dysfunction and to remove inflammatory mediators.[77]

14. Use short-acting narcotics and propofol for sedation to allow for early extubation.

D. **Postoperative considerations**

1. Select medications to provide short-acting anxiolysis and sedation that either allow the patient to awaken and be extubated within hours of its discontinuation (propofol) or while still being given (dexmedetomidine).

2. Provide adequate analgesia without producing respiratory depression (continuous IV morphine, NSAIDs, epidural analgesia).

3. Use antihypertensive medications, rather than sedatives, to control hypertension.

4. Administer volume judiciously to optimize hemodynamics, and then use diuresis once hemodynamics have stabilized to eliminate extravascular lung water.

5. Have a higher threshold for blood transfusions (hematocrit in the low 20s) except in elderly patients or those with hypotension, tachycardia, or oxygenation issues, in whom a higher hematocrit may be beneficial.

6. Initiate aggressive management of postoperative bleeding with low threshold for reexploration to minimize use of blood products, which can lead to increased pulmonary morbidity including TRALI.[35–37]

7. Initiate hyperglycemia protocol to reduce risk of sternal wound infection (see Appendix 6).[72,78]

VIII. Ventilatory Weaning and Extubation in the Immediate Postoperative Period

A. **Criteria for weaning**. Weaning a patient from the ventilator depends on the ability and desire of the nursing and medical staffs to identify when the patient is ready to be weaned, and their willingness to initiate weaning when indicated, no matter what time of the day or night, not when it is convenient to do so. The criteria for weaning are noted in Table 10.3.

B. **Method of weaning after short-term ventilation**

1. Minimize sedation or use dexmedetomidine.

2. Maintain the FIO_2 at 0.5 or below with PEEP of no more than $5-7.5$ cm H_2O. If the patient still requires a higher level of PEEP, weaning is usually not indicated. If oxygenation is satisfactory, lower the PEEP in $2.5-5$ cm H_2O increments to 5 cm H_2O and initiate weaning.

Table 10.3 • *Weaning Criteria from Mechanical Ventilation*

Initial Postoperative Period

1. Awake with stimulation

2. Adequate reversal of neuromuscular blockade

3. Chest tube drainage <50 mL/h

4. Core temperature $>35.5\,°C$

5. Hemodynamic stability

    a. Cardiac index >2.2 L/min/m^2

    b. Blood pressure stable at $100-140$ systolic on/off meds

    c. Heart rate <120 bpm

    d. No arrhythmias

6. Satisfactory arterial blood gases (ABGs) on full ventilation

    a. $PaO_2/FIO_2 >150$ ($PO_2 >75$ torr on FIO_2 of 0.5)

    b. $PCO_2 <50$ torr

    c. pH $7.30-7.50$

Prolonged Ventilation

1. Underlying disease process has resolved

2. Awake, oriented with adequate mental alertness to initiate an inspiratory effort

3. Hemodynamic stability on no vasoactive drugs

4. Hemoglobin and metabolic status are optimized

5. Satisfactory ABGs as above (many studies recommend $PaO_2/FIO_2 >200$) with respiratory rate <35/min

6. Rapid shallow breathing index (respiratory rate/tidal volume in liters) <100

Table 10.4 • Failure Criteria During Weaning from the Ventilator

1. Somnolence, agitation, or diaphoresis
2. Systolic blood pressure increases by more than 20/min or to over 160 mm Hg
3. Heart rate changes by more than 20% in either direction or to over 120 bpm
4. Acute need for vasoactive medication
5. Arrhythmias develop or become more frequent
6. Respiratory rate increases more than 10 breaths/min or to over 35/min for 5 minutes
7. PaO_2 falls to less than 60 torr on FiO_2 of 0.5 or SaO_2 falls to less than 90%
8. PCO_2 rises above 50 torr with respiratory acidosis (pH < 7.30)

---

3. Weaning is usually accomplished in the SIMV mode. The IMV rate is reduced by two breaths every 30 minutes with observation of the SaO_2. If the patient is alert with good respiratory efforts, he/she may be immediately placed on CPAP of 5 cm H_2O. If the ABGs and respiratory mechanics are acceptable after a 30–60 minute spontaneous breathing trial (SBT) on either T-piece or CPAP of 5 cm H_2O (see extubation criteria below), the endotracheal tube is removed.

4. Weaning should be stopped and ventilation resumed at a higher rate when there are clinical signs that it is not being tolerated. These signs are noted in Table 10.4.

5. **Note:** A rise in PA pressures is often the first hemodynamic abnormality noted in the patient who is not tolerating weaning very well. Tachypnea is the first clinical sign of ineffective weaning.

C. **Extubation criteria** include the weaning criteria listed in Table 10.3 as well as the additional considerations noted in Table 10.5.

D. Extubation may be accomplished from CPAP or T-piece. Although oxygenation may be slightly better during a CPAP than a T-piece trial, post-extubation oxygenation is frequently better in patients weaned with T-piece because the PaO_2 declines less than in patients who were extubated from CPAP.[79]

E. Additional considerations

1. Some patients get very agitated when sedatives are weaned. Even though adequate ABGs may be maintained, agitated patients are frequently given more sedation throughout the night with another attempt at weaning in the morning. Steps noted on page 394 may be taken if the patient is breathing dyssynchronously with the ventilator. Gradual weaning of sedation, substituting dexmedetomidine for propofol, assurance from the nurses that "you're doing well", and then a very rapid wean to CPAP and extubation is often the best course for these patients.

2. If the patient was very difficult to intubate in the operating room, it is essential to ensure that the ABGs and respiratory mechanics are satisfactory before extubation. Extubation in the middle of the night should be performed cautiously in these patients. An individual experienced in difficult intubations should be present. A flexible laryngoscope, video laryngoscope, or bronchoscope should also be available.

Table 10.5 • Extubation Criteria

Initial Postoperative Period

1. Awake without stimulation

2. Acceptable respiratory mechanics

   a. Negative inspiratory force >25 cm H_2O

   b. Tidal volume >5 mL/kg

   c. Vital capacity >10–15 mL/kg

   d. Spontaneous respiratory rate <24/min

3. Acceptable arterial blood gases (ABGs) on 5 cm or less of CPAP or PSV

   a. PaO_2 >70 torr on FiO_2 of 0.5 or less

   b. PCO_2 <48 torr

   c. pH 7.32–7.45

Prolonged Ventilation

1. Comfortable breathing pattern without diaphoresis, agitation or anxiety; respiratory rate <35/min

2. Adequate mental status to protect the airway, initiate a cough, and raise secretions

3. Hemodynamic tolerance of the weaning process as delineated in Table 10.3

4. Respiratory mechanics and ABGs as above

5. A cuff leak >110 mL with the cuff deflated

3. Elderly patients and those with more advanced cardiac disease or hepatic dysfunction often take longer to awaken from anesthesia even if sedatives are not administered. This may reflect slow metabolism of medications administered intraoperatively or may occasionally represent transient obtundation from borderline cerebral hypoperfusion during surgery or other causes. It is important to resist the temptation to reverse narcotic effect with naloxone. This medication can precipitate severe pain, anxiety, hypertension, dysrhythmias, and bleeding, and may result in recurrent respiratory depression when its effects have worn off. Similarly, flumazenil to reverse benzodiazepines should be avoided early in the postoperative period. Keep in mind that the offset of propofol is significantly greater when doses producing deep sedation are used.[48]

4. However, if a patient fails to awaken after 24–36 hours and the question arises as to whether this represents a stroke, encephalopathy, or simply residual sedation, one might consider the cautious use of a reversal agent to sort out the nature of the problem. Naloxone (Narcan) may be given in 0.1–0.2 mg IV increments every 3 minutes. Flumazenil is given in a dose of 0.2 mg IV over 30 seconds, followed by doses of 0.3 mg, then 0.5 mg every 30 seconds, if necessary, to a maximum of 3 mg in one hour.

5. Many patients, especially those who have received supplemental narcotics, will demonstrate excellent respiratory mechanics when stimulated, but then drift off

to sleep and become apneic. Constricted pupils may be noted in patients with persistent narcotic effect. These patients are not yet ready for weaning and extubation. Do not confuse comfortable breathing with persistent narcotic or sedative effect.

IX. Post-Extubation Respiratory Care (Table 10.6)

A. After extubation, the patient's breathing pattern, SaO_2, and hemodynamics must be observed carefully. Occasionally, especially in the patient who was difficult to intubate, laryngeal stridor may be prominent and may require use of racemic epinephrine, steroids, or even reintubation. Failure to demonstrate a "cuff leak" during positive-pressure ventilation when the cuff is deflated usually indicates laryngotracheal edema that may cause upper airway obstruction after extubation. This phenomenon is uncommon after short-term intubation, but may be noted after several days of mechanical ventilation (see page 422).

B. Because the median sternotomy incision is associated with moderate discomfort and decreased chest wall compliance, patients tend to splint, take shallow breaths, and cough poorly. Oxygenation may be compromised by fluid overload and atelectasis from poor inspiratory effort. It is advisable to supply 40−70% humidified oxygen by face mask for a few days.

C. If the patient has borderline oxygenation, higher levels of oxygen may need to be provided or some form of noninvasive ventilation utilized to improve oxygenation and avoid reintubation.[80,81]

    1. A non-rebreather mask covers the patient's nose and mouth and is attached to a reservoir bag which is continuously filled with oxygen at a rate of 8−15 L/min. The patient inhales oxygen from the reservoir bag and then exhales through a one-way valve to the atmosphere, thus ensuring that little exhaled gas or room air is inspired during the next breath. Partial rebreather masks lack the one-way valve, but ensure a higher FiO_2 than a simple face mask because of a tighter fit and the oxygen reservoir bag.

Table 10.6 • Post-Extubation Respiratory Care

1. Monitor pulse oximetry

2. Place on face mask, nasal cannula, or BiPAP mask to achieve $SaO_2 > 90\%$

3. Adequate analgesia (morphine, ketorolac)

4. Chest x-ray after pleural tubes are removed

5. Incentive spirometer/deep breaths q1−2h; use cough pillow

6. Mobilization as soon as possible; frequent repositioning in bed

7. Compression stockings (T.E.D.) for VTE prophylaxis; consider Venodyne boots or SC heparin if high-risk

8. Aggressive diuresis once hemodynamically stable

9. Bronchodilators for bronchospasm (consider steroids if severe COPD)

10. Antibiotics for a positive sputum culture

2. Bilevel positive airway pressure (BiPAP) noninvasive ventilation delivers preset inspiratory and expiratory positive airway pressure. It is superior to incentive spirometry in improving oxygenation in the first few postoperative days.[82] It has also been shown to prevent the increase in extravascular lung water associated with the weaning process that is noted in patients placed on nasal cannula after extubation.[83]

3. Continuous positive airway pressure (CPAP) provides a continuous level of positive airway pressure without any ventilatory support. Nasal CPAP masks are helpful in patients with cardiogenic pulmonary edema by preventing alveolar collapse, redistributing intra-alveolar fluid, improving pulmonary compliance, and reducing the pressure of breathing.[84] A study of prophylactic nasal CPAP of 10 cm H_2O for at least 6 hours showed that it improved oxygenation better than CPAP for 10 minutes every 4 hours, with a lower incidence of pneumonia and reintubation.[85] However, another study found noninvasive pressure support ventilation (NIPSV) superior to CPAP in preventing atelectasis after surgery.[86]

D. Upon transfer to the floor, most patients benefit from use of supplemental oxygen via nasal cannula for a few days. Monitoring of SaO_2 by pulse oximetry is helpful in patients with borderline oxygenation, especially during ambulation. The patient should be mobilized and encouraged to cough and take deep breaths. A cooperative patient who can actively participate in these maneuvers can generally prevent atelectasis and pulmonary complications, but additional support is commonly necessary in elderly patients and those with significant chest wall discomfort. A "cough pillow" should be used to brace the chest during deep breathing and coughing to minimize discomfort and splinting.

1. An incentive spirometer is very beneficial in maintaining the functional residual capacity (FRC) and preventing atelectasis, although its effectiveness in preventing postoperative pulmonary complications is unclear.[87] A literature review showed that CPAP, BiPAP, or intermittent positive-pressure breathing (IPPB) produced better pulmonary function and oxygenation than incentive spirometry, although the incidence of complications was comparable. However, none of these was more effective than preoperative patient education.[88] One study showed that the same benefit could be derived from taking 30 deep breaths without mechanical assistance as from use of a blow bottle device or inspiratory resistance positive expiratory pressure mask.[89]

2. Chest physical therapy may be helpful in patients with significant underlying lung disease, borderline pulmonary function, or copious secretions, but otherwise is of little additional benefit.[90] Albuterol administered via nebulizer is frequently beneficial in patients with bronchospasm.

E. Although dysphagia with difficulty swallowing foods is unusual in patients intubated for less than 48 hours, it is not uncommon following a longer duration of intubation. Careful attention must be paid to the patient's initial oral intake to observe for potential aspiration. Patients who require longer periods of intubation usually require a full swallowing evaluation before initiating oral intake (see page 696).[91,92]

F. Once the patient is hemodynamically stable and no longer needs volume administration to maintain intravascular volume, aggressive diuresis with intravenous furosemide, either with intermittent bolus doses or a continuous infusion, should be initiated to eliminate excess extravascular lung water. Diuretics are continued until the patient has reached his/her preoperative weight and can be weaned from nasal cannula with an acceptable SaO_2 (>90% on room air).

G. Satisfactory analgesia is very helpful in improving the patient's respiratory effort. Initially, intravenous morphine is given, either as bolus doses or as an infusion, and is supplemented by an NSAID, such as ketorolac 15–30 mg IV or IM. Subsequently, most patients do well with oral narcotics such as oxycodone or hydrocodone with acetaminophen. Patients with significant pain issues may benefit from patient-controlled analgesia (PCA) pumps that provide morphine, fentanyl, or remifentanil.[52,53] Alternatively, a fentanyl patch (Duragesic) can be used in patients with persistent pain despite opioid use. A common dose is 25 µg/h, which is the dose delivered by a 10 cm^2 patch. Note that the fentanyl plasma concentration is increased by amiodarone.

H. Elastic graduated compression (anti-embolism) stockings (GCS) should be used routinely for patients after surgery to reduce the risk of venous thromboembolism (VTE). Mobilization is probably more important in reducing this risk. If the patient remains in the ICU and is sedated or poorly mobilized, sequential or intermittent pneumatic compression devices (IPC), such as the Venodyne system, should be used.[93] A recommendation for early initiation of heparin therapy for VTE prophylaxis is controversial, especially because of the potential risk of developing a hemopericardium and delayed tamponade.[94,95] The 2008 ACCP recommendation is to use **either** low-molecular-weight heparin (usually enoxaparin 40 mg qd) **or** low-dose unfractionated heparin (5000 units SC bid), **or** "optimally used" bilateral GCS or IPC for patients at high risk for VTE.[96]

X. Acute Respiratory Insufficiency/Short-Term Ventilatory Support

A. Prolonged mechanical ventilation beyond 48 hours is necessary in about 5–10% of patients undergoing open-heart surgery.[18,19] It may be necessary until hemodynamic issues or transient pleuropulmonary insults, such as pulmonary edema, have resolved. It may also be indicated for patients without intrinsic pulmonary problems who are sedated, obtunded, or sustain neurologic insults. These patients may have adequate gas exchange but need an endotracheal tube for airway protection.

B. Acute respiratory insufficiency characterized by inadequate oxygenation (PaO_2 <60 torr with an FiO_2 of 0.5 or PaO_2/FiO_2 ≤120) or ventilation (PCO_2 >50 torr) during mechanical ventilatory support occurs in up to 10% of patients undergoing surgery on cardiopulmonary bypass.[17] This usually results from a severe perioperative cardiopulmonary insult (such as a long duration of CPB or postcardiotomy low cardiac output syndrome) that is superimposed on preexisting lung disease. Predisposing factors to acute pulmonary dysfunction are essentially the same as those that are predictive of the need for prolonged ventilatory support (see pages 396–398).

1. Predisposing factors to acute pulmonary dysfunction immediately after surgery include advanced age, significant COPD, active smoking history, obesity (BMI >30 kg/m^2), diabetes, a mean PA pressure ≥20 mm Hg, depressed left ventricular function (stroke volume index ≤30 mL/m^2), low serum albumin, a history of cerebrovascular disease and clinical CHF.[17]

2. Intraoperative factors include emergency surgery and CPB time ≥140 minutes. The latter is often associated with a significant inflammatory response, due to which patients usually receive a significant amount of volume during and after surgery.

3. The development of acute respiratory insufficiency is associated with more renal dysfunction, gastrointestinal and neurologic complications, nosocomial infections, and the need for prolonged mechanical ventilatory support.[18] The development of multisystem organ problems explains the high mortality rate of postoperative respiratory failure, which averages 20−25%.

4. Several logistic models have been created which are predictive of prolonged ventilatory failure (>72 hours).[19,20] One simple model found that the combination of a Parsonnet score >7 (Table 3.9, page 158) with a poor ejection fraction, age >65 with pulmonary hypertension, or an emergency reoperation for bleeding or cardiac arrest predicted 50% of patients requiring prolonged ventilation (>24 hours). A more sophisticated bedside model is noted in Figure 10.2.[19]

C. "Acute lung injury" defined by poor oxygenation is a clinical spectrum that ranges from a transient phenomenon with low risk to that of ARDS, which carries a very high mortality rate. In most patients with a PaO_2/FiO_2 ratio <200−300 immediately after surgery, a short period of ventilatory support while the patient is hemodynamically supported and diuresed usually results in improvement in oxygenation and the requirement for very short-term ventilation. In contrast, acute lung injury may progress to a chronic phase of ventilatory dependence in fewer than 5% of patients. It is also more likely in older patients with preexisting pulmonary, cardiac, or renal problems that compromise postoperative recovery or when postoperative care is complicated by stroke, bleeding, and multiple blood transfusions.[18,19] Chronic respiratory insufficiency/ventilator dependence will be discussed in section XI (pages 413−418).

D. Etiology. During the first 48 hours, oxygenation problems predominate and can produce tissue hypoxia. Inadequate ventilation (hypercapnia) at this time is usually the result of a mechanical problem.

1. Inadequate O_2 delivery and ventilation (mechanical problems)

    a. Ventilator malfunction

    b. Improper ventilator settings: low FiO_2, inspiratory flow rate, tidal volume, or respiratory rate

    c. Endotracheal tube problems: cuff leak, incorrect endotracheal tube placement (larynx, mainstem bronchus, esophagus), kinking or occlusion of the tube

2. Low cardiac output states leading to mixed venous desaturation, venous admixture, and hypoxemia

3. Pulmonary problems

    a. Atelectasis or lobar collapse

    b. Pulmonary edema

        i. Cardiogenic from fluid overload and/or left ventricular dysfunction, hemodilution on pump with reduced colloid oncotic pressure.

        ii. Noncardiogenic from pulmonary endothelial injury with increased microvascular permeability. This may be related to activation of complement, neutrophils, and macrophages with release of inflammatory mediators associated with extracorporeal circulation. This problem is more prominent as the duration of bypass lengthens and is more common in patients receiving multiple blood transfusions.[32]

    c. Pneumonia

    d. Intrinsic pulmonary disease (COPD), bronchospasm, or air trapping

    e. Blood transfusions: microembolization, transfusion of proinflammatory mediators, TRALI

  4. Intrapleural problems

    a. Pneumothorax

    b. Hemothorax or pleural effusion

  5. Metabolic problems: shivering leading to increased peripheral oxygen extraction

  6. Pharmacologic causes: drugs that inhibit hypoxic pulmonary vasoconstriction (nitroglycerin, nitroprusside, calcium channel blockers, ACE inhibitors)[97]

E. The acute development of shortness of breath or an abrupt change in ABGs after an uneventful early postoperative course should raise suspicion of the following problems:

  1. Pneumothorax, possibly tension

  2. Atelectasis or lobar collapse from poor inspiratory effort or mucus plugging

  3. Aspiration pneumonia

  4. Acute pulmonary edema (from myocardial ischemia, LV dysfunction, or undetected renal insufficiency)

  5. Delayed tamponade causing a low cardiac output syndrome

  6. Pulmonary embolism

F. **Manifestations**

  1. Tachypnea (rate >30 breaths/min) with shallow breaths

  2. Paradoxical inward movement of the abdomen during inspiration ("abdominal paradox")

  3. Agitation, diaphoresis, obtundation, or mental status changes

  4. Tachycardia or bradycardia

  5. Arrhythmias

  6. Hypertension or hypotension

G. **Assessment and management** of acute respiratory insufficiency during mechanical ventilation (Table 10.7).[98]

  1. **Examine the patient:** auscultate for bilateral breath sounds and listen over the stomach to make sure the tube has not slipped into the larynx or been placed in the esophagus.

  2. **Increase the FIO_2 to 1.0** until the causative factors have been identified. **Manually ventilate** with a resuscitation bag (Ambu) if ventilator malfunction is suspected. This not only provides ventilation but also permits an assessment of pulmonary compliance. **Note:** Make sure the gas line on the bag is attached to the oxygen (green) and not the room air (yellow) connector and the gas has been turned on.

  3. **Ensure adequate alveolar ventilation**

    a. **Check ventilator function** and settings and optimize the following:

      i. Tidal volume

      ii. Ventilator trigger sensitivity

Table 10.7 • Management of Acute Ventilatory Insufficiency

1. Examine patient, ventilator settings and function, ABGs, and chest x-ray

2. Hand ventilate with 100% oxygen; increase FiO_2 on ventilator until problem is sorted out

3. Ensure alveolar ventilation by correcting mechanical problems (adjust ventilator, reposition endotracheal tube, insert chest tube)

4. Assess and optimize hemodynamics

5. Add PEEP in 2.5–5 cm H_2O increments while decreasing FiO_2 to 0.5 or less; serially evaluate cardiac outputs at higher levels of PEEP to ensure optimal systemic oxygen delivery

6. Consider sedation or paralysis if patient-ventilator dyssynchrony not improved by change in ventilator settings

7. Treat identifiable problems

    a. Diuretics for pulmonary edema

    b. Antibiotics for pneumonia

    c. Bronchodilators for bronchospasm

    d. Transfusion for low hematocrit (<26%)

8. Chest physiotherapy

9. Begin nutritional supplementation

---

    iii. Inspiratory flow rate. Patients with COPD may have significant air trapping which produces an autoPEEP effect. This is noted when inspiration commences before expiratory airflow is completed, resulting in positive airway pressure at the end of expiration. It can exacerbate the adverse hemodynamic effects of PPV, cause barotrauma, and impair patient triggering of assisted ventilation. Steps that can be taken to eliminate this problem are discussed on pages 420–421.

  b. Obtain a chest x-ray to look for any of the potential etiologic factors listed above; specifically note any mechanical problems that can be corrected by simple repositioning of the endotracheal tube or chest tube insertion.

  c. Repeat the ABGs

  d. Note: An acute increase in peak inspiratory pressure may signify the development of a pneumothorax, although it can also result from severe bronchospasm, flash pulmonary edema, mainstem intubation, or an obstructed airway (copious secretions, the patient biting the endotracheal tube).

  4. Assess and optimize hemodynamic status. A Swan-Ganz pulmonary artery catheter is useful in assessing the patient's fluid status and cardiac output. The latter can also be assessed less invasively using a FloTrac device, which measures continuous cardiac outputs from an arterial line, or using an esophageal Doppler. A low cardiac output reduces oxygen delivery, lowers the mixed venous oxygen saturation, and increases venous admixture, further decreasing the PaO_2. Inotropic support or diuresis may be indicated to improve oxygenation. An echocardiogram may be helpful in identifying a contributory problem, such as significant LV or RV dysfunction, cardiac tamponade, mitral regurgitation, or a recurrent ventricular septal defect.

5. **Alveolar recruitment** maneuvers that increase the mean airway pressure can open previously closed alveoli to increase the surface area for oxygen exchange and prevent early airway closure. This will decrease intrapulmonary shunting by improving ventilation to perfused areas. It will also redistribute lung water from the alveoli to the perivascular interstitial space, although it does not decrease extravascular lung water content.

   a. A baseline level of 5 cm H_2O of **PEEP** is usually added to the circuit for all patients admitted to the ICU. This substitutes for the loss of the "physiologic PEEP" of normal breathing caused by the endotracheal tube. This level of PEEP is well tolerated by the heart, but probably does little to improve oxygenation.[47]

   b. PEEP is added in increments of 2.5−5 cm H_2O up to 10 cm H_2O or greater to improve oxygenation and allow weaning of the FIO_2 to less than 0.5. With low mean airway pressures, intrapulmonary shunting may result from inadequate ventilation of perfused alveoli, and increasing the FIO_2 alone will often be ineffective in improving oxygenation if the shunt exceeds 20%. This problem can be overcome by increasing the tidal volume and the level of PEEP. Furthermore, using an $FIO_2 > 0.5$ for several days can produce alveolar-capillary damage, alveolar collapse, and stiff, noncompliant lungs (so-called "oxygen toxicity").

   c. Caution must be exercised when using high levels of PEEP because it will accentuate the adverse effects of PPV on hemodynamics by creating high positive airway and intrathoracic pressures.[99] Increasing levels of PEEP reduce venous return, increase pulmonary vascular resistance (PVR) which can depress RV performance, and will lead to decreased LV filling and a reduced cardiac output in the hypovolemic patient. Thus, adding PEEP could be counterproductive because it may actually reduce oxygen transport and tissue oxygenation, lower the mixed venous oxygen saturation, and increase admixture, further decreasing the PaO_2. Volume infusion is necessary to counteract these effects before increasing the level of PEEP. The optimal level of PEEP can be determined by observation of the arterial waveform and serial assessments of cardiac function while adjustments are being made.

   d. One study showed that although oxygenation may be comparably improved by using a high level of CPAP (40 cm H_2O) or a high level of PEEP (20 cm H_2O), the latter is usually associated with more stable hemodynamics.[100]

   e. Adding high levels of PEEP to patients with severe COPD results in increased transmission of airway pressure to the lungs, resulting in overdistention of alveoli that are highly compliant and poorly perfused, resulting in increased V/Q shunting and possibly producing endothelial damage and progressive hypoxia.

   f. In patients with intrinsic pulmonary disease, and especially ARDS, the PVR may be elevated and the lungs less compliant. Increasing levels of PEEP may produce RV failure and dilatation, shifting the interventricular septum and compromising filling and compliance of the left ventricle. In these patients, volume infusion must be given cautiously.

g. High levels of PEEP can result in "barotrauma" (pneumothorax, subcutaneous emphysema, or pneumomediastinum), which can compromise ventilation and produce acute hemodynamic embarrassment. Barotrauma is caused by alveolar overdistention, and is attributable more directly to the severity of the underlying lung disease than to the peak airway pressure. Nonetheless, modes of ventilation that provide lower tidal volumes have been used in patients with ARDS to improve oxygenation.[101]

h. **Note:** Care must be exercised when suctioning a patient on high levels of PEEP. Oxygenation can become very marginal when PEEP has been temporarily discontinued. A PEEP valve should be used during manual ventilation if the patient's oxygenation is dependent on PEEP.

i. The interpretation of pressure tracings from a pulmonary artery catheter is influenced by PEEP. The measured CVP, PA, and left atrial pressures are elevated, but transmural filling pressures, which determine the gradient for venous return, are decreased, because pressure is transmitted through the lungs to the pleural space. A general rule is that the true pulmonary capillary wedge pressure (PCWP) is equal to the measured pressure minus one-half of the PEEP level at end-expiration (minus one-quarter if lung compliance is decreased). Another way of assessing the PCWP is the "index of transmission":[99]

$$\text{Index of transmission} = (\text{end-inspiratory PCWP} - \text{end-expiratory PCWP})/$$
$$(\text{plateau airway pressure} - \text{total PEEP})$$

$$\text{Transmural PCWP} = \text{end-expiratory PCWP}$$
$$- (\text{index of transmission} \times \text{total PEEP})$$

j. In situations in which the alveolar pressure exceeds that in the pulmonary vessels (e.g., during hypovolemia), the PCWP will reflect the intra-alveolar pressure and not the left atrial pressure.

6. **Sedation** with/without paralysis often improves gas exchange by improving the efficiency of ventilation. It can relax the diaphragm and chest wall and reduce the energy expenditure or "oxygen cost" of breathing. A sedation protocol (Figure 10.3) with titration of drug effect using a sedation scale, such as the Ramsay scale or the Richmond Agitation Sedation Scale (RASS) (Tables 10.8 and 10.9), should be utilized to optimize patient comfort.[102–104] It is generally preferable to use propofol or dexmedetomidine if it is anticipated that a short additional period of ventilatory support is required. Otherwise, fentanyl may be used to reduce pain and anxiety. Lorazepam is probably the least beneficial medication to use because it is associated with a higher rate of delirium in the ICU.[63,104]

7. Additional supportive measures include the following:

a. **Diuresis** (usually with IV furosemide) usually improves oxygenation in the early postoperative period when pulmonary interstitial edema may impair gas exchange. Depending on the patient's hemodynamic stability and renal function, a continuous infusion of IV furosemide (10–20 mg/h) can be used to promote a steady diuresis.

b. The patient's chest x-ray should be reviewed and cultures obtained of pulmonary secretions. Indiscriminate use of antibiotics should be discouraged, but broad-

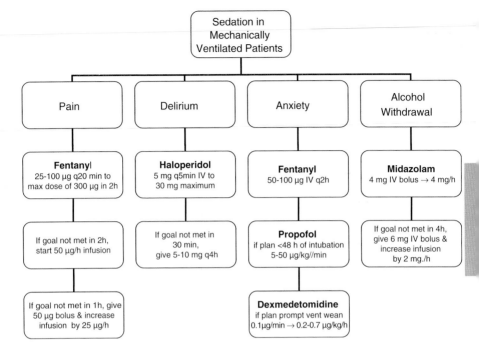

Figure 10.3 • Algorithm for sedation in the ICU.

spectrum antibiotics can be initiated if there is suspicion of an infectious component to the patient's borderline pulmonary function. The antibiotics should then be modified depending on culture sensitivities.

c. **Bronchodilators,** such as albuterol, are useful for patients with increased airway resistance that may be compromising their ventilatory or hemodynamic status. Steroids may be useful for the patient with severe COPD (see page 428).

Table 10.8 • Ramsay Scale	
Sedation Level	**Description**
1	Anxious and agitated
2	Cooperative, tranquil, oriented
3	Responds only to verbal commands
4	Asleep with brisk response to light stimulation
5	Asleep without response to light stimulation
6	Nonresponsive

Table 10.9 • Richmond Agitation Sedation Scale (RASS)

Target RASS	RASS Description
+4	Combative, violent, danger to staff
+3	Pulls or removes tubes or catheters; aggressive
+2	Frequent nonpurposeful movement, fights ventilator
+1	Anxious, apprehensive, but not aggressive
0	Alert and calm
−1	Awakens to voice (eye opening/contact) >10 sec
−2	Light sedation, briefly awakens to voice (eye opening/contact) <10 sec
−3	Moderate sedation, movement or eye opening. No eye contact
−4	Deep sedation, no response to voice, but movement or eye opening to physical stimulation
−5	Unarousable, no response to voice or physical stimulation

    d. Measures to prevent atrial fibrillation should be considered since patients with intrinsic lung disease or postoperative respiratory failure are more predisposed to the development of postoperative arrhythmias, which can compromise hemodynamic performance. Cardioselective β-blockers can be used safely even in patients with bronchospasm. Short-term use of amiodarone is rarely associated with idiosyncratic acute respiratory failure and should not deter its use in patients with COPD.[105,106]

    e. Blood transfusions can be given to treat anemia if the hematocrit is less than 26%. Despite the intuitive logic that blood transfusions should improve blood oxygen content and tissue oxygen delivery and should potentially reduce the duration of mechanical ventilation, there is little benefit, and even a detriment, to a liberal transfusion policy.[107,108] Transfused red cells have a low level of 2,3-DPG and thus initially have poor oxygen-carrying capacity, they transmit proinflammatory mediators that can worse pulmonary function, and they are immunosuppressive, increasing the risk of nosocomial infection.[35]

    f. Bronchoscopy may be beneficial when postural drainage and suctioning are unable to resolve atelectasis because of the presence of tenacious secretions.

8. Methods of mechanical ventilation for patients requiring prolonged ventilatory support are discussed in section XII (pages 418–421).

XI. Chronic Respiratory Failure/Ventilator Dependence

A. Etiology. The inability to wean the patient from the ventilator within a few days after surgery may be caused by problems that impair oxygenation ("hypoxemic respiratory failure)" and/or produce primary ventilatory insufficiency ("hypercapneic respiratory failure"). Although many patients can be weaned after a few days of additional ventilatory support once contributing factors have been treated, a few will progress to a phase of ventilator dependence. Although consensus conferences consider "prolonged mechanical ventilation" to be >21 days in duration,[109] the STS considers it to be >24 hours from the time the patient arrives in the ICU. Most studies of cardiac surgery patients use either ventilation times >24 h or >48 h as the definition. Nonetheless, any patient who cannot be weaned within a few days of surgery should be managed so as to achieve extubation as soon as is feasible. The mortality rate associated with the need for prolonged ventilation for just 5 days after cardiac surgery is approximately 20–25% with death commonly resulting from multisystem organ failure.

1. **Hypoxia.** The persistence of oxygenation problems beyond 48 hours usually indicates severe hemodynamic compromise or an acute parenchymal lung problem. These are frequently superimposed on preexisting problems, such as preoperative acute pulmonary edema, pulmonary hypertension, or COPD. The primary causes of hypoxemia are:

   a. Hemodynamic instability, especially a low cardiac output state that requires multiple pressors. This increases the oxygen cost of breathing and can produce both hypoxemia and hypercarbia.

   b. Parenchymal problems:

      i. Interstitial pulmonary edema, either noncardiogenic (capillary leak or sepsis) or cardiogenic (CHF)

      ii. Pneumonia

      iii. Lower airway obstruction (bronchitis, secretions, bronchospasm) often associated with COPD

2. Adult respiratory distress syndrome **(ARDS)** represents a nonspecific diffuse acute lung injury with inflammation of the lung parenchyma. It is associated with noncardiogenic pulmonary edema from increased microvascular permeability. The lungs become stiff and noncompliant with severe impairment to gas exchange from alveolar-capillary damage, interstitial edema, and atelectasis. ARDS can produce both oxygenation and ventilatory failure.[110,111]

   a. CPB has been implicated as a causative factor of ARDS because it produces a systemic inflammatory response. Neutrophil-initiated pulmonary dysfunction with oxygen free-radical generation is suspected to be the mechanism of this injury. However, since ARDS develops in fewer than 1% of patients undergoing open-heart surgery, other important contributory factors must be present. Factors such as older age, smoking, and hypertension have been associated with the development of ARDS, but they are very common comorbidities in surgical patients.[32,111]

   b. Although the pathophysiology of ARDS appears to be noncardiogenic in nature, most patients developing the syndrome have compromised cardiac function. The major risk factors for the development of postoperative ARDS are reoperations, perioperative shock, increasing number of blood transfusions, emergency surgery, poor LV function, and advanced NYHA class. It might be inferred that the capillary leak associated with CPB may be worse in patients in poor clinical condition, especially if there is perioperative hemodynamic compromise, and these patients are more prone to develop this highly lethal syndrome. Subsequently, any additional insult, such as pneumonia, sepsis, cardiogenic pulmonary edema from LV dysfunction or renal failure, or multiple transfusions, will lead to progressive respiratory deterioration, multisystem organ failure, and death.

3. Transfusion-related acute lung injury **(TRALI)** is similar in appearance to ARDS with noncardiogenic pulmonary edema resulting from increased microvascular permeability. It is most likely an immune-mediated phenomenon with interaction between donor plasma antibodies and recipient leukocyte antigens.[37] This may then result in the release of cytotoxic substances that damage lung tissue. The definition of TRALI includes a PaO_2/FiO_2 <300 along with the development of pulmonary infiltrates within 6 hours of transfusion. This carries a much more favorable prognosis than ARDS, but should still be distinguished from the more benign postoperative scenario of hypoxemia in patients who may have received transfusions that does not satisfy this definition.

4. **Hypercarbia.** Primary ventilatory failure is caused by an imbalance between ventilatory capacity and demand and is the most common reason for failure to wean from the ventilator.[112] The patient is incapable of generating the respiratory effort necessary to sustain the "work of breathing", a term that refers to the work necessary to overcome the impedance to ventilation produced by the disease process and the resistance of the ventilator circuitry. Contributory factors include:

   a. Increased ventilatory demand with increased CO_2 production and O_2 demand
      i. Sepsis (which also impairs oxygen uptake), fever, chills
      ii. Pain, anxiety
      iii. Catabolic states
      iv. Carbohydrate overfeeding
      v. Increased dead space (COPD)
      vi. Reduced lung compliance – pneumonia, pulmonary edema
      vii. Increased resistance – bronchospasm, airway inflammation
   b. Decreased respiratory drive
      i. Altered mental status from medications, stroke, delirium, or encephalopathy
      ii. Sleep deprivation
   c. Decreased respiratory muscle function
      i. Significant obesity
      ii. Ventilatory muscle weakness from protein malnutrition, medications (neuromuscular blockers, aminoglycosides, steroid myopathy), dynamic hyperinflation, disuse myopathy, or critical illness polyneuropathy
      iii. Metabolic abnormalities (hypophosphatemia, hyper- or hypomagnesemia, hypokalemia, hypocalcemia, hypothyroidism)
      iv. Diaphragmatic paralysis from phrenic nerve injury. This may be caused by the use of iced slush within the pericardial well during cardioplegic arrest. Unilateral paralysis usually does not cause ventilatory insufficiency unless

there is severe underlying lung disease. Bilateral paralysis may require prolonged ventilatory support, although recovery can usually be anticipated within a year.[113] Diaphragmatic plication can improve pulmonary function when the patient is severely compromised by this problem.[114]

    d. The transition from mechanical to spontaneous ventilation with conversion from positive to negative intrapleural pressure increases LV afterload. This increases metabolic and cardiac demands and may not be tolerated by patients with limited cardiac reserve.

B. **Clinical manifestations** of ventilator dependence that often indicate inability to wean include:

    1. Tachypnea (rate >30 breaths/min) with shallow breaths

    2. Paradoxical inward movement of the abdomen during inspiration ("abdominal paradox")

C. **Management** involves selecting an appropriate means of ventilation (see section XII, pages 418–421) while identifying the factors that may be contributing to ventilator dependence.[98,115,116] Measures should be taken to optimize cardiac performance, improve the respiratory drive and neuromuscular competence, and reduce the respiratory load by improving intrinsic pulmonary function and reducing the minute ventilation requirement (Table 10.10). As these issues are being addressed, it is important to identify when a patient is ready for weaning or discontinuation of ventilatory support. One study suggested that there was a trigger point of recovery

---

Table 10.10 • Supportive Measures in Patients with Chronic Ventilatory Failure

1. Select appropriate mode of ventilatory support

2. Suction PRN and prevent aspiration

3. Optimize hemodynamic status

4. Provide adequate analgesia but avoid oversedation and neuromuscular blockers; use intermittent interruption of sedatives rather than a continuous infusion

5. Provide adequate nutrition, preferably with low carbohydrate enteral feedings

6. Optimize metabolic and electrolyte status (thyroid, hematocrit, glucose, magnesium, phosphate)

7. Specific considerations:

    a. Bronchodilators/steroids for bronchospasm

    b. Antibiotics for infections/antipyretics for fever

    c. Diuresis for fluid overload

    d. Drain any pleural effusions

    e. Specific measures to prevent ventilator-associated pneumonia

8. Physical therapy and repositioning to prevent decubitus ulcers

9. Stress ulcer prophylaxis with sucralfate or a proton-pump inhibitor

10. Consider tracheostomy if anticipate prolonged ventilatory support > 2 weeks

usually related to an improvement in respiratory mechanics that indicates when fairly rapid weaning is feasible in patients with chronic respiratory failure.[117]

1. **Improve hemodynamic status** with inotropic support. Pulmonary vasodilators, such as nitroprusside and nitroglycerin, should generally be avoided because they can increase intrapulmonary shunting by preventing hypoxic vasoconstriction. Milrinone is beneficial by providing inotropic, lusitropic (relaxant), and vasodilator effects that can improve RV and LV function.

2. **Improve respiratory drive and neuromuscular competence**

   a. Avoid oversedation and neuromuscular blockers. Daily interruption of sedation is associated with more rapid weaning from ventilatory support than a continuous sedative infusion.[118–120]

   b. Provide adequate nutrition to achieve positive nitrogen balance and improve respiratory muscle strength and immune competence. Most patients fare well with standard tube feedings, but in patients with significant hypercarbia, low-carbohydrate tube feedings (Pulmocare) should be considered. Overfeeding with carbohydrates or fats can increase CO_2 production and the respiratory quotient (RQ), which will add to the ventilatory burden. The RQ represents the CO_2 output/O_2 uptake and is normally 0.8.

   c. Select the appropriate mode of ventilatory support to reduce the work of breathing and train the respiratory muscles to support spontaneous ventilation.[115] Avoid prolonged periods of spontaneous ventilation until the patient appears ready for a weaning trial. In patients with severe oxygen desaturation, use of the prone position may improve oxygenation and allow for earlier weaning.[121]

   d. Optimize acid–base, electrolyte, and endocrine (thyroid) status. Metabolic alkalosis and hypothyroidism inhibit the central respiratory drive. Correct potassium, magnesium, and phosphate levels. Correct profound anemia.

   e. Initiate physical therapy.

   f. Evaluate diaphragmatic motion during fluoroscopy ("sniff test"). Diaphragmatic plication may improve respiratory function in patients with ventilator dependence caused by unilateral diaphragmatic dysfunction.

3. **Reduce the respiratory load**

   a. Reduce impedance to ventilation

      i. Give bronchodilators or steroids for bronchospasm (see pages 427–428).

      ii. Employ chest physical therapy, frequent repositioning, and suctioning to mobilize and aspirate secretions and prevent atelectasis.

      iii. Consider tracheostomy (see pages 417–418).

   b. Improve lung compliance

      i. Antibiotics for pneumonia

      ii. Diuretics for fluid overload and pulmonary edema

      iii. Thoracentesis or tube thoracostomy for pleural effusions

      iv. Prevent abdominal distention with nasogastric suction or metoclopramide

   c. Reduce the minute ventilation requirement

      i. Provide adequate analgesia for pain and sedatives for anxiety. Excessive sedation must be avoided because it inhibits the central respiratory drive.

    ii. Administer antipyretics for fever to reduce metabolic demand.

   iii. Treat infections (sepsis, pneumonia) with appropriate antibiotics to minimize antibiotic resistance.

   iv. Avoid overfeeding to lower CO_2 production.

4. Take steps to prevent **ventilator-associated pneumonia** (VAP) or initiate appropriate treatment once it develops.

  a. VAP is common in patients who are older, receive more blood transfusions or require reexploration, are undergoing reoperations, ascending aortic, or emergent surgery, are taking steroids, require inotropic support, or require more prolonged duration of ventilation. It is noted in up to 45% of patients on mechanical ventilation for over 48 hours and is associated with a mortality rate around 40%.[122–126]

  b. Basic strategies involve using oral intubation and attempting extubation as soon as feasible, adequate hand washing by the healthcare team, keeping the patient semi-recumbent, draining condensates from the ventilator circuit, maintaining adequate cuff pressure to prevent aspiration, avoiding gastric overdistention, using oro- rather than nasogastric tubes, initiating enteral feedings when feasible to provide adequate nutritional support, and using continuous subglottic suctioning. Oropharyngeal cleansing with 0.12–2% chlorhexidine reduces the risk of VAP.[127]

  c. Stress ulcer prophylaxis should be achieved using sucralfate rather than antacids or H_2 antagonists that raise gastric pH. Proton pump inhibitors have been found to be very effective in reducing the risk of stress-related bleeding, but some studies have shown an increased risk of nosocomial pneumonia compared with H_2 blockers,[128] while others have not found this to be the case.[129]

  d. The use of selective digestive decontamination to reduce the incidence of lower respiratory tract infection is controversial and not routinely recommended.[126,130] There is evidence that the combination of topical oropharyngeal agents, drugs given down the nasogastric tube (tobramycin, polymyxin, and amphotericin), and intravenous antibiotics (broad-spectrum cephalosporins) can reduce the incidence of VAP in surgical patients, but this strategy may lead to the emergence of antibiotic-resistant strains.

  e. Organisms causing early- and late-onset VAP are usually different. Early-onset VAP often responds to empiric monotherapy (such as ceftriaxone) until specific culture results are available. Late-onset VAP is commonly caused by *Enterobacter*, *Pseudomonas*, or MRSA, and usually requires initial combination therapy with antibiotics such as ceftazidime, ciprofloxacin, and vancomycin.[126]

5. Tracheostomy should be performed to reduce the risk of laryngeal damage and swallowing dysfunction if it is anticipated that the patient may require mechanical ventilatory support for more than 2 weeks. A tracheostomy reduces airway resistance and glottic trauma, improves the ability to suction the lower airways, lowers the risk of sinusitis (although it probably does not reduce the risk of VAP), improves patient comfort and mobility, often allows the patient to eat, and generally makes the patient look and feel better. It commonly leads to earlier decannulation than standard endotracheal intubation.

    a. Avoidance of tracheostomy is reasonable when it is anticipated that extubation might be accomplished within 7–10 days. One study of patients on ventilatory support for 3 days found clinical parameters suggesting the absence of major organ system problems to be predictive of successful weaning by the 10th postoperative day. These included a Glasgow coma score of 15, urine output >500 mL/24 h, absence of acidosis (bicarbonate ≥20 mmol/L), no requirement for epinephrine or norepinephrine, and absence of lung injury.[131]

    b. The traditional concept has been that tracheostomy should be delayed for at least 2–3 weeks after a median sternotomy to decrease the risk of deep sternal wound infection (DSWI). Studies present conflicting results on whether a percutaneous or surgical tracheostomy or its timing influences the risk of DSWI. It is likely that the increased risk noted in some studies is related to the severity of illness producing respiratory failure and other associated complications rather than the tracheostomy itself.[131–137]

    c. A percutaneous dilatational tracheostomy performed at the bedside has a low complication rate that may include bleeding, posterior tracheal laceration, tube obstruction from hematoma or tracheal edema of the posterior wall, and stomal infection. The incidence of late tracheal stenosis is lower than that of a surgical tracheostomy.

XII. Methods of Ventilatory Support[112,115]

    A. Full ventilatory support is required when the patient remains anesthetized and sedated after surgery. It is also required for the patient with acute or chronic respiratory failure while underlying disease processes are treated and nutrition is optimized. Ventilatory support is initially provided using volume- or pressure-controlled ventilation. Inadequate support may lead to ventilatory muscle fatigue, whereas excessive support may lead to muscle atrophy, so settings for each patient must be individualized.

    B. Positive-pressure ventilation improves ventilation/perfusion matching to increase the efficiency of gas exchange. It also reduces the work of breathing in the sedated and/or paralyzed patient. However, weaning from ventilatory support should be initiated as soon as feasible to minimize the potential complications of prolonged ventilatory support that contribute to its high mortality. These include:[18,99]

      1. Pulmonary effects (barotrauma, acute lung injury, ventilator-associated pneumonia), diaphragmatic atrophy, respiratory muscle weakness (polyneuropathy), and diminished mucociliary clearance

      2. Hemodynamic compromise

      3. Gastrointestinal issues: stress ulceration, hypomotility and intolerance of tube feedings, splanchnic hypoperfusion, swallowing difficulties after extubation

      4. Renal dysfunction and fluid retention

      5. Increased intracranial pressure (from reduced cerebral venous flow)

      6. Disordered sleep and delirium

    C. **Volume-limited modes**. Most patients are initially placed on "volume ventilators" that deliver a preset tidal volume. A limit is set on the peak pressure to avoid barotrauma. Patients with noncompliant stiff lungs or bronchospastic airways can be difficult to ventilate in this mode because some of the preset tidal volume may not be delivered once the peak pressure limit is reached. This system is best for patients with normal or increased compliance (emphysema).

1. Ventilator settings should be selected to provide a minute ventilation of 8–10 L/min. These include a respiratory rate of 10–12/min and a tidal volume of 8–10 mL/kg (<6 mL/kg for low tidal volume ventilation for ARDS).[101] 5 cm of PEEP is routinely added. Adjustments may be made based upon ABGs, but the plateau airway pressure should ideally be maintained <30 cm H_2O.

2. **Assist/control (A/C) ventilation** delivers a preset tidal volume when triggered by the patient's inspiratory effort (a demand valve senses a negative airway deflection) or at preset intervals if no breath is taken. The rate should generally be set about 4 breaths below the patient's spontaneous rate or at 10–12 breaths/min before the patient begins spontaneous breathing. If the patient is out of synchrony with the ventilator or hyperventilates, a significant respiratory alkalosis or acidosis may occur. This mode of ventilation is best used only when the patient requires significant ventilator support and should not be used for weaning. In fact, the patient's efforts may persist despite the machine's superimposed breath, leading to increased respiratory muscle fatigue.

3. **Controlled mandatory ventilation (CMV)** will provide a positive-pressure breath to the patient at a preset tidal volume and rate. This should also be used only during the temporary period of full ventilator support because it will lead to respiratory muscle deconditioning.

4. **Intermittent mandatory ventilation (IMV).** In the IMV mode, the patient's spontaneous inspiration will generate a tidal volume consistent with his or her effort and the machine will deliver a full tidal volume at a designated rate.

5. **Synchronized intermittent mandatory ventilation (SIMV).** In the SIMV mode, the patient breathes spontaneously and, at preset intervals, the next spontaneous breath is augmented by a full tidal volume from the ventilator. Since the ventilator's breath is synchronized to the patient's efforts, high peak pressures are avoided and breathing is more comfortable. Flow-by triggering is used such that the ventilator provides a breath when the return flow is less than the delivered flow. This results in decreased work of breathing. Because many of the patient's efforts are not augmented, SIMV should not be used during the early phase of chronic ventilatory support because it increases the work of breathing more than A/C ventilation. However, it is an excellent mode for ventilatory weaning in that it produces good patient-ventilator synchrony, preserves respiratory muscle function, and produces a low airway pressure. A low level of pressure support can be added to decrease the work of spontaneous breathing.

D. **Pressure-limited (cycled) ventilation.** Pressure ventilators deliver gas flow up to a set peak airway pressure limit at a preset respiratory rate. The amount of gas flow delivered (the tidal volume) depends upon the compliance of the lungs, airway resistance, and tubing resistance. This ensures delivery of a more consistent tidal volume to patients with increased airway resistance (bronchospasm, restrictive lung disease). It is best avoided in patients with emphysema, in whom overinflation of the lungs can occur at low pressures. The peak airway pressure is constant but generally lower than with volume-limited ventilation. It may produce more homogeneous gas distribution, improved gas exchange, better patient-ventilator synchrony, and perhaps earlier weaning from mechanical ventilation than volume-limited ventilation. However, there is little evidence that it improves oxygenation or the work of breathing.[98] Pressure-limited ventilation can be delivered in the A/C, CMV, or IMV (SIMV) mode.

1. **Pressure-limited A/C** allows the patient's inspiratory effort to trigger pressure-limited breaths in addition to those delivered at the set respiratory rate and pressure.

2. **Pressure-limited CMV** (pressure-controlled ventilation or PCV) is a time-cycled mode of ventilation that provides no additional ventilation above that delivered by the preset peak airway pressure and respiratory rate. PCV at a level of 20 cm H_2O provides full ventilatory support with a tidal volume of about 8–10 mL/kg. This is used in a similar manner to volume-controlled CMV in the patient who is not initiating any spontaneous breaths.

3. **Pressure-limited IMV** allows the patient to take spontaneous unassisted breaths in addition to ventilation provided at the set rate and pressure limit.

E. **Pressure support ventilation (PSV)** is a flow-limited system that provides ventilation only as triggered by the patient's efforts. It will then deliver inspiratory pressure until the inspiratory flow falls below about 25% of its peak value. The tidal volume delivered following the patient's inspiratory effort depends on the selected level of pressure support and inspiratory flow rate, lung compliance and airway resistance, and the resistance of the circuitry. PSV is best used to provide partial support as the patient is weaned from the ventilator (see pages 424–425) since it cannot provide any support unless the patient triggers a breath.

F. No matter which mode of ventilation is selected, attention must be paid to avoiding high peak inspiratory pressures. This can produce barotrauma as well as hemodynamic compromise by impeding venous return and impairing ventricular function. The inspiratory plateau pressure (IPP), which is the peak pressure at the end of inspiration, should be maintained at less than 35 cm H_2O. Means of lowering the IPP include lowering of the level of PEEP, lowering the tidal volume, or decreasing the inspiratory flow rate to increase the inspiratory:expiratory (I:E) ratio.

1. Low tidal volume ventilation has been used in patients with ARDS. It is believed that alveolar overdistention can produce changes in endothelial cell permeability and produce barotrauma and noncardiogenic pulmonary edema. Low tidal volume ventilation (5–6 mL/kg) may improve oxygenation with permissive hypercapnia, and has been associated with reduced mortality in patients with ARDS.[101]

2. Decreasing the inspiratory flow rate increases the inspiratory flow time and may decrease peak pressures. However, if the expiratory time is too short to allow for full exhalation, as may occur in patients with bronchospastic airways, the next breath may be "stacked" on top of the previous one, producing lung hyperinflation and the autoPEEP effect.[99] Inspiration will commence before expiratory airflow is completed, resulting in positive airway pressure at the end of expiration. This may impair patient triggering of assisted ventilation. This problem can be overcome by taking steps to improve the expiratory phase of ventilation:

   a. Increasing the inspiratory flow rate (tidal volume/inspiratory flow time)

   b. Decreasing the I:E ratio

    c. Treating conditions that increase expiratory flow resistance, such as bronchospasm

    d. Decreasing the respiratory rate or tidal volume

    e. Adding PEEP to the ventilator settings

  3. Patient-ventilator dyssynchrony occurs when the phase of respiration differs between the patient and the ventilator. The patient appears to be fighting the ventilator, becomes short of breath, and tires out from the increased work of breathing. Although patient-related factors, such as delirium, may be contributory, ventilator adjustments can usually overcome the problem. For example, ineffective triggering or too long an inspiratory time (i.e., the tidal volume is too high for the inspiratory flow rate) may cause dyssynchrony.[98]

G. Noninvasive positive-pressure ventilation (NIPPV) can be used as a means of avoiding intubation in patients with acute respiratory decompensation.[138] It can also facilitate earlier extubation in patients in whom standard criteria are not quite met. The primary advantage is the avoidance of the risks of intubation, including laryngotracheal trauma, sinusitis, and respiratory tract infections.

  1. Generally, an oronasal mask with a soft silicone seal is used to improve patient comfort, although it can make the patient feel claustrophobic. A bilevel positive airway pressure (BiPAP) device is commonly used because it is leak-tolerant, allows for rebreathing, and is more effective in lowering the PCO_2. The term BiPAP is usually used for these devices, but this is actually the trademark of a ventilator manufactured by Respironics, Inc.

  2. The oxygen flow rate is adjusted to achieve an SaO_2 >90%. Generally, it is not possible to exceed an FIO_2 of 0.5, so if the patient is severely hypoxic, intubation will usually be necessary.

  3. The ventilator is set in a pressure-limited mode with an initial pressure of 8–10 cm H_2O and gradually increased to a maximum of 20 cm H_2O. This limits the maximal inspiratory time and improves patient–ventilator synchrony. The expiratory pressure is set at 5 cm H_2O.

  4. Use of dexmedetomidine is very helpful in reducing patient agitation during NIPPV for hypoxia because it does not produce respiratory depression.[139]

XIII. Weaning from the Ventilator[112,116,140,141]

  A. Once it is decided that a patient no longer requires full ventilatory support, a means of weaning the patient from the ventilator should be selected. Intuitively, the gradual reduction of ventilatory support using either IMV or PSV should allow for strengthening of the respiratory muscles and a successful wean. However, studies of weaning modalities have shown that this strategy does not expedite the weaning process, and in fact may delay it. Thus, a common practice is to decide when withdrawal of support might be possible and then place the patient on a T-tube trial of spontaneous ventilation.

  B. Practical aspects of weaning and extubation

    1. It is essential to address and treat all the potentially correctable causes of respiratory failure. Once this has been accomplished, weaning can be initiated if the criteria noted in Table 10.3 are met. Generally, weaning should not be considered if the patient has insufficient oxygenation (PaO_2 <55 torr).

2. The use of sedatives during mechanical ventilation is usually necessary to reduce the patient's anxiety and minute ventilation requirements.[102–104] However, continuous IV sedation depresses the patient's sensorium and respiratory drive and can delay the weaning process. Thus, a sedation protocol with daily awakening and administering sedatives only as necessary should expedite the weaning process.[118–120]

3. No matter which technique is used for weaning (T-piece, SIMV, or PSV), a spontaneous breathing trial (SBT) is performed using T-piece or a low level of CPAP or PSV for no more than 2 hours. All of these techniques are associated with fairly comparable extubation outcomes.[142]

   a. If the patient appears to be weaning satisfactorily with a comfortable breathing pattern and mental status, adequate hemodynamics and ABGs (Tables 10.3 and 10.5), extubation can be accomplished. Additional concerns include the ability to protect the airway, initiate a cough and raise secretions. The necessity to suction more than every 2 hours for excessive secretions may preclude extubation.

   b. One of the criteria often used to predict the possibility of post-extubation stridor and the need for reintubation is the "cuff leak" test. A crude way of doing this is to deflate the endotracheal tube cuff and feel how much of the delivered breath exits around the tube. One objective method involves recording the difference between the inspiratory tidal volume and the average of several expiratory tidal volumes with the cuff deflated. A cuff leak <110 mL may be predictive of post-extubation stridor, although some studies have found this assessment a very insensitive and inaccurate predictor of stridor.[143,144] One of the problems with this method is that some of the inspiratory volume may also leak with the cuff down, so the cuff leak volume may be spuriously high since it may measure both inspiratory and expiratory leak.[145] A third method is the "percent cuff leak", which measures the difference between the exhaled tidal volume with the cuff up and down, divided by the exhaled volume with the cuff up. Values less than 10% are predictive of stridor and the need for reintubation.[146]

   c. If there are concerns about post-extubation stridor, especially in patients intubated >6 days, steroids may be of benefit in reducing laryngeal edema. Most studies suggest that this must be started at least 4 hours and possibly 12–24 hours prior to planned extubation. Regimens include methylprednisolone 20–40 mg IV q4–6 h or dexamethasone 4 mg IM q6h.[147–149]

   d. If the patient does not satisfy extubation criteria after a SBT, 24 hours of full ventilation is recommended before another attempt at weaning. If the next attempt is unsuccessful, pressure-support weaning is probably better than T-piece or SIMV weaning.[139] It is estimated that about 10% of patients will still require reintubation even if they meet extubation criteria.

4. Noninvasive positive-pressure ventilation using BiPAP can improve oxygenation in many patients after extubation. It may be used to provide ventilatory support if the patient is extubated even though standard criteria are not met. If the patient has evidence of pulmonary edema, mask CPAP usually suffices.[138]

C. Predictors of weaning success

1. Several predictors of weaning success have been evaluated, but the easiest and arguably most sensitive predictor of a successful ventilatory wean is a "rapid shallow breathing index" (RSBI) of less than 100 breaths/min.[150-152] The RSBI is the ratio of the respiratory rate/tidal volume in liters during spontaneous ventilation for 1 minute. If the RSBI is <100, a weaning trial should be attempted because the estimated rate of successful weaning is greater than 80%. An RSBI >100 does not preclude weaning, since about 50% of such patients can be weaned and extubated. Generally, however, if the RSBI exceeds 100 and the patient's respiratory rate is greater than 38 during a brief SBT, the likelihood of a successful wean is quite low. One study found that extubation failure was most likely when the RSBI was >57, the patient was in positive fluid balance within the 24 hours before extubation, or pneumonia was present at the time of extubation.[153]

2. Maintenance of satisfactory oxygenation with comfortable breathing usually predicts successful extubation. These include markers such as a PaO_2 >60 torr on an FiO_2 <0.35, a PaO_2/FiO_2 ratio >200 or A-a gradient <350 torr on 100% oxygen.

3. Careful observation of the patient's breathing pattern is very important in assessing weaning success. Evidence of tachypnea, increased respiratory effort, or change in hemodynamics (especially an increase in PA pressure if a Swan-Ganz catheter is in place) often suggest that the patient is not tolerating the weaning process (Table 10.4).

D. T-piece weaning

1. T-piece weaning traditionally involved alternating periods of full support (rest) with increasing periods of independent spontaneous ventilation (stress) to theoretically increase the strength and endurance of the respiratory muscles. However, the sudden transition to a complete workload may not be well tolerated in the early phase of recovery from severe ventilatory failure and may result in profound respiratory muscle fatigue.

2. However, once contributing factors to a patient's ventilatory dependence have been addressed and it is ascertained that weaning should be attempted, an SBT of 30 minutes to 2 hours can be used to see if the patient satisfies the criteria for extubation. T-piece weaning in this fashion appears to be the most rapid method of achieving extubation.[140,142]

E. Synchronous intermittent mandatory ventilation (SIMV) weaning

1. With SIMV, the mandatory breaths are patient-triggered, thus avoiding over-inflation and improving the patient's comfort. During the weaning process, the IMV rate is gradually decreased and the patient assumes a greater proportion of the minute ventilation. Since the energy expenditure of the respiratory muscles increases as the IMV rate is lowered, lowering of the IMV rate during the day can be coupled with complete rest at night to avoid muscle fatigue.

2. Patient effort increases in proportion to both the ventilator-assisted breaths and spontaneous breaths.[140] Respiratory muscle rest does not occur during the mandatory breath and this may induce respiratory muscle fatigue. Although

SIMV uses a demand trigger valve, use of a flow-by system provides adequate gas flow to minimize the work of breathing. When the patient can maintain spontaneous ventilation for a prolonged period of time and satisfies standard criteria, extubation can be accomplished.

3. The use of pressure support concomitantly with IMV can also reduce the work of breathing during the patient's spontaneous respirations. Weaning can be accomplished by initially reducing the IMV rate and subsequently reducing the level of pressure support. The duration of spontaneous ventilation on progressively lower levels of pressure support or CPAP is then extended and the patient is extubated.

4. Rapid SIMV weaning is usually used immediately after surgery to achieve early extubation. However, most studies have shown that SIMV weaning is the least effective means of weaning a chronically ventilated patient.[112,140,152]

F. Pressure support ventilation (PSV) weaning[115,140]

1. With PSV, the patient's spontaneous inspiration triggers the ventilator to deliver gas flow to the circuit until a selected amount of inspiratory pressure is achieved ("patient-triggered" and "pressure-limited"). If the patient does not trigger the ventilator, no breath is delivered. Airway pressure remains constant by automatic adjustment of the flow rate as long as the patient maintains an inspiratory effort. Inspiratory gas flow stops when the inspiratory flow rate falls below 25% of the peak inspiratory flow rate, and exhalation is then allowed to occur passively. Modifications of this system include "volume support", with which the PSV level is automatically adjusted to provide a preset tidal volume, and "volume assured pressure support", with which additional volume is given to provide a preset tidal volume, even if the pressure rises.

2. The patient's own effort determines the respiratory rate, the inspiratory time and flow rate (tidal volume/inspiratory time), and the expiratory time. The tidal volume received depends on the level of PSV, the patient's respiratory effort, and any airway resistance. As long as the inspiratory flow is adequate, higher levels of support will reduce the work of breathing, especially since it can overcome any impedance in the system (small endotracheal tube, bronchospasm, secretions) to initiate ventilation. Thus, PSV generally results in more comfortable breathing for the patient. By reconditioning the respiratory muscles to assume more spontaneous ventilation without producing excessive energy expenditure, PSV may expedite the weaning process.

3. PSV results in lower peak airway pressures, slower respiratory rates, and higher tidal volumes than other modes of ventilation. Thus, it is beneficial for the patient who is out of synchrony with the ventilator ("fighting the ventilator"). However, if the patient has COPD, the inspiratory phase may be prolonged and the patient may try to expire during late inspiration from the ventilator. This may induce patient discomfort but can be counteracted by reducing the level of pressure support or converting to pressure control to provide a shorter inspiratory phase.

4. Weaning is accomplished by progressively lowering the levels of PSV and observing the patient for fatigue and other parameters indicative of intolerance of the weaning process (Table 10.4). Weaning options include:

a. Increasing the duration of spontaneous ventilation with lower levels of PSV during the daytime ("sprinting") with full support of higher levels of PSV at night. If the patient tolerates PSV for 12 hours, the level of PSV is gradually reduced by 2 cm H_2O intervals daily or every other day, and the tidal volume and respiratory rate are assessed. Extubation is accomplished when the patient is able to breathe comfortably for 2 hours at low levels of PSV (around 6–8 cm H_2O support).

b. PSV with IMV. A level of partial PSV support is selected and the IMV rate is gradually decreased. When the IMV rate has been reduced to less than 4 breaths/min, the PSV level is decreased as discussed above.

c. If the failure criteria noted in Table 10.4 are noted, PSV should be titrated to achieve a respiratory rate <25/min and an additional period of support should be provided before another attempt at weaning.

5. Potential disadvantages of PSV

a. PSV requires an intact respiratory drive to trigger the ventilator. Inadequate ventilation will result if the patient is apneic or has an unstable neurologic status, respiratory drive, or mechanics.

b. Cardiac output may be compromised because airway pressure is always positive. With IMV weaning, there is a phase of negative intrathoracic pressure that can augment venous return.

c. Shallow tidal volumes from poor inspiratory effort may lead to atelectasis.

d. A gas leak in the system may prevent PSV from being terminated, producing persistently high airway pressures and hemodynamic compromise.

e. In-line nebulizers (for bronchodilators) are in the inspiratory limb and may make it difficult for the patient to initiate a breath to trigger PSV.

XIV. Other Respiratory Complications

A. Respiratory complications can occur during the period of mechanical ventilation, soon after extubation, or later during convalescence on the postoperative floor. The management of these complications must be individualized, taking the patient's overall medical condition, the extent and nature of the surgical procedure, the precipitating factors, and the phase of recovery into consideration. The management of pneumothorax, pleural effusions, chylothorax, and bronchospasm are discussed here. Pulmonary embolism, diaphragmatic dysfunction, and pneumonia are discussed in Chapter 13.

B. **Pneumothorax.** If the pleural space is entered at the time of surgery, a chest tube should be placed for evacuation of air and fluid. Occasionally, a small pneumothorax will be noted on an early postoperative chest x-ray, often related to passage of a sternal wire through the pleura. If small, this may be managed conservatively, but it may potentially enlarge with the use of positive-pressure ventilation and therefore must be carefully reassessed. A chest tube should be placed for a larger pneumothorax. Less commonly, a pneumothorax will be absent on the initial x-ray but evident on subsequent films. A small pneumothorax noted after extubation or after chest tube removal can generally be observed and monitored by serial x-rays if the patient is asymptomatic.

1. Always consider the possibility of a pneumothorax (possibly tension) when ABGs deteriorate or hemodynamic instability develops for no obvious reason after several hours of stability. The first sign is often a sudden increase in the peak inspiratory pressure, indicated by repeated alarming of the ventilator.

2. Evidence of an air leak in the chest drainage system may indicate loose connections, rather than a leak from the lung. However, chest tubes should never be removed until it is confirmed that an air leak is not the result of an intrapleural or parenchymal problem. Air leaks gradually resolve in the vast majority of patients within a few days. If not, placement of a new pleural tube through the lateral chest wall should be considered. Use of a Heimlich valve may allow the patient to be discharged with an active air leak.

3. Progressive subcutaneous emphysema may develop if air exits under positive pressure where the pleura has been violated. In patients with severe emphysema or bronchospastic airways, it may result from alveolar rupture. However, it may result from visceral pleural injury at the time of surgery, no matter how small. Subcutaneous emphysema may occur when the chest tubes are still in place (usually when they are kinked), but it more commonly occurs after they have been removed. A pneumothorax may or may not be present. Management usually requires placement of unilateral or bilateral chest tubes, and, if the emphysema is severe, performing decompressing skin incisions in the upper chest or neck.

4. A chest x-ray should always be performed after the removal of pleural chest tubes. A small pneumothorax (<20%) can be observed with serial films. However, aspiration of the pleural space or placement of a new chest tube is indicated for a larger pneumothorax or if the patient is symptomatic.

C. **Pleural effusions** are noted postoperatively in approximately 60% of patients undergoing cardiac surgery and are more common when the pleural cavity has been entered for ITA takedown.[154] This usually results from oozing of blood and serous fluid from the chest wall. However, a hemothorax may develop if blood spills over from the pericardial space. An effusion developing on the right side is more commonly serous in nature from fluid overload.

1. **Prevention.** Adequate drainage of opened pleural cavities at the time of surgery should reduce the incidence of bloody effusions, but the optimal positioning of chest tubes in the most dependent portion of the pleural space is often not accomplished. This is especially true after ministernotomy incisions. Leaving a silastic (Blake) drain in the pleural cavity for several days after surgery has been shown to lower the incidence of late pleural effusions.[155]

2. A hemothorax may develop if significant mediastinal bleeding drains into an opened pleural cavity. This may prove beneficial in avoiding cardiac tamponade, but should be suspected in the patient with hemodynamic instability, a falling hematocrit, filling pressures that fail to rise with volume (although they may rise if tamponade is also developing), and increasing peak inspiratory pressures on the ventilator. A supine chest x-ray may demonstrate more opacification on one side than the other, but the degree of hemothorax may be difficult to determine. If it cannot be well defined by chest x-ray, a CT scan is helpful. However, compared with an upright chest x-ray, a CT scan tends to overestimate the size of an effusion that may be clinically insignificant. Echocardiography can also identify a large left pleural effusion.

3. A large pleural effusion can produce atrial or ventricular diastolic collapse and cardiac tamponade even in the absence of a pericardial effusion.[156,157] These findings can be confirmed by echocardiography.

4. Most patients with pleural effusions are asymptomatic, and in the vast majority of cases, small effusions resolve within a few months, either with use of diuretics (especially right-sided effusions) or spontaneously. However, patients with underlying lung disease or moderate effusions may develop dyspnea. In these situations, a thoracentesis is indicated either in the hospital or during a follow-up visit. This can usually be performed safely based upon evaluation of a chest x-ray, but ultrasound-guided thoracentesis may be helpful in improving localization for needle placement.[158] Chest tube placement may be considered for large effusions in the early postoperative period, when blood is more likely to have accumulated.

5. Postpericardiotomy syndrome may contribute to the development of recurrent serous or serosanguineous effusions. This should be managed initially by use of NSAIDs or steroids, but may require a thoracentesis for symptom relief.

D. **Chylothorax** is a rare complication of surgery caused by interruption of lymphatic tributaries of the thoracic duct in the left upper mediastinum. It is most likely to occur during proximal mobilization of the left ITA near the subclavian vessels or during aortic arch surgery.

1. **Manifestations.** If early drainage is significant, turbulent milky fluid may be noted in the chest tubes that is exacerbated by dietary fat. More commonly, an enlarging left pleural effusion will be noted after the chest tubes have been removed.

2. **Diagnosis.** Examination of the pleural fluid will reveal chyle, which is sterile, with large quantities of lymphocytes and a high level of triglycerides (>110 mg/dL). Staining with Sudan III can distinguish chyle from purulent fluid.

3. **Treatment.** Conservative treatment with chest tube drainage, elimination of fat from the diet, and use of medium-chain triglycerides (which comes as an oral oil to be mixed with fruit juices) is recommended initially. If drainage persists for more than a few days, use of octreotide (Sandostatin) 100 µg SC q8h is highly successful in terminating the leak.[159,160] If this fails, thoracoscopic clipping, coagulation, or ligation can be performed.[161]

E. **Bronchospasm** can occur at the termination of surgery and can produce difficulty with sternal closure. Severe bronchospasm and air trapping developing in the ICU can produce difficulties with mechanical ventilation as well as hemodynamic problems that can mimic cardiac tamponade. Modification of the ventilator circuit to increase the inspiratory flow rate will decrease the inspiration:expiration (I:E) ratio, allowing more time for exhalation, and should decrease the autoPEEP effect. Bronchospasm can be precipitated by fluid overload, drug reactions, blood product transfusions, or the use of β-blockers, and it can occur in patients with or without known COPD or bronchospastic airways. Treatment involves the following:

1. Inhalational bronchodilators delivered by metered dose inhaler (MDI) or nebulizer are helpful during mechanical ventilation as well as after extubation. They can reduce bronchospasm and reduce dynamic hyperinflation of the lung, the latter perhaps contributing more to symptomatic improvement. Short-acting β_2-agonists combined with anticholinergic (muscarinic) medications (such as ipratroprium) provide superior benefit to individual medications alone.[162-164]

2. Commonly used fast-acting bronchodilators:
   a. Short-acting β_2-agonists:
      i. Albuterol (Ventolin, Proventil) 0.5 mL of 0.5% solution (2.5 mg) in 3 mL normal saline q6h or two puffs q6h
      ii. Levalbuterol (Xopenex) 0.63 mg in 3 mL normal saline q8h (three times daily); it can also be given as two inhalations q4−6h through a pressured MDI
   b. Anticholinergics: Ipratroprium (Atrovent) 2.5 mL of 0.02% (0.5 mg) in 2.5 mL normal saline q6−8h or two puffs q4−6h
   c. Combination preparations of albuterol and ipratroprium provide the best bronchodilation. Duoneb contains albuterol 3 mg/ipratropium bromide 0.5 mg given in 3 mL normal saline up to four times a day. The Combivent MDI provides 100 µg of albuterol and about 20 µg of ipratroprium with two inhalations given four times a day.
3. Other bronchodilators
   a. Racemic epinephrine can be used in patients with laryngospasm around the time of endotracheal extubation. It is usually given as 0.5 mL of a 0.25% solution in 3.5 mL normal saline and can be given every 4 hours.
   b. An intravenous infusion of low-dose epinephrine is an excellent choice for inotropic support for low cardiac output syndrome because it provides bronchodilatory effects. Since it is also a strong positive chronotrope, it must be used cautiously when sinus tachycardia is present.
   c. Phosphodiesterase inhibitors (aminophylline preparations) have potential cardiac toxicity at higher doses (arrhythmias, tachycardia) and are therefore best avoided unless the patient has refractory bronchospasm.
4. Corticosteroids are frequently beneficial when bronchospasm is refractory to the above measures. They may increase airway responsiveness to other β_2-agonists. Dosing regimens involve no more than 2 weeks of treatment.[164] Two of these protocols are the following:
   a. Methylprednisolone (SoluMedrol) 0.5 mg/kg IV q6h × 3 days, then prednisone 0.5 mg/kg q12h × 3 days, then 0.5 mg/kg qd × 4 days (10-day total course)
   b. Methylprednisolone 125 mg IV q6h × 3 days, then prednisone 60 mg qd × 4 days, then 40 mg qd × 4 days, then 20 mg qd × 4 days (15-day total course)
5. **Note:** β-blockers are generally contraindicated during episodes of bronchospasm. However, patients with a history of bronchospastic airways can frequently tolerate the selective β-blockers, such as esmolol, metoprolol, and atenolol.

References

1. Meade MO, Guyatt G, Butler R, et al. Trials comparing early vs late extubation following cardiovascular surgery. Chest 2001;120:445S–53S.
2. Cheng DCH, Karski J, Peniston C, et al. Early tracheal extubation after coronary artery bypass graft surgery reduces costs and improves resource use. A prospective, randomized, controlled trial. *Anesthesiology* 1996;85:1300–10.
3. Reis J, Mota JC, Ponce P, Costa-Pereira A, Guerreiro M. Early extubation does not increase complication rates after coronary artery bypass graft surgery with cardiopulmonary bypass. *Eur J Cardiothorac Surg* 2002;21:1026–30.
4. Roosens C, Heerman J, De Somer F, et al. Effects of off-pump coronary surgery on the mechanics of the respiratory system, lung, and chest wall: comparison with extracorporeal circulation. *Crit Care Med* 2002;30:2430–7.
5. Polese G, Lubli P, Mazzucco A, Luzzani A, Rossi A. Effects of open heart surgery on respiratory mechanics. *Intensive Care Med* 1999;25:1092–9.
6. Ng CS, Wan S, Yim AP, Arifi AA. Pulmonary dysfunction after cardiac surgery. *Chest* 2002;121:1269–77.
7. Cox CM, Ascione R, Cohen AM, Davies IM, Ryder IG, Angelini GD. Effect of cardiopulmonary bypass on pulmonary gas exchange: prospective randomized study. *Ann Thorac Surg* 2000;69:140–5.
8. Taggart DP. Respiratory dysfunction after cardiac surgery: effects of avoiding cardiopulmonary bypass and the use of bilateral internal mammary arteries. *Eur J Cardiothorac Surg* 2000;18:31–7.
9. Guizilini S, Gomes WJ, Faresin SM, et al. Influence of pleurotomy on pulmonary function after off-pump coronary artery bypass grafting. *Ann Thorac Surg* 2007;84:817–22.
10. Foghsgaard S, Gazi D, Bach K, Hansen H, Schmidt TA, Kjaergard HK. Minimally invasive aortic valve replacement reduces atelectasis in cardiac intensive care. *Acute Card Care* 2009;11:169–72.
11. Wheatley GH 3rd, Rosenbaum DH, Paul MC, et al. Improved pain management outcomes with continuous infusion of a local anesthetic after thoracotomy. *J Thorac Cardiovasc Surg* 2005;130:464–8.
12. Ogus H, Selimoglu O, Basaran M, et al. Effect of intrapleural analgesia on pulmonary function and postoperative pain in patients with chronic obstructive pulmonary disease undergoing coronary artery bypass graft surgery. *J Cardiothorac Vasc Anesth* 2007;21:816–9.
13. Cislaghi F, Condemi AM. Corona A. Predictors of prolonged mechanical ventilation in a cohort of 5123 cardiac surgical patients. *Eur J Anaesthesiol* 2009;26:396–403.
14. Legare JF, Hirsch GM, Buth KJ, MacDougall C, Sullivan JA. Preoperative prediction of prolonged mechanical ventilation following coronary artery bypass grafting. *Eur J Cardiothorac Surg* 2001;20:930–6.
15. Suematsu Y, Sato H, Ohtsuka T, Kotsuka Y, Araki S, Takamoto S. Predictive risk factors for delayed extubation in patients undergoing coronary artery bypass grafting. *Heart Vessels* 2000;15:214–20.
16. Branca P, McGaw P, Light R. Factors associated with prolonged mechanical ventilation following coronary artery bypass surgery. *Chest* 2001;119:537–46.
17. Rady MY, Ryan T, Starr NJ. Early onset of acute pulmonary dysfunction after cardiovascular surgery: risk factors and clinical outcome. *Crit Care Med* 1997;25:1831–9.
18. Filsoufi F, Rahmanian PB, Castillo JG, Chikwe J, Adams DH. Logistic risk model predicting postoperative respiratory failure in patients undergoing valve surgery. *Eur J Cardiothorac Surg* 2008;34:953–9.
19. Reddy SLC, Grayson AD, Griffiths EM, Pullan DM, Rashid A. Logistic risk model for prolonged ventilation after adult cardiac surgery. *Ann Thorac Surg* 2007;84:528–36.
20. Dunning J, Au J, Kalkat M, Levine A. A validated rule for predicting patients who require prolonged ventilation post cardiac surgery. *Eur J Cardiothorac Surg* 2003;24:270–6.
21. Hachenberg T, Tenling A, Nyström SO, Tyden H, Hedenstierna G. Ventilation-perfusion inequality in patients undergoing cardiac surgerry. *Anesthesiology* 1994;80:509–19.
22. Hagl C, Harringer W, Gohrbandt B, Haverich A. Site of pleural drain insertion and early postoperative pulmonary function following coronary artery bypass grafting with internal mammary artery. *Chest* 1999;115:757–61.

23. Gilbert TB, Barnas GM, Sequeira AJ. Impact of pleurotomy, continuous positive airway pressure, and fluid balance during cardiopulmonary bypass on lung mechanics and oxygenation. *J Cardiothorac Vasc Anesth* 1996;10:844–9.

24. Hurlbut D, Myers ML, Lefcoe M, Goldbach M. Pleuropulmonary morbidity: internal thoracic artery versus saphenous vein graft. *Ann Thorac Surg* 1990;50:959–64.

25. O'Brien JW, Johnson SH, VanSteyn SJ, et al. Effects of internal mammary artery dissection on phrenic nerve perfusion and function. *Ann Thorac Surg* 1991;52:182–8.

26. Vargas FS, Terra-Filho M, Hueb W, Teixeira LR, Cukier A, Light RW. Pulmonary function after coronary bypass surgery. *Respir Med* 1997;91:629–33.

27. Shenkman Z, Shir Y, Weiss YG, Bleiberg B, Gross D. The effects of cardiac surgery on early and late pulmonary functions. *Acta Anaesthesiol Scand* 1997;41:1193–9.

28. Iyem H, Islamoglu F, Yagdi T, et al. Effects of pleurotomy on respiratory sequelae after internal mammary artery harvesting. *Tex Heart Inst J* 2006;33:116–21.

29. Merino-Ramirez MA, Juan G, Ramón M, et al. Electrophysiologic evaluation of phrenic nerve and diaphragm function after coronary bypass surgery: prospective study of diabetes and other risk factors. *J Thorac Cardiovasc Surg* 2006;132:530–6.

30. Yamazaki K, Kato H, Tsujimoto S, Kitamura R. Diabetes mellitus, internal thoracic artery grafting, and the risk of an elevated hemidiaphragm after coronary artery bypass surgery. *J Cardiothorac Vasc Anesth* 1994;8:437–40.

31. Daganou M, Dimopoulou I, Michalopoulos N, et al. Respiratory complications after coronary artery bypass surgery with unilateral or bilateral internal mammary artery grafting. *Chest* 1998;113:1285–9.

32. Asimakopoulos G, Smith PLC, Ratnatunga CP, Taylor KM. Lung injury and acute respiratory distress syndrome after cardiopulmonary bypass. *Ann Thorac Surg* 1999;68:1107–15.

33. Insler SR, O'Connor MS, Leventhal MJ, Nelson DR, Starr NJ. Association between postoperative hypothermia and adverse outcome after coronary artery bypass surgery. *Ann Thorac Surg* 2000;70:175–81.

34. Ng CS, Arifi AA, Wan S, et al. Ventilation during cardiopulmonary bypass: impact on cytokine response and cardiopulmonary function. *Ann Thorac Surg* 2008;85:154–62.

35. Koch C, Li L, Figueroa P, Mihaljevic T, Svensson L, Blackstone EH. Transfusion and pulmonary morbidity after cardiac surgery. *Ann Thorac Surg* 2009;88:1410–8.

36. Marik PE, Corwin HL. Acute lung injury following blood transfusion: expanding the definition. *Crit Care Med* 2008;36:3080–4.

37. Toy P, Popovsky MA, Abraham E, et al. Transfusion-related acute lung injury: definition and review. *Crit Care Med* 2005;33:721–6.

38. Society of Thoracic Surgeons Blood Conservation Guidelines Task Force, Ferraris VA, Ferraris SP, Saha SP, et al. Perioperative blood transfusion and blood conservation in cardiac surgery: the Society of Thoracic Surgeons and the Society of Cardiovascular Anesthesiologists clinical practice guideline. *Ann Thorac Surg* 2007;83(5 suppl):S27–86.

39. Yamagishi T, Ishikawa S, Ohtaki A, Takahashi T, Ohki S, Morishita Y. Obesity and postoperative oxygenation after coronary artery bypass grafting. *Jpn J Thorac Cardiovasc Surg* 2000;48:632–6.

40. Tripp HF, Bolton JW. Phrenic nerve injury following cardiac surgery: a review. *J Card Surg* 1998;13:218–23.

41. Turker G, Goren S, Sahin S, Korfali G, Sayan E. Combination of intrathecal morphine and remifentanil infusion for fast-track anesthesia in off-pump coronary artery bypass surgery. *J Cardiothorac Vasc Anesth* 2005;19:708–13.

42. Lena P, Balarac N, Lena D, et al. Fast-track anesthesia with remifentanil and spinal analgesia for cardiac surgery: the effect on pain control and quality of recovery. *J Cardiothorac Vasc Anesth* 2008;22:536–42.

43. Toraman F, Evrenkaya S, Yuce M, Göksel O, Karabulut H, Alhan C. Fast-track recovery in noncoronary cardiac surgery patients. *Heart Surg Forum* 2005;8:E61–4.

44. Guggenberger H, Schroder TH, Vontheim R, et al. Remifentanil or sufentanil for coronary surgery: comparison of postoperative respiratory impairment. *Eur J Anaesthesiol* 2006;23:832–40.

45. Rathgeber J, Schorn B, Falk V, Kazmaier S, Speigel T, Burchardi H. The influence of controlled mandatory ventilation (CMV), intermittent mandatory ventilation (IMV) and biphasic intermittent positive airway pressure (BIPAP) on duration of intubation and consumption of analgesics and sedatives. A prospective analysis of 596 patients following adult cardiac surgery. *Eur J Anaesthesiol* 1997;14:576–82.

46. Kazmaier S, Rathgeber J, Buhre W, et al. Comparison of ventilatory and haemodynamic effects of BIPAP and S-IMV/PSV for postoperative short-term ventilation in patients after coronary artery bypass grafting. *Eur J Anaesthesiol* 2000;17:601–10.

47. Michalopoulos A, Anthi A, Rellos K, Geroulanos S. Effects of positive end-expiratory pressure (PEEP) in cardiac surgery patients. *Respir Med* 1998;92:858–62.

48. Barr J, Egan TD, Sandoval NF, et al. Propofol dosing regimens for ICU sedation based upon an integrated pharmacokinetic-pharmacodynamic model. *Anesthesiology* 2001;95:324–33.

49. Herr DL, Sum-Ping ST, England M. ICU sedation after coronary artery bypass graft surgery: dexmedetomidine-based versus propofol-based sedation regimens. *J Cardiothorac Vasc Anesth* 2003;17:576–84.

50. Riker RR, Shehabi Y, Bokesch PM, et al. Dexmedetomidine vs midazolam for sedation of critically ill patients: a randomized trial. *JAMA* 2009;301:489–99.

51. Ruokonen E, Parviainen I, Jakob SM, et al. Dexmedetomidine versus propofol/midazolam for long-term sedation during mechanical ventilation. *Intensive Care Med* 2009;35:282–90.

52. Gurbet A, Goren S, Sahin S, Uchunkaya N, Korfali G. Comparison of analgesic effects of morphine, fentanyl, and remifentanil with intravenous patient-controlled analgesia after cardiac surgery. *J Cardiothorac Vasc Anesth* 2004;18:755–8.

53. Baltali S, Turkoz A, Bozdogan N, et al. The efficacy of intravenous patient-controlled remifentanil versus morphine anesthesia after coronary artery surgery. *J Cardiothorac Vasc Anesth* 2009;23:170–4.

54. Bojar RM, Rastegar H, Payne DD, et al. Methemoglobinemia from intravenous nitroglycerin: a word of caution. *Ann Thorac Surg* 1987;43:332–4.

55. Suematsu Y, Sato H, Ohtsuka T, Kotsuka Y, Araki S, Takamoto S. Predictive risk factors for pulmonary oxygen transfer in patients undergoing coronary artery bypass grafting. *Jpn Heart J* 2001;42:143–53.

56. Montes FR, Sanchez SI, Giraldo JC, et al. The lack of benefit of tracheal extubation in the operating room after coronary artery bypass surgery. *Anesth Analg* 2000;91:776–80.

57. Nicholson DJ, Kowalski SE, Hamilton GA, Meyers MP, Serrette C, Duke PC. Postoperative pulmonary function in coronary artery bypass graft surgery patients undergoing early tracheal extubation: a comparison between short-term mechanical ventilation and early extubation. *J Cardiothorac Vasc Anesth* 2002;16:27–31.

58. Canver CC, Chanda J. Intraoperative and postoperative risk factors for respiratory failure after coronary bypass. *Ann Thorac Surg* 2003;75:853–8.

59. Yende S, Wunderink R. Causes of prolonged mechanical ventilation after coronary artery bypass surgery. *Chest* 2002;122:245–52.

60. Rajakaruna C, Rogers CA, Angelini GD, Ascione R. Risk factors for and economic implications of prolonged ventilation after cardiac surgery. *J Thorac Cardiovasc Surg* 2005;130:1270–7.

61. Murthy SC, Arroliga AC, Walts PA, et al. Ventilatory dependency after cardiovascular surgery. *J Thorac Cardiovasc Surg* 2007;134:484–90.

62. Lauruschkat AH, Arnrich B, Albert AA, et al. Diabetes mellitus as a risk factor for pulmonary complications after coronary bypass surgery. *J Thorac Cardiovasc Surg* 2008;135:1047–53.

63. Pandharipande PP, Pun BT, Herr DL, et al. Effect of sedation with dexmedetomidine vs lorazepam on acute brain dysfunction in mechanically ventilated patients: the MENDS randomized controlled trial. *JAMA* 2007;298:2644–53.

64. Ngaage DL, Martins E, Orkell E, et al. The impact of the duration of mechanical ventilation on the respiratory outcome in smokers undergoing cardiac surgery. *Cardiovasc Surg* 2002;10:345–50.

65. Hulzebos EHJ, Helders PJM, Favie NJ, De Bie RA, de la Riviere AB, Van Meeteren NLU. Preoperative intensive inspiratory muscle training to prevent postoperative pulmonary complications in high-risk patients undergoing CABG surgery. A randomized clinical trial. *JAMA* 2006;296:1851–7.

66. Stein R, Maia CP, Silveira AD, Chiappa GR, Myers J, Ribeiro JP. Inspiratory muscle strength as a determinant of functional capacity early after coronary artery bypass graft surgery. *Arch Phys Med Rehabil* 2009;10:1685–91.

67. Karaiskos TE, Palatianos GM, Triantafillou CD, et al. Clinical effectiveness of leukocyte filtration during cardiopulmonary bypass in patients with chronic obstructive pulmonary disease. *Ann Thorac Surg* 2004;78:1339–44.

68. Boodram S, Evans E. Use of leukocyte-depleting filters during cardiac surgery with cardiopulmonary bypass: a review. *J Extra Corpor Technol* 2008;40:27–42.

69. Boodhwani M, Nathan HJ, Mesana TG, Rubens FD, on behalf of the Cardiotomy Investigators. Effects of shed mediastinal blood on cardiovascular and pulmonary function: a randomized, double-blind study. *Ann Thorac Surg* 2008;86:1167–74.

70. Whitlock RP, Chan S, Devereaux PJ, et al. Clinical benefit of steroid use in patients undergoing cardiopulmonary bypass: a meta-analysis of randomized trials. *Eur Heart J* 2008;29:2592–600.

71. Chaney MA, Durazo-Arvizu RA, Nikolov MP, Blakeman BP, Bakhos M. Methylprednisolone does not benefit patients undergoing coronary artery bypass grafting and early tracheal extubation. *J Thorac Cardiovasc Surg* 2001;121:561–9.

72. Lazar HL, McDonnell M, Chipkin SR, et al. The Society of Thoracic Surgeons practice guidelines series: blood glucose management during adult cardiac surgery. *Ann Thorac Surg* 2009;87:663–9.

73. Chen HH, Sundt TM, Cook DJ, Heublein DM, Burnett JC Jr. Low dose nesiritide and the preservation of renal function in patients with renal dysfunction undergoing cardiopulmonary-bypass surgery: a double-blind placebo-controlled pilot study. *Circulation* 2007;116(suppl II):I-134–8.

74. Landoni G, Biondi-Zoccai, GG, Marino G, et al. Fenoldopam reduces the need for renal replacement therapy and in-hospital death in cardiovascular surgery: a meta-analysis. *J Cardiothorac Vasc Anesth* 2008;22:27–33.

75. Cogliati AA, Vellutini R, Nardini A, et al. Fenoldopam infusion for renal protection in high-risk cardiac surgery patients: a randomized clinical study. *J Cardiothorac Vasc Anesth* 2007;21:847–5.

76. Haase M, Haase-Fielitz A, Bellomo R, et al. Sodium bicarbonate to prevent increases in serum creatinine after cardiac surgery: a pilot double-blind, randomized trial. *Crit Care Med* 2009;37:39–47.

77. Huang H, Yao T, Wang W, et al. Continuous ultrafiltration attenuates the pulmonary injury that follows open heart surgery with cardiopulmonary bypass. *Ann Thorac Surg* 2003;76:136–40.

78. Swenne CL, Lindholm C, Borowiec J, Schnell AE, Carlsson M. Peri-operative glucose control and development of surgical wound infections in patients undergoing coronary artery bypass graft. *J Hosp Infect* 2005;61:201–12.

79. Jones DP, Byrne P, Morgan C, Fraser I, Hyland R. Positive end-expiratory pressure vs T-piece. Extubation after mechanical ventilation. *Chest* 1991;100:1655–9.

80. De Santo LS, Bancone C, Santarpino G, et al. Noninvasive positive-pressure ventilation for extubation failure after cardiac surgery: pilot safety evaluation. *J Thorac Cardiovasc Surg* 2009;137:342–6.

81. Lellouche F. Noninvasive ventilation in patients with hypoxemic acute respiratory failure. *Curr Opin Crit Care* 2007;13:12–9.

82. Matte P, Jacquet L, Van Dyck M, Goenen M. Effects of conventional physiotherapy, continuous positive airway pressure and non-invasive ventilatory support with bilevel positive airway pressure after coronary artery bypass grafting. *Acta Anaesthesiol Scand* 2000;44:75–81.

83. Gust R, Gottschalk A, Schmidt H, Bottiger BW, Bohrer H, Martin E. Effects of continuous (CPAP) and bi-level positive airway pressure (BiPAP) on extravascular lung water after extubation of the trachea in patients following coronary artery bypass grafting. *Intensive Care Med* 1996;22:1345–50.

84. Vital FM, Saconato H, Ladeira MT, et al. Non-invasive positive pressure ventilation (CPAP or bilevel NPPV) for cardiogenic pulmonary edema. *Cochrane Database Syst Rev* 2008;3:CD005351.

85. Zarbock A, Mueller E, Netzer S, Gabriel A, Feindt P, Kindgen-Milles D. Prophylactic nasal continuous positive airway pressure following cardiac surgery protects from postoperative pulmonary complications: a prospective, randomized, controlled trial in 500 patients. *Chest* 2009;135:1252–9.

86. Pasquina P, Merlani P, Granier JM, Ricou B. Continuous positive airway pressure versus noninvasive pressure support ventilation to treat atelectasis after cardiac surgery. *Anesth Analg* 2004;99:1001–8.

87. Overend TJ, Anderson CM, Lucy SD, Bhatia C, Jonsson BI, Timmermans C. The effect of incentive spirometry on postoperative pulmonary complications. A systematic review. *Chest* 2001;120:971–8.

88. Freitas ER, Soares BG, Cardoso JR, Atallah AN. Incentive spirometry for preventing pulmonary complications after coronary artery bypass graft. *Cochrane Database Syst Rev* 2007;3:CD004466.

89. Westerdahl E, Lindmark B, Eriksson T, Hedenstierna G, Tenling A. The immediate effects of deep breathing exercises on atelectasis and oxygenation after cardiac surgery. *Scand Cardiovasc J* 2003;37:363–7.

90. Pasquina P, Tramèr MR, Walder B. Prophylactic respiratory physiotherapy after cardiac surgery: systematic review. *BMJ* 2003;327:1379–81.

91. Barquist E, Brown M, Cohn S, Lundy D, Jackowski J. Postextubation fiberoptic endoscopic evaluation of swallowing after prolonged endotracheal intubation: a randomized, prospective trial. *Crit Care Med* 2001;29:1710–3.

92. Barker J, Martino R, Reichardt B, Hickey EJ, Ralph-Edwards A. Incidence and impact of dysphagia in patients receiving prolonged endotracheal intubation after cardiac surgery. *Can J Surg* 2009;52:119–24.

93. Ramos R, Salem BI, De Pawlikowski MP, Coordes C, Eisenberg S, Leidenfrost R. The efficacy of pneumatic compression stockings in the prevention of pulmonary embolism after cardiac surgery. *Chest* 1996;109:82–5.

94. Close V, Purohit M, Tanos M, Hunter S. Should patients post-cardiac surgery be given low molecular weight heparin for deep-vein thrombosis prophylaxis? *Interact Cardiovasc Thorac Surg* 2006;5:624–9.

95. Jones HU, Mulestein JB, Jones KW, et al. Early postoperative use of unfractionated heparin or enoxaparin is associated with increased surgical re-exploration for bleeding. *Ann Thorac Surg* 2005;80:519–22.

96. Geerts WH, Bergqvist D, Pineo GF, et al. Prevention of venous thromboembolism. American College of Chest Physicians evidence-based clinical practice guidelines (8th edition). *Chest* 2008;133:381S–453S.

97. Tsai BM, Wang M, Turrentine MW, Mahomed Y, Brown JW, Meldrum DR. Hypoxic pulmonary vasoconstriction in cardiothoracic surgery: basic mechanisms to potential therapies. *Ann Thorac Surg* 2004;78:360–8.

98. Schmidt SL, Hyzy RC. Overview of mechanical ventilation. www.utdol.com version 17.2, 2009.

99. Garrison G, Hyzy RC. Physiologic and pathophysiologic consequences of mechanical ventilation. www.utdol.com version 17.2, 2009.

100. Celebi S, Köner O, Menda F, Korkut K, Suzer K, Cakar N. The pulmonary and hemodynamic effects of two different recruitment maneuvers after cardiac surgery. *Anesth Analg* 2007;104:384–90.

101. Malhotra A. Low-tidal-volume ventilation in the acute respiratory distress syndrome. *N Engl J Med* 2007;357:1113–20.

102. Shapiro MB, West MA, Nathens AB, et al. V. Guidelines for sedation and analgesia during mechanical ventilation: general overview. *J Trauma* 2007;63:945–50.

103. Sessler CN, Varney K. Patient-focused sedation and analgesia in the ICU. *Chest* 2008;133:552–65.

104. Gommers D, Bakker J. Medications for analgesia and sedation in the intensive care unit: an overview. *Crit Care* 2008;12(suppl 3):S4 (available at ccforum.com/content/12/S3/S4).

105. Kuralay E, Cingöz F, Kiliç S, et al. Supraventricular tachyarrhythmias prophylaxis after coronary artery surgery in chronic obstructive pulmonary disease patients (early amiodarone prophylaxis trial). *Eur J Cardiothorac Surg* 2004;25:224–30.

106. Kaushik S, Hussain A, Clarke P, Lazar HL. Acute pulmonary toxicity after low-dose amiodarone therapy. *Ann Thorac Surg* 2001;72:1760–1.

107. Hébert PC, Blajchman MA, Cook DJ, et al. Do blood transfusions improve outcomes related to mechanical ventilation? *Chest* 2001;119:1850–7.

108. Spiess BD. Choose one: damned if you do/damned if you don't! *Crit Care Med* 2005;33:1871–3.

109. MacIntyre NR, Epstein SK, Carson S, Scheinhorn D, Christopher K, Muldoon S. Management of patients requiring prolonged mechanical ventilation. Report of a NAMDRC Consensus Conference. *Chest* 2005;128:3937–54.

110. Milot J, Perron J, Lacasse Y, Letourneau L, Cartier PC, Maltais F. Incidence and predictors of ARDS after cardiac surgery. *Chest* 2001;119:884–8.

111. Asimakoipoulos G, Taylor KM, Smith PL, Ratnatunga CP. Prevalence of acute respiratory distress syndrome after cardiac surgery. *J Thorac Cardiovasc Surg* 1999;117:620–1.

112. MacIntyre NR, Cook DJ, Ely EW Jr, et al. Evidence-based guidelines for weaning and discontinuing ventilatory support. A collective task force facilitated by the American College of Chest Physicians; The American Association for Respiratory Care; and the American College of Critical Care Medicine. *Chest* 2001;120:375S–95S.

113. Elefteriades J, Singh M, Tang P, et al. Unilateral diaphragm paralysis: etiology, impact, and natural history. *J Cardiovasc Surg (Torino)* 2008;49:289–95.

114. Versteegh MI, Braun J, Voigt PG, et al. Diaphragm plication in adult patients with diaphragm paralysis leads to long-term improvement of pulmonary function and level of dyspnea. *Eur J Cardiothorac Surg* 2007;32:449–56.

115. Bozyk P, Hyzy RC. Modes of mechanical ventilation. www.utdol.com version 17.2, 2009.

116. Manthous CA, Schmidt GA, Hall JB. Liberation from mechanical ventilation. A decade of progress. *Chest* 1998;114:886–901.

117. Herlihy JP, Koch SM, Jackson R, Nora H. Course of weaning from prolonged mechanical ventilation after cardiac surgery. *Tex Heart Inst J* 2006;33:122–9.

118. Kollef MH, Levy NT, Ahrens TS, Schaiff R, Prentice D, Sherman G. The use of continuous IV sedation is associated with prolongation of mechanical ventilation. *Chest* 1998;114:541–8.

119. Schweickert WD, Gehlbach BK, Pohlman AS, Hall JB, Kress JP. Daily interruption of sedative medications and complications of critical illness in mechanically ventilated patients. *Crit Care Med* 2004;32:1272–6.

120. Mehta S, Burry L, Martinez-Motta JC, et al. A randomized trial of daily awakening in critically ill patients managed with a sedation protocol: a pilot trial. *Crit Care Med* 2008;36:2092–9.

121. Maillet JM, Thierry S, Brodaty D. Prone positioning and acute respiratory distress syndrome after cardiac surgery: a feasibility study. *J Cardiothorac Vasc Anesth* 2008;22:414–7.

122. Hortal J, Giannella M, Pérez MJ, et al. Incidence and risk factors for ventilator-associated pneumonia after major heart surgery. *Intensive Care Med* 2009;35:1518–25.

123. Hortal J, Muñoz P, Cuerpo G, et al. Ventilator-associated pneumonia in patients undergoing major heart surgery: an incidence study in Europe. *Crit Care* 2009;13:R80.

124. Pawar M, Mehta Y, Khurana P, Chaudhary A, Kulkarni V, Trehan N. Ventilator-associated pneumonia: incidence, risk factors, outcome, and microbiology. *J Cardiothorac Vasc Anesth* 2003;17:22–8.

125. Isakow W, Kollef MH. Preventing ventilator-associated pneumonia: an evidence-based approach of modifiable risk factors. *Semin Respir Crit Care Med* 2006;27:5–17.

126. American Thoracic Society; Infectious Diseases Society of America. Guidelines for the management of adults with hospital-acquired, ventilator-associated, and healthcare-associated pneumonia. *Am J Respir Crit Care Med* 2005;171:388–416.

127. Tantipong H, Morkchareonpong C, Jaiyinde S, Thamlikitkul V. Randomized controlled trial and meta-analysis of oral decontamination with 2% chlorhexidine solution for the prevention of ventilator-associated pneumonia. *Infect Control Hosp Epidemiol* 2008;29:131–6.

128. Miano TA, Reichert MG, Houlse TT, MacGregor DA, Kincaid EH, Bowton DL. Nosocomial pneumonia risk and stress ulcer prophylaxis. A comparison of pantoprazole vs ranitidine in cardiothoracic surgery patients. *Chest* 2009;136:440–7.

129. Steinberg KP. Stress-related mucosal disease in the critically ill patient: risk factors and strategies to prevent stress-related bleeding in the intensive care unit. *Crit Care Med* 2002;30(6 Suppl):S362–4.

130. Kollef MH. Selective digestive decontamination should not be routinely employed. *Chest* 2003;123:464S–8.

131. Trouillet JL, Combes A, Vaissier E, et al. Prolonged mechanical ventilation after cardiac surgery: outcome and predictors. *J Thorac Cardiovasc Surg* 2009;138:948–53.

132. Ngaage DL, Cale AR, Griffin S, Guvendik L, Cowen ME. Is post-sternotomy percutaneous dilatation tracheostomy a predictor for sternal wound infections? *Eur J Cardiothorac Surg* 2008;33:1076–81.

133. Byhahn C, Rinne T, Halbig S, et al. Early percutaneous tracheostomy after median sternotomy. *J Thorac Cardiovasc Surg* 2000;120:329–34.

134. Stamenkovic SA, Morgan IS, Pontefract DR, Campanella C. Is early tracheostomy safe in cardiac patients with median sternotomy incisions? *Ann Thorac Surg* 2000;69:1152–4.

135. Curtis JJ, Clark NC, McKenney CA, et al. Tracheostomy: a risk factor for mediastinitis after cardiac operation. *Ann Thorac Surg* 2001;72:731–4.

136. Rahmanian PB, Adams DH, Castillo JG, Chikwe J, Filsoufi F. Tracheostomy is not a risk factor for deep sternal wound infection after cardiac surgery. *Ann Thorac Surg* 2007;84:1984–92.

137. Force SD, Miller DL, Petersen R, et al. Incidence of deep sternal wound infections after tracheostomy in cardiac surgery patients. *Ann Thorac Surg* 2005;80:618–22.

138. Liesching T, Kwok H, Hill NS. Acute applications of noninvasive positive pressure ventilation. *Chest* 2003;124:699–713.

139. Takasaki Y, Kido T, Semba K. Dexmedetomidine facilitates induction of noninvasive positive pressure ventilation for acute respiratory failure in patients with severe asthma. *J Anesth* 2009;23:147–50.

140. Jubran A, Tobin MJ. Methods of weaning from mechanical ventilation. www.utdol.com version 17.2, 2009.

141. MacIntyre N. Discontinuing mechanical ventilatory support. *Chest* 2007;132:1049–56.

142. Esteban E, Alía I, Tobin MJ, et al. Effect of spontaneous breathing trial duration on outcome of attempts to discontinue mechanical ventilation. Spanish Lung Failure Cooperative Group. *Am J Respir Crit Care Med* 1999;159:512–8.

143. Engoren M. Evaluation of the cuff-leak test in a cardiac surgery population. *Chest* 1999;116:1029–31.

144. Kriner EJ. Shafazand S, Colice GL. The endotracheal tube cuff-leak test as a predictor for postextubation stridor. *Respir Care* 2005;50:1632–8.

145. Prinianakis G, Alexopoulou C, Mamidakis E, Kondili E, Georgopoulos D. Determinants of the cuff-leak test: a physiological study. *Crit Care* 2005;9:R24–31.

146. Sandhu RS, Pasquale MD, Miller K, Wasser TE. Measurement of endotracheal tube cuff leak to predict postextubation stridor and need for reintubation. *J Am Coll Surg* 2000;190:682–7.

147. Jaber S, Jung B, Chanques G, Bonnet F, Marret E. Effects of steroids on reintubation and post-extubation stridor in adults: meta-analysis of randomized controlled trials. *Crit Care* 2009;13:R49.

148. Roberts RJ, Welch SM, Devlin JW. Corticosteroids for prevention of postextubation laryngeal edema in adults. *Ann Pharmacother* 2008;42:686–91.

149. Lee CH, Peng MJ, Wu CL. Dexamethasone to prevent postextubation airway obstruction in adults: a prospective, randomized, double-blind, placebo-controlled trial. *Crit Care* 2007;11:R72.

150. Jubran A, Tobin MJ. Predictors of weaning outcome. www.utdol.com version 17.2, 2009.

151. Yang KL, Tobin MJ. A prospective study of indexes predicting the outcome of trials of weaning from mechanical ventilation. *N Engl J Med* 1991;324:1445–50.

152. Meade M, Guyatt G, Sinuff T, et al. Trials comparing alternative weaning modes and discontinuation assessments. *Chest* 2001;120:425S–37S.

153. Frutos-Vivar F, Ferguson MD, Esteban A, et al. Risk factors for extubation failure in patients following a spontaneous breathing trial. *Chest* 2006;130:1664–71.

154. Light RW, Rogers JT, Moyers JP, et al. Prevalence and clinical course of pleural effusions at 30 days after coronary artery and cardiac surgery. *Am J Respir Crit Care Med* 2002;166:1567–71.

155. Payne M, Magovern GJ Jr, Benckart DH, et al. Left pleural effusion after coronary artery bypass decreases with a supplemental pleural drain. *Ann Thorac Surg* 2002;73:149–52.

156. Kopterides P, Lignos M, Papanikolaou S, et al. Pleural effusion causing cardiac tamponade: report of two cases and review of the literature. *Heart Lung* 2006;35:66–7.

157. Bilku RS, Bilku DK, Rosin MD, Been M. Left ventricular diastolic collapse and late regional cardiac tamponade postcardiac surgery caused by large left pleural effusion. *J Am Soc Echocardiogr* 2008;21:978.e9-11.

158. Feller-Kopman D. Ultrasound-guided thoracentesis. *Chest* 2006;129:1709–14.

159. Kilic D, Sahin E, Gulcan O, Bolat B, Turkoz R, Hatipoglu A. Octreotide for treating chylothorax after cardiac surgery. *Tex Heart Inst J* 2005;32:437–9.

160. Barili F, Polvani G, Topkara VK, et al. Administration of octreotide for management of postoperative high-flow chylothorax. *Ann Vasc Surg* 2007;21:90–2.

161. Takeo S, Yamazaki K, Takagi M, Nakashima A. Thoracoscopic ultrasonic coagulation of thoracic duct in management of postoperative chylothorax. *Ann Thorac Surg* 2002;74:263–5.

162. The COMBIVENT Inhalation Solution Study Group. Routine nebulized ipratropium and albuterol together are better than either alone in COPD. *Chest* 1997;112:1514–21.

163. Celli BR. Update on the management of COPD. *Chest* 2008;133:1451–62.

164. Stoller JK. Acute exacerbations of chronic obstructive pulmonary disease. *N Engl J Med* 2002;346:988–94.

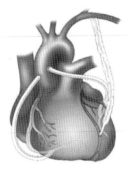

CHAPTER 11

Cardiovascular Management

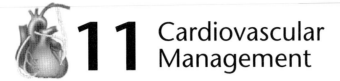

11 Cardiovascular Management

The achievement of satisfactory hemodynamic performance is the primary objective of postoperative cardiac surgical management. Optimal cardiac function ensures adequate perfusion and oxygenation of other organ systems and improves the chances for an uneventful recovery from surgery. Even brief periods of cardiac dysfunction can lead to impairment of organ system function, leading to potentially life-threatening complications. This chapter presents the basic concepts in cardiovascular management and then reviews the evaluation and management of the low cardiac output syndrome, hypertension, coronary spasm, perioperative myocardial infarction, cardiac arrest, and rhythm disturbances that can contribute to compromised cardiovascular function.

I. Basic Principles

The important concepts of postoperative cardiac care are those of cardiac output, tissue oxygenation, and the ratio of myocardial oxygen supply and demand. Ideally, one should strive to obtain a cardiac index greater than 2.2 $L/min/m^2$ with a normal mixed venous oxygen saturation while optimizing the oxygen supply:demand ratio.

A. **Cardiac output** is determined by the stroke volume and heart rate ($CO = SV \times HR$). The stroke volume is equal to the left ventricular end-diastolic volume (LVEDV) minus the left ventricular end-systolic volume (LVESV) and is calculated by dividing the cardiac output by the heart rate. The three major determinants of stroke volume are preload, afterload, and contractility.

1. **Preload** refers to the LV end-diastolic fiber length and is generally considered to reflect left-sided ventricular volume at end-diastole (the LVEDV). Although this can be estimated by echocardiography, preload is more commonly assessed by a measurement of left-sided filling pressures using a pulmonary artery (Swan-Ganz) catheter. These include the pulmonary artery diastolic (PAD) pressure and pulmonary capillary wedge pressure (PCWP). The left atrial pressure (LAP) provides a more precise approximation of the LV end-diastolic pressure (LVEDP) but requires placement of a catheter directly into the left atrium at the time of surgery. The relationship between filling pressures and volumes is determined by ventricular compliance.

   a. The PAD pressure generally correlates with the PCWP, and in most patients "wedging" of the catheter is unnecessary. However, the PAD may be higher than

Manual of Perioperative Care in Adult Cardiac Surgery, 5th Edition. By Robert M. Bojar.
Published 2011 by Blackwell Publishing Ltd.

the PCWP in patients with preexisting pulmonary hypertension or intrinsic pulmonary disease, in whom there is an increased transpulmonary gradient (equal to the PA mean pressure minus the PCWP). In these patients, the PAD will underestimate the LV volume status, yet wedging of the catheter is not recommended because of an increased risk of PA rupture.

b. Filling pressures must be interpreted cautiously in the early postoperative period.[1,2] The PAD and PCW pressures often correlate poorly with the LVEDV early after surgery because of altered ventricular compliance from myocardial edema resulting from cardiopulmonary bypass (CPB) and the use of cardioplegia solutions.[3] Furthermore, the release of various inflammatory substances during bypass and the administration of blood products may increase the pulmonary vascular resistance (PVR).

c. A stiff, hypertrophied left ventricle noted in patients with hypertension or aortic stenosis has reduced ventricular compliance and frequently manifests diastolic dysfunction coming off bypass. These patients usually require high filling pressures to achieve adequate ventricular filling. In contrast, the dilated, volume-overloaded heart may be highly compliant, with an elevated LVEDV at lower pressures.[3]

d. For patients with relatively normal ventricular function, many centers do not use Swan-Ganz catheters and rely upon central venous pressure (CVP) measurements to assess preload. Although this is an inaccurate means of assessing preload in the diseased heart, it gives a fairly good approximation of left-heart filling in the normal heart.[4] Generally, if the CVP exceeds 15–18 mm Hg, inotropic support is indicated. If the patient has other signs of low cardiac output (poor oxygenation, tapering urine output, acidosis), insertion of a Swan-Ganz catheter will allow for a more objective evaluation of the problem.

2. **Afterload** refers to the left ventricular systolic wall tension, which is related to the intraventricular systolic pressure and wall thickness. It is determined by both the preload (Laplace's law relating radius to wall tension) and the systemic vascular resistance (SVR) against which the heart must eject after the period of isovolumic contraction. The SVR can be calculated from measurements obtained from the Swan-Ganz catheter (Table 11.1). It should be kept in mind that the equation to calculate SVR is based on the cardiac output, not the cardiac index. Thus, it will be higher in the smaller patient at a comparable cardiac index. The use of vasodilators to lower the SVR may improve the stroke volume, often in combination with volume infusions and inotropic agents.

3. **Contractility** is the intrinsic strength of myocardial contraction at constant preload and afterload. However, it can be improved by increasing preload or heart rate, decreasing the afterload, or using inotropic medications.

a. Contractility generally reflects systolic function as assessed by the ejection fraction, but is only indirectly related to the cardiac output. For example, the cardiac output generated by a dysfunctional dilated ventricle with a poor ejection fraction may be comparable to or greater than that generated by a normal sized heart with a normal ejection fraction, especially if a significant tachycardia is present. Conversely, a low cardiac output does not necessarily imply that ventricular function is impaired. It may be noted with slow heart rates, with hypovolemia, and with a small, hypertrophied ventricle.

Table 11.1 • Hemodynamic Formulas

Formula	Normal values
Cardiac output (CO) and index (CI)	
$CO = SV \times HR$	4–8 L/min
$CI = CO/BSA$	2.2–4.0 L/min/m²
Stroke volume (SV)	
$SV = CO\,(L/min) \times \dfrac{1000\,(mL/L)}{HR}$	60–100 mL/beat (1 mL/kg/beat)
Stroke volume index (SVI)	
$SVI = SV/BSA$	33–47 mL/beat/m²
Mean arterial pressure (MAP)	
$MAP = DP + \dfrac{(SP - DP)}{3}$	70–100 mm Hg
Systemic vascular resistance (SVR)	
$SVR = \dfrac{MAP - CVP}{CO} \times 80$	800–1200 dyne-s/cm⁵
Pulmonary vascular resistance (PVR)	
$PVR = \dfrac{PAP - PCWP}{CO} \times 80$	50–250 dyne-s/cm⁵
Left ventricular stroke work index (LVSWI)	
$LVSWI = SVI \times (MAP - PCWP) \times 0.0136$	45–75 g/M/m²/beat

BSA = body surface area; HR = heart rate; DP = diastolic pressure; SP = systolic pressure; CVP = central venous pressure; PAP = mean pulmonary artery pressure; PCWP = pulmonary capillary wedge pressure.

b. Nonetheless, the state of contractility is usually inferred from an analysis of the cardiac output and filling pressures, based upon which steps can be taken to optimize hemodynamic performance. In cardiac surgery patients, the cardiac output is usually obtained by thermodilution technology using a Swan-Ganz catheter and bedside computer. A measured aliquot of volume is infused into the CVP port of the catheter and the thermister near the tip measures the pattern of temperature change from which the computer calculates the cardiac output. A continuous cardiac output catheter is frequently used during off-pump surgery and can provide frequent in-line assessments of the cardiac output. The FloTrac device (Edwards Lifesciences) calculates the cardiac output from the energy of the arterial pressure waveform and is helpful when thermodilution assessment appears inaccurate or the PA catheter has been removed.[5]

B. Tissue oxygenation

1. Oxygen transport to tissues is the basic principle upon which hemodynamic support should be based. It is determined by the cardiac output (CO), the hemoglobin (Hb) level, and the arterial oxygen saturation (SaO_2). This is represented by the equation:

$$O_2 \text{ delivery} = CO(Hb \times \% \text{ sat})(1.39) + (PaO_2)(0.0031)$$

where 1.39 is the mL of oxygen transported per gram of Hb and 0.0031 is the solubility coefficient of oxygen dissolved in solution (mL/torr of PaO_2).

2. It should be noted in this equation that the majority of oxygen transported to the tissues is in the form of oxygen bound to Hb, not that dissolved in solution. Thus, one of the major factors lowering O_2 delivery in the postoperative period is a low hematocrit. Increasing the Hb level by 1 g/dL can increase blood oxygen content by 1.39 vol%, whereas an increase in PaO_2 of 100 torr will only transport an additional 0.3 vol% of oxygen.

3. Studies have suggested that the safe lower limit for hematocrit in the early postoperative period to maintain adequate tissue oxygenation is probably around 22–24% in the stable, elective patient.[6] Since this may reduce tissue oxygen delivery to less than 60% of normal, it is imperative that arterial oxygen saturation be close to 100% and cardiac output be optimized to achieve adequate O_2 delivery. Once an arterial saturation of 90% has been achieved, there is little additional benefit of maintaining a high FIO_2 and PaO_2.

4. The threshold for administering blood transfusions has increased with the understanding that patients may fair better postoperatively with hematocrits under 30%.[7] Furthermore, the morbidity associated with blood transfusions has also become more apparent. Transfusions contain proinflammatory cytokines, low levels of 2,3-DPG with increased hemoglobin affinity for oxygen, and are associated with an increased risk of respiratory complications, wound infections, and mortality.[8–10] Despite these concerns, it is a fairly universal practice to transfuse patients to a hematocrit over 25% when they are elderly, frail, have poor ventricular function, borderline respiratory function, hypotension, tachycardia, ischemic ECG changes, or a metabolic acidosis.

5. **Mixed venous oxygen saturation** (SvO_2) can be used to assess the adequacy of tissue perfusion and oxygenation, aiming for an SvO_2 >60%. PA catheters using reflective fiberoptic oximetry are available to monitor the SvO_2 in the pulmonary artery on a continuous basis. Intermittent SvO_2 measurements can be obtained from blood samples from the distal PA port of the Swan-Ganz catheter. A change of 10% in the SvO_2 can occur before any change is noted in hemodynamic parameters. Despite its theoretical benefit, several studies have suggested that the SvO_2 is an unreliable and insensitive predictor of the cardiac output. However, when analyzed in conjunction with other hemodynamic parameters, trends in the SvO_2 offer insight into cardiac performance and tissue oxygen delivery.[11]

   a. In the postoperative cardiac surgical patient, a fall in SvO_2 generally reflects decreased oxygen delivery or increased oxygen extraction by tissues and is suggestive of a reduction in cardiac output. However, other constantly changing factors that affect oxygen supply and demand may also influence SvO_2 and must be taken into consideration. These include shivering, pain, agitation, temperature, anemia, alteration in FIO_2, and the efficiency of alveolar gas exchange. The Fick equation, which uses the arteriovenous oxygen content difference to determine cardiac output, can be rearranged as follows:

$$SvO_2 = SaO_2 - \frac{VO_2}{Hb \times 1.39 \times CO} \times 10$$

where:

SvO_2 = mixed venous oxygen saturation

SaO_2 = arterial oxygen saturation

VO_2 = oxygen consumption

normal PvO_2 = 40 torr and SvO_2 = 75%

normal PaO_2 = 100 torr and SaO_2 = 99%

b. This equation indicates that a decrease in SvO_2 may result from a decrease in SaO_2, cardiac output, or hemoglobin level, or an increase in oxygen consumption.

c. When the arterial O_2 saturation is normal (SaO_2 > 95%), a PvO_2 < 30 torr or an SvO_2 <60% suggests the presence of a decreased cardiac output and the need for further assessment and therapeutic intervention. Conversely, a rise in SvO_2 reflects less oxygen extraction as seen with hypothermia, sepsis, or intracardiac or significant peripheral arteriovenous shunting. When an elevated SvO_2 is noted, oxygen delivery or utilization may be impaired and an otherwise "normal" cardiac output may be insufficient to provide adequate tissue oxygenation.

6. When the cardiac index exceeds 2.2 L/min/m^2 and the arterial oxygen saturation is adequate (>95%), it may be inferred that oxygen delivery to the tissues is satisfactory. Thus, SvO_2 measurements to assess oxygen delivery are not necessary. However, there are a few situations in which calculation of tissue oxygenation may be valuable in assessing cardiac function:

a. When the thermodilution cardiac output is unreliable (tricuspid regurgitation, improperly positioned Swan-Ganz catheter) or cannot be obtained (Swan-Ganz catheter has not been placed or cannot be placed, such as in the patient with a mechanical tricuspid valve or central venous thrombosis, or has been removed).[12]

b. When the thermodilution cardiac output may seem spuriously low and inconsistent with the clinical scenario (malfunctioning Swan-Ganz catheter or incorrect calibration of computer). A normal SvO_2 indicates that the cardiac output is sufficient to meet tissue metabolic demands.

c. When the cardiac output is marginal, in-line assessment of trends in the mixed venous oxygen saturation can provide up-to-date information on the relative status of cardiac function.

C. Myocardial oxygen supply and demand

1. Myocardial O_2 demand (mvO_2) is influenced by factors similar to those that determine the cardiac output (afterload, preload, heart rate, and contractility). Reducing afterload will generally improve cardiac output with a decrease in mvO_2, whereas an increase in any of the other three factors will improve cardiac output at the expense of an increase in mvO_2. *Preoperative* management of the patient with ischemic heart disease is primarily directed towards minimizing O_2 demand.[13]

2. **Myocardial O_2 supply** is determined by coronary blood flow, the duration of diastole, the coronary perfusion pressure, the Hb level, and the arterial oxygen saturation. When complete revascularization has been achieved, *postoperative* management is directed towards optimizing factors that improve O_2 supply and, to a lesser degree, minimize an increase in O_2 demand.

   a. A heart rate of 80–90 bpm should be achieved and excessive tachycardia and arrhythmias must be avoided.

   b. An adequate perfusion pressure (mean arterial pressure > 80 mm Hg) should be maintained, taking care to avoid both hypotension and hypertension.

   c. Ventricular distention and wall stress (i.e., afterload) should be minimized by avoiding excessive preload, reducing the SVR, and using inotropic medications to improve contractility.

   d. The hematocrit should be maintained at a safe level. Although an increased level of hemoglobin should improve oxygen delivery, transfusions carry inherent risks. In general, myocardial ischemia should not occur in the well-protected, revascularized heart unless the hematocrit drops into the low 20s.

   e. Ischemic ECG changes suggest that coronary blood flow may not be adequate. This may result from stenosis, thrombus, or spasm in a native vessel or bypass graft or incomplete revascularization. If ECG changes are noted, immediate attention and possible reevaluation by catheterization are indicated.

II. Low Cardiac Output Syndrome

A. General comments

1. The achievement of a satisfactory cardiac output is the primary objective of postoperative cardiovascular management. Hemodynamic norms for the patient recovering uneventfully from cardiac surgery are a cardiac index (CI) greater than 2.0 L/min/m^2, a PCWP or PAD pressure below 20 mm Hg, and a heart rate below 100 bpm. The patient should have warm, well-perfused extremities with an excellent urine output.[14]

2. Low cardiac output states are more common in patients with advanced age, LV systolic or diastolic dysfunction (e.g., low ejection fraction or cardiac output, LVEDP > 20 mm Hg), longer durations of aortic cross-clamping or CPB, re-operations, concomitant CABG-valve operations, mitral valve surgery, and patients with chronic kidney disease.[15–18] Diastolic dysfunction is a particularly difficult problem to treat at the conclusion of bypass and usually requires pharmacologic support for a low output state.[19] Increased lactate release after 5 minutes of reperfusion is an independent predictor of a low cardiac output. It suggests that there is delayed recovery of aerobic metabolism, perhaps as a result of inadequate myocardial protection.[20]

3. Myocardial function generally declines for about 6–8 hours following surgery, presumably from ischemia/reperfusion injury with use of cardioplegic arrest, before returning to baseline within 24 hours.[3,21] Temporary inotropic support is often required during this period to optimize hemodynamic performance. Drugs used to provide support at the conclusion of CPB should generally be continued for this brief period of time and can be weaned once the cardiac output is satisfactory.

4. When marginal ventricular function is present in the anesthetized or sedated patient, the compensatory mechanisms normally present in the awake patient that can augment cardiac output are blunted. These include sympathetic autonomic stimulation and endogenous catecholamine production that can increase heart rate, contractility, and arterial and venous tone, elevating both preload and afterload. All of these factors may improve cardiac output or systemic blood pressure, but they may also increase myocardial oxygen demand at a time when asymptomatic ischemia is commonly present.[22]

5. When these compensatory mechanisms are not present in the sedated patient, therapeutic intervention is necessary to improve the cardiac output. It is imperative to intervene before or at the first sign of clinical manifestations of a low cardiac output syndrome. These include:

   a. Poor peripheral perfusion with pale, cool extremities and diaphoresis

   b. Pulmonary congestion and poor oxygenation

   c. Impaired renal perfusion and oliguria

   d. Metabolic acidosis

6. The use of invasive monitoring to continuously evaluate a patient's hemodynamic status allows for appropriate therapeutic interventions to be undertaken before these advanced clinical signs become apparent. Nonetheless, subtle findings, such as a progressive tachycardia or cool extremities, should alert the astute clinician to the fact that the patient needs more intensive management. Intervention is indicated for a low cardiac output state, defined as a cardiac index below $2.0 \, L/min/m^2$, usually associated with left-sided filling pressures exceeding 20 mm Hg and an SVR exceeding 1500 dyne-s/cm^5. It cannot be overemphasized that observing trends in hemodynamic parameters, rather than absolute numbers, is important when evaluating a patient's progress or deterioration.

7. A general scheme for the management of postoperative hemodynamic problems is presented in Table 11.2.

Table 11.2 • Management of Hemodynamic Problems

BP	PCW	CO	SVR	Plan
↓	↓	↓	↓	Volume
N	↑	N	↑	Venodilator or diuretic
↓	↑	↓	↑	Inotrope
↑	↑	↓	↑	Vasodilator
↑↓	↑	↓	↑	Inotrope/vasodilator/IABP
↓	N	N ↑	↓	α-agent

↑ increased; ↓ decreased; N normal; ↑↓ variable

B. Etiology. A low cardiac output state may result from abnormal preload, contractility, heart rate, or afterload. It may also be noted in patients with satisfactory systolic function but marked left ventricular hypertrophy and diastolic dysfunction.[23]

   1. Decreased left ventricular preload

   a. Hypovolemia (bleeding, vasodilation from warming, vasodilators, narcotics, or sedatives)

   b. Cardiac tamponade

   c. Positive-pressure ventilation and PEEP

   d. Right ventricular dysfunction (RV infarction, pulmonary hypertension)

   e. Tension pneumothorax

   2. Decreased contractility

   a. Low ejection fraction

   b. Myocardial "stunning" from transient ischemia/reperfusion injury or myocardial ischemia; perioperative infarction

   i. Poor intraoperative myocardial protection

   ii. Incomplete myocardial revascularization

   iii. Anastomotic complications/graft thrombosis

   iv. Native coronary artery or graft spasm

   v. Evolving infarction at time of surgery

   c. Hypoxia, hypercarbia, acidosis

   3. Tachy- and bradyarrhythmias

   a. Tachycardia with reduced cardiac filling time

   b. Bradycardia

   c. Atrial arrhythmias with loss of atrial contraction

   d. Ventricular arrhythmias

   4. Increased afterload

   a. Vasoconstriction

   b. Fluid overload and ventricular distention

   c. Left ventricular outflow tract obstruction following mitral valve repair or replacement (from struts or retained leaflet tissue)

   5. Diastolic dysfunction with impaired relaxation and high filling pressures

   6. Syndromes associated with cardiovascular instability and hypotension

   a. Sepsis (hypotension from a reduction in SVR; hyperdynamic with a high cardiac output early and myocardial depression at a later stage)

   b. Anaphylactic reactions (blood products, drugs)

   c. Adrenal insufficiency (primary or in the patient on preoperative steroids)

   d. Protamine reactions

C. Assessment (concerns noted in parentheses)

   1. Bedside physical examination: breath sounds, jugular venous distention, murmurs, warmth of extremities, and peripheral pulses (cool extremities, weak pulses, distended neck veins)

2. Hemodynamic measurements: assess filling pressures and determine the cardiac output with a Swan-Ganz catheter; calculate SVR; measure SvO_2 (low cardiac output, high filling pressures, high SVR, low SvO_2)

3. Arterial blood gases (hypoxia, hypercarbia, acidosis/alkalosis) hematocrit (anemia), and serum potassium (hypo- or hyperkalemia)

4. ECG (ischemia, arrhythmias, conduction abnormalities)

5. Chest x-ray (pneumothorax, hemothorax, position of the endotracheal tube or intra-aortic balloon)

6. Urinary output (oliguria)

7. Chest tube drainage (mediastinal bleeding)

8. Two-dimensional echocardiography is very helpful when the cause of a low cardiac output syndrome is unclear. Along with hemodynamic measurements, it can help identify whether it is related to LV systolic or diastolic dysfunction, RV systolic dysfunction, or cardiac tamponade. **Transesophageal echocardiography (TEE)** provides better and more complete information than a transthoracic study and can be readily performed in the intubated patient. It should always be considered when the clinical picture is consistent with tamponade but a transthoracic study is inconclusive.[24]

D. **Treatment** (Table 11.3)

1. Ensure satisfactory **oxygenation** and **ventilation** (see Chapter 10).

2. Treat **ischemia** or **coronary spasm** if suspected to be present. Myocardial ischemia often responds to intravenous nitroglycerin (NTG) but may require further investigation if it persists. Coronary spasm (see page 516) can be difficult to diagnose but usually responds to IV NTG and/or a calcium channel blocker, such as sublingual nifedipine or IV diltiazem.

3. Optimize **preload** by raising filling pressures with volume infusion to a PCWP or PAD pressure of about 18–20 mm Hg. This may be all that is necessary to achieve a satisfactory cardiac output. Volume infusion is preferable to atrial pacing for improving cardiac output because it produces less metabolic demand on the recovering myocardium.[25]

   a. The ideal left-sided filling pressures can be determined from a review of pre- and intraoperative hemodynamic data and an understanding of the patient's cardiac pathophysiology. Filling pressures will differ once the patient is anesthetized due to alterations in loading conditions and autonomic tone. They will subsequently be affected by reduced ventricular compliance at the termination of CPB. Direct visual inspection of the heart, evaluation of TEE images, and measurement of cardiac outputs at this time will usually indicate the appropriate filling pressures for optimal ventricular filling and cardiac performance.

   b. For example, a PCWP around 15–18 mm Hg is usually best for patients with preserved LV function. In contrast, a PCWP in the low 20s may be necessary to achieve adequate preload in patients with poor LV function, a stiff hypertrophied ventricle with diastolic dysfunction, a small LV chamber (mitral stenosis or after resection of a left ventricular aneurysm), or preexisting pulmonary hypertension from mitral valve disease. Ventricular size and compliance should be kept in mind when deciding whether additional volume is the next appropriate step in the patient with marginal cardiac function.[3]

Table 11.3 • Management of Low Cardiac Output Syndrome

1. Look for non-cardiac correctable causes (respiratory, acid–base, electrolyte)
2. Treat ischemia or coronary spasm
3. Optimize preload (PCWP or LA pressure of 18–20 mm Hg)
4. Optimize heart rate at 90–100 bpm with pacing
5. Control arrhythmias
6. Assess cardiac output and start inotrope if cardiac index is less than 2.0 L/min/m²
   - Epinephrine unless arrhythmias or tachycardia
   - Dopamine (if low SVR) or dobutamine (if high SVR)
   - Milrinone/inamrinone
7. Calculate SVR and start vasodilator if SVR over 1500
   - Nitroprusside if high filling pressures, SVR, and blood pressure
   - Nitroglycerin if high filling pressures or evidence of coronary ischemia or spasm
8. If SVR is low
   - Norepinephrine if marginal cardiac output
   - Phenylephrine if satisfactory cardiac output
   - Vasopressin 0.01–0.07 units/min if satisfactory cardiac output
9. Blood transfusion if hematocrit less than 26%
10. IABP if refractory to pharmacologic intervention
11. Ventricular assist device if no response to the above

c. The response to volume infusion may be variable (see postoperative scenario described on pages 312–315). Failure of filling pressures to rise with volume may result from the capillary leak that is present during the early postoperative period. It may also result from vasodilation associated with rewarming or the use of medications with vasodilator properties, such as propofol or narcotics. It is more common in the volume-overloaded compliant ventricle. However, it may also reflect the beneficial attenuation of peripheral vasoconstriction that is attributable to an improvement in cardiac output caused by the volume infusion. As the SVR and afterload gradually decrease, the cardiac output may improve further without an increase in preload.

d. A rise in filling pressures without improvement in cardiac output may adversely affect myocardial performance as well as the function of other organ systems. At this point, inotropic support is usually necessary. Thus, careful observation of the response to volume infusion is imperative.

   i. Excessive preload increases left ventricular wall tension and may exacerbate ischemia by increasing myocardial oxygen demand and decreasing the transmyocardial gradient (aortic diastolic minus LV diastolic pressure) for coronary blood flow. It may also impair myocardial contractility.

ii. Excessive preload may lead to interstitial edema of the lungs, resulting in increased extravascular lung water, ventilation/perfusion abnormalities, and hypoxemia.

iii. Excessive preload in the patient with right ventricular dysfunction may impair myocardial blood flow to the RV, resulting in progressive ischemia. A distended RV may contribute to left ventricular dysfunction because of overdistention and septal shift that impairs LV distensibility and filling.

iv. The presence of RV or biventricular dysfunction may also cause systemic venous hypertension which may reduce perfusion pressure to other organ systems. This may affect the kidneys (causing oliguria), the gastrointestinal (GI) tract (causing splanchnic congestion, jaundice, or ileus), or the brain (contributing to altered mental status).

v. Thus, the temptation must be resisted to administer additional volume to the failing heart with high filling pressures. **Excessive preload *must* be avoided because it may lead to deterioration, rather than improvement, in hemodynamic performance.**

4. Stabilize the **heart rate and rhythm**. All attempts should be made to achieve atrioventricular synchrony with a heart rate of 90–100 bpm. This may require atrial (AOO or AAI) or atrioventricular (DDD or DVI) pacing. These modalities take advantage of the 20–30% improvement in cardiac output provided by atrial contraction that will not be achieved with ventricular pacing alone. This is especially important in the hypertrophied ventricle. Temporary biventricular pacing may be beneficial in improving hemodynamics (both systolic and diastolic function) in patients with impaired ventricular function, especially with prolonged AV conduction (wide QRS complex).[26–28] However, this may provide primarily a short-term hemodynamic benefit with no impact on clinical outcome.[29] Antiarrhythmic drugs should be used as necessary to control ventricular ectopy or slow the response to atrial fibrillation (AF).

5. **Improve contractility** with inotropic agents. This should be based on an understanding of the α, β, or nonadrenergic hemodynamic effects of vasoactive medications and their anticipated effects on preload, afterload, heart rate, and contractility. These medications and a strategy for their selection are noted on pages 457–472.

   a. The use of inotropic agents in the early postoperative period may seem paradoxical in that augmented cardiac output is being achieved at the expense of an increase in oxygen demand (e.g., increased heart rate and contractility). However, the major determinant of oxygen demand is the pressure work that the left ventricle must perform. This is reflected by the afterload, which is determined by preload and SVR. Inotropic drugs that are used to increase contractility do not necessarily increase oxygen demand in the failing heart because they reduce preload, afterload, and frequently the heart rate as a result of improved cardiac function.

   b. If the cardiac output remains low despite pharmacologic support, physiologic support with an **intra-aortic balloon pump** (IABP) should be considered strongly. If the patient cannot be weaned from bypass or has hemodynamic evidence of severe ventricular dysfunction despite maximal medical therapy and the IABP, use of **a circulatory assist device** should be considered. This is discussed starting on page 478.

6. **Reduce afterload** with vasodilators if the cardiac output is marginal while carefully monitoring systemic blood pressure to avoid hypotension. Vasodilators must be used cautiously when the cardiac index is very poor, because an elevated SVR from intense vasoconstriction is often a compensatory mechanism in low cardiac output states to maintain central perfusion. If the calculated SVR exceeds 1500 dyne-s/cm^5, vasodilators may be indicated either alone or in combination with inotropic medications.

7. It is essential to integrate all hemodynamic parameters when determining whether a patient is or is not doing well. For example, the blood pressure may be high when the heart is not performing well, the cardiac output may be acceptable when the heart is struggling, and the cardiac output can be low even when ventricular function is normal.

   a. The presence of a satisfactory or elevated blood pressure (BP) is not necessarily a sign of good cardiac performance. Blood pressure is related directly to **both** the cardiac output and the systemic vascular resistance (BP = CO × SVR). In the early postoperative period, myocardial function may be marginal despite normal or elevated blood pressure because of an elevated SVR resulting from augmented sympathetic tone and peripheral vasoconstriction. Vasodilators can be used to reduce afterload in the presence of elevated filling pressures, thus reducing myocardial ischemia and improving myocardial function. However, **withdrawal of inotropic support in the hypertensive patient should be considered only after a satisfactory cardiac output has been documented.** Otherwise, acute deterioration may ensue.

   b. One should not be deceived into concluding that myocardial function is satisfactory when the cardiac output is "adequate" but is being maintained by fast heart rates at low stroke volumes.

      i. Although sinus tachycardia is often related to the use of catecholamines or even milrinone, it is often an ominous sign of acute myocardial ischemia or infarction, and it may render the borderline heart ischemic. The stroke volume index (SVI) is an excellent method of assessing myocardial function, because it assesses how much blood the heart is pumping each beat. Unless the patient is hypovolemic, a low SVI (less than 30 mL/beat/m^2) indicates poor myocardial function for which inotropic support is usually indicated. Although β-blockers would theoretically be beneficial to control tachycardia in the injured or ischemic heart, they are poorly tolerated in the presence of LV dysfunction and should be use cautiously, if at all.

      ii. Sinus tachycardia may represent a beneficial compensatory mechanism for a small stroke volume in a patient with a small left ventricular chamber (following LV aneurysm resection or mitral valve replacement for mitral stenosis). In these situations, an attempt to slow the heart rate pharmacologically may compromise the cardiac output significantly. Not infrequently, sinus tachycardia is a means of compensating for hypovolemia and quickly resolves after fluid administration.

      iii. Tachycardia may also be present in patients with left ventricular hypertrophy and diastolic dysfunction, especially after aortic valve replacement for aortic stenosis. In these situations, the cardiac output may be low despite preserved ventricular function because of a small noncompliant LV chamber. β-blockers or calcium channel blockers can be used to slow the heart rate after adequate volume replacement has been achieved, but must be used with extreme caution. Use of a medication with lusitropic (relaxant) properties, such as milrinone or nesiritide, may be helpful.

    iv. Tachycardia accompanying a large stroke volume is often seen in young patients with preserved ventricular function. It can be treated safely with a β-blocker, such as esmolol.

  c. The cardiac output may be marginal when the patient is hypovolemic (even if LV function is normal) and does not develop a compensatory tachycardia. This is noted in patients who were well β-blocked prior to surgery and in those who require pacing at the conclusion of the operation. Pacing up to a rate of 90 bpm and a moderate volume infusion are invariably successful in improving the cardiac output in this situation. If the cardiac output is not acceptable once the filling pressures are satisfactory, an inotrope should be added. The common temptation to continue to administer fluid once the filling pressures are elevated may be more harmful than helpful to the struggling heart.

8. **Maintain blood pressure**

  a. If the patient has **a satisfactory cardiac output but a low systemic resistance and low blood pressure**, the filling pressures are often low and a moderate volume infusion should improve the blood pressure. This scenario is common in sedated patients receiving medications that have potent vasodilator properties. It is also common in patients who had been taking certain medications preoperatively, such as the angiotension-converting enzyme (ACE) inhibitors, angiotensin receptor blockers (ARBs), calcium channel blockers, and amiodarone (which blocks sympathetic stimulation by α and β blockade).

    i. If hypotension persists after volume infusion, an α-agent should be used to increase the systemic vascular resistance. Norepinephrine (NE) is the preferred drug when the cardiac output is marginal because it has β-agonist properties, whereas phenylephrine is a pure α-agonist and is best used only if the cardiac output is satisfactory. Some patients respond better to norepinephrine than phenylephrine, and others just the reverse.

    ii. Although NE does induce renal vasoconstriction, it generally has little adverse effect on renal function.[30–32] Furthermore, if NE is effective in raising the systemic pressure, it does not affect intestinal mucosal perfusion or the splanchnic oxygen supply:demand ratio.[33] Thus, unless the patient remains hypotensive in a low cardiac output state, concerns about impaired regional perfusion are mitigated.

    iii. When catecholamine-resistant hypotension persists despite a satisfactory cardiac output, it may represent a condition of autonomic failure termed "vasoplegia". This may be a consequence of the systemic inflammatory response (although it has been noted after off-pump surgery as well) and may be related to nitric oxide-induced vasodilation. It has been shown that levels of vasopressin are low in most normotensive patients after bypass but are inappropriately low in patients with "vasodilatory shock". **Arginine vasopressin** acts on vasomotor V_1 and renal V_2 receptors and, given in a dose of 0.01–0.07 units/min, can restore blood pressure in these patients. Such low doses may suffice because patients with vasodilatory shock tend to be hypersensitive to its effects. Concerns when using vasopressin include the following:

- Vasopressin does improve renal perfusion in that it constricts the efferent rather than the afferent arterioles, in contradistinction to the effects of α-agents on renal perfusion. However, one study suggested that it increased the glomerular filtration rate, resulting in an increase in the filtered load of sodium, but also increased renal oxygen extraction and impaired renal oxygenation.[34]

- It induces intestinal and gastric mucosal vasoconstriction; thus if the cardiac output remains marginal, mesenteric ischemia is more likely to occur.[35]

- It does not provide any inotropic support, so any improvement in ventricular function is related to an improvement in perfusion pressure. Thus, it must be used with caution in patients with persistent low cardiac output states.

- It is beneficial in patients with low SVR and pulmonary hypertension as it does not produce a significant alteration in PA pressures.[36]

- It may induce vasospasm in ITA grafts.[37]

iv. An alternative to the use of vasopressin is **methylene blue** 1.5 mg/kg, which inhibits guanylate cyclase activation by nitric oxide. It has been reported to be beneficial in reducing morbidity and mortality in patients with postbypass vasoplegia.[38–40]

b. **If the patient has a persistently low blood pressure and cardiac output** despite volume infusions and adequate filling pressures, inotropic support should be initiated or increased, anticipating a rise in systemic blood pressure. If this does not occur, an IABP may be required to improve the cardiac output. Frequently, an α-agent must also be added simultaneously to augment the blood pressure, and norepinephrine is preferable because it provides some β effects. Sometimes, use of an α-agent to improve coronary perfusion pressure leads to an improvement in cardiac output. As noted above, vasopressin is best avoided when the cardiac output is marginal because it is a pure vasoconstrictor with no inotropic properties and may compromise splanchnic blood flow.

c. Correct **anemia** with blood transfusions. The hematocrit is usually maintained above 24% in the postoperative period, but transfusions should be considered for persistent hypotension, hemodynamic instability, metabolic acidosis, or evidence of myocardial ischemia.

E. **Right ventricular failure and pulmonary hypertension** (also see pages 317–318 and 327–328)

1. A low cardiac output state may be the result of RV failure, producing inadequate filling of the left heart. Patients may be predisposed to RV dysfunction because of preexisting conditions, such as:

a. Right coronary artery (RCA) disease or severe coronary disease in a left-dominant circulation

b. RV infarction secondary to a proximal RCA occlusion

c. Pulmonary hypertension (PH) of any cause: most commonly this is associated with mitral/aortic disease or severe LV dysfunction, but may result from severe lung disease (cor pulmonale) or primary pulmonary hypertension. In patients with PH undergoing heart transplantation, the donor heart may not be able to acutely adapt to long-standing pulmonary hypertension, especially if undersized with a prolonged ischemic time, and RV failure will ensue.

2. RV systolic dysfunction may also occur in patients with no known preexisting RV problems. It may be attributable to:

   a. Poor myocardial protection, usually due to poor collateral circulation with an occluded RCA or due to exclusive use of retrograde cardioplegia

   b. Prolonged ischemic times/myocardial stunning

   c. Inadvertent RCA distribution ischemia (obstruction of a coronary ostium during aortic valve replacement, kinking of the RCA ostial button in aortic root replacements)

   d. Coronary embolism from air (usually in valve operations), thrombi, or particulate matter (in reoperative CABG or valve operations)

   e. Systemic hypotension causing RV hypoperfusion

   f. Acute pulmonary hypertension (increased PVR and RV afterload) from:
   - Vasoactive substances associated with blood product transfusions and CPB
   - Severe LV dysfunction
   - Protamine reaction ("catastrophic pulmonary vasoconstriction")
   - Hypoxemia and acidosis
   - Tension pneumothorax

   g. RV pressure overload: intrinsic pulmonary disease, acute respiratory distress syndrome, pulmonary embolism

3. Isolated RV dysfunction is characterized by a high RA/PCW pressure ratio, although this is usually unreliable when LV dysfunction is also present. RV ejection fraction thermodilution catheters and echocardiography are very helpful in assessing the status of RV function. However, the presence of significant tricuspid regurgitation in these patients may render thermodilution cardiac outputs unreliable. Thus, alternative means of assessing cardiac output, such as a mixed venous oxygen saturation or the FloTrac system, may be necessary.

4. RV dysfunction may contribute to progressive LV dysfunction due to ventricular interdependence. When the RV dilates, it shifts the interventricular septum leftward, impairing LV distensibility. Progressive LV dysfunction may then reduce systemic perfusion pressure, causing RV ischemia, and may elevate PA pressures and RV afterload.

5. The goals of treatment are to optimize RV preload, ensure AV conduction, maintain systemic perfusion pressure, improve RV contractility, reduce RV afterload by reducing PVR, and optimize left ventricular function (Table 11.4).

   a. **RV preload** must be raised cautiously to avoid the adverse effects of RV dilatation on RV myocardial blood flow and LV function. It is generally taught that cardiac output can be improved by volume infusions in patients sustaining RV infarctions with compromised RV function. However, the RA pressure should not be

Table 11.4 • Management of Right Ventricular Failure

1. Optimize preload with CVP of 18–20 mm Hg

2. Ensure AV conduction

3. Maintain adequate systemic perfusion pressure with vasoactive medications or an IABP

4. Reduce RV afterload (PVR) and improve RV contractility

   a. Correct hypothermia, hypoxemia, hypercarbia, acidosis

   b. Select inotropes with vasodilator properties (milrinone, inamrinone, low-dose epinephrine, dobutamine, isoproterenol)

   c. Nesiritide

   d. Use a pulmonary vasodilator

      • Inhaled nitric oxide

      • Inhaled epoprostenol

      • Inhaled iloprost

5. Optimize left ventricular function

6. Mechanical circulatory assist (RVAD) if no response to the above

increased to more than 20 mm Hg. If no improvement in cardiac output ensues when volume is given to reach this pressure, additional volume infusions should be avoided. Volume overload of the right ventricle contributes to progressive deterioration of RV function, impairment of LV filling, and systemic venous hypertension.

b. AV conduction is essential.

c. Systemic perfusion pressure must be maintained while trying to avoid medications that can also increase PVR. Maintaining adequate perfusion of the RV may require **IABP** support.[41]

d. Correction of hypothermia, hypoxemia, and respiratory acidosis by hyperventilation will decrease the PVR (acidosis rather than hypercarbia is most deleterious).

e. Inotropic medications that can support RV and LV function and also reduce the pulmonary artery pressure should be selected.[42]

   i. The phosphodiesterase (PDE) inhibitors, **milrinone** and **inamrinone**, are very beneficial in improving RV contractility and reducing PA pressures, although they are usually associated with systemic hypotension that requires an α-agent to support the SVR. Unfortunately, the use of α-agents may also increase the PVR. Dobutamine may produce similar effects to those of the PDE inhibitors. The combination of IV milrinone with oral sildenafil produces a synergistic reduction in PVR.[42]

   ii. Isoproterenol may be the most effective drug to improve RV contractility. It use must be tempered by the possibility of inducing a significant tachycardia.

   iii. Dobutamine is an effective inotrope that improves RV contractility in patients with RV failure, although it has little effect on pulmonary hemodynamics.

   iv. Levosimendan (see page 467) exhibits similar inotropic effects to dobutamine, but is more effective in reducing RV afterload. Clinical experience with this medication in patients with RV failure is limited, but it holds promise.[43]

f. **Pulmonary vasodilators** should also be considered.

   i. **Nitroso dilators**, including nitroglycerin and nitroprusside, may be effective in reducing PA pressures, but nitroglycerin is usually associated with a reduction in cardiac output and nitroprusside primarily reduces the SVR. Thus, they may be beneficial in patients with moderate PH and RV dysfunction, but have relatively limited applications in patients with severe RV dysfunction. They have been supplanted by other more potent and selective pulmonary vasodilators.

   ii. **Nesiritide** is a synthetic B-type natriuretic peptide (BNP) that has no direct inotropic effect, but it exhibits a lusitropic effect that reduces PA pressures and to some degree systemic pressures. Thus it indirectly improves the cardiac output. It has been shown to improve outcomes in high-risk patients undergoing mitral valve surgery.[44] It also improves renal perfusion and exerts a powerful diuretic effect that achieves a synergistic effect when used with the loop diuretics.[45] It is given as a $2\,\mu g/kg$ IV bolus over 1 minute followed by an infusion of $0.01-0.03\,\mu g/kg/min$ (see further discussion of nesiritide on pages 466–467).

   iii. **Inhaled nitric oxide (iNO)** is a selective pulmonary vasodilator that can decrease RV afterload and augment RV performance with minimal effect on SVR, thus maintaining systemic perfusion pressure.[46] The usual dose is 10–40 ppm administered via the ventilatory circuit. The circuit must be designed to optimally mix O_2 and NO to generate a low level of NO_2, which is toxic to lung tissue. Measurements of the concentraton of NO in the inhalation limb and NO_2 in the exhalation limb of the ventilatory circuit by chemiluminescence are essential during delivery. Ideally, a scavenger system should be attached to the exhaust port of the ventilator. Although iNO is quite effective, it is very expensive, somewhat cumbersome to use, and potentially toxic if not appropriately monitored. When pulmonary hypertension and RV failure are severe enough to warrant use of iNO, operative mortality rates are very high (>60% for most patients), except those receiving iNO after heart transplantation.[47]

     • iNO does not increase intrapulmonary shunting. It may reverse the hypoxic vasoconstriction that is frequently noted with other pulmonary vasodilators (such as nitroprusside) and may improve the PaO_2/FiO_2 ratio.[48]

     • When pulmonary hypertension is refractory to nitric oxide, as may be noted in valve patients, the addition of dipyridamole 0.2 mg/kg IV may reduce RV afterload.[49] Dipyridamole blocks the hydrolysis of cyclic GMP (cGMP) in vascular smooth muscle and may also attenuate rebound pulmonary hypertension noted after nitric oxide withdrawal.

This phenomenon may be the result of elevated endothelin-1 levels induced by NO administration.[50]

- NO in the bloodsteam is rapidly metabolized to methemoglobin (metHb) and levels should be monitored. Methemoglobinemia is rarely noted in adults, but can be a significant problem in young children.

- NO should be weaned slowly to prevent a rebound increase in PVR. A general guideline is to decrease the dose no more than 20% every 30 minutes. Inhalation can be stopped once 6 ppm is reached.

- A comparative study of iNO and milrinone in patients with pulmonary hypertension upon separation from bypass showed that iNO was associated with lower heart rates, better RV ejection fraction, and less requirement for phenylephrine to support systemic resistance.[51]

- Other studies have shown that iNO, prostacyclin, and iloprost were all effective in lowering PA pressures and improving RV function.[52,53]

iv. **Prostaglandin and prostacyclin analogs** are potent pulmonary vasodilators that have been used primarily to assess vascular reactivity in patients awaiting heart transplantation. However, they are also beneficial in reducing PA pressure and improving RV function in patients with severe pulmonary hypertension during and after various types of cardiac surgery (usually mitral valve surgery and cardiac transplantation).

- **Epoprostenol** (prostacyclin, PGI_2 [Flolan]) is both a pulmonary and very strong systemic vasodilator when administered intravenously because it is not inactivated by the lungs. However, inhaled PGI_2 is a very effective short-acting selective pulmonary vasodilator that can improve RV performance without affecting SVR. It may also improve oxygenation by decreasing ventilation/perfusion mismatch. Studies have reported use of a single 60 μg inhalation in the operating room or a continuous inhalation using either a weight-based protocol (up to 50 ng/kg/min, at which dose some systemic vasodilation may occur) or a concentration-based protocol, giving 8 mL/h of a 20 μg/mL solution. There is complete reversal of effect about 25 minutes after inhaled PGI_2 is stopped.[54–56]

- **Iloprost** (Ventavis) is a synthetic prostacyclin analog that also reduces PVR and increases cardiac output with little effect on blood pressure or SVR. It can be given in an aerosolized dose of 25–50 μg during and after surgery. Its hemodynamic effect lasts 1–2 hours after a single administration. Comparative studies have shown it to be superior to both iNO and nitroglycerin in reducing PVR while also improving cardiac output.[52,57–59] Additional advantages over iNO are its lower cost, lack of toxic metabolites, and ease of administration.

- **PGE_1** is an effective pulmonary vasodilator at a dose of 0.03–0.2 μg/kg/min, but at doses greater than 0.1 μg/kg/min, systemic vasodilation may occur. This can be offset by the infusion of epinephrine directly into a left atrial line.[60,61] This medication is rarely used because of the availability of the prostacyclin analogs.

- A comparative study of iNO (40 ppm), PGE_1 (0.1 μg/kg/min) and NTG (3–5 μg/kg/min) in patients with pulmonary hypertension after cardiac surgery showed that all three medications were capable of reducing PVR. However, iNO increased cardiac output without systemic vasodilation, PGE_1 increased cardiac output and improved RV performance with systemic vasodilation, and NTG reduced SVR without any hemodynamic improvement.[62] This study demonstrated the advantages of the inhaled pulmonary vasodilators over several systemically administered medications.

    v. **Sildenafil** is a PDE type V inhibitor that prevents the degradation of cGMP and reduces pulmonary vascular tone. Given in oral doses of 25–50 mg bid–qid, it has been used to wean patients off intravenous or inhaled pulmonary vasodilator support.[63,64]

  g. **Endothelin receptor antagonists** have been used in patients with primary pulmonary hypertension and may also prove beneficial in postoperative patients with elevated PA pressures and RV dysfunction. The utility and role of these medications has yet to be delineated. Available medications include bosentan, which can be taken orally, and tezosentan, which is administered parenterally.

  h. If RV dysfunction persists despite use of inotropic support, pulmonary vasodilators, and an IABP, implementation of mechanical assistance with a right ventricular assist device may be necessary.

F. **Diastolic dysfunction** is a common cause of congestive heart failure (CHF) in hypertensive patients, and can pose hemodynamic problems after surgery when ventricular compliance is affected by use of CPB and cardioplegia. It is most prominent after a prolonged period of cardioplegic arrest, especially in the small hypertrophied heart.

  1. Diastolic dysfunction is caused by decreased diastolic compliance, often with an inappropriate tachycardia.[65] The end result is a low cardiac output syndrome with a small left ventricular chamber at end-diastole yet high left-sided filling pressures. The stiffness of the heart is usually evident on echocardiogram, which may confirm normal systolic function even though the patient is in a low output state.

  2. This problem can be difficult to manage and often results in end-organ dysfunction, such as renal failure, that progresses until the diastolic dysfunction improves (see page 317). Although inotropic drugs are frequently given, they are of little benefit. In contrast, ACE inhibitors may improve diastolic compliance; lusitropic drugs, such as the calcium channel blockers, magnesium, nesiritide, and milrinone, may improve ventricular relaxation; and bradycardic drugs, such as β-blockers or calcium channel blockers, can be used for an inappropriate tachycardia. Aggressive diuresis may also be beneficial in reducing myocardial edema that might contribute to reduced compliance.

III. Inotropic and Vasoactive Drugs

A. General comments

  1. A variety of vasoactive medications are available to provide hemodynamic support for the patient with marginal myocardial function.[14] They should be chosen carefully to achieve a satisfactory cardiac index (>2.2 $L/min/m^2$) and blood pressure once adequate filling pressures have been achieved. The selection of a particular drug depends on an understanding of its mechanism of action and limitations to its use (see page 468 for recommendations on drug selection). The catecholamines exert their effects on α- and β-adrenergic receptors. They elevate levels of intracellular cyclic AMP (cAMP) by β-adrenergic stimulation of adenylate cyclase. In contrast, the phosphodiesterase (PDE) inhibitors (milrinone, inamrinone) elevate cAMP levels by inhibiting cAMP hydrolysis. Elevation of cAMP augments calcium influx into myocardial cells and increases contractility.

a. α_1 and α_2 stimulation result in increased systemic and pulmonary vascular resistance. Cardiac α_1-receptors increase contractility and decrease the heart rate.

b. β_1 stimulation results in increased contractility (inotropy), heart rate (chronotropy), and conduction (dromotropy).

c. β_2 stimulation results in peripheral vasodilation and bronchodilation.

2. The net effects of medications that share α and β properties usually depend on the dosage level and are summarized in Table 11.5.

3. Concomitant use of several medications with selective effects may minimize the side effects of higher doses of individual medications. For example:

a. Inotropes with vasoconstrictive (α) properties can be combined with vasodilators to improve contractility while avoiding an increase in SVR (e.g., norepinephrine with nitroprusside).

b. Inotropes with vasodilator properties can be combined with α-agonists to maintain SVR (e.g., milrinone with neosynephrine or norepinephrine).

c. Catecholamines can be combined with the PDE inhibitors to provide synergistic inotropic effects while achieving pulmonary and systemic vasodilation (e.g., epinephrine with milrinone).

d. α-agents can be infused directly into the left atrium to maintain SVR while a pulmonary vasodilator is infused into the right heart.

4. The benefits of most vasoactive medications are noted when adequate blood levels are achieved in the systemic circulation. Thus, these medications should be given into the central circulation via controlled infusion pumps rather than peripherally. Although higher levels can be reached by drug infusion into the left atrium to avoid pulmonary vascular effects and reduce drug inactivation by the lungs, this is an uncommon practice.

5. The standard mixes and dosage ranges are listed in Table 11.6.

B. Epinephrine

1. Hemodynamic effects

a. Epinephrine is a potent β_1-inotropic agent that increases cardiac output by an increase in heart rate and contractility. At doses less than 2 μg/min (<0.02–0.03 μg/kg/min), it has a β_2 effect that produces mild peripheral vasodilation, but the blood pressure is usually maintained or elevated by the increase in cardiac output. At doses greater than 2 μg/min (>0.03 μg/kg/min), α effects will increase the SVR and raise the blood pressure. Metabolic acidosis may also be noted at low doses of epinephrine when α effects are not evident.

b. Epinephrine has strong β_2 properties that produce bronchodilation.

c. Although epinephrine may contribute to arrhythmias or tachycardia, studies have shown that epinephrine given at a dose of 2 μg/min causes less tachycardia than dobutamine given at a dose of 5 μg/kg/min.[66]

Table 11.5 • Hemodynamic Effects of Vasoactive Medications

Medication	SVR	HR	PCW	CI	MAP	MvO$_2$
Dopamine	↓↑	↑↑↑	↓↑	↑	↓↑	↑
Dobutamine	↓	↑↑↑	↓	↑	↓↔↑	↑↔
Epinephrine	↓↑	↑↑	↓↑	↑	↑	↑
Milrinone/ Inamrinone	↓↓	↑	↓	↑	↓	↓↑
Isoproterenol	↓↓	↑↑↑↑	↓	↑	↓↑	↑↑
Calcium chloride	↑	↔	↑	↑	↑↑	↑
Norepinephrine	↑↑	↑↑	↑↑	↑	↑↑↑	↑
Phenylephrine	↑↑	↔	↑	↔	↑↑	↔↑
Vasopressin	↑↑	↔	↑	↔	↑↑↑	↔↑
Nesiritide	↓	↔	↓↓	↑*	↓	↓↓

↑ increased; ↓ decreased; ↔ no change; ↓↑ variable effect. The relative effect is indicated by the number of arrows.

Note:
1. The effect may vary with dosage level (particularly dopamine and epinephrine, in which case the effect seen at low dose is indicated by the first arrow).
2. For some medications, an improvement in MAP may occur from the positive inotropic effect despite a reduction in SVR.
3. The effects of inamrinone, milrinone, and calcium are not mediated by α and β receptors.

*indirect effect.

    d. Epinephrine delivered through a left atrial line produces a higher cardiac index with less increase in PVR, but in cases of RV dysfunction, the PDE inhibitors are preferable.[60]

  2. Indications

    a. Epinephrine is usually the first-line drug for a **borderline cardiac output** in the absence of tachycardia or ventricular ectopy. It is very helpful in the hypertrophied heart that often takes a while to recover adequate systolic function after cardioplegic arrest. Epinephrine is extremely effective and has very low cost.

    b. It is especially helpful in **stimulating the sinus node** mechanism when the intrinsic heart rate is slow. It is frequently beneficial in improving the atrium's responsiveness to pacing at the conclusion of bypass.

    c. Bronchospasm may respond well to epinephrine, especially when an inotrope is also required.

    d. Anaphylaxis (protamine reaction)

    e. Resuscitation from cardiac arrest

  3. Starting dose is 1 μg/min (about 0.01 μg/kg/min) with a mix of 1 mg/250 mL. Dosage can be increased to 4 μg/min (about 0.05 μg/kg/min). Higher doses are rarely indicated in patients following cardiac surgery.

Table 11.6 • Mixes and Dosage Ranges for Vasoactive Medications

Medication	Mix	Dosage Range
Dopamine	400 mg/250 mL	2–20 µg/kg/min
Dobutamine	500 mg/250 mL	5–20 µg/kg/min
Epinephrine	1 mg/250 mL	1–4 µg/min (0.01–0.05 µg/kg/min)
Milrinone	20 mg/200 mL	50 µg/kg bolus, then 0.375–0.75 µg/kg/min
Inamrinone	200 mg/200 mL	0.75 mg/kg bolus, then 10–15 µg/kg/min
Isoproterenol	1 mg/250 mL	0.5–10 µg/min (0.0075–0.1 µg/kg/min)
Norepinephrine	4 mg/250 mL	1–50 µg/min (0.01–0.5 µg/kg/min)
Phenylephrine	40 mg/250 mL	5–150 µg/min (0.05–1.5 µg/kg/min)
Vasopressin	40 units/80 mL	0.01–0.07 units/min
Nesiritide	1.5 mg/100 mL	2 µ/kg bolus, then 0.01–0.03 µg/kg/min

Note: x milligrams placed in 250 mL gives a infusion rate of x micrograms (mg divided by 100) in 15 drops of solution. For example, a 200 mg/250 mL mix gives a drip of 200 µg in 15 drops. 60 microdrops = 1 mL. 15 drops/min = 15 mL/h.

Note: the final volume of the mix reflects the total volume; thus for inamrinone, 50 mL of inamrinone is added to 150 mL to achieve a total volume of 200 mL. For all of the other medications, the drug volume is very small.

C. **Dopamine**

1. **Hemodynamic effects** depend on the dosage administered, although plasma levels and effects may not correlate with the infused dose.

   a. At doses of 2–3 µg/kg/min, dopamine has a selective "dopaminergic" effect that reduces afferent arteriolar tone in the kidney, with an indirect vasoconstrictive effect on efferent arterioles. The net effect is an increase in renal blood flow, glomerular filtration rate, and urine output. The diuretic effect may also be attributable to effects on renal tubular function as well as some inotropic effect, since there may be some activation of α_1- and β_1-receptors at this level.[67] This can produce a profound tachycardia. There is also a mild β_2 effect which decreases SVR and may reduce the blood pressure. Despite use of low-dose dopamine to improve urine output, it has not been shown that it can prevent or alter the natural history of acute kidney injury once it develops, and it is not recommended to preserve renal function during surgery.[68,69]

   b. At doses of 3–8 µg/kg/min, dopamine exhibits a β_1 inotropic effect that improves contractility, and, to a variable degree, a chronotropic effect that increases heart rate and the potential for arrhythmogenesis. It also has a dromotropic effect that increases AV conduction during atrial fibrillation/flutter.[70]

   c. At doses greater than 8 µg/kg/min, there are increasing inotropic effects, but also a predominant α effect that occurs directly and by endogenous release of norepinephrine. This raises the SVR, systemic blood pressure, and filling pressures, and may adversely affect myocardial oxygen consumption and ventricular function. Concomitant use of a vasodilator, such as nitroprusside, to counteract these α effects allows for the best augmentation of cardiac output. The dopaminergic effect may still be present despite the vasoconstrictive effects.[14]

2. Indications

   a. Dopamine may be considered a first-line drug for a **low cardiac output state**, especially when the SVR is low and the blood pressure is marginal. Its use may be limited by the development of a profound tachycardia, even at very low doses, and occasionally by excessive urine output. In these situations, another inotrope should be selected.

   b. It is beneficial in **improving urine output** in patients with or without preexisting renal dysfunction.[67] Nonetheless, the "renoprotective" effect of dopamine during open-heart surgery and in the early postoperative course is controversial, with most studies suggesting it has no demonstrable benefit in preserving renal function.[68,69]

3. Starting dose is 2 µg/kg/min with a mix of 400 mg/250 mL. Dosage can be increased to 20 µg/kg/min.

D. Dobutamine

1. Hemodynamic effects

   a. Dobutamine is a positive inotropic agent with a strong β_1 effect that increases heart rate in a dose-dependent manner and also increases contractility. It also exhibits mild vasodilatory β_2 effects that tend to offset a mild vasoconstrictive α_1 effect, resulting in a reduction in SVR, although one study suggested just the opposite effect on SVR.[71] Most commonly, diastolic filling pressures are reduced and blood pressure is maintained by improved cardiac performance.

   b. Dobutamine has been compared with other inotropic agents in several studies.

     i. Dobutamine and dopamine increase myocardial oxygen demand to a comparable degree, but only dobutamine is able to match this increase with augmented myocardial blood flow.[72] This favorable effect on the myocardial supply:demand ratio is offset to some degree, however, by the development of tachycardia. Other studies have shown that, in contrast to dopamine, dobutamine reduces left ventricular wall stress and oxygen demand by lowering preload and afterload.[73] This is particularly evident in volume-overloaded hearts (valve replacement for mitral or aortic regurgitation).[74]

     ii. Dobutamine causes more tachycardia than epinephrine.[66]

     iii. Dobutamine and the PDE inhibitors provide comparable hemodynamic support, although dobutamine is associated with more hypertension, tachycardia, and a greater chance of triggering atrial fibrillation.[75]

2. Indications

   a. Dobutamine is most useful when the **cardiac output is marginal and there is a mild elevation in SVR**. Its use is usually restricted by development of a tachycardia.

    b. It is a moderate **pulmonary vasodilator** and may be helpful in improving RV function and lowering RV afterload.

    c. It has a synergistic effect in improving cardiac output when used with a PDE inhibitor (milrinone/inamrinone). This combination is commonly used in patients awaiting cardiac transplantation.

  3. **Starting dose** is 5 µg/kg/min using a mix of 500 mg/250 mL. Dosage can be increased to 20 µg/kg/min.

E. **Milrinone (Primacor) and Inamrinone (Inocor)**

  1. **Hemodynamic effects**

    a. These are phosphodiesterase (PDE) III inhibitors that can best be described as "inodilators".[76] They improve cardiac output by reducing systemic and pulmonary vascular resistance and by exerting a moderate positive inotropic effect. There is usually a modest increase in heart rate, a lowering of filling pressures, and a moderate reduction in systemic blood pressure. Thus, they generally are associated with a reduction in myocardial oxygen demand. They also lower coronary vascular resistance.[77,78] Although the unloading effect produced by the decrease in SVR may contribute a great deal to their efficacy, an α-agent (phenylephrine or norepinephrine) is frequently required to maintain systemic blood pressure. PDE inhibitors increase cyclic AMP levels, which causes relaxation of myofilaments, and this lusitropic effect improves ventricular compliance after bypass.[79] However, some studies suggest that these drugs do not exhibit lusitropic properties and have no effect on diastolic dysfunction in unselected patients.[80,81]

    b. Additive effects on ventricular performance are noted when these medications are combined with one of the catecholamines, such as epinephrine, dobutamine, or dopamine, due to differing sites of action.

    c. Milrinone and inamrinone provide comparable hemodynamic effects, and have been compared with dobutamine in several studies. The increase in cardiac output is similar to that achieved with dobutamine, but dobutamine is associated with a greater increase in heart rate and a higher incidence of atrial and ventricular arrhythmias.[75] Consequently, dobutamine may increase myocardial oxygen demand and the risk of periperative infarction.

    d. The tachycardia produced by the PDE inhibitors may be offset by the use of β-blockers without compromising the beneficial inotropic effects.[82]

  2. **Indications**

    a. These are generally second-line medications that should be used for a **persistent low cardiac output state** despite use of one of the catecholamines or when their use is limited by tachycardia. However, a preemptive bolus of milrinone given on pump significantly reduces the need for any catecholamine in the immediate perioperative period.[83]

    b. They are particularly valuable in patients with **right ventricular dysfunction** associated with an elevation in PVR, such as patients with pulmonary hypertension from mitral valve disease or those awaiting and following cardiac transplantation.

    c. Their lusitropic (relaxant) properties may be of value in patients with significant **diastolic dysfunction** that may contribute to a low output state, even with preserved systolic function.

3. **Advantages and disadvantages**

   a. PDE inhibitors have long elimination half-lives of 1.5–2 hours for milrinone and 3.6 hours for inamrinone. The half-lives are even longer in patients with low cardiac output states, being 2.3 and 4.8 hours, respectively, for patients in CHF. Thus, an intraoperative bolus can be used to terminate bypass and provide a few hours of additional inotropic support without the need for a continuous infusion.

   b. Because the hemodynamic effects persist for several hours after the drug infusion is discontinued (in contrast to the short duration of action of the catecholamines), the patient must be observed carefully for deteriorating myocardial function for several hours as their effects wear off.

   c. Inamrinone has been associated with the development of thrombocytopenia. Therefore, platelet counts must be monitored on a daily basis. In contrast, thrombocytopenia is very rare with milrinone, which is often used for weeks at a time in patients awaiting transplantation.[84]

   d. PDE inhibitors vasodilate arterial conduits. Thus, they may prove beneficial in a patient with suspected coronary or graft spasm who requires inotropic support.[77,78]

4. **Starting doses**

   a. Milrinone: 50 μg/kg IV bolus over 10 minutes, followed by a continuous infusion of 0.375–0.75 μg/kg/min of a 20 mg/200 mL solution. Note that because of its long half-life, it takes up to 6 hours to reach a steady-state level if not given with a loading dose.

   b. Inamrinone: 0.75 mg/kg bolus over 10 minutes, followed by a continuous infusion of 10–15 μg/kg/min with a mix of 200 mg/200 mL. When given during surgery, a 1.5 mg/kg bolus is usually required to achieve a satisfactory plasma concentration.

F. **Isoproterenol**

1. **Hemodynamic effects**

   a. Isoproterenol has a strong β_1 effect that increases cardiac output by a moderate increase in contractility and a marked increase in heart rate with a slight β_2 effect that lowers SVR. The increased myocardial O_2 demand caused by the tachycardia limits its usefulness in coronary bypass patients. Isoproterenol may produce ischemia out of proportion to its chronotropic effects, and it also predisposes to ventricular arrhythmias.

   b. Isoproterenol's β_2 effect lowers PVR and reduces right-heart afterload.

   c. There is a strong β_2 bronchodilator effect.

2. **Indications**

   a. **Right ventricular dysfunction** associated with an elevation in PVR. Isoproterenol is both an inotrope and a pulmonary vasodilator and thus is helpful in supporting RV function following mitral valve surgery in patients with pulmonary hypertension. Because it causes a profound tachycardia, it has generally been replaced by the PDE inhibitors. However, it is still commonly used following heart transplantation to reduce PVR, improve RV function, and produce ventricular relaxation.

    b. Bronchospasm when an inotrope is required.

    c. Bradycardia in the absence of functioning pacemaker wires. It is commonly used after heart transplantation to maintain a heart rate of 100–110 bpm.

  3. Starting dose is 0.5 μg/min with a mix of 1 mg/250 mL. It can be increased to about 10 μg/min (usual dosage range is 0.0075–0.1 μg/kg/min).

G. Norepinephrine (Levophed)

  1. Hemodynamic effects

    a. Norepinephrine (NE) is a powerful catecholamine with both α- and β-adrenergic properties. Its predominant α effect raises SVR and blood pressure, while the β_1 effect increases both contractility and heart rate.

    b. By increasing afterload and contractility, NE increases myocardial oxygen demand and may prove detrimental to the ischemic or marginal myocardium. Although it may also cause regional redistribution of blood flow, studies suggest that renal and intestinal perfusion are maintained if the systemic blood pressure improves.[30–33] Furthermore, the addition of dobutamine has been shown to improve gastric mucosal perfusion in patients receiving NE.[85]

    c. Note: There is a tendency to think that NE is providing only an α effect, but it does possess strong β properties. Thus, it should be anticipated that both the cardiac output and heart rate will fall when the drug is weaned.

  2. Indications

    a. Norepinephrine is primarily indicated when the patient has a marginally **low cardiac output with a low blood pressure caused by a low SVR.** This is often noted when the patient warms and vasodilates. Use of a pure α-agent is feasible if the cardiac index exceeds 2.5 L/min/m^2, but NE can provide some inotropic support if the cardiac index is borderline. If the cardiac index is below 2.0 L/min/m^2, another inotrope should probably be used in addition to norepinephrine.

    b. It is frequently effective in raising the blood pressure when little effect has been obtained from phenylephrine (and vice versa).

    c. It has been used as an inotrope to improve cardiac output in conjunction with a vasodilator, such as phentolamine or sodium nitroprusside, to counteract its α effects.

  3. Starting dose is 1 μg/min (about 0.01 μg/kg/min) with a mix of 4 mg/250 mL. The dose may be increased as necessary to achieve a satisfactory blood pressure. Higher doses (probably >20 μg/min or >0.2 μg/kg/min) most likely will reduce visceral and peripheral blood flow, frequently producing a metabolic acidosis.

H. Phenylephrine (Neo-Synephrine)

  1. Hemodynamic effects

    a. Phenylephrine is a pure α-agent that increases SVR and may cause a reflex decrease in heart rate. Myocardial function may be compromised if an excessive increase in afterload results. However, it is frequently improved by an elevation in coronary perfusion pressure that resolves myocardial ischemia.

    b. Phenylephrine has no direct cardiac effects.

2. **Indications**

   a. Phenylephrine is indicated only to **increase the SVR when hypotension coexists with a satisfactory cardiac output**. This is commonly noted at the termination of bypass or in the ICU when the patient warms and vasodilates. If the blood pressure remains low after volume infusions, yet the cardiac output is satisfactory, phenylephrine can be used to maintain a systemic blood pressure around 100–110 mm Hg. Significantly higher pressures should be avoided to minimize the adverse effects of an elevated SVR on myocardial function.

   b. Phenylephrine can be used **preoperatively to treat ischemia** by maintaining perfusion pressure while nitroglycerin is used to reduce preload.

3. **Advantages and disadvantages**

   a. Patients often become refractory to the effects of phenylephrine after several hours, necessitating a change to norepinephrine. Conversely, some patients respond very poorly to norepinephrine and have an immediate blood pressure response to low-dose phenylephrine.

   b. By providing no cardiac support other than an increase in central perfusion pressures, phenylephrine has limited indications.

   c. **Note:** Be very careful when administering an α-agent to the patient whose entire revascularization procedure is based on arterial grafts, as it may provoke spasm.

4. **Starting dose** is 5 μg/min with a mix of 40 mg/250 mL. The dosage can be increased as necessary to maintain a satisfactory blood pressure. The usual dosage range is 0.05–1.5 μg/kg/min.

I. **Vasopressin**. See pages 451–452.

J. **Calcium chloride**

1. **Hemodynamic effects**

   a. Calcium chloride's primary effect is to increase the SVR and the mean arterial pressure.[86] It has little effect on the heart rate. It produces a transient improvement in systolic function at the termination of CPB, although it may increase ventricular stiffness, suggesting it produces transient diastolic dysfunction.[87]

   b. One study showed that $CaCl_2$ produces a transient inotropic effect if hypocalcemia is present and a more sustained increase in SVR, independent of the calcium level.[88]

   c. A study that compared epinephrine and calcium chloride upon emergence from CPB showed that both increased the mean arterial pressure, but only epinephrine increased the cardiac output, suggesting that calcium did not provide any inotropic support.[89] Although this study did not find any beneficial or negative effect of combining these two medications, another one did suggest that calcium salts may attenuate the cardiotonic effects of catecholamines, such as dobutamine or epinephrine, but have little effect on the efficacy of inamrinone.[90]

2. **Indications**

   a. Frequently used **at the termination of CPB to augment systemic blood pressure** by either a vasoconstrictive or positive inotropic effect.

   b. **To support myocardial function or blood pressure on an emergency basis** until further assessment and intervention can be undertaken. **Note:** Calcium is not recommended for routine use during a cardiac arrest.

   c. **Hyperkalemia** (K^+ >6.0 mEq/L).

3. **Usual dose** is 0.5–1 g slow IV bolus.

K. Triiodothyronine (T_3)

  1. Hemodynamic effects

    a. Thyroid hormone (triiodothyronine or T_3) exerts a positive inotropic effect by increasing aerobic metabolism and synthesis of high-energy phosphates. It causes a dose-dependent increase in myocyte contractile performance that is independent of and additive to β-adrenergic stimulation.[91]

    b. Most patients have reduced levels of free T_3 for up to 3 days following operations on CPB.[92,93] Routine adminstration of T_3 to maintain normal levels produces a transient improvement in cardiac output, lowers troponin release, and lowers SVR.[94] However, multiple studies have indicated that it does not influence outcomes and cannot be recommended for routine use.[95−98] However, significant improvement in hemodynamics has been noted in patients with impaired ventricular function, many of whom could not be weaned from bypass on multiple inotropes until T_3 was administered.[99]

    c. Note: Calcium channel blockers have been shown to interfere with the action of T_3.

    d. There is some evidence that postoperative atrial fibrillation is more common in patients with subclinical hypothyroidism and low T_3 levels, and that administration of T_3 may reduce the incidence of postoperative AF.[100−102]

  2. Indications

    a. T_3 may be indicated to provide inotropic support as a salvage step when CPB cannot be terminated with maximal inotropic support and an IABP.

    b. T_3 is helpful in improving donor heart function in brain-dead patients when ventricular function is depressed.

  3. Usual dose is 10−20 μg, although some studies have used a bolus of 0.8 μg/kg followed by an infusion of 0.12 mcg/kg/h for 6 hours.[96]

L. Other modalities to treat low cardiac output

  1. Nesiritide is a recombinant B-type natriuretic peptide that has been used primarily in patients with decompensated heart failure. It decreases sympathetic stimulation and inhibits the neurohormonal response (i.e., activation of the renin−angiotensin− aldosterone system and endothelin) noted in patients with heart failure. By inference, these same changes may be seen in patients with postcardiotomy ventricular dysfunction and elevated PA pressures.

    a. Nesiritide produces balanced vasodilation resulting in a decrease in preload (PA pressure) and afterload (SVR). It indirectly increases cardiac output and does so with no increase in heart rate or myocardial oxygen demand. It exhibits lusitropic (relaxant) properties, dilates native coronary arteries and arterial conduits, and has no proarrhythmic effects.

    b. Nesiritide dilates the renal afferent and efferent arterioles, producing an increase in glomerular filtration. It thus has a strong diuretic and natriuretic effect that is synergistic with that of the loop diuretics.

    c. Clinical studies in cardiac surgical patients have shown improved hemodynamics in high-risk patients undergoing mitral surgery, similar outcomes as milrinone in patients with LV dysfunction, less deterioration in renal function and possibly improved long-term survival in patients with low ejection fractions undergoing CABG, and mitigation of renal deterioration in patients with preexisting renal dysfunction.[44,103−107]

d. Indications

  i. Postcardiotomy low output states associated with systolic or diastolic dysfunction, especially when associated with pulmonary hypertension and RV dysfunction. Nesiritide should be considered if problems persist despite a catecholamine and PDE inhibitor, and it may be considered in place of the latter.

  ii. Prophylactic infusion during CPB in patients with preexisting renal dysfunction to optimize renal protection.

  iii. Improvement in postoperative diuresis in patients with renal dysfunction if unresponsive to loop diuretics and intravenous thiazides.[45]

e. Starting dose. Nesiritide is given in a dose of $2 \mu g/kg$ over 1 minute followed by an infusion of $0.01-0.03 \mu g/kg/min$. It has a rapid onset of action with most of its hemodynamic effects noted within the first 30 minutes. Although its half-life is only 18 minutes, hypotension may persist for hours after the infusion is discontinued. It may be given through a peripheral IV and does not require intensive monitoring.

2. **Glucose–insulin–potassium (GIK)** has been demonstrated to have an inotropic effect on the failing myocardium after cardioplegic arrest. It provides metabolic support to the myocardium by increasing anaerobic glycolysis, lowering free fatty acid levels, preserving intracellular glycogen stores, and stabilizing membrane function. The mixture contains 50% glucose, 80 units/L of regular insulin, and 100 mEq/L of potassium infused at a rate of 1 mL/kg/h.[108]

3. **Levosimendan** is a calcium-sensitizing "inodilator" that has been used for patients with decompensated heart failure and has been further evaluated in the management of cardiac surgical patients.[109]

  a. Mechanisms and effects. Levosimendan improves cardiac function by both inotropic and vasodilatory effects. The positive inotropic effect results from sensitizing myofilaments to calcium without increasing intracellular calcium levels. It also has coronary, pulmonary, and systemic vasodilator effects by opening ATP-dependent potassium channels in vascular smooth muscle. Thus, it improves cardiac output by increasing stroke volume with little increase in heart rate, by reducing afterload from its vasodilating effects, and to a slight degree by lusitropic effects. Given at high doses, it may require use of an α-agent to counteract systemic vasodilation. The one major difference between levosimendan and other inotropes is the enhancement of contractility without an increase in myocardial oxygen demand. At low doses, it is not arrhythmogenic. The half-life is $70-80$ hours, so it has a long-lasting effect after administration.

  b. Indications. Levosimendan is useful in improving hemodynamics in patients with anticipated postcardiotomy RV and LV dysfunction and in facilitating weaning from bypass.[110] In patients with RV dysfunction, it decreases PVR and improves RV contractility (better than dobutamine in one study).[111] An infusion started prior to bypass (with or without a loading dose of $24 \mu g/kg$) is very effective in reducing troponin leakage (suggesting a cardioprotective effect), reducing the need for additional inotropic support, maintaining an improved cardiac output, and reducing mortality. These findings were noted when comparing levosimendan vs. placebo, levosimendan + dobutamine vs. milrinone + dobutamine, and levosimendan used alone vs. milrinone + dobutamine.[111-116]

   c. Starting dose. It is given as a 12–24 µg/kg loading dose over 10 minutes, followed by a continuous infusion of 0.1 µg/kg/min.

4. **Dopexamine** is a synthetic catecholamine that stimulates dopaminergic receptors as well as β_2- and, to a lesser extent, β_1-adrenergic receptors. It provides an inotropic effect by inhibiting neuronal uptake of catecholamines and it also increases heart rate in a dose-related manner. It decreases SVR, improves renal and splanchnic perfusion, and may improve ITA flow.[117] It also decreases PVR and can improve RV function. Its effects are fairly equivalent to those of dobutamine, although it may cause more tachycardia, and it may be superior to dopamine.[118-120] It is given as an infusion of 1–4 µg/kg/min. This drug was not approved for use in the United States as of late 2010.

5. **Enoximone** is a PDE inhibitor with hemodynamic effects similar to those of milrinone and inamrinone. It decreases systemic, pulmonary, and coronary resistance, and has a positive inotropic effect with minimal alteration in heart rate. The degree of vasodilation may be less than that of the other drugs, but an α-agent is frequently required to offset the vasodilation caused by a bolus injection. It is not associated with the development of thrombocytopenia. In a study comparing it with dobutamine, enoximone was shown to reduce troponin release and the need for additional inotropes.[121] When given in combination with esmolol during and after surgery for 24 hours, advantages included a reduction in heart rate and an increase in cardiac output compared with use of enoximone alone.[122] It has also been used in an oral form to allow for weaning a patient off IV inotropic support.[123] Enoximone is given as a 0.5–1.0 mg/kg bolus at the termination of bypass followed by a continuous infusion of 2.5 µg/kg/min. This drug was not approved for use in the United States as of late 2010.

M. **Recommended strategy for selection of vasoactive medications**

1. The selection of a vasoactive medication should be based on several factors:

   a. An adequate understanding of the underlying cardiac pathophysiology derived from hemodynamic measurements and echocardiography.

   b. Knowledge of the α, β, or nonadrenergic hemodynamic effects of the medications and their anticipated influence on preload, afterload, heart rate, and contractility.

2. Vasoactive medications are usually started in the operating room and maintained for about 6–12 hours while the heart recovers from the period of ischemia/reperfusion. The doses are adjusted as the patient's hemodynamic parameters improve. Occasionally, when the heart demonstrates persistent "stunning" or has sustained a perioperative infarction, pharmacologic support and/or an IABP may be necessary for several days.

3. When the cardiac index is satisfactory (>2.2 L/min/m^2) but the blood pressure is low, an α-agent should be selected. Phenylephrine is commonly used in the operating room, but norepinephrine is probably a better drug to use in that it provides some β effects that are beneficial during the early phase of myocardial recovery. Systolic blood pressure need only be maintained around 100 mm Hg (mean pressure >80 mm Hg) to minimize the increase in afterload. If neither of

these medications suffices, vasopressin should be utilized.[36] Occasionally, a simple bolus of 1−2 units of vasopressin overcomes the initial vasoplegic state after pump and minimizes the subsequent need for an α-agent.

4. When the cardiac index remains marginal (<2.0 L/min/m^2) after optimizing volume status, heart rate, and rhythm, an inotropic agent should be selected. The first-line drugs are usually epinephrine, dobutamine, or dopamine. The major limitation to their use is the development of tachycardia, which tends to be less prominent with low-dose epinephrine, which is usually the drug of first choice. At inotropic levels, dopamine and epinephrine tend to raise SVR, whereas dobutamine's effect on SVR is variable but usually not significant. If a satisfactory cardiac output has been achieved and the blood pressure is elevated, addition of a vasodilator is beneficial. If the blood pressure is low, an α-agent can be added.

5. If the cardiac output still remains suboptimal despite moderate doses of drugs (epinephrine 2−3 μg/min [0.03−0.04 μg/kg/min], dobutamine 10 μg/kg/min, or dopamine 10 μg/kg/min), a second drug should be used. The PDE inhibitors exhibit additive effects to those of the catecholamines and should be selected. These medications lower the SVR and may cause a modest tachycardia. They commonly require the use of norepinephrine to maintain SVR, although blood pressure may be maintained by the improvement in cardiac function. If norepinephrine is used, its β effect may further improve contractility, but it can also increase the heart rate. Its α effect usually has minimal effect on organ system perfusion if a satisfactory cardiac output can be achieved, but it can compromise flow in arterial conduits (such as the ITA or radial artery). If the cardiac index remains marginal despite the use of two medications, an IABP should be inserted.

6. If the patient cannot be weaned from bypass and has hemodynamic evidence of persistent cardiogenic shock (CI <1.8 L/min/m^2, PCWP >20 mm Hg) despite medications and the IABP, a circulatory assist device should be considered.

7. **Note:** It is not uncommon for the cardiac output to fall to below 1.8−2.0 L/min/m^2 during the first 4−6 hours after surgery, which represents the time of maximal myocardial depression. The dose of an inotrope may need to be increased transiently or, less frequently, another one added if the cardiac output does not improve with volume infusion. However, it is the **persistence of a low output state** beyond this time that raises concern, especially if there is any evidence of myocardial ischemia on ECG, rising filling pressures out of proportion to fluid administration, oliguria, or a progressive metabolic acidosis. An IABP may need to be inserted in the ICU if these problems are present. However, in the absence of any specific identifiable problem, most patients will gradually improve, and one should not be overly alarmed by transient drops in cardiac output or respond too aggressively. If there is any concern, echocardiography is helpful in assessing whether ventricular dysfunction or cardiac tamponade is causing the low output state, and can direct management appropriately.

8. **Note:** Use of α-agents can be dangerous in patients receiving radial artery grafts or when multiple grafts are based on ITA inflow. It is preferable to reduce the dose of the vasodilating drug (diltiazem or nitroglycerin used to prevent spasm), rather than increase the dose of a vasoconstricting medication if hypotension is noted.

N. Vasoactive medications provide specific hemodynamic benefits, but their use may be limited by the development of adverse effects. Nearly all of the catecholamines will increase myocardial oxygen demand by increasing heart rate and contractility. Other side effects that may necessitate changing to or addition of another medication include:

1. Arrhythmogenesis and tachycardia (epinephrine, isoproterenol, dobutamine, dopamine)

2. Vasoconstriction and poor renal, splanchnic, and peripheral perfusion (norepinephrine, phenylephrine, vasopressin)

3. Vasodilation requiring α-agents to support systemic blood pressure (milrinone, inamrinone)

4. Excessive urine output (dopamine)

5. Thrombocytopenia (inamrinone)

6. Cyanide and thiocyanate toxicity (nitroprusside)

7. Methemoglobinemia (nitroglycerin)

O. **Weaning of vasoactive medications**

1. Once the cardiac output and blood pressure have stabilized for a few hours, vasoactive medications should be weaned. α-agents should generally be weaned first. Their use should ideally be restricted to increasing the SVR to support blood pressure when the cardiac output is satisfactory. However, there are circumstances when α-agents are required to maintain cerebral and coronary perfusion in the face of a poor cardiac output. In these desperate life-saving situations, the resultant intense peripheral vasoconstriction can compromise organ system and peripheral perfusion, causing renal, mesenteric, and peripheral ischemia, acidosis, and frequently death.

    a. In the routine patient, SVR and blood pressure increase when myocardial function improves, narcotic effects abate, and sedatives, such as propofol, have been discontinued. As the patient awakens and develops increased intrinsic sympathetic tone, α-agents can be stopped.

    b. When milrinone, inamrinone, or an IABP is used to support myocardial function, an α-agent is frequently required to counteract the unloading effect and decreased SVR that is achieved. It may not be possible to wean the α-agent before the patient has been weaned from one of these medications or the IABP, because the patient may become hypotensive despite an excellent cardiac output. It is usually necessary to wean the α-agent in conjunction with the weaning of the other modalities.

    c. An occasional patient who has sustained a small perioperative infarction will have an excellent cardiac output but a low SVR. This requires temporary α support until the blood pressure improves spontaneously. Such support may be required for several days.

2. The stronger positive inotropes with the most potential detrimental effects on myocardial metabolism should be weaned next. Those that possess α properties should be decreased to doses at which these effects do not occur. If an IABP is present, it should not be removed until the patient is on a low dose of only one inotrope, unless complications of the IABP develop. Otherwise, weaning of the IABP should usually be deferred.

a. The catecholamines should be weaned first to low doses. If the patient is on multiple drugs, epinephrine should be weaned to a low dose (2 μg/min or less) to avoid any α effects. Then dobutamine (which lacks significant α effects) and dopamine should be weaned to doses less than 10 μg/kg/min. At this dose, the α effects of dopamine should dissipate but the β effects will be maintained.

b. Milrinone and inamrinone are second-line drugs and are usually weaned off with the patient still supported by low doses of catecholamines. These medications have few deleterious effects on myocardial function, but often require the use of α-agents. Thus, concomitant weaning of these medications is generally recommended before terminating the infusion of a catecholamine.

  i. Because of their long half-lives, the PDE inhibitors should be stopped hours before the withdrawal of other major support modalities (IABP). The dose is halved and then discontinued a few hours later if hemodynamics remain stable. The cardiac output must be monitored to observe for potential deterioration in myocardial function that may occur several hours after the infusion has been stopped. Occasionally, the patient may require the reinstitution of inotropic support at that point.

  ii. Early discontinuation of inamrinone (or conversion to milrinone) should also be considered when the patient develops progressive thrombocytopenia. It is not always clear whether this is caused by this medication or by other coexisting problems, such as heparin-induced thrombocytopenia or IABP-induced platelet destruction.

  iii. If the patient has a significant tachycardia from a catecholamine, the PDE inhibitor may be used exclusively (although often with an α-agent), and thus would be the last medication discontinued.

c. IABP removal may be performed once the patient is on low doses of inotropic support, such as epinephrine at 1 μg/min or dobutamine or dopamine at 5 μg/kg/min.

d. The requirement for vasoactive medications in patients on circulatory assist devices depends on the extent of support provided and the function of the unsupported ventricle. In patients receiving univentricular support, inotropic medications may be necessary to improve the function of the unassisted ventricle. Patients with biventricular support are usually given only α-agents or vasopressin to support systemic resistance. If the device is being used for temporary support, rather than as a bridge to transplantation, inotropes may be given to assess cardiac reserve when flows are transiently reduced. If ventricular function is recovering, an inotrope, such as milrinone, can be given to provide support after removal of the device, if necessary.

3. Vasodilators are commonly used during the early phase of postoperative recovery to reduce blood pressure when the patient is hypothermic, vasoconstricted, and hypertensive. They are weaned as the patient vasodilates to maintain a systolic blood pressure of 100–120 mm Hg.

   a. Vasodilators may also be used alone or in conjunction with inotropic medications to improve myocardial function by lowering the SVR. In this situation, they are weaned concomitantly with the inotropes, depending on the cardiac output and the blood pressure. Sodium nitroprusside has a very short half-life, clevidipine's duration of action is only about 5–15 minutes, but nicardipine has a duration of action of 4–6 hours.

b. In patients with preexisting hypertension, conversion from intravenous anti-hypertensives to oral agents can be tricky. Some patients require significant doses of multiple drugs to control their blood pressure, only to become hypotensive when the drugs take effect and sympathetic stimulation and the hormonal response to surgery abate. The initial drug is usually a β-blocker (unless the patient is bradycardic), which is routinely used for prophylaxis of atrial fibrillation. An ACE inhibitor or angiotensin receptor blocker is then added, starting at a low dose if not used before or at a lower dose than used preoperatively. Intravenous hydralazine can be used on a prn basis until higher doses of medications take effect.

IV. Intra-aortic Balloon Counterpulsation

Intra-aortic balloon counterpulsation provides hemodynamic support and/or control of ischemia both before and after surgery.[124–126] In contrast to most inotropic agents, the intra-aortic balloon pump (IABP) provides physiologic assistance to the failing heart by decreasing myocardial oxygen demand and improving coronary perfusion. Although it is an invasive device with several potential complications, it has proven invaluable in improving the results of surgery in high-risk patients and allowing for the survival of many patients with postcardiotomy ventricular dysfunction.

A. **Indications**

1. Ongoing ischemia refractory to medical therapy or hemodynamic compromise prior to urgent or emergent surgery.

2. Prophylactic placement for high-risk patients with critical coronary disease (usually left main disease) or severe left ventricular dysfunction – usually following cardiac catheterization, but occasionally at the beginning of surgery.[127–129]

3. High-risk patients undergoing off-pump surgery to maintain hemodynamic stability during lateral wall or posterior wall grafting.[130]

4. Unloading for cardiogenic shock or mechanical complications of myocardial infarction (acute mitral regurgitation, ventricular septal rupture).

5. Postcardiotomy low cardiac output syndrome unresponsive to moderate doses of multiple inotropic agents. The survival rate for patients in this category is only about 70%. IABP has proven successful in patients with predominantly RV failure as well.[41]

6. Postoperative myocardial ischemia.

7. Acute deterioration of myocardial function to provide temporary support or serve as a bridge to transplantation.

B. **Contraindications**

1. Aortic regurgitation

2. Aortic dissection

3. Severe aortic and peripheral vascular atherosclerosis (balloon can be inserted via the ascending aorta during surgery).

C. Principles

1. It reduces the impedance to LV ejection ("unloads the heart") by rapid deflation just before ventricular systole.

2. It increases diastolic coronary perfusion pressure by rapid inflation just after aortic valve closure and improves ITA and graft diastolic flow.[131]

3. This sequence reduces the time-tension index (systolic wall tension) and increases the diastolic pressure-time index, favorably altering the myocardial oxygen supply: demand ratio.

4. The IABP may also improve left ventricular diastolic function after surgery.[132]

5. The utility of IABP in patients with predominantly RV failure is most likely based upon improvement in RV perfusion from diastolic augmentation along with improvement in LV function from unloading.[41]

D. Insertion techniques

1. The IABP is placed through the femoral artery with the balloon situated just distal to the left subclavian artery so as not to impair flow into the left internal thoracic artery (Figure 11.1). Generally, a 40 cc balloon is selected for most patients, reserving smaller (25 or 34 cc) balloons (which have a shorter balloon length) for smaller patients, usually women.

2. Percutaneous insertion is performed by the Seldinger technique, placing the balloon through a sheath (as small as 7.5 Fr) and over a guidewire. The sheath can be left in place or removed from the artery (especially if the femoral artery is small). Sheathless systems can minimize the reduction in flow in femoral vessels and are preferable in patients with peripheral vascular disease and diabetes, but shearing of the balloon during placement can occur in patients with significant

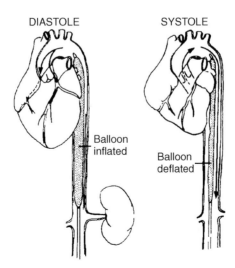

DIASTOLE   SYSTOLE

Balloon inflated

Balloon deflated

Figure 11.1 • The intra-aortic balloon is positioned just distal to the left subclavian artery. Balloon inflation occurs in early diastole and improves coronary perfusion pressure. Deflation occurs just before systole to reduce the impedance to left ventricular ejection. (Reproduced with permission from Maccioli et al., *J Cardiothorac Anesth* 1988;2:365–73.)

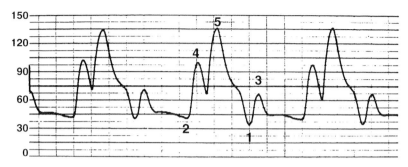

Figure 11.2 • Intra-aortic balloon tracing at 1:2 inflation ratio. Note that the balloon aortic end-diastolic pressure (1) is lower than the patient's aortic end-diastolic pressure (2), and that the balloon-assisted peak systolic pressure (3) is lower than the systolic pressure that is generated without a preceding assisted beat (4). These changes reflect a decreased impedance to ejection during systole. Coronary perfusion pressure is increased by diastolic augmentation achieved by balloon inflation (5).

iliofemoral disease.[133] Percutaneous insertion is associated with a significant risk of limb ischemia in patients with known peripheral vascular disease. Although insertion of the IABP can be performed blindly in the OR or at the bedside, preoperative placement is usually performed in the cardiac cath lab using fluoroscopy to visualize the wire and the eventual location of the balloon. This may allow for placement through a tortuous iliofemoral system, which otherwise might be fraught with danger. During surgery, the position of the balloon catheter can be identified by TEE.

3. Surgical insertion can be accomplished by exposing the femoral artery and placing the balloon through a sidearm graft or directly into the vessel through an arteriotomy or a percutaneous sheath.

4. Alternative cannulation sites in patients with severe aortoiliac disease include the ascending aorta, subclavian artery, and brachial artery.[134,135]

E. **IABP timing** is performed from the ECG or the arterial waveform.

1. ECG: input to the balloon console is provided from skin leads or the bedside monitor. Inflation is set for the peak of the T wave at the end of systole with deflation set just before or on the R wave. The use of bipolar pacing eliminates the interpretation of pacing spikes as QRS complexes by the console.

2. Arterial waveform: inflation should occur at the dicrotic notch with deflation just before the onset of the aortic upstroke. This method is especially useful in the operating room, where electrocautery may interfere with the ECG signal.

3. A typical arterial waveform during a 1:2 ratio of IABP inflation is demonstrated in Figures 11.2 and 11.3. This shows the systolic unloading (decrease in the balloon-assisted systolic and diastolic pressures) and the diastolic augmentation that are achieved with the IABP.

4. Appropriate timing of inflation and deflation is essential. Proper timing should improve stroke volume and reduce LV end-systolic volume and pressure. Early inflation may decrease stroke volume due to the abrupt increase in LV afterload during late systolic ejection. Late deflation will increase afterload during early

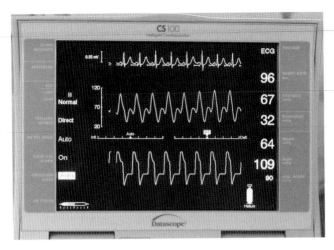

Figure 11.3 • IABP monitor showing the ECG, arterial pressure tracing with balloon augmentation, and balloon inflation/deflation pattern.

ejection and decrease afterload during late ejection. This may increase stroke volume but also increase stroke work.[136]

F. IABP problems and complications

1. **Inability to balloon.** Once the balloon is situated properly and has unwrapped, satisfactory ballooning should be achieved by proper timing of inflation and deflation. However, unsatisfactory ballooning can occur in the following situations.

   a. Unipolar atrial pacing. This produces a large atrial pacing spike that can be interpreted by the console as a QRS complex leading to inappropriate inflation. Use of bipolar pacing eliminates this problem. Most monitoring equipment suppresses pacing signals.

   b. Rapid rates. Some balloon consoles are unable to inflate and deflate fast enough to accommodate heart rates over 150 (usually when there is a rapid ventricular response to atrial fibrillation). Augmentation can be performed with a 1:2 ratio.

   c. Arrhythmias. Atrial and ventricular ectopy can disrupt normal inflation and deflation patterns and must be treated.

   d. Volume loss from the balloon detected by the console monitor alarms. This indicates a leak in the system, either at the connectors or from the balloon itself. Volume loss may also indicate that the balloon has not unwrapped properly, preventing proper inflation.

   e. Balloon rupture. When blood appears in the balloon tubing, the balloon has perforated. Escape of gas (usually helium) from the balloon into the bloodstream can occur. **The balloon must be removed immediately.** Difficulty with removal (balloon entrapment) may be encountered if thrombus has formed within the balloon. Most consoles have alarms that will call attention to this problem and prevent the device from inflating.

2. **Vascular complications**

    a. Catastrophic complications, such as aortic dissection or rupture of the iliac artery or aorta, are very uncommon. Paraplegia can result from development of a periadventitial aortic hematoma or embolization of atherosclerotic debris.[137,138]

    b. Embolization to visceral vessels, especially the mesenteric and renal arteries, can occur in the presence of significant aortic atherosclerosis, although balloon placement usually does not affect mesenteric flow.[139–141] Cerebral embolization can occur if there are mobile atheromas in the proximal descending thoracic aorta.[142] Renal ischemia may occur if the balloon is situated too low and inflates below the level of the diaphragm.[143]

    c. Distal ischemia is the most common complication of indwelling balloons, occurring in about 10–15% of patients. It is more likely to occur when the IABP remains in place longer and in patients with impaired ventricular function.[144] It is more common in patients who are older, female (small femoral arteries), diabetic, or have peripheral vascular disease, especially involving the iliofemoral system. Thrombosis near the insertion site or distal thromboembolism can also occur. Use of intravenous heparin (maintaining a PTT of 1.5–2 times control) is advisable to minimize ischemic and thromboembolic problems if the balloon remains in place for more than a few days after surgery. Otherwise, patients have a low-grade coagulopathy in the early postoperative period and anticoagulation is not necessary.

    d. The presence of distal pulses or Doppler signals must be assessed in all patients with an IABP. This should be compared with a preoperative peripheral pulse examination. Not infrequently, cool extremities with weak signals are noted in the early postoperative period from peripheral vasoconstriction that may be associated with a low cardiac output state, hypothermia, or use of vasopressors. This should resolve when the patient warms and myocardial function improves. However, persistent ischemia jeopardizes the viability of the distal leg. Options at this time include:

      i. Removing the sheath from the femoral artery if the balloon has been placed percutaneously.

      ii. Removing the balloon if the patient appears to be hemodynamically stable. If adequate distal perfusion cannot be obtained, femoral exploration is indicated.

      iii. Removing the balloon and placing it in the contralateral femoral artery (if that leg has adequate perfusion) if the patient is IABP-dependent. Using as small a caliber balloon as possible with sheath removal is essential.

      iv. Considering placement of a transthoracic balloon.

3. **Thrombocytopenia.** The mechanical action of persistent inflation and deflation will destroy circulating platelets. It is not always clear whether progressive thrombocytopenia is caused by the IABP or by medications that the patient may be receiving, such as heparin or inamrinone. Platelet counts must be checked on a daily basis.

G. Weaning of the IABP

1. IABP support can be withdrawn when the cardiac output is satisfactory on minimal inotropic support (usually 1 µg/min of epinephrine or 5 µg/kg/min of either

dopamine or dobutamine). However, earlier removal may be indicated if complications develop, such as leg ischemia, balloon malfunction, thrombocytopenia, or infection.

2. Weaning is initiated by decreasing the inflation ratio from 1:1 to 1:2 for about 2–4 hours, and then to 1:3 or 1:4 (depending on which console device is used) for 1–2 more hours. Once it is determined that the patient can tolerate a low inflation ratio with stable hemodynamics, the IABP should be removed. Remember that the IABP produces efficient unloading, and the blood pressure noted on the monitor is lower during balloon assistance than with an unassisted beat (actually the diastolic pressure is higher, but the true systolic pressure is lower). Thus, visual improvement in blood pressure with weaning of the IABP is not, by itself, a sensitive measure of the patient's progress. If there is an anticipated delay in removal of more than a few hours for manpower reasons or because of the need to correct a coagulopathy, the ratio should be increased to at least 1:2 to prevent thrombus formation.

3. The operative mortality for patients receiving a prophylactic IABP is less than 5%, but it rises to about 30% for patients requiring postcardiotomy support.[145] One study showed that the most significant correlate of operative mortality was a serum lactate level >10 mmol/L during the first 8 hours of support (100% mortality). Additional poor prognostic signs were a metabolic acidosis (base deficit >10 mmol/L), mean arterial pressure < 60 mm Hg, urine output < 30 mL/h for 2 hours, and the requirement for high doses of epinephrine or norepinephrine (>10 µg/min) during the early postoperative period.[146]

H. IABP removal techniques

1. Balloons inserted by the percutaneous technique can usually be removed percutaneously. This is performed by compressing the groin distal to the insertion site as the balloon is removed, allowing blood to flush out the skin wound for several heart beats, and then compressing just proximal to the skin hole where the arterial puncture site is located (Figure 11.4). Pressure must be maintained for at least 45 minutes to ensure satisfactory thrombus formation at the puncture site. **Note:** It

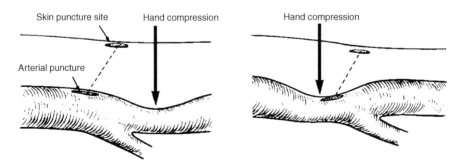

Figure 11.4 • Technique of percutaneous balloon removal. Initial compression is held below the level of the arterial puncture site to allow for flushing of blood. However, subsequent pressure should be maintained over the arterial puncture site to prevent bleeding. Note that the hole in the artery lies more cephalad than the hole in the skin. (Modified with permission from Rodigas & Finnegan, *Ann Thorac Surg* 1985;40:80–1.)

is important to resist the temptation to remove manual pressure and peek to see if hemostasis is achieved. This can be counterproductive and flush away immature clot that is sealing the vessel. Improved surface hemostasis may be obtained using the D-STAT Dry (Vascular Solutions) hemostatic bandage, which contains bovine thrombin.

2. **Note:** Coagulation parameters must be checked and corrected before percutaneous removal or the patient may require groin exploration for persistent hemorrhage or a false aneurysm.

3. Surgical removal should be considered in patients with small or diseased vessels and in those with very weak pulses or Doppler signals with the balloon in place. The need for a thrombectomy and embolectomy may be anticipated in these patients. If the IABP has been in place for more than 5 days, percutaneous removal can be performed, but there is a greater chance that surgical repair of the femoral artery may be required.

V. Circulatory Assist Devices

A. If a patient cannot be weaned from cardiopulmonary bypass despite maximal pharmacologic support and use of an IABP, consideration should be given to placement of a circulatory assist device.[147] These devices provide flow to support the systemic and/or pulmonary circulation while resting the heart, allowing it to undergo metabolic and functional recovery. In some cases, weaning and removal of the device may be possible after several days of recovery. In others, weaning is not possible and bridging to transplantation or destination therapy with a longer-term device must be considered. Some of the more popular devices that can be used for short or long-term support are discussed on pages 484–493.

B. **Clinical conditions** that may benefit from assist devices include:

1. Post-cardiotomy ventricular dysfunction refractory to maximal medical therapy and an IABP

2. Acute myocardial infarction with cardiogenic shock. Percutaneous LVADs can provide superior hemodynamics to use of an IABP, although improved outcomes have not been universally noted.[148,149] Depending on the extent and location of the infarct, right, left, or biventricular assist may be indicated.

3. Supporting high-risk interventions in the cath lab

4. Resuscitation from cardiac arrest[150]

5. Patients with class IV CHF and deteriorating clinical status: temporary support may be useful in patients with myocarditis, but bridging to transplantation or destination therapy with long-term devices may be indicated for patients with chronic heart failure.

C. **Left ventricular assist devices (LVADs)**

1. LVADs provide systemic perfusion while decompressing the left ventricle. LV wall stress is reduced by about 80% with a 40% decrease in myocardial oxygen demand. LVAD flow is dependent on adequate intravascular volume and right ventricular function. Although volume unloading might be superior with pulsatile pumps, left ventricular pressure unloading is comparable with pulsatile and nonpulsatile (centrifugal or axial flow) pumps.[151,152]

Table 11.7 • Indications for Circulatory Assist Devices

1. Complete and adequate cardiac surgical procedure
2. Correction of all metabolic problems (ABGs, acid–base, electrolytes)
3. Inability to wean from bypass despite maximal pharmacologic therapy and use of IABP
4. Cardiac index <1.8 L/min/m²

LVAD	RVAD	BiVAD
Systolic BP < 90 mm Hg	Mean RAP > 20 mm Hg	LAP > 20 mm Hg
LAP > 20 mm Hg	LAP < 15 mm Hg	RAP > 20–25 mm Hg
SVR > 2100 dyne-s/cm⁵	No tricuspid regurgitation	No tricuspid regurgitation
Urine output < 20 mL/h		Inability to maintain LVAD flow > 2.0 L/min/m² with RAP > 20 mm Hg

LVAD, left ventricular assist device; RVAD, right ventricular assist device; BiVAD, biventricular assist devices; RAP, right atrial pressure; LAP, left atrial pressure.

2. **Indications** (Table 11.7). The general indications for LVAD insertion are the presence of a cardiac index <1.8 L/min/m² with a systolic BP <80 mm Hg and a PCWP or left atrial pressure (LAP) >20 mm Hg on maximal medical support and an IABP. In the postcardiotomy patient, an extensive delay in initiating VAD support increases the risk of multisystem organ failure and death.[153] Any of the clinical situations listed in section B with primarily LV failure may benefit from LVAD insertion.

3. **Contraindications.** When the indications for LVAD placement are present, critical elements of decision making include whether there is a reasonable chance of recovery, whether the patient is a candidate for transplantation or destination therapy if there is little chance for recovery, whether RVAD placement is also indicated, or whether placement is contraindicated based upon noncardiac comorbidities. Generally, one must consider the patient's age and general medical condition, the status of RV function, noncardiac organ system function (neurologic, pulmonary, renal, hepatic), and other medical issues (infectious, vascular disease, diabetes), in making this critical decision. Risk factor models to assess survivability after LVAD implantation are helpful in reaching the appropriate decision.[154]

4. **Technique.** Drainage is provided from the left atrium or left ventricular apex with return of blood to the aorta (Figure 11.5). A left atrial catheter may be inserted for accurate monitoring of left-sided filling pressures.

5. **Management** during LVAD support
   a. LVAD flow is initiated to achieve a systemic flow of 2.2 L/min/m² with an LA pressure of 10–15 mm Hg. Pulsatile devices have an automatic mode that ejects a full stroke volume once the reservoir or bladder is full, although other triggering

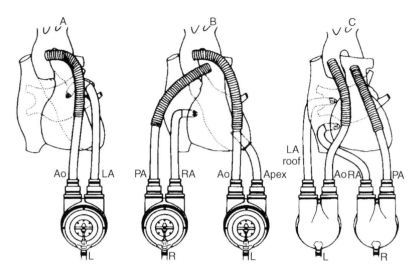

Figure 11.5 • Cannulation techniques for ventricular assist devices. (A) LVAD with left atrial and aortic cannulation. (B) BiVAD setup. The RVAD consists of right atrial and pulmonary artery cannulation. The LVAD cannulation sites are the left ventricular apex (the most common site) and the aorta. (C) BiVAD setup with LVAD drainage from the roof of the left atrium. The Thoratec device is demonstrated in this diagram, but the cannulation sites are similar for nearly all assist devices. (Reprinted with permission of the Massachusetts Medical Society from Farrar et al., *N Engl J Med* 1988;318:333–40.)

    modes are available. The flow rate of centrifugal or axial flow devices can be preset on a console, with limitations to flow being hypovolemia, improper position of the drainage catheter, or RV failure. Adequacy of tissue perfusion can be assessed by mixed venous oxygen saturations.

  b. To decrease myocardial oxygen demand and allow for ventricular recovery, vasoactive medications should be used only as necessary to support RV function or increase systemic resistance to maintain a mean arterial pressure >75 mm Hg. α-agents or vasopressin may be necessary because LVAD patients commonly manifest "vasodilatory shock".[155]

  c. Heparinization is recommended to achieve a PTT of 2–2.5 times normal or an ACT of 185–200 seconds for most short-term assist devices (Abiomed BVS 5000 and AB 5000 ventricles) once perioperative bleeding has ceased. An infusion of 500 units/hour of heparin usually suffices, although most patients become heparin-resistant. For pump flows < 3 L/min or during weaning attempts, the PTT and ACT should be increased to 2.5–3 times normal and 250–300 seconds, respectively. Anticoagulation is also required in patients with bioprosthetic or mechanical valves.

  d. Anticoagulation recommendations for other longer-term devices are noted below under each system.

  e. For patients in whom temporary support is anticipated, left ventricular function is assessed by transesophageal echocardiography (TEE) after at least 48 hours of support. However, weaning is rarely possible before 5 days of support. Flow is reduced in 0.5 L/min intervals every 5 minutes to 2 L/min with careful observation of regional and global wall motion, filling pressures, and systemic pressure. Low-dose inotropic support can be initiated during the weaning process. If adequate recovery has occurred, full flow is resumed, and soon thereafter the patient can be brought to the operating room for device explantation. Again the heart is observed for a short period of time at low flow with or without low-dose inotropic support. If recovery appears adequate, the device is removed.

   f. Note that external compressions during ventricular fibrillation are contraindicated with the Abiomed AB 5000 and HeartMate XVE devices, but can be performed with other systems, including percutaneous and continuous flow devices.

6. **Overall results.** The mortality rate associated with VAD usage for postcardiotomy support depends on how aggressively one approaches a low output syndrome. Because of the high incidence of bleeding and other organ system problems associated with VADs, there is often a reluctance to insert the device "prematurely", because in the majority of cases the heart will gradually improve with time on pharmacologic and IABP support without organ system sequelae. Thus, although there is concern that complications associated with premature VAD insertion could compromise outcomes, an early, aggressive approach to VAD insertion may lower mortality rates, not just because the patient might have survived without its use, but because it might avoid the adverse sequelae of a prolonged low cardiac output syndrome in some patients.

   a. A seminal study from 1999 showed that patients who required two or three inotropes to separate from CPB had mortality rates of 42% and 80%, respectively. Insertion of an Abiomed LVAD within 3 hours of the first attempt to wean from bypass still resulted in an operative mortality of 60%; however, further delay in insertion was associated with a high risk of multisystem organ failure and a 100% mortality.[153]

   b. In general, it has been estimated that weaning can be accomplished in about 50% of patients receiving LVADs for postcardiotomy support with 25–30% of patients surviving to be discharged from the hospital (i.e., an operative mortality of 70–75%). Improved survival may be noted in patients with preserved RV function, no evidence of a perioperative MI, and recovery of LV function within 48–72 hours. In two fairly recent studies from experienced centers in Europe, postcardiotomy survival with LVAD support was about 50%.[156,157]

   c. If ventricular function does not recover after a week of support with a short-term device, a longer-term device should be considered as a bridge to transplantation. Survival following transplantation is similar to that of patients not requiring mechanical assist.[158]

D. Right ventricular assist devices (RVADs)

1. RVADs provide pulmonary blood flow while decompressing the right ventricle.[159] RV failure may result from RV infarction, worsening of preexisting RV dysfunction caused by pulmonary hypertension, or poor intraoperative protection. One of the main contributing factors to RV dysfunction is an elevation in PVR, which can often be attributed to proinflammatory cytokines and microembolization from multiple blood product transfusions.

2. Achieving satisfactory systemic flow rates depends on having adequate intravascular volume and LV function. Although isolated RV failure may occur, it is more commonly associated with left ventricular failure in the postcardiotomy period and may be evident after an LVAD has been implanted (see BiVADs, below).

3. **Indications** (Table 11.7). RVAD insertion is indicated when there is evidence of severe RV dysfunction with a high CVP (usually >20 mm Hg) and inability to maintain a satisfactory cardiac output despite maximal pharmacologic therapy (usually epinephrine/milrinone and an IABP). Evidence of vasopressor-refractory low cardiac output syndrome with hypotension, oliguria, and lactic acidosis is highly predictive of mortality; therefore, early RVAD placement should be considered in such a patient.[41]

4. **Technique.** Drainage is provided from the right atrium with return of desaturated blood to the pulmonary artery (Figure 11.5).

5. **Management** during RVAD support

   a. RVAD flow is initiated to achieve a flow rate of 2.2 L/min/m^2, increasing the LA pressure to 15 mm Hg while maintaining an RA pressure of 5–10 mm Hg. Most pulsatile devices function automatically, ejecting the full stroke volume once the device reservoir is full. Centrifugal and axial flow pump systems can be modified to provide RV support. Inability to achieve satisfactory flow rates may indicate hypovolemia, improper position of the drainage catheter, or cardiac tamponade that compresses the right atrium. If intravascular volume is adequate and tamponade is not present, systemic hypotension may be the result of impaired LV function that may require inotropic, IABP, or LVAD support. It may also result from systemic vasodilation that requires use of an α-agent or vasopressin. TEE is helpful in evaluating the status of LV function in patients on RVAD support.

   b. Pulmonary vasodilators, including milrinone, inhaled nitric oxide, epoprostenol, iloprost, or sildenafil may be beneficial in reducing pulmonary artery pressures and RV afterload, allowing for recovery of RV function.[160]

   c. The requirement for heparinization is similar to that for LVADs.

   d. Assessment of myocardial recovery by TEE and weaning of the device are similar to LVADs.

6. **Overall results.** Patients receiving RVADs for postcardiotomy support have a poor prognosis. Weaning has been accomplished in about 35% of patients, with 25% of patients surviving to be discharged from the hospital.

E. **Biventricular assist devices (BiVADs)**

1. BiVADs provide support of both the pulmonary and systemic circulations (but do not provide oxygenation) and can function during periods of ventricular fibrillation.

   a. The necessity for biventricular assist in patients receiving pulsatile LVADs is about 35%, because left ventricular decompression often unmasks RV dysfunction by increasing septal shift and RV stroke work. The necessity for RVAD placement is less with continuous-flow devices than with pulsatile VADs because continuous-flow devices produce less LV unloading, resulting in less septal shift and better preservation of RV mechanics.[161–163]

b. Numerous studies have evaluated predictors for RV failure and the necessity for BiVAD assist in patients receiving LVADs. These factors include preexisting RV dysfunction with low RV stroke work index, a high CVP or CVP/PCW pressure ratio > 0.63, preoperative ventilatory support, abnormal hepatic or renal function, and a requirement for multiple vasoactive drugs to maintain flow. Additionally, RV function may deteriorate if the PVR is increased from blood product transfusions, or if RV ischemia is exacerbated by systemic hypotension. [163–165]

c. Pulmonary vasodilators may be benefical in reducing RV afterload after LVAD implantation and may obviate the need to place an RVAD. [160]

2. **Indications.** See Table 11.7.

3. **Technique.** BiVAD support incorporates the techniques noted above for LVAD and RVAD connections (Figure 11.5). Usually BiVAD support is provided using either the Abiomed BVS 5000 system, the Abiomed BV 5000 ventricles, or the Thoratec pneumatic VADs. Occasionally, in patients being bridged to transplantation, one of the HeartMate devices may be placed, anticipating the need for only LVAD assist, only to find that biventricular assist becomes necessary when RV failure or intractable arrhythmias occur.

4. **Management** during BiVAD support

   a. Sequential manipulations of RVAD and LVAD flow are used to achieve a systemic flow rate of 2.2 L/min/m^2. The RVAD flow is increased to raise the LA pressure to 15–20 mm Hg, and then the LVAD flow is increased to reduce the LA pressure to 5–10 mm Hg. Once filling of these pulsatile devices is accomplished, they function in a fill-to-empty mode. Inability to achieve satisfactory flow rates usually indicates hypovolemia, tamponade, or catheter malposition on either side. Left- and right-sided flow rates may differ because of varying contributions of the native ventricles to pulmonary or systemic flow.

   b. Heparin requirements are similar to those noted above for LVADs.

   c. Assessment of recovery and weaning are similar to the methods described for RVAD and LVAD devices.

5. **Overall results.** The requirement for biventricular support has an adverse effect on survival. In a report from the Cleveland Clinic, 70% died on support and 30% survived to receive transplants. [166] These poor results reflect the adverse impact of biventricular failure on survival.

F. **Extracorporeal membrane oxygenation (ECMO)**

1. ECMO is a form of extracorporeal life support (ECLS) that serves as an alternative to ventricular assist devices. The system employs a membrane oxygenator, centrifugal pump, heat exchanger, oxygen blender, and a heparin-coated circuit. The latter provides a more biocompatible surface that minimizes platelet activation and the systemic inflammatory response, and reduces or eliminates the heparin requirement. This allows the ECMO circuit to be used for several days.

2. **Indications.** ECMO is indicated for the short-term treatment of severe postcardiotomy ventricular dysfunction with or without hypoxemia. Criteria for use are similar to those for left ventricular or biventricular assist. In many patients requiring VAD support, the duration of CPB is quite long due to the delay in deciding to proceed with VAD support, often resulting in both cardiogenic and noncardio-

genic pulmonary edema that impairs oxygenation.[167–169] ECMO can also be used emergently in patients sustaining cardiac arrest and in patients with severe hypoxemic ARDS, while the lung recovers from the inciting pathologic insult.[170,171]

3. **Technique.** At the conclusion of surgery, the same cannulation setup used for CPB is maintained (right atrium and aorta). If ECMO is considered subsequently, it may be established with venous drainage from the internal jugular vein or femoral vein with return of blood to the femoral artery through a side graft to allow for distal perfusion or to the axillary or carotid artery. An IABP is frequently inserted as well to improve coronary perfusion since the ECMO circuit is providing nonpulsatile flow. Percutaneous femorofemoral bypass may be used to resuscitate a patient from cardiac arrest.

4. **Management.** Maximal medical support is essential to optimize the results of ECMO. Some of the essential elements are:

   a. Optimizing preload to provide pulmonary perfusion

   b. Supporting SVR with α-agents or vasopressin

   c. Aggressive use of pulmonary vasodilators for pulmonary hypertension

   d. Early and aggressive use of renal replacement therapy

   e. Avoidance of anticoagulation

   f. Use of low tidal volume ventilation

5. If the patient has suffered a severe neurologic insult or is not considered a candidate for transplantation, ECMO is usually terminated after 48 hours. If the heart does not recover after up to 1 week of ECMO support, a clinical decision must be made about conversion to long-term support. Careful assessment of neurologic, pulmonary, hepatic, and renal status is essential. It is sometimes difficult to ascertain whether the patient has survivable or nonsurvivable organ system dysfunction that might contraindicate LVAD implantation.

6. **Results.** The results of ECMO depend on the indication for its use and the degree of organ system failure at the time it is initiated. Patients in whom it is implanted for a cardiac arrest fare poorly, although one report found a 31% survival in patients undergoing emergent ECMO for prolonged cardiac arrest.[170] Patients who develop multisystem organ failure before ECMO is initiated or who develop acute renal failure requiring dialysis have a very high mortality rate.[172] Of patients receiving ECMO for postcardiotomy cardiogenic shock, approximately 40–50% will die on ECMO support, while 40–50% can be weaned, but less than half of those will survive to be discharged. Thus, the operative mortality rate for patients requiring ECMO for postcardiotomy support averages around 60–70%.[169,173,174] Somewhat improved results have recently been reported from China, with hospital mortality rates of around 45% for patients requiring postoperative ECMO support.[175,176] With an aggressive strategy of transplanting patients bridged from ECMO to long-term devices, about 25% may survive to transplantation.

G. **Devices available to provide ventricular assist**

   1. **General concepts**

      a. Short-term partial support for high-risk percutaneous coronary intervention (PCI) or cardiogenic shock is best provided with percutaneously inserted systems.

b. Surgically implantable continuous-flow (centrifugal, axial) or pulsatile pumps are generally used for short-term postcardiotomy support, although the percutaneous systems can also be used, with either percutaneous or direct catheter insertion. If myocardial recovery does not occur, a clinical decision can then be made, based primarily upon the patient's neurologic function and organ system recovery, whether a device capable of longer-term support should be implanted as either a bridge to transplantation or destination therapy. Thus these devices are implanted as a "bridge to decision".[177]

c. Nonpulsatile continuous-flow pumps (centrifugal or axial flow) were initially recommended only for short-term support (7–10 days) because of concerns that device design and lack of pulsatility would contribute to hemolysis and end-organ damage with longer-term use. Furthermore, it was assumed that they might not be as effective as pulsatile pumps in pressure and volume unloading the heart. However, it has been demonstrated that unloading is just as efficient and organ system recovery is just as likely as with pulsatile pumps.[152,153,179] Therefore, the latter have now been supplanted in most centers by continuous-flow devices, which are smaller, have more durability, and can be used for long-term support.[178,179]

2. **Percutaneous support** devices are most commonly used in patients undergoing high-risk PCI and patients with cardiogenic shock from an acute MI. The two most popular devices are the Tandem Heart and the Impella LP 2.5.[148,180]

a. The **TandemHeart (PTVA)** system (CardiacAssist, Inc.) is a continuous-flow centrifugal pump that can provide up to 4 L/min flow (Figure 11.6). It consists of a 21 Fr transseptal cannula that is placed percutaneously through the femoral vein and positioned across the atrial septum into the left atrium. Blood drains into a dual-chamber pump which uses an impeller to pump the blood back to the patient through 15 or 17 Fr cannulas placed into one or both femoral arteries. Anticoagulation with heparin to achieve a PTT of 2.5–3 times normal (65–80 seconds) or an ACT >200 seconds is recommended. This device can also be used as an LVAD for postcardiotomy support with direct LA or LV and aortic cannulation or as an RVAD for postcardiotomy support or cardiogenic shock from an RV infarct with percutaneous or direct placement of cannulas into the RA and PA.[181–183]

b. The **Impella LP 2.5** (Abiomed) is a 12 Fr catheter-based miniaturized rotary blood pump that is inserted via the femoral artery and positioned across the aortic valve into the left ventricle (Figure 11.7). The axial-flow device withdraws blood from the distal end of the catheter in the LV and pumps it into the ascending aorta. Although the Impella LP 2.5 can only provide partial support with 2.5 L/min flow, it is capable of reducing cardiac work and increasing cardiac output. It is most applicable during high-risk PCI.[180]

3. **Short-term devices: nonpulsatile centrifugal pumps** are the most readily available, inexpensive and easy-to-use systems for uni- or biventricular short-term support. They are labor-intensive in that they require fairly constant attention to flow rates. Their use is usually limited to about 1–2 weeks, at which time conversion to long-term devices may be necessary if recovery does not occur.

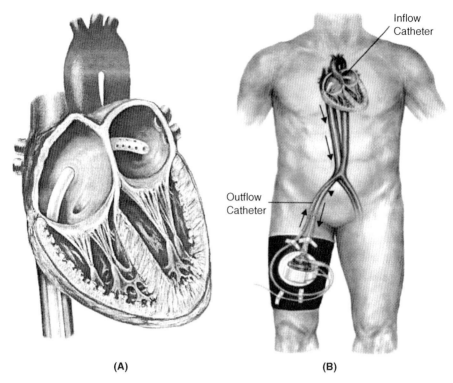

(A)   **(B)**

Figure 11.6 • The Tandem Heart percutaneous ventricular assist (PTVA) system. A cannula is introduced into the femoral vein and passed transseptally into the left atrium. The arterial return cannula is placed in the femoral artery.

a. **BioMedicus** centrifugal pumps are routinely used for CPB and are not approved for use as assist devices. However, in the absence of more sophisticated devices, they can be used successfully to provide a brief period of uni- or biventricular support until other devices can be implanted. These systems are also used in ECMO circuits. Similarly, the **Sarns Delphin centrifugal pump** has been used successfully for LVAD support. One report of 35 patients receiving the Sarns pump for postcardiotomy support found that more than 70% of patients could be weaned, with a 52% hospital survival rate.[184]

b. The **TandemHeart PTVA system** (see above) can be used for patients in cardiogenic shock and postcardiotomy RV or LV dysfunction for temporary support or as a "bridge to a bridge".

c. The **Levitronix Centrimag** is a centrifugal pump that uses a magnetically levitated rotor to propel blood forward. This system avoids friction to minimize blood trauma and can be used for several months of support, although the motor and external circuit may need to be changed after 6 weeks. It uses the standard cannulas and sites for uni- or biventricular assist. Heparinization to a PTT of 60–100 seconds is recommended.[185]

Impella®
Micro-Axial Flow Pump

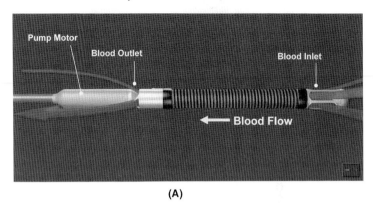

(A)

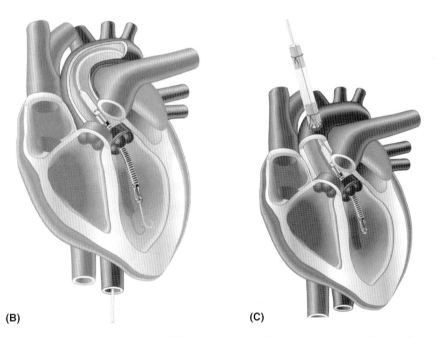

(B)   **(C)**

Figure 11.7 • The Impella devices. (A) The basic design of the catheter with an inlet that lies within the left ventricle and an outlet within the ascending aorta, next to which is located the rotary pump. (B) The Impella 2.5 device (12 Fr diameter) and Impella 5 (21 Fr diameter) devices have similar designs and are placed percutaneously to lie across the aortic valve. (C) The Impella LD device is placed through a graft sewn to the ascending aorta.

d. The **Arrow CorAide** was developed at the Cleveland Clinic and has been modified as a "Dexaide" for RV assist. It is an implantable centrifugal pump that has been designed to avoid blood stagnation and mechanical wear, which should improve its durability and nonthrombogenicity. The inlet cannula is placed through the LV apex with a graft sewn to the ascending aorta. The device sits just above the diaphragm near the LV apex and the drive line exits the the right upper quadrant of the abdomen. This device can provide up to 8 L/min of flow. Long-term anticoagulation with warfarin and antiplatelet drugs is recommended.[186]

4. **Short-term devices: pulsatile pumps**

   a. The **Abiomed BVS 5000** system is a pulsatile pneumatic device that is located at the patient's bedside (Figure 11.8). Specially designed catheters provide venous return to the pump, and a catheter with an integral graft is sewn to the outflow vessel. The RVAD system involves catheter drainage from the right atrium with return of blood to the pulmonary artery. LVAD support involves drainage from the left atrium or LV apex with return flow to the aorta. Ejection occurs once the bladder into which the blood drains has reached a designated volume. The device can generally be used for up to 2 weeks, at which time the decision can be made about conversion to a long-term device. Anticoagulation with heparin is necessary (see page 480). One of the drawbacks is the formation of fibrinous clot in the outflow chamber that may give rise to thromboembolism.[187]

   b. The Abiomed AB5000 ventricles and the Thoratec VAD can be used for short-term or long-term support (see section on long-term devices, below).

5. **Long-term devices: nonpulsatile continuous flow pumps** use axial flow technology with a nonpulsatile rotary pump that withdraws blood from the left ventricle and expels it into the aorta. These devices are preload- and afterload-sensitive and can provide unloading comparable to that of pulsatile devices. However, in contrast, the degree of unloading can be prescribed, such that excessive LV unloading that can lead to RV failure can be minimized. These devices are effective in maintaining organ system perfusion and can be used as long-term bridges or destination therapy.

   a. The **Impella LP 5.0** is a microaxial pump that is similar in principle to the Impella LP 2.5 but can provide up to 5 L/min flow. The cannula is larger (21 Fr vs. 12 Fr), although the catheter size of both devices is 9 Fr. It may be placed via the femoral artery or the right axillary artery.[188,189] The Impella LD is a shorter version of this device and is inserted via a graft sewn to the ascending aorta (Figure 11.7C).

   b. The **Thoratec Heartmate II** is a continuous flow device with a rotary pump that can provide up to 10 L/min flow. The inflow cannula is placed through the LV apex and the outflow cannula is sewn to the ascending aorta (Figure 11.9). The pump is inserted in a preperitoneal pocket with a drive line exiting the right upper quadrant. Early anticoagulation with heparin has been used, but can contribute to bleeding and is probably not essential. The patient is then maintained on warfarin with a target INR around 2.0. This device is an excellent bridge to transplantation and has also been used for destination therapy.[190,191]

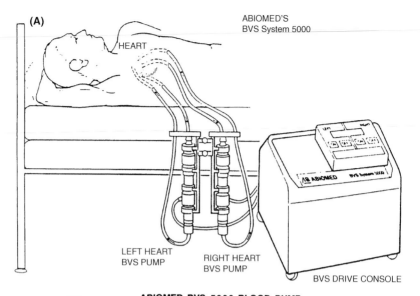

(A) ABIOMED'S
BVS System 5000

HEART

LEFT HEART
BVS PUMP

RIGHT HEART
BVS PUMP

BVS DRIVE CONSOLE

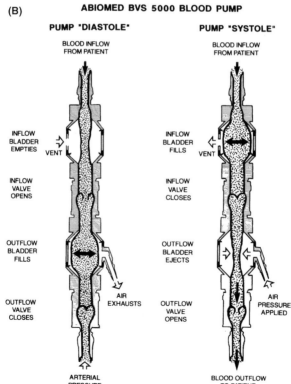

(B) **ABIOMED BVS 5000 BLOOD PUMP**

PUMP "DIASTOLE"

BLOOD INFLOW
FROM PATIENT

INFLOW
BLADDER
EMPTIES

VENT

INFLOW
VALVE
OPENS

OUTFLOW
BLADDER
FILLS

AIR
EXHAUSTS

OUTFLOW
VALVE
CLOSES

ARTERIAL
PRESSURE

PUMP "SYSTOLE"

BLOOD INFLOW
FROM PATIENT

INFLOW
BLADDER
FILLS

VENT

INFLOW
VALVE
CLOSES

OUTFLOW
BLADDER
EJECTS

AIR
PRESSURE
APPLIED

OUTFLOW
VALVE
OPENS

BLOOD OUTFLOW
TO PATIENT

Figure 11.8 • The Abiomed BVS 5000 System. (A) The devices are located at the patient's bedside and are connected to the drive console for pneumatic activation. (B) A cross-sectional view of the heart pumps during systole and diastole. (Courtesy of Abiomed, Inc.).

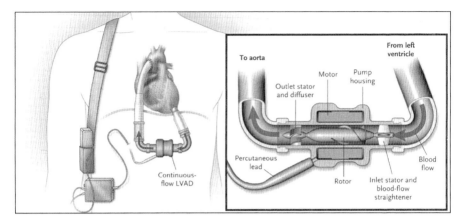

Figure 11.9 • The Thoratec HeartMate II device is a continuous-flow pump interposed between a cannula placed into the left ventricular apex and a graft sewn to the ascending aorta. (Reprinted with permission from Slaughter et al., *N Engl J Med* 2009;361:2241–51. Copyright © 2009 Massachusetts Medical Society. All rights reserved.)

    c. The **Jarvik 2000** is fairly similar in concept to the HeartMate II, providing axial flow and rotary pump technology with LV apical and aortic cannulation (Figure 11.10A). It has shown good durability with a low risk of complications in early trials and has been used as a bridge to transplantation, but may eventually be approved for destination therapy.[191,192]

    d. The **Micromed Heart Assist 5 (DeBakey)** is also similar in concept to the other continuous-flow pumps (Figure 11.10B). It has been miniaturized as well for pediatric implantation.[193] Early experience has shown excellent bridging to transplantation with comparable post-transplant survival to pulsatile devices.

6. Long-term devices: pulsatile systems

    a. The **Abiomed AB5000** ventricle resembles the Thoratec pneumatic VAD system (described below) in providing a pneumatically driven device that lies on the abdominal wall (Figure 11.11). The device includes an Angioflex membrane and proprietary trileaflet valves. This system avoids the extensive tubing and bedside arrangement of the BVS 5000 device. It can be used for uni- or biventricular support. Initial anticoagulation with heparin with subsequent use of warfarin to achieve an INR of 2 is recommended to reduce the risk of thromboembolism.

    b. The **Thoratec VAD** is a pulsatile pneumatic paracorporeal device that lies on the abdominal wall with the patient tethered only by the pneumatic drive line. Cannulation is similar to that of the Abiomed systems with specially designed catheters and grafts to provide drainage and blood return. These cannulas can be attached to one or two separate units to provide uni- or biventricular support. This device can provide long-term temporary support and can be used as a bridge

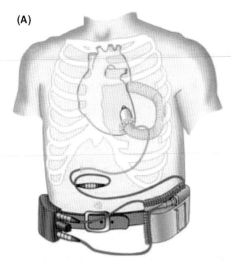

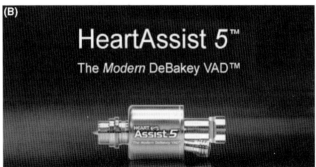

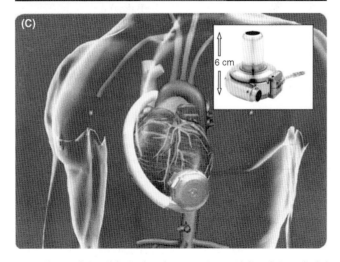

Figure 11.10 • (A) The Jarvik 2000 device has the pump inserted directly into the left ventricular apex with return of blood into the descending aorta. (B) The DeBakey Heart Assist device is similar to the HeartMate with a cannula inserted into the LV apex and the axial flow device lying outside the heart. This device has been miniaturized for pediatric use. (C) The HeartWare device is inserted into the LV apex. The insert demonstrates the small size of this device.

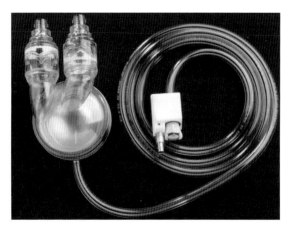

Figure 11.11 • The Abiomed AB5000 ventricle attached to a pneumatic drive line. (Courtesy of Abiomed, Inc.)

to transplantation. It also requires full anticoagulation. Its use has generally been supplanted by the Abiomed BV 5000, which has more modern design and ease of use.

c. The **Thoratec HeartMate VE** is an implantable, pulsatile, electric device that can provide only left ventricular assist (Figure 11.12). Blood drains from the LV apex through a porcine valve into the device, which then ejects a stroke volume when the chamber is filled or at a fixed rate. Because the device has a unique textured surface, aspirin alone is sufficient to minimize the risk of thromboembolism. Early heparinization and warfarin are recommended for patients with prosthetic valves. If the patient has a mechanical aortic valve, it should be covered or sewn shut to prevent thromboembolism from the valve surface.

   i. This device has been used as a bridge to transplantation and was evaluated in the REMATCH trial which showed its benefit for destination therapy with a 1-year survival of just over 50%.[194,195] Its primary deficiencies are deterioration of the porcine valves resulting in regurgitation into the device (with rapid filling and an increase in the ejection rate), and the development of drive-line infections.

   ii. If a patient receiving a HeartMate subsequently requires RVAD support, the Abiomed AB5000 ventricle is usually used. If BiVAD support is indicated from the outset, the Abiomed BV 5000 ventricles are placed to support both ventricles.

d. A number of other devices are being investigated to provide bridging and destination therapy. Among those are the **CardioWest** total artificial heart and the **AbioCor TAH** (Abiomed).[196,197] The critical design features to improve success rates include biocompatibility to reduce the risk of thromboembolism and blood element damage and improved transcutaneous energy transmission systems to reduce the risk of infection.

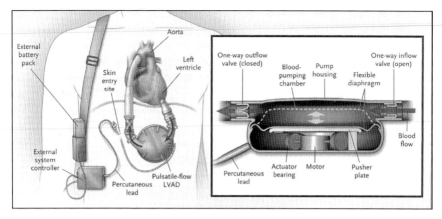

Figure 11.12 • Thoratec HeartMate VE (vented electric) LVAD system. The device rests in a preperitoneal pocket in the left upper quadrant. Blood enters the device through an apical cannulation site and is pumped through a graft sewn to the ascending aorta. Porcine valves are incorporated into inflow and outflow grafts. (Reprinted with permission from Slaughter et al., *N Engl J Med* 2009;361:2241–51. Copyright © 2009 Massachusetts Medical Society. All rights reserved.)

H. Complications. Continuing improvements in technology and perioperative care have reduced, but not eliminated, some of the complications associated with the long-term use of circulatory assist devices. These include the following:

1. **Mediastinal bleeding.** Despite reversal of anticoagulation, a substantial percentage of patients (up to 60%) require reexploration for evacuation of mediastinal clot that can cause tamponade (manifested by inadequate drainage into the device).[198] Contributing factors include coagulopathies related to long durations of CPB in postcardiotomy patients, the large amount of dead space around the catheters in the mediastinum, often an open chest, and the use of early anticoagulation to minimize thrombus formation within the devices. Although early anticoagulation is desirable, it must be withheld if bleeding is still present. Fibrinolysis and platelet dysfunction are common with LVADs as well.[199]

2. **Mediastinitis and sepsis.** Between 40% and 50% of patients receiving VADs develop nosocomial infections, many of which are device-related, and some of which are not. They most commonly originate at the drive-line exit site that is used for energy transmission. Because long-term antibiotic usage is commonplace, resistant organisms are often identified. In addition, many patients are debilitated and malnourished and have numerous intravascular and other invasive catheters that can become colonized. Although the infection risk is lowest with implantable devices that allow for primary wound closure, bacteremia is still very common, being noted in about 45% of patients in a study at the Cleveland Clinic.[200] The most common organisms are *Staphylococcus aureus* and coagulase-negative staph, *Candida*, and *Pseudomonas aeruginosa*. Infection is

associated with a significantly increased mortality, especially so in the case of fungal endocarditis, which occurs in about 20% of patients. If this develops, antifungal therapy along with either device removal and replacement or urgent transplantation may lead to a successful result. Drive-line site infections are very common with long durations of LVAD assistance and may compromise long-term survival.[201] Generally, however, infections are controllable and do not influence the results of transplantation.[202]

3. **Thromboembolism** resulting in stroke has become less of a problem with newer device designs and better refinement of anticoagulation requirements. Patients with mechanical aortic valves should have them covered with tissue or sewn shut to prevent thromboembolism.

4. **Malignant ventricular arrhythmias** may develop as a result of myocardial ischemia, infarction, or the use of catecholamines. BiVADs function during ventricular fibrillation, as can LVADs as long as the PVR is not high. If LVAD flow cannot be maintained, the patient may require placement of an RVAD. Fibrillation may foster thrombus formation in the ventricles and should be treated aggressively. Early cardioversion should also be considered to prevent RV injury from prolonged fibrillation.[203] Chest compressions can be used for percutaneous and continuous flow devices, but are contraindicated for the pulsatile devices (Abiomed AB 5000 and HeartMate XVE).

5. **Renal failure** is usually caused by prolonged episodes of hypotension or low cardiac output prior to insertion of a VAD. It generally returns to the patient's baseline after VAD implantation, except when there is evidence of other organ system failure (especially hepatic) or infection. Early aggressive treatment with renal replacement therapy (usually with continuous venovenous hemofiltration) should be considered. The mortality rate for patients with persistent renal failure on VAD support is very high.

6. **Respiratory failure** is usually attributable to a prolonged duration of CPB, sepsis, and use of multiple blood products.

7. **Vasodilatory shock** due to inappropriately low levels of vasopressin is not uncommon in patients requiring placement of LVADs. In fact, vasopressin hypersensitivity may be noted. Use of arginine vasopressin up to 0.1 units/min effectively increases mean arterial pressure in these patients.[155]

8. **Heparin-induced thrombocytopenia** (HIT) is common in VAD recipients, with an incidence of 26% in one report.[204] Although this report did not note adverse outcomes using heparin for transplantation, another report did in fact find the development of HIT to be associated with adverse outcomes. Use of an alternative anticoagulation regimen during transplantation and for device thromboprophylaxis would appear to be a reasonable approach unless the time from diagnosis to transplantation exceeds 2–3 months.[204,205]

9. Patients receiving LVADs become immunologically sensitized and have a reduced rate of transplantation due to crossmatch issues. Furthermore, they have a higher risk of rejection. However, after transplantation, survival appears to be similar to that of nonbridged recipients who are not sensitized. Immunomodulatory treatment with intravenous immunoglobulins and cyclophosphamide may be beneficial in offsetting the problems associated with sensitization.[206]

VI. Systemic Hypertension

A. General comments

1. Systemic hypertension is fairly common after open-heart surgery. In the immediate postoperative period, it usually results from vasoconstriction due to systemic hypothermia, enhanced sympathetic nervous system activity, and altered baroreceptor sensitivity. Postoperative hypertension is more common in patients with chronic hypertension, diabetes, vascular disease, and chronic kidney disease.

2. Hypertension more commonly results from elevated systemic vascular resistance than from hyperdynamic myocardial performance. Therefore, it is imperative that cardiac hemodynamics be assessed before therapeutic interventions are initiated. **One should never assume that hypertension is the result of hyperdynamic cardiac performance.** Withdrawal of inotropic support when hypertension is due to intense vasoconstriction may precipitate rapid hemodynamic deterioration if the cardiac output is marginal.

3. Treatment is indicated to maintain the systolic blood pressure <140 mm Hg or the mean arterial pressure <90 mm Hg. Aggressive treatment is warranted to minimize the potential adverse effects of hypertension. These include an increase in afterload, which increases systolic wall stress and can precipitate myocardial ischemia and impair ventricular function, and the potential for mediastinal bleeding, suture-line disruption, aortic dissection, and stroke.

B. Etiology

1. The hormonal milieu of cardiopulmonary bypass, including elevated levels of norepinephrine and vasopressin and an altered renin–angiotensin system, increases autonomic tone and induces a hyperadrenergic state

2. Vasoconstriction from hypothermia, vasopressors, or a low cardiac output state

3. Fever, anxiety, pain, agitation and awakening when sedatives wear off

4. Abnormal arterial blood gases (hypoxia, hypercarbia, acidosis)

5. Pharyngeal manipulation (readjusting an endotracheal tube, placing a nasogastric tube or echo probe)

6. Hyperdynamic ventricles, especially in patients with left ventricular hypertrophy

7. Altered baroreceptor function, following combined CABG–carotid endarterectomy

8. Severe acute hypoglycemia

C. Assessment

1. Careful patient examination, especially for breath sounds and peripheral perfusion

2. Assessment of cardiac hemodynamics

3. Measurement of arterial blood gases, serum potassium, hematocrit

4. Review of chest x-ray and 12-lead ECG

5. Note: Don't forget to check the chest drainage unit for the amount of mediastinal bleeding!

D. Treatment.[207] Systolic pressure should be maintained between 100 and 130 mm Hg (mean arterial pressure around 80–90 mm Hg). The objective is to reduce the SVR sufficiently enough to lower myocardial oxygen demand without compromising coronary perfusion pressure. A secondary benefit is frequently an improvement in

myocardial function. Ideally, an antihypertensive agent should prevent myocardial ischemia without adversely affecting heart rate, AV conduction, or myocardial contractility. When used in the early postoperative period, it should have rapid onset and offset of action in the event of changes in hemodynamics.

1. Ensure satisfactory oxygenation and ventilation.

2. Use vasodilator medications if the cardiac output is satisfactory (see section VII, below).

3. Provide inotropic support along with vasodilators if the cardiac output is marginal (cardiac index <2.0 L/min/m^2).

4. Sedate with propofol 25–50 µg/kg/min, midazolam 2.5–5.0 mg IV, or morphine 2.5–5.0 mg IV. Sedation is usually an appropriate first step in the fully ventilated patient when extubation is not imminently planned. However, antihypertensive drugs rather than sedatives are preferable to allow for early extubation.

5. Control shivering with meperidine 25–50 mg IV or pharmacologic paralysis (always with sedation).

VII. Vasodilators and Antihypertensive Medications

A. **General comments**

1. A variety of medications can be used to control systemic hypertension (Table 11.8). Their hemodynamic effects depend on the patient's intravascular volume and myocardial function, and the site at which they exert their antihypertensive action. Vasodilators may reduce blood pressure by increasing venous capacitance (reducing preload) or decreasing arterial resistance (which reduces afterload and usually preload as well). Other antihypertensive medications reduce blood pressure by inhibiting central adrenergic discharge or exerting a negative inotropic effect, a property also shared by several of the vasodilators. Thus, a careful cardiac assessment is required to ensure that the appropriate medication is selected.

2. Antihypertensive medications are most commonly used during the early phase of postoperative recovery when the patient is hypothermic, vasoconstricted, and hypertensive. They are weaned off as the patient vasodilates in order to maintain a systolic blood pressure of 100–130 mm Hg. Vasodilators may also be used alone or in conjunction with inotropic medications to improve myocardial function by lowering SVR.

3. The most commonly used medication in the ICU is sodium nitroprusside, although other intravenous medications, such as nitroglycerin, calcium channel blockers (clevidipine or nicardipine), β-blockers (continuous infusion of esmolol or labetalol), ACE inhibitors (enalaprilat), or fenoldopam can also be considered in selected situations.

4. Most patients without chronic hypertension will exhibit only transient hypertension after surgery and usually do not require antihypertensive therapy after 24 hours. For those with a history of hypertension, oral medications must be initiated before transfer from the ICU. The appropriate choice depends on the patient's hemodynamic status and renal function (see pages 505–506).

Table 11.8 • Mixes and Dosage Ranges for Common Intravenous Antihypertensive Medications

Medication	Mix	Dosage range
Nitroprusside	50 mg/250 mL	0.1–8 µg/kg/min
Nitroglycerin	50 mg/250 mL	0.1–10 µg/kg/min
Calcium channel blockers		
Clevidipine	50 mg/100 mL	1–6 mg/h
Nicardipine	50 mg/250 mL	5–15 mg/h
Diltiazem	250 mg/250 mL	0.25 mg/kg over 2 min, then 0.35 mg/kg over 2 min, then 5–15 mg/h
Verapamil	120 mg/250 mL	0.1 mg/kg bolus over 2 minutes, then 2–5 µg/kg/min
Beta-blockers		
Esmolol	2.5 g/250 mL	0.25–0.5 mg/kg/min bolus then 50–200 µg/kg/min
Labetalol	200 mg/200 mL	1–4 mg/min
Enalaprilat		0.625–1.25 mg IV over 5 min
Hydralazine		10–20 mg IV q6h
Fenoldopam	10 mg/250 mL	0.05–0.1 µg/kg/min initial infusion, up to 0.8 µg/kg/min

B. Sodium nitroprusside (SNP)

1. **Hemodynamic effects**

   a. SNP primarily relaxes arterial smooth muscle and reduces SVR and PVR. It has a lesser effect on venous capacitance that will also reduce preload. The overall effect is a reduction in systemic blood pressure and filling pressures, often resulting in an improvement in left ventricular function. Maintenance or improvement in cardiac output usually requires a modest volume infusion to restore filling pressures to an optimal level. The approach is: "optimize preload → reduce afterload → restore preload". The development of a reflex tachycardia during SNP infusion usually reflects hypovolemia.

   b. SNP is a very dangerous drug which always requires close monitoring with an indwelling arterial cannula. It has a very rapid onset of action (within seconds) and can lower the blood pressure precipitously. Fortunately, its effects dissipate within 1–2 minutes.

2. **Indications**

   a. **To control systemic hypertension** caused by an increase in SVR. SNP is an excellent drug to use if cardiac function is marginal, filling pressures are elevated, and SVR is high.

b. **To improve myocardial function** when the SVR is elevated, usually when systemic hypertension is present. The best results are often obtained with concomitant inotropic support.

3. The usual **starting dose** is 0.1 µg/kg/min with a mix of 50 mg/250 mL. The bottle must be wrapped in aluminum foil to prevent metabolic breakdown from light. The dose is gradually increased to a maximum of 8 µg/kg/min.

4. **Adverse effects**

   a. Potentiation of myocardial ischemia by:

      i. A reduction in diastolic perfusion pressure. If filling pressures do not decrease when systemic perfusion pressure falls, the diastolic transmyocardial gradient for coronary blood flow will be reduced, potentially producing myocardial ischemia.

      ii. Producing a coronary steal syndrome by dilating resistance vessels in the coronary circulation and shunting of blood away from ischemic zones.[208]

      iii. Causing a reflex tachycardia.

   b. Reflex increase in contractility and dp/dt; in a patient with an aortic dissection, this mandates concomitant use of a β-blocker.

   c. Inhibition of hypoxic vasoconstriction, which produces ventilation/perfusion mismatch and hypoxia.

   d. Tachyphylaxis to its vasodilating effects.

   e. **Cyanide toxicity.** Nitroprusside is metabolized to cyanide, which is then converted to thiocyanate in the liver. Cyanide toxicity, manifested by metabolic acidosis and an elevated mixed venous PO_2, may occur when large doses (>8 µg/kg/min) are given for several days (cumulative dose >1 mg/kg over 12−24 hours) or if hepatic dysfunction is present. The risk of developing cyanide toxicity may be accelerated following surgery using CPB.[208] Moderate cyanide toxicity is treated by converting the cyanide to thiocyanate for its excretion by the kidneys:

      i. Sodium bicarbonate for metabolic acidosis in doses of 1 mEq/kg

      ii. Sodium thiosulfate 150 mg/kg IV (approximately 12.5 g in a 50 mL D5W solution given over 10 minutes)

   f. **Thiocyanate toxicity** (level > 5 mg/dL) may develop from chronic use of SNP especially when there is impaired renal excretion of this metabolite. It is manifested by dyspnea, vomiting, and mental status changes with dizziness, headache, and loss of consciousness. **Treatment** of both severe cyanide and thiocyanate toxicity involves use of nitrite preparations to induce methemoglobin (metHb) formation. The metHb combines with cyanide to form cyanmethemoglobin, which is nontoxic.

      i. Amyl nitrite inhalation of 1 ampule over 15 seconds.

      ii. Sodium nitrite 5 mg/kg IV slow push. This is usually given at a rate of 2.5 mL/min of a 3% solution to a total of 10−15 mL. One-half of this dose can be used subsequently if toxicity recurs.

      iii. Sodium thiosulfate in the dose noted above can then be administered to convert the cyanide that is gradually dissociated from cyanmethemoglobin into thiocyanate for excretion.

C. Nitroglycerin (NTG)

1. Hemodynamic effects

    a. NTG is primarily a venodilator that lowers blood pressure by reducing preload, filling pressures, stroke volume, and cardiac output. If filling pressures are satisfactory, NTG will maintain aortic diastolic perfusion pressure, although at high doses some arterial vasodilation does occur. In the presence of hypovolemia or a marginal cardiac output, NTG should be avoided, because it will lower cardiac output further and produce a reflex tachycardia.

    b. NTG dilates coronary conductance vessels and improves blood flow to ischemic zones.[209]

    c. NTG is rapid-acting with an onset of action of 2–5 minutes and a duration of action of 10–20 minutes.

2. Indications

    a. Hypertension in association with myocardial ischemia or high filling pressures

    b. ECG changes of **myocardial ischemia**; NTG is useful prior to surgery in conjunction with phenylephrine to maintain coronary perfusion pressures.

    c. Coronary spasm

    d. Pulmonary hypertension, to reduce right ventricular afterload and improve RV function

3. Starting dose

is $0.1\,\mu g/kg/min$ with a mix of $50\,mg/250\,mL$. The dose can be titrated up to $10\,\mu g/kg/min$. The dose used prophylactically to prevent radial artery spasm is only $5–10\,\mu g/min$. NTG must be administered through non-polyvinyl chloride (PVC) tubing because PVC tubing absorbs up to 80% of the NTG.

4. Adverse effects.

Nitroglycerin is metabolized by the liver to nitrites, which oxidize hemoglobin to metHb. Methemoglobinemia and impaired oxygen transport can occur if the patient receives extremely high doses of IV NTG (over $10\,\mu g/kg/min$) for several days or has renal or hepatic dysfunction. The diagnosis is suggested by the presence of chocolate-brown blood and a lower oxygen saturation measured by oximetry than one would expect from the PaO_2. It can be confirmed by an elevated metHb level (>1% of total hemoglobin). Symptoms (cyanosis, progressive weakness, and acidosis) are usually not noted until the metHb level exceeds 15–20%. The treatment is intravenous methylene blue 1 mg/kg of a 1% solution.[210]

D. Calcium channel blockers (CCBs)

1. Hemodynamic and electrophysiologic effects

    a. The calcium channel blockers control hypertension by relaxing vascular smooth muscle and producing peripheral vasodilation. The various CCBs have differing effects on cardiovascular hemodynamics and electrophysiology (Table 11.9). Use of these medications during the perioperative period has been shown to reduce the incidence of myocardial infarction, ischemia, and supraventricular arrhythmias, and may also improve survival.[211]

    b. Other effects may include coronary vasodilation, negative inotropy, a reduction in sinoatrial (SA) nodal automaticity (slowing the sinus mechanism), and slowing of AV nodal conduction (decreasing the ventricular rate response to atrial tachyarrhythmias).

Table 11.9 • Effects of Calcium Channel Blockers

	Clevidipine	Nicardipine	Diltiazem	Verapamil	Nifedipine	Amlodipine
Inotropy	0	0	↓	↓↓	0 ↑	0
Heart rate	0	0 ↑	↓↓	↓↓	↑	0
AV conduction	0	0	↓↓	↓↓	0	0
Systemic resistance	↓↓↓	↓↓↓	↓↓	↓↓	↓↓	↓↓
Coronary vascular resistance	↓↓	↓↓↓	↓↓	↓↓	↓↓	↓↓

0, no effect; ↑ increased; ↓ decreased. The relative effect is indicated by the number of arrows.

2. **Indications**
   a. Use as a first-line drug for control of **postoperative hypertension.** Clevidipine and nicardipine lack a negative inotropic effect and can be used independent of the cardiac output; in contrast, other CCBs, which might be used for other primary indications (vasospasm or rate control in atrial fibrillation), have negative inotropic properties.
   b. Treatment of **coronary vasospasm**
   c. Prevention of **radial artery spasm**
   d. **Slowing the ventricular response** to atrial fibrillation/flutter (diltiazem)
3. **Clevidipine** is a very short-acting CCB that relaxes arterial vascular smooth muscle without producing myocardial depression. It has an immediate onset of action and a duration of action of 5–15 minutes. It is metabolized by blood and tissue esterases and therefore is safe to use in patients with renal or hepatic dysfunction.[212]
   a. **Indications.** An excellent first-line drug for control of early postoperative hypertension because it has a rapid onset of action with achievement of a target blood pressure usually within 6 minutes. It minimizes blood pressure fluctuations and has rapid offset of action in the event of hemodynamic problems.
   b. **Dosage.** It is given in an initial dose of 1–2 mg/h; if the blood pressure remains elevated, the dose can be doubled every 90 seconds; as the blood pressure approaches the target range, the dose should be adjusted in smaller increments every 5–10 minutes. The usual maintenance dose is 4–6 mg/h. It comes premixed with a concentration of 0.5 mg/mL in 50 mL or 100 mL bottles.
   c. **Advantages.** The ECLIPSE trial showed that clevidipine was more effective than SNP or NTG in maintaining the BP within a target range, and when the blood pressure range was narrowed, it was also more effective than nicardipine in

minimizing BP excursions. Interestingly, there was a trend towards lower mortality compared with SNP, but outcomes were otherwise comparable with all four drugs.[213]

4. **Nicardipine** selectively relaxes arterial smooth muscle, reducing the SVR. It lacks a negative inotropic effect, produces a minimal increase in heart rate, and has no effect on AV conduction. It has a rapid onset of action, but has a half-life of about 45 minutes and a duration of action of 4–6 hours.

   a. **Indications**

      i. An excellent first-line drug for control of hypertension in the hemodynamically stable patient because of a rapid onset of action, selective arterial vasodilation, and minimal cardiac effects. The only concern is its long duration of action in the event of hemodynamic changes.

      ii. Radial artery spasm prophylaxis in a dose of 0.25 μg/kg/min.[214] Prophylaxis may be optimized by combining nicardipine with nitroglycerin.[215] However, one study of preexisting vasospasm in coronary artery conduits found that nicardipine added to NTG caused no more vasodilation than NTG alone.[216]

   b. **Dosage.** It is given with an initial dose of 5 mg/h using a mix of 50 mg/ 250 mL; the rate is then increased by 2.5 mg/h every 5–15 minutes to a maximum dose of 15 mg/h.

   c. Advantages over SNP

      i. It has a rapid onset of action and provides more stable BP control than SNP.

      ii. It is not a venodilator that reduces preload, and does not produce a reflex tachycardia.

      iii. It does not produce a coronary steal and is a potent coronary vasodilator that can improve distribution of blood to ischemic zones. It has been shown to decrease the extent and duration of postoperative ischemia compared with NTG.[217]

   d. Disadvantages

      i. The long offset of action can be problematic in the hemodynamically unstable patient.

      ii. It does increase ventilation/perfusion mismatch and can produce hypoxemia.

5. **Diltiazem** reduces systemic blood pressure by lowering the SVR, but also has significant cardiac effects that limit its use as an antihypertensive agent. It depresses systolic function by a negative inotropic effect, slows the heart rate, and suppresses AV conduction.

   a. **Indications**

      i. **Slowing the ventricular response** to atrial fibrillation. Diltiazem slows AV conduction and can produce heart block; therefore, pacemaker backup should be available when it is administered intravenously. **Note:** The patient's blood pressure and cardiac output are often marginal when atrial fibrillation develops and there is often some reluctance to use diltiazem for rate control. However, a reduction in ventricular response will usually improve stroke volume and blood pressure. If the blood pressure is marginal, a pure α-agent may be given along with diltiazem. If the blood pressure is unacceptably low, then cardioversion should be performed.

　　ii. Prevention of **radial artery spasm**

　　iii. Treatment of **coronary artery spasm** (diltiazem is a potent coronary vasodilator)

　　iv. **Systemic hypertension** when there is another indication for its use (such as radial artery prophylaxis or slowing the ventricular response to AF).

　b. **Dosage.** An IV bolus of 0.25 mg/kg IV is given over 2 minutes, which may be followed by a repeat bolus of 0.35 mg/kg 15 minutes later. A continuous infusion is then started at a rate of 5–15 mg/h with a 250 mg/250 mL mix.

6. **Verapamil** reduces systemic blood pressure by lowering SVR, but it also has significant cardiac effects that depress contractility, slow the heart rate, and depress AV conduction. In the early postoperative period, indications for its use are similar to those for diltiazem, which is preferentially used. The IV dosage is a 0.1 mg/kg IV bolus followed by a 2–5 µg/kg/min continuous infusion of a 120 mg/250 mL mix.

7. **Nifedipine** is a potent arterial vasodilator that lowers blood pressure by reducing SVR, and may also increase cardiac output because of a baroreceptor-mediated reflex tachycardia and a slight reflex increase in cardiac inotropy and AV conduction. It is also a potent coronary vasodilator and is beneficial in treating coronary spasm. Although it has been shown to be an effective antihypertensive drug, it has a long duration of action (6–8 hours) and is rarely used in the ICU.

8. **Amlodipine** is an oral CCB that reduces SVR and blood pressure and may improve cardiac output due to a decrease in afterload. It has no negative inotropic effects and no effect on the SA node or AV nodal conduction. It produces a gradual decrease in blood pressure that persists for 24 hours after an oral dose. Thus, it is indicated for the long-term control of blood pressure. Because it is an effective antispasmodic agent, it is frequently used for the prevention of radial artery spasm in a 5 mg daily dose.

E. **β-blockers**

1. **Hemodynamic effects**

　a. In contrast to the vasodilating drugs, β-blockers reduce blood pressure primarily by their negative inotropic and chronotropic effects. They reduce contractility, lowering the stroke volume and cardiac output, and also slow the heart rate by depressing the SA node. Their antihypertensive activity may also be attributable to a decrease in central sympathetic outflow and suppression of renin activity.

　b. β-blockers slow AV conduction and can precipitate heart block. Pacemaker backup should be available when IV β-blockers are given. This electrophysiologic effect is beneficial in reducing the ventricular rate response to atrial tachyarrhythmias.

2. **Indication.** β-blockers can be used to control postoperative systolic hypertension associated with a satisfactory cardiac output. They are especially beneficial in the hyperdynamic, tachycardic heart that is often noted in patients with normal

LV function and/or LV hypertrophy. **Note:** Intravenous β-blockers should be avoided in hypertensive patients with compromised cardiac output.

3. **Esmolol** is a cardioselective, ultrafast, short-acting β-blocker with an onset of action of 2 minutes, reaching a steady-state level in 5 minutes, and with reversal of effect in 10−20 minutes. Because of its very short duration of action, esmolol is the β-blocker of choice in the ICU for transient hypertension control.

   a. Esmolol is contraindicated in the hypertensive patient with low cardiac output. Frequently, blood pressure and cardiac output are maintained by fast heart rates at low stroke volumes. Use of esmolol in this circumstance will often reduce blood pressure and cardiac output by a negative inotropic effect with little reduction in heart rate. Even in patients with an excellent cardiac output, the reduction in blood pressure is generally more pronounced than the decrease in heart rate.

   b. Esmolol can be used safely in the patient with a history of bronchospasm because of its cardioselectivity.

   c. **Dosage.** Because patients tend to be very sensitive to esmolol in the immediate postoperative period, an initial dose of 0.25 mg/kg or less can be given to determine its effect on heart rate and blood pressure. If an adequate antihypertensive effect is not achieved, a repeat bolus dose up to 0.5 mg/kg can be given and a maintenance infusion of 50−100 μg/kg/min started. Additional bolus doses can be given with an increase in the infusion rate by 50 μg/kg/min to a maximum infusion rate of 200 μg/kg/min of a 2.5 g/250 mL mix.

4. **Labetalol** has both α- and β-blocking properties as well as a direct vasodilatory effect. The ratio of β:α effects is 3:1 for the oral form and 7:1 for the intravenous form. In the postoperative cardiac surgical patient, IV labetalol reduces blood pressure primarily by its negative inotropic and chronotropic effects. The α-blocking effect prevents reflex vasoconstriction.[218]

   a. The onset of action for IV labetalol is rapid with a maximum blood pressure response at 5 minutes for a bolus injection and 10−15 minutes for a continuous infusion. Since the approximate duration of action is 6 hours, labetalol is useful when a **longer-acting antihypertensive drug** is desired. It is a very useful medication for the patient with an **aortic dissection,** both pre- and postoperatively.

   b. **Dosage.** Labetalol is given as a 0.25 mg/kg bolus over 2 minutes with subsequent doses of 0.5 mg/kg every 15 minutes until effect is achieved (to a total dose of 300 mg). Alternatively, a continuous IV infusion can be given at a rate of 1−4 mg/min, mixing 40 mL of the 5 mg/mL solution in 160 mL (200 mg/ 200 mL).

5. **Metoprolol** is a cardioselective β-blocker that is given routinely in oral form for atrial fibrillation prophylaxis (starting at 25 mg bid). It can be supplemented by 5 mg doses IV every 5 minutes for three doses if rapid AF does occur. With IV usage, the onset of action is 2−3 minutes with a peak effect in 20 minutes and a duration of action up to 5 hours. It is rarely used intravenously for hypertension control, but is beneficial in reducing systolic hypertension postoperatively in increasing oral doses as long as the heart rate remains above 60 bpm and the patient has adequate cardiac function.

F. Enalaprilat

1. Enalaprilat is an intravenous ACE inhibitor that inhibits activation of the renin–angiotensin system and also blunts the increase in other vasoactive substances that normally rise with CPB (catecholamines, endothelin, and atrial natriuretic peptide).

2. Enalaprilat reduces blood pressure by producing balanced arterial and venous vasodilation, reducing both preload and afterload without a reflex increase in heart rate. It thus may reduce myocardial oxygen demand while producing an improvement in cardiac performance in patients with impaired LV function. It also does not produce hypoxic vasoconstriction, and has no effect on gas exchange and oxygen delivery.[219] It may also have some beneficial effects on postoperative renal function.[220]

3. **Indication.** Because of its long duration of action, this drug can be considered in the hemodynamically stable patient with depressed ventricular function who has persistent hypertension in the ICU but is unable to take oral medications. It can subsequently be converted to the oral ACE inhibitors.

4. **Dosage.** Enalaprilat is given in a dose of 0.625–1.25 mg IV over 5 minutes q6h, which produces an initial clinical response in 15 minutes with a peak effect in 4 hours. If the initial response is unsatisfactory, a second dose may be given after 1 hour.

G. Hydralazine

1. Hydralazine is a direct arteriolar vasodilator that decreases SVR and systemic blood pressure. The reduction in afterload may improve myocardial function, but is usually accompanied by a compensatory tachycardia.

2. **Indication.** Hydralazine is most commonly used as a prn drug when adequate blood pressure control has not been achieved as the patient is being converted from IV to oral antihypertensive medications. Often a patient is started back on a lower dose of preoperative medications but has persistent hypertension for a few days that subsequently abates. Use of prn hydralazine allows the clinican to avoid being too aggressive with the reinstitution of higher-dose or multiple medications that might otherwise precipitate hypotension when the transient hyperadrenergic state improves.

3. **Dosage.** The usual dose is 10 mg IV q15 minutes until effect and them q6h prn. Less commonly it is given in a dose of 20–40 mg IM. The onset of action after IV injection is about 5–10 minutes with a peak effect at 20 minutes and a duration of action of 3–4 hours.

H. Fenoldopam mesylate

1. Fenoldopam is a dopamine (DA_1) receptor agonist that is a rapid-acting peripheral and renal vasodilator with onset of action of 5 minutes and a duration of action of <30 minutes. Its antihypertensive effect is accompanied by a reflex tachycardia, an increase in stroke volume index, and an increase in cardiac index.[221,222] It also lowers PVR, with potential theoretical benefits in patients with preexisting RV dysfunction. Its beneficial effect on renal function is related to dilatation of renal afferent arterioles, resulting in an increase in renal blood flow. It also produces hypokalemia, either through a direct drug effect or enhanced K^+–Na^+ exchange.

2. **Indication.** This drug is rarely used for postoperative hypertension, but, if used for renoprotection during surgery, the dose could be increased to immediately control severe hypertension when rapid onset of effect is necessary.

3. **Dosage.** A continuous infusion is given starting at 0.05–0.1 μg/kg/min using a 10 mg/250 mL mix. The dose may be increased in 0.05–0.1 μg/kg/min increments every 15 minutes until effect is achieved to a maximum rate of 0.8 μg/kg/min. The dose used to provide a renoprotective effect (0.1 μg/kg/min) generally does not produce systemic hypotension.

I. **Selection of the appropriate antihypertensive medication in the postoperative cardiac surgical patient**

1. When filling pressures are normal or slightly elevated and the cardiac output is marginal, a selective arterial vasodilator with minimal cardiac effects is the best selection. **Clevidipine** is a very short-acting drug that is able to achieve a target blood pressure fairly rapidly and has a rapid offset of action in the event of hemodynamic compromise. **Nitroprusside** is both an arterial and a venous dilator, so it is effective in reducing elevated filling pressures and improving cardiac output while it lowers the blood pressure. In patients with low filling pressures, volume infusion may be necessary to prevent a precipitous drop in blood pressure. Because SNP is so powerful, more caution is necessary in initiating the infusion to avoid overshoot, and thus it tends to take longer to achieve a target blood pressure. The efficacy of **nicardipine** is similar to clevidipine, but its longer duration of action may prove detrimental if used during a period of hemodynamic instability. With any of these medications, use of additional inotropic support must be considered if the cardiac output is marginal and does not improve with reduction in afterload.

2. When filling pressures are high and the cardiac output is satisfactory, a venodilator, such as **nitroglycerin,** may be beneficial. This will reduce venous return, filling pressures, stroke volume, cardiac output, and blood pressure. It may be beneficial if there is evidence of myocardial ischemia. However, nitroglycerin is best avoided when hypovolemia or a marginal cardiac output is present.

3. When the heart is hyperdynamic with adequate filling pressures, a high cardiac output, and frequently a tachycardia, a β-blocker with negative inotropic and chronotropic properties, such as **esmolol,** should be selected. Any of the calcium channel blockers, including those with negative chronotropic properties, such as **diltiazem,** can also be selected in that they may improve myocardial oxygen metabolism, especially when there is evidence of ischemia.

4. Once the patient is able to tolerate oral medications, the IV medications should be weaned while monitoring the blood pressure response to oral medications. It is most appropriate to restart the medications the patient was taking before surgery, but others should be considered under certain circumstances.

   a. β-blockers (**metoprolol** 25–75 mg PO bid) are initiated in virtually all patients to reduce the incidence of atrial fibrillation and may also control blood pressure. They can be used effectively when the patient has a fast sinus mechanism. In patients with impaired LV function, **carvedilol,** which is an α- and β-blocker, can be started at a dose of 3.125 mg twice daily and increased up to 25 mg twice daily as tolerated.

b. The next choice is usually an **ACE inhibitor,** such as lisinopril 5–10 mg PO qd or ramipril 1.25 mg bid. This should be considered for all patients with poor ventricular function (ejection fraction <35%) but must be used cautiously in patients with renal dysfunction.[223] If the patient cannot tolerate an ACE inhibitor (usually because of a cough), an angiotensin receptor blocker (**ARB**) can be chosen.

c. The third choice is usually a **calcium channel blocker,** such as amlodipine (Norvasc), diltiazem, or verapamil, which are alternative choices for spasm prophylaxis in patients receiving radial artery grafts. Diltiazem is useful as an antihypertensive when utilized to control the ventricular response to atrial fibrillation.

d. Long-acting **nitrates** are alternative coronary vasodilators that can be used in patients receiving radial artery grafts and may also provide an antihypertensive benefit.

VIII. Cardiac Arrest

A. Cardiac arrest is a serious and dreaded complication of any cardiac operation that can occur unexpectedly at the conclusion of surgery, during transport from the operating room, in the ICU, or later during convalescence on the floor. It must be managed immediately by standard American Heart Association (AHA) ACLS protocols and, if not immediately successful, by open-chest massage. Prompt and aggressive CPR is essential to restore satisfactory cardiac function and hopefully prevent severe neurologic sequelae from compromising the results of a successful resuscitation. The mortality rate for patients sustaining a cardiac arrest after cardiac surgery has ranged from 30% to 75% in different series.[224–226] Survival is most likely when bleeding is the predisposing cause – patients arresting from ventricular arrhythmias caused by a myocardial infarction or pump failure are less likely to survive.[226]

B. Basic and ACLS recommendations[227] should be followed for patients sustaining a cardiac arrest outside of an ICU setting, with consideration given to early resternotomy if resuscitation is unsuccessful and the patient is within 10 days of surgery. However, a modified protocol is indicated in ICU patients, in whom initial pacing or defibrillation should be attempted before initiating cardiac compressions (Figure 11.13).[228] In these extensively monitored patients, early cardioversion is likely to be successful. In patients with excessive bleeding or tamponade, early resternotomy within 10 minutes is likely to improve survival. In other patients, it will allow for performance of internal massage, which is nearly twice as effective as external compressions in increasing the cardiac output and coronary perfusion pressure.[229]

A: Establish an airway

B: Manually ventilate the patient with positive-pressure ventilation (8–10/min)

C: Provide circulation by chest compressions (100/min) (only after three attempts at defibrillation [VT/VF] in ICU patients or attempted pacing for asystole). Uninterrupted chest compressions are essential to optimize perfusion and should be performed as long as necessary or until the chest can be opened; if an Ambu bag is not available, aim for a compression ventilation ratio of 15:2; place intravenous lines if not present.

D: Defibrillate for VF/pulseless ventricular tachycardia (VT)

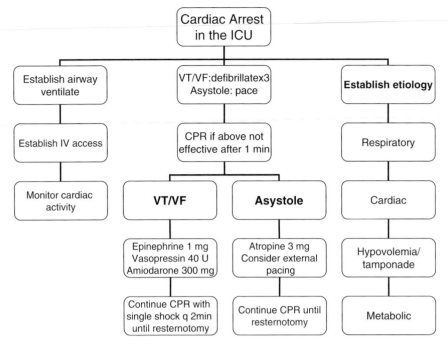

Figure 11.13 • A simplified algorithm for the management of a cardiac arrest in the ICU. Note that up to three defibrillations for VF or pacing for asystole should be attempted within the first minute prior to initiating external compressions in a patient with a witnessed arrest in the ICU.

C. **Etiology and assessment.** While resuscitation is under way, an evaluation should be undertaken to determine the possible cause of the cardiac arrest (Table 11.10). The most common causes of non-VF arrests in cardiac surgical patients are cardiac tamponade, marked hypovolemia from bleeding, asystole from pacing failure, and tension pneumothorax.

1. Listen to the chest, check the ventilator function, ABGs, acid–base and electrolyte status. If the patient is not intubated, secure an airway first, administer oxygen, and then intubate. Do **not** try to intubate before delivering oxygen by face mask because this may prolong the period of hypoxemia. This assessment may indicate whether the patient has:

   • Severe ventilatory or oxygenation disturbance (hypoxia, hypercarbia from pneumothorax, endotracheal tube displacement, acute pulmonary embolism)

   • Severe acid–base and electrolyte disturbances (acidosis, hypo- or hyperkalemia)

2. Check the chest tube drainage and review the chest x-ray. These may indicate whether there is:

   • Acute impairment of venous return (tension pneumothorax, cardiac tamponade, occasionally with sudden cessation of massive bleeding)

   • Acute hypovolemia (massive mediastinal bleeding)

Table 11.10 • Most Common Causes of Postoperative Cardiac Arrest

Cause	Treatment
Hypovolemia	Volume infusions
Hypoxia	Hand ventilation with 100% O_2
Hydrogen ion acidosis	Sodium bicarbonate
Hyperkalemia	Calcium chloride, glucose/insulin/ bicarbonate drip
Hypokalemia	KCl infusion
Hypothermia	Warming blankets
Tamponade	Pericardiocentesis, subxiphoid exploration, or emergency sternotomy
Tension pneumothorax	Needle decompression, chest tube
Thrombosis (myocardial infarction)	IABP, emergency cardiac catheterization
Thrombosis (pulmonary embolism)	Anticoagulation, embolectomy, IVC umbrella

Tablets
  Drug overdose
  Digoxin toxicity
  β-blockers, calcium channel blockers
	
	Gastric lavage, activated charcoal
	Digibind
	Inotropic support, pacing

3. Assess whether inotropes, vasopressors, or vasodilators are being administered at the correct rate. There may potentially be:
   - Inadvertent cessation of inotropic support
   - Profound vasodilation from bolusing of nitroprusside
4. Examine the cardiac monitor and ECG. These may reveal:
   - Third-degree heart block (may occur spontaneously or if AV pacing fails in a patient with complete heart block)
   - Acute ischemia (graft thrombosis, coronary spasm)
   - Ventricular tachyarrhythmias (ventricular tachycardia or fibrillation)
   D. **Treatment.** Cardiac surgery patients are usually extensively monitored in the ICU, and ventilation can be provided immediately by Ambu bags present at the bedside. Many patients are still intubated and most arrests are "witnessed". Thus immediate resuscitation using ICU protocols should be used. On the floor, most patients are only monitored by telemetry and many arrests are not "witnessed". Thus, immediate resuscitation using standard ACLS protocols should be used.
      1. **Hand ventilate** with an Ambu bag with 100% oxygen at a rate of 8–10/min; listen for bilateral breath sounds. Intubate after establishing an adequate airway after a brief period of satisfactory manual ventilation. Perform endotracheal

suctioning for a potential tube or airway obstruction. If the latter is present, it is best to remove the tube, hand ventilate, and have an experienced individual reintubate the patient.

2. **In any patient sustaining a cardiac arrest after cardiac surgery refractory to the protocols listed below, emergency resternotomy for open-chest resuscitation should be considered immediately and performed within 10 minutes of the arrest** as this has been shown to improve survival.

   a. Emergency resternotomy is a life-saving procedure in patients with bleeding or tamponade as it will allow for evacuation of blood and control of bleeding. Invariably, immediate hemodynamic improvement will be noted if the patient has been fluid resuscitated. In patients with other causes of cardiac arrest, such as myocardial ischemia from graft occlusion or primary arrhythmic events, internal massage is much more effective than external compressions.[229]

   b. Emergency resternotomy is still feasible up to 10 days after surgery and should also be considered in nonsurgical causes of postoperative cardiac arrest.[228]

   c. Emergency reexploration for cardiac arrest can be problematic in patients whose surgery was performed through a minimally invasive thoracotomy approach. A full sternotomy is usually required to perform effective cardiac massage and it has been recommended that sternal saws be available in the ICU for use by an experienced surgeon if internal massage is indicated.[228]

3. **Ventricular tachycardia or fibrillation (VT/VF)** can be identified on a monitor and confirmed by lack of a pulse.

   a. **ICU patients. Three attempts at defibrillation** with 200 joules (biphasic) or 360 joules (monophasic) should be performed, all **within 1 minute of arrest**. If the patient remains in VT/VF or has severe hypotension after 1 minute, **then external chest compressions** at a rate of 100/min should be commenced. Preparations should be made for an emergency resternotomy, which should then be performed as soon as possible. The rationale for delaying external massage is that it can cause disruption of the sternal closure, injury to bypass grafts, or damage to the ventricular myocardium from prosthetic valves. This potential damage can be minimized if compressions are **delayed for a very short period of time (<1 minute)** to prepare and use the defibrillator or attach the pacing wires to a pacemaker in cases of asystole or bradycardia. After subsequent defibrillations, it is advisable to continue CPR briefly since the initial rhythm may be slow and not generate much pressure, but will improve.

   b. **Floor patients or unwitnessed arrests. External compressions** should be started **immediately** while the defibrillation equipment is readied. **Defibrillation** should be done as soon as possible and then repeated every 2 minutes, if necessary. It is recommended that CPR be resumed immediately after each defibrillation, with assessment of the rhythm on the monitor and palpation for a pulse during CPR and for no more than 10 seconds with CPR stopped. If the patient is not monitored, CPR should be continued for 2 minutes before checking for a pulse. After 2 minutes of CPR, defibrillation should be attempted again. Since most patients respond fairly promptly to defibrillation

Table 11.11 • Drug Doses Used During Cardiac Arrest

Vasopressin	40 units IV push × 1 dose
Epinephrine (1:1000)	1 mg IV push, repeat doses q3–5 minutes
Amiodarone	300 mg IV push; can give 150 mg q5 min to total 2.2 g/24h
Lidocaine	1–1.5 mg/kg bolus, followed by 0.5–0.75 mg/kg boluses every 5–10 minutes to total dose of 3 mg/kg
Magnesium sulfate	1–2 g in 10 mL D5W
Atropine	1 mg IV push with repeat doses of 1 mg q3–5 min to total dose of 0.04 mg/kg

and an emergency sternotomy can be accomplished fairly readily, the AHA recommendation to wait 2 minutes between defibrillations may produce an unnecessay delay that may compromise the potential for successful resuscitation and it is therefore not recommended.

c. Initial medications are given after three unsuccessful shocks within the first minute in ICU patients or after two attempts for floor patients (Table 11.11).

- **Vasopressin** 40 units IV as a single dose provides comparable or superior efficacy to epinephrine in promoting return of spontaneous circulation.[230]

- **Epinephrine** 1 mg IV push (10 mL of 1:10,000 solution) should be given if VT/VF persists or recurs after defibrillation. It may be repeated every 3–5 minutes.

- If the cardiac arrest occurs outside of the ICU setting and intravenous access is not immediately available, epinephrine, vasopressin, and lidocaine are effective when given down an endotracheal tube at 2–2.5 times the usual IV dose diluted in 10 mL of normal saline. Note that ACLS protocols recommend the intraosseous route as second choice, but this requires a special rigid needle from an access kit.

- Although vasopressin or epinephrine is recommended as an initial pharmacologic adjunct, they can potentially cause more harm (severe hypertension) than good and the European guidelines advise against their routine use.[228]

d. Antiarrhythmic drugs may improve the success of defibrillation and should be used for persistent/recurrent VT/VF despite three shocks. Defibrillation should be repeated after each dose of medication.

- **Amiodarone** should be given first in a bolus dose of 300 mg; a dose of 150 mg may be repeated every 3–5 minutes to a maximum dose of 2.2 g IV/24 h. It is then given as an infusion of 1 mg/min for 6 hours, then 0.5 mg/min for 18 hours with conversion to oral dosing if necessary.

- **Lidocaine** may be given for refractory VT/VF as a 1–1.5 mg/kg bolus followed by 0.5–0.75 mg/kg boluses twice every 5–10 minutes to a total dose of 3 mg/kg.

- **Magnesium sulfate** 1–2 g in 10 mL of D5W IV may be helpful for torsades de pointes, especially if hypomagnesemia is suspected.
- Although amiodarone is universally recommended as the preferred drug, there is little evidence that it improves hospital survival!

4. **Asystole or pulseless electrical activity (PEA)** (pacing spikes or QRS complex with no detectable pulse). Note that a paced patient who develops PEA may have underlying VF. The pacer may need to be turned off to identify this rhythm.

   - Initiate immediate epicardial pacing by connecting the patient's atrial and ventricular pacing wires to a pacing box, which should be available at the bedside or nearby. The pacemaker should be set in the DDD mode at a rate of 90 beats/min. The default emergency setting of VOO can be used initially but will be less effective since it will only pace the ventricle.
   - With a witnessed arrest, CPR may be delayed 1 minute while the pacing wires are connected. If successful **pacing with a documented pulse** cannot be achieved **within 1 minute** of a witnessed arrest, **external compressions must be started.** Compressions should be started immediately in patients with an unwitnessed arrest.
   - Attempt **transcutaneous pacing** after the resuscitation is under way.
   - **Epinephrine** bolus 1 mg IV (10 mL of a 1:10,000 solution) every 3–5 minutes; an infusion of 2–10 µg/min can be used for bradycardia.
   - **Vasopressin** one dose of 40 units IV can be given instead of epinephrine.
   - **Atropine** 1 mg IV with repeat doses of 1 mg every 3–5 minutes to a total dose of 0.04 mg/kg (European guidelines suggest one dose of 3 mg via a central line).[228]

5. **Bradycardia** that is unresponsive to epicardial pacing
   - **Atropine** 0.5 mg IV with repeat doses of 0.5–1.0 mg every 3–5 minutes to a total dose of 3 mg
   - Attempt **transcutaneous** pacing
   - **Epinephrine** 2–10 µg/min (1 mg/250 mL mix)
   - **Dopamine** infusion 2–10 µg/kg/min (400 mg/250 mL mix)

6. **Tachycardia with pulses** may be well tolerated at a rate less than 150 bpm, but at higher rates the patient may develop chest pain, altered mental status, or hypotension.

   a. If unstable – perform synchronized cardioversion with 200–360 joules.

   b. **Stable with narrow QRS** usually represents a supraventricular mechanism.
      - **Regular rhythm** – give adenosine 6 mg IV push and may repeat with 12 mg IV doses twice; if conversion occurs, this probably represents a reentry supraventricular tachycardia; if the rhythm does not convert, it may represent atrial flutter, ectopic atrial tachycardia, or junctional tachycardia that should be managed with diltiazem and/or β-blockers.
      - **Irregular rhythm** may be atrial fibrillation/flutter or multifocal atrial tachycardia that should be managed with IV diltiazem and/or β-blockers.

    c. Stable with wide complex QRS is usually VT or AF with aberrancy.

- **Regular rhythm** is most likely VT and should be treated by amiodarone 150 mg IV over 10 minutes with synchronized cardioversion; if it represents SVT with aberrancy, it should be treated with adenosine.
- **Irregular rhythm** is most commonly AF with aberrancy, to be treated with diltiazem and/or β-blockers; less common are AF with WPW syndrome (use amiodarone), polymorphic VT, or torsades de pointes (magnesium).

7. **Persistent hypotension.** Reestablishment of satisfactory myocardial blood flow is the most important element in a successful resuscitation. Because coronary perfusion occurs during compression "diastole" (i.e., when the aortic pressure exceeds the right atrial pressure), elevation of SVR and coronary perfusion pressure is critical. This is best achieved with medications that have predominantly α effects (epinephrine in high doses) or strong vasoconstrictor properties (vasopressin). Patients with a cardiac etiology to their arrest will often benefit from placement of an IABP.

8. **Controversial medications during cardiac arrest**

    a. Sodium bicarbonate should not be given routinely for the attended arrest during which excellent ventilation and cardiac compressions are achieved. Administration of $NaHCO_3$ reduces SVR and compromises cerebral perfusion, creates extracellular alkalosis that shifts the oxygen–hemoglobin dissociation curve to the left inhibiting oxygen release to tissues, exacerbates central venous acidosis, inactivates catecholamines administered during an arrest, and can produce hypernatremia and hyperosmolarity. Its use should be guided by the results of ABGs drawn every 10 minutes during the arrest. It is given in doses of 1 mEq/kg, with half the dose readministered 10 minutes later if ABGs are not available.

    b. Calcium chloride is not routinely recommended during a cardiac arrest as it may contribute to intracellular damage. Doses of 5–10 mL of a 10% solution can be given for hyperkalemia, hypocalcemia, or calcium channel blocker toxicity.

9. **Post-arrest care.** Virtually all patients following an arrest should be monitored and assessed in the ICU. Most will stabilize if an immediately treatable cause has been identified. If the chest has been opened, it may be closed in the ICU if provisions are available. Otherwise, it is beneficial to return the patient to the operating room for further evaluation and chest closure. Most patients will require mechanical ventilatory support, and use of sedatives can confound a neurologic evaluation. Once the patient's hemodynamics, arterial blood gases, acid–base status, and electrolyte and glucose status have improved, early weaning of sedation is recommended. Myocardial stunning is common and an immediate post-arrest assessment of myocardial function by echocardiography may be misleading as to whether the arrest was caused by a primary cardiac event. Similarly, cardiac biomarkers may be elevated from ischemia and defibrillation and not necessarily reflect myocardial damage preceding the arrest. However, placement of an IABP is very beneficial when a myocardial insult is suspected and cardiac catheterization should be considered if there are any associated ECG changes prior to or following the arrest. Patients suffering VF/VT arrests with known impairment of LV function should be further evaluated by an electrophysiologist, and implantation of an implantable cardioverter-defibrillator (ICD) should be considered.

IX. Perioperative Myocardial Infarction

Despite advances in myocardial protection, use of off-pump procedures, and refinements in surgical technique, a small percentage of patients will sustain a perioperative myocardial infarction (PMI).[231] Depending on the degree of myocardial necrosis, a PMI may be of little consequence to the patient or it may result in a low output state, CHF, or malignant arrhythmias. A hemodynamically significant infarction invariably results in increased perioperative mortality and reduced long-term survival. Studies suggest that cardiac enzyme elevations beyond threshold levels also correlate with impaired survival.[232–240]

A. **Predisposing factors**

1. Left main or diffuse three-vessel disease

2. Preoperative ischemia or infarction. This includes ST-elevation infarctions (STEMIs), acute coronary syndromes, or evidence of ongoing ischemia, often following a failed PCI.

3. Poor LV systolic and diastolic function (low ejection fraction, CHF, LVEDP >15 mm Hg, LVH)

4. Reoperations, which predispose to atheroembolism of debris or to graft thrombosis

5. Coronary endarterectomy

6. Long aortic cross-clamp period

B. **Mechanisms**

1. Prolonged ischemia during anesthetic induction or before the establishment of coronary reperfusion. This is usually caused by tachycardia, hypertension/hypotension, or ventricular distention, but may occasionally result from damage to grafts during reoperation or embolization down a stenotic vein graft.

2. Inadequate myocardial protection or ischemia/reperfusion injury following cardioplegic arrest. Research into the biochemical mechanism of PMI suggests that this insult is caused by activation of the Na^+–H^+ exchanger leading to intracellular calcium accumulation, cell contracture, and cell death. Prophylactic use of a Na^+–H^+ exchange inhibitor, such as cariporide, in the perioperative period has been shown to reduce the incidence of PMI.[241]

3. Incomplete revascularization

4. Graft flow problems from anastomotic stenosis, graft spasm, or thrombosis

5. Native coronary vasospasm

6. Coronary air or particulate embolization (usually from patent but atherosclerotic vein grafts during reoperations)

C. **Diagnosis.** The diagnosis of a PMI is usually entertained by the **combination** of new ECG changes (new ST changes or Q waves), evidence of new regional or global wall motion abnormalities by echocardiography, and elevation of cardiac specific markers. However, several factors must be considered before concluding that myocardial necrosis has occurred.

1. Postcardiotomy ventricular dysfunction may suggest the development of a PMI, but often represents a prolonged period of reversible myocardial depression ("stunning") that can recover after several days of pharmacologic or mechanical support. However, the persistence of new regional wall motion abnormalities on serial evaluations is more consistent with the occurrence of a PMI.

2. Significant ST elevation on a postoperative ECG suggests a problem with graft flow and an evolving infarction (Figure 8.2, page 321). New Q waves on the ECG are noted in about 5% of patients after surgery, but in many cases are not associated with significant enzyme elevation and therefore may be of little consequence. These "false positive" Q waves may be associated with areas of altered depolarization or unmasking of old infarcts.[237,242] The persistence of ST segment depression, deep T wave inversions, ventricular tachyarrhythmias, or a new bundle branch block for over 48 hours suggests some degree of myocardial injury, especially if associated with new regional wall motion abnormalities. T wave inversions, in particular, are commonly noted days to weeks after surgery when there has been no other evidence of PMI.

3. Virtually all open-heart operations are associated with an elevation in cardiac biomarkers, and this correlates with the extent of global ischemia. Less elevation after off-pump surgery, which avoids cannulation, global ischemic arrest, and ventricular fibrillation, and higher levels after valve and combined valve-CABG surgery are consistent with this concept.[234,243] The significance of enzyme elevation must be put into the context of its relationship to adverse outcomes. Clearly, there is a spectrum of myocardial damage that may result from cardiac surgery, and the definition of a **significant** PMI is based on the premise that enzyme levels beyond a certain threshold level are associated with more myocardial necrosis and adverse outcomes.

   a. Creatine kinase-MB fractions have traditionally been used to assess the degree of myocardial necrosis. Two studies of CABG patients found CK-MB fractions of > 40 ng/L and > 100 ng/mL (> 8–20 times the upper limit of normal [ULN]) to be predictive of adverse events, but the development of Q waves alone was not.[237,238] Pooled data from numerous studies found that a CK-MB > 5–8 times ULN predicted an increased risk of death at 40 months.[240] The 2008 Society of Thoracic Surgeons (STS) data specifications defined an early postoperative MI as an elevation of CK-MB levels to > 5 × ULN with or without the development of Q waves. However, these specifications did not incorporate troponin levels, evidence of graft occlusion, or loss of myocardial function into the definition.

   b. Troponin is a very sensitive and specific marker for myocardial injury, often suggesting a PMI when elevations are simply those expected after a routine cardiac operation. Numerous studies have evaluated the correlation of troponin levels with adverse cardiac events, operative mortality, and survival, with variable results. Average troponin I (TnI) levels following uncomplicated CABGs without ECG changes have ranged from 6 to 18 ng/mL in several studies.[232–234,244,245] However, TnI levels > 8–15 ng/mL measured 12–24 hours postoperatively did correlate with adverse events and hospital death.[233–235,244] One report indicated that for every 50 ng/L increase in TnI, the odds of operative death increased by 40%.[232] Another study identified increased short- and long-term mortality with the following higher quartiles of troponin levels at 24 hours: 0–2.19, 2.20–4.3, 4.31–8.48, and > 8.49 ng/mL.[236] Thus, although the threshold levels for clinical significance may differ, most studies concur that the greater the elevation in troponin, the greater the risk of adverse outcomes.

   c. Based upon an analysis of the literature, a joint task force of four major cardiology societies[246] offered an expert consensus on the definition of a perioperative MI, which has been incorporated into the 2011 STS data specifications. A PMI is defined as an elevation of biomarkers (either CK or troponin) to > 5 × the 99th percentile of the normal reference range during the first 72h after a CABG *plus:*

1. New pathological Q waves or LBBB *or*
2. Angiographically documented new graft or native coronary artery occlusion *or*
3. Imaging evidence of new loss of viable myocardium

D. Presentation and treatment

1. **Intraoperative ischemia.** Identification of new regional wall motion abnormalities by transesophageal echocardiography is a sensitive means of assessing intraoperative myocardial ischemia. These changes precede evidence of ischemia noted with Swan-Ganz monitoring (elevation of PA pressures) or the ECG (ST segment elevation). Aggressive treatment to reduce myocardial oxygen demand and maintain perfusion pressure is essential to lower the risk of PMI. Placement of an IABP prior to going on bypass can often reduce the risk of surgery in patients with ongoing ischemia. In patients undergoing reoperative surgery, avoiding manipulation of patent but diseased grafts is essential to prevent atheroembolism.

2. **Postcardiotomy low cardiac output syndrome with/without ECG evidence of ischemia.** Although enzyme elevation is more prominent with a longer duration of aortic clamping, fastidious attention to myocardial protection should offset the adverse effects of prolonged cross-clamping. The occurrence of severe postcardiotomy ventricular dysfunction, whether caused by ischemia, "stunning", or an infarction, requires careful evaluation and treatment.

   a. If myocardial dysfunction or ischemia is noted in the operating room at the conclusion of CPB, the adequacy of the operative procedure should be assessed. Supplemental grafts or graft revision may be necessary. IABP or circulatory assist devices may be indicated in addition to pharmacologic support.

   b. If ECG changes are detected upon arrival in the ICU (especially ST changes), intravenous NTG or calcium channel blockers (if spasm is suspected) should be given. Emergency coronary angiography with possible PCI or surgical graft revision should be strongly considered. An IABP is helpful in temporarily improving coronary perfusion and reducing the workload of the heart.

   c. Management of a hemodynamically significant MI involves supportive care until arrhythmias and hemodynamic instability resolve. Cardiac output should be optimized in standard fashion, but care must be taken to avoid excessive volume infusions and tachycardia that may increase myocardial oxygen demand and worsen an ischemic insult. Use of milrinone or placement of an IABP will minimize oxygen consumption. It is difficult to treat the sinus tachycardia that frequently accompanies a low cardiac output state because it usually represents a compensatory mechanism to maintain cardiac output. Sinus tachycardia is frequently a sign of an "injured heart" and can perpetuate myocardial ischemia and damage. It can only be treated once the cardiac output improves.

3. **Good cardiac output but low SVR.** The patient sustaining a small PMI may have a normal cardiac output accompanied by systemic hypotension. This syndrome

usually requires use of an α-agent for several days to maintain an adequate systemic blood pressure until the SVR returns to normal.

4. **Persistent ventricular ectopy** may reflect ischemia, infarction, or reperfusion of previously ischemic muscle. It may be treated short-term with lidocaine or with amiodarone. β-blockers are generally used for their antiarrhythmic effect in patients with preserved ventricular function. However, nonsustained or sustained ventricular tachycardia occurring in patients with impaired ventricular function often requires electrophysiologic testing, use of amiodarone, and placement of an ICD.

5. Some patients will have an infarction diagnosed by electrocardiographic, enzymatic, or functional criteria but will have no clinical or hemodynamic sequelae. These patients do not require any special treatment, but should be maintained on β-blockers.

E. **Prognosis**

1. An uncomplicated infarction generally does not influence operative mortality or long-term survival. Despite a return of ventricular function to baseline, the heart may fail to demonstrate functional improvement during exercise. However, studies do suggest a correlation between the level of enzyme elevation and reduced survival.[232–240] Most of these studies did not correlate early hemodynamic performance with the level of enzyme elevation.

2. A hemodynamically significant MI (i.e., one presenting as a low cardiac output syndrome or malignant arrhythmias) does increase operative mortality and decrease long-term survival.[247]

3. The prognosis following a perioperative infarction is determined primarily by the adequacy of revascularization and the residual ejection fraction. One study reported that the prognosis for patients sustaining an MI with an ejection fraction >40% and with complete revascularization was comparable to patients not developing a perioperative infarction.[248]

X. Coronary Vasospasm

A. Vasospasm has become increasingly recognized as a cause of postoperative morbidity and mortality following coronary artery bypass grafting. It can affect normal coronary arteries, bypassed vessels, saphenous vein grafts, or arterial grafts (ITA, radial, gastroepiploic artery).[249,250]

B. **Etiology** may be related to enhanced α-adrenergic tone, use of α-agents such as phenylephrine to support blood pressure, endothelial dysfunction from reduced nitric oxide production, hypothermia, hypomagnesemia, or CCB withdrawal.[251] It has also been associated with the administration of 5-HT$_3$ antagonists, such as ondansetron (Zofran), which is commonly prescribed for postoperative nausea.[252]

C. **Diagnosis** of vasospasm can be extremely difficult to confirm and requires further evaluation to differentiate it from other more common clinical conditions with similar manifestations. The usual presentation is ST elevation consistent with ischemia, often with a low cardiac output state, hypotension, ventricular arrhythmias, or heart block.

D. **Evaluation**

1. An ECG will usually show localized, and occasionally diffuse, ST elevations, although these findings are more commonly associated with a compromise of graft flow, usually at an anastomosis. As noted, spasm may occur in native coronary arteries (unbypassed or beyond an anastomosis) as well as in arterial and rarely venous conduits. Spasm is most

common in radial artery grafts, but is usually mitigated by the prophylactic use of perioperative vasodilators.

2. Echocardiography will usually demonstrate an area of hypokinesis which corresponds to the ECG changes, but it is not diagnostic of spasm.

3. Coronary angiography may be necessary to make the appropriate diagnosis if there is no response to IV therapy with coronary vasodilators. It will usually demonstrate sluggish flow through grafts, diffuse spasm, and poor flow into distal native vessels. Resolution of spasm with intracoronary nitroglycerin or a calcium channel blocker (verapamil) confirms the diagnosis.[215] Differentiation from technical problems at the anastomosis can be difficult due to poor flow. If there is little response to pharmacologic intervention, reexploration may be indicated.

E. **Treatment** involves hemodynamic support and initiation of medications that can reverse the vasospasm. Improvement in ECG changes is consistent with spasm, but does not eliminate the possibility of some compromise of graft flow from surgical issues.

1. Optimize oxygenation and correct acidosis.

2. Optimize hemodynamic parameters. If an inotrope is indicated, a PDE inhibitor is the best choice because it is a potent vasodilator of the ITA and perhaps of native vessels as well.

3. Correct hypomagnesemia (**magnesium sulfate** 1–2 g in 10 mL of D5W IV).

4. Start **IV nitroglycerin** at 0.5 μg/kg/min and raise as tolerated.

5. Select a **calcium channel blocker** (use low-dose unless the patient is hypertensive):

   a. IV diltiazem drip: 0.25 mg/kg IV bolus over 2 minutes, followed by a repeat bolus of 0.35 mg/kg 15 minutes later. A continuous infusion is then given at a rate of 5–15 mg/h using a 250 mg/250 mL mix.

   b. IV verapamil drip: 0.1 mg/kg bolus, followed by a 2–5 μg/kg/min infusion of a 120 mg/250 mL mix (most likely to cause hypotension).

   c. IV nicardipine 5 mg/h with a mix of 50 mg/250 mL; the dose can increased by 2.5 mg/hr every 5–15 minutes to a maximum dose of 15 mg/h, if tolerated.

6. If the patient does not improve and/or ECG changes persist, emergency cardiac catheterization is indicated to identify and possibly correct the problem. During catheterization, intracoronary nitroglycerin and verapamil are usually successful in reversing spasm.

7. Once the patient has stabilized, an oral coronary vasodilator is recommended. These include isosorbide mononitrate sustained release (Imdur) 20 mg qd, nifedipine 30 mg q6h, diltiazem CD 180 mg QD, or amlodipine 5 mg qd.

8. Statins may prove of benefit in reducing spasm.[253]

XI. Pacing Wires and Pacemakers

A. General comments

1. The use of cold cardioplegic arrest is commonly associated with temporary sinus node or AV node dysfunction. Placement of two temporary right atrial and two right ventricular epicardial pacing wire electrodes is beneficial in many patients to optimize hemodynamics at the conclusion of bypass and for several hours in the ICU (Figure 11.14). Pacing wires are also useful in the event that medications used to control atrial fibrillation precipitate advanced AV block. They can also be used

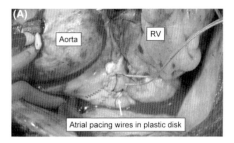

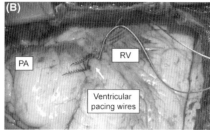

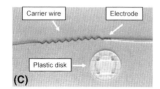

Figure 11.14 • (A) Atrial pacing wires (Medtronic 6500) are placed into a plastic disk that is sewn low on the right atrial free wall, permitting contact of the electrodes with the atrial wall. (B) The two ventricular wires are sewn superficially over the right ventricular free wall. (C) Close up of the pacing wire demonstrating the plastic carrier wire adjacent to the electrode and the plastic disk into which the atrial wires are placed. PA; pulmonary artery; RV; right ventricle.

for overdrive pacing and they have diagnostic utility in delineating unusual rhythm problems.

2. Reluctance to routinely place wires during surgery is based on concerns that bleeding and tamponade may complicate their removal. This is nearly always associated with removal of ventricular wires, and although very uncommon, can be life-threatening. Nonetheless, although most surgeons will place ventricular wires, many tend to avoid placement of atrial pacing wires. Bleeding is rare with their removal unless they are directly sewn to the right atrium. Placing the wires into a plastic button sewn low on the right atrial free wall will virtually never result in bleeding with wire removal (Medtronic model 6500 wires). The benefits of atrial pacing in bradycardic patients with left ventricular hypertrophy or dysfunction can be significant.

3. To define whether pacing wire placement should be performed routinely, one study found that 15% of patients needed pacing to terminate bypass, but less than 10% of patients required temporary pacing postoperatively.[254] However, placement of at least one ventricular pacing wire is essential, and the risk:benefit ratio of atrial pacing wires suggests that they should be placed routinely as well.

B. **Diagnostic uses.** When the exact nature of an arrhythmia cannot be ascertained from a 12-lead ECG, atrial electrograms (AEGs) are helpful in making the appropriate diagnosis. Atrial pacing wires can be used to record atrial activity in both unipolar and bipolar modes. With suitably equipped monitors, these recordings can be obtained simultaneously with standard limb leads to distinguish among atrial and junctional arrhythmias and differentiate them from more life-threatening ventricular arrhythmias. Simultaneous ECG and AEG tracings for each of the most commonly encountered postoperative arrhythmias are provided in section XII, starting on page 529. The technique for obtaining atrial wire tracings is either of the following:

1. A multichannel recorder can be used to print simultaneous monitor ECGs and AEGs. Most monitoring systems have cartridges with three leads for recording the AEG: two of them represent the arm leads and are connected with alligator clips to

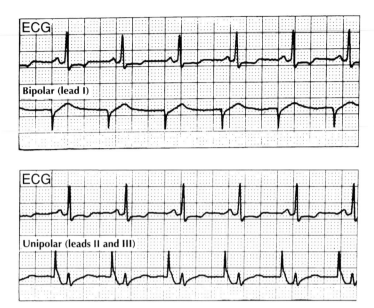

Figure 11.15 • Sinus rhythm in simultaneous monitor leads and AEGs. In the upper tracing, note that the bipolar AEG (lead I) produces predominantly an atrial complex with essentially no visible ventricular complex. In contrast, the unipolar tracing (leads II and III) at the bottom shows both a large atrial wave and a smaller ventricular complex.

the atrial pacing wires; the third represents a left leg lead and is attached to an electrode pad over the patient's flank. When the monitor channel for the AEG is set on lead I, a bipolar AEG is obtained (Figure 11.15). This shows a large atrial complex and a very small or undetectable ventricular complex. When the AEG monitor channel is set on leads II or III, a unipolar atrial electrogram is obtained. This demonstrates a large atrial and slightly smaller ventricular complex.

2. When a standard ECG machine is used, the two arm leads are connected to the atrial wires with alligator clips, and the leg leads are attached to the right and left legs. A bipolar AEG will be recorded in lead I and a unipolar AEG in leads II or III. Alternatively, the atrial wires can be connected to the V leads. Bipolar AEGs give a better assessment of atrial activity than unipolar AEGs and can distinguish between sinus tachycardia and atrial arrhythmias. However, because the AEG and standard ECG tracings are not obtained simultaneously, a unipolar tracing is required to differentiate sinus from junctional tachycardia because it can demonstrate the relationship between the larger atrial and smaller ventricular complexes.

C. Therapeutic uses

1. Optimal hemodynamics are achieved at a heart rate of around 90 bpm in the immediate postoperative period. Use of temporary pacing wires attached to an external pulse generator (Figure 11.16) to increase the heart rate is preferable to the use of positive chronotropic agents that have other effects on myocardial function. Atrial or AV pacing will nearly always demonstrate superior hemodynamics to ventricular pacing. Since AV delay is often prolonged after bypass, shortening it

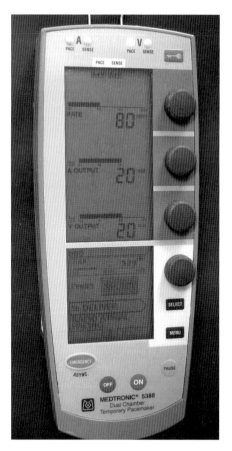

Figure 11.16 • The Medtronic model 5388 external pacemaker. This device can be used to provide pacing in a variety of modes, including AAI, DVI, DDD, and VVI pacing. It also has rapid atrial pacing capabilities.

artificially using AV pacing can improve hemodynamics, especially in patients with impaired ventricular function.[255]

2. Biventricular pacing using leads placed during surgery will improve LV systolic and diastolic function compared with RA-RV pacing in patients with AV block who have LV dysfunction. Benefit is greatest in patients who also have a wide QRS complex.[26–28]

3. Reentrant rhythms can be terminated by rapid pacing. Rapid atrial pacing can terminate type I atrial flutter (flutter rate less than 350/min) and other paroxysmal supraventricular tachycardias. Rapid ventricular pacing can terminate VT.

D. **Pacing nomenclature**

1. The sophistication and reprogrammability of permanent pacemaker systems led to the establishment of a joint nomenclature by the North American Society of Pacing and Electrophysiology (NASPE) and the British Pacing and Electrophysiology Group (BPEG). This nomenclature classifies pacemakers by their exact mode of function (Table 11.12).

Table 11.12 • Pacemaker Identification Codes

			Code Positions		
I	**II**	**III**	**IV**	**V**
Chamber paced	Chamber sensed	Response to sensing	Programmability/rate response	Antitachyarrhythmia functions
O – none	O – none	O – none	O – none	O – none
A – atrium	A – atrium	T – triggers pacing	R – rate-reponsive	P – antitachycardia pacing
V – ventricle	V – ventricle	I – inhibits pacing	P – simple programmable	S – shock
D – dual	D – dual	D – triggers and inhibits pacing	M – multiprogrammable	D – dual (pace and shock)
S – single chamber	S – single chamber		C – communicating	

Table 11.13 • Temporary Pacing Modes Used After Heart Surgery

Code positions			Description
I	II	III	
A	O	O	Asynchronous atrial pacing
A	A	I	Atrial demand pacing
V	V	I	Ventricular demand pacing
D	V	I	AV sequential pacing (ventricular demand)
D	D	D	AV sequential pacing (both chambers sense)

A, atrium; V, ventricle; D, both chambers; I, inhibits; O, does not apply.

2. Use of the first three letters is helpful in understanding the temporary pacemaker systems that are used after cardiac surgical procedures (Table 11.13). The most common modes are AOO (asynchronous atrial pacing), VVI (ventricular demand pacing), DVI (AV sequential pacing), and DDD (AV sequential demand pacing).

E. **Atrial pacing**

1. Atrial bipolar pacing is achieved by connecting both atrial electrodes to the pacemaker. This produces a smaller pacing stimulus artifact on a monitor than unipolar pacing and can often be difficult to detect even in multiple leads (Figure 11.17). It does, however, prevent IABP consoles from misinterpreting large pacing spikes as QRS complexes.

2. Atrial pacing can also be achieved using transesophageal electrodes or a pacing catheter placed through "paceport" Swan-Ganz catheters. These are particularly beneficial during minimally invasive surgery.[256]

3. Pacing is usually accomplished in the AOO or AAI mode. The usual settings include a pulse amplitude of 10–20 mA in the asynchronous mode (insensitive to the ECG signal), set at a rate faster than the intrinsic heart rate. With the Medtronic 5388 external pacemaker, AAI demand pacing may be accomplished if atrial sensing is satisfactory.

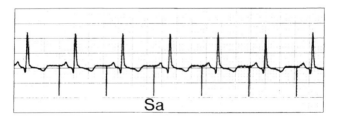

Figure 11.17 • Atrial pacing at a rate of 95 bpm. The atrial pacing stimulus artifact (Sa) is well seen in this tracing, but is frequently difficult to identify on the monitor. The height of the atrial pacing spike may be increased on the monitor for better visualization, or it may be decreased to prevent problems with ECG interpretation or intra-aortic balloon tracking.

4. **Indications.** Atrial pacing requires the ability to capture the atrium as well as normal conduction though the AV node. It is ineffective during atrial fibrillation/flutter.

   a. Sinus bradycardia or desire to increase the sinus rate to a higher level

   b. Suppression of premature ventricular complexes: set at a rate slightly faster than the sinus mechanism

   c. Suppression of premature atrial complexes or prevention of atrial fibrillation (with dual-site atrial pacing)

   d. Slow junctional rhythm

   e. Overdriving supraventricular tachycardias (atrial flutter, paroxysmal atrial or AV junctional reentrant tachycardia). Rapid atrial pacing can interrupt a reentrant circuit and convert it to sinus rhythm or a nonsustained rhythm, such as atrial fibrillation, which may terminate spontaneously.

5. **Technique of overdrive pacing**

   a. Overdrive pacing is accomplished using pacemakers that can produce rates as high as 800/min. When attaching pacemaker wires to the generator, **be absolutely certain** that the atrial wires, not the ventricular wires, are being attached. Pacing initially 10–15 beats/min above the ventricular rate will confirm that the ventricle is not being paced, which can occur when atrial pacing wires are placed close to the ventricle.

   b. The patient must be attached to an ECG monitor during rapid atrial pacing. Bipolar pacing should be used to minimize distortion of the atrial complex. Pacing spikes are often best identified by evaluation of lead II.

   c. Turn the pacer to full current (20 mA) and to a rate about 10 beats faster than the tachycardia or flutter rate. When the atrium has been captured, increase the rate slowly until the morphology of the flutter waves changes (atrial complexes become positive). This is usually about 20–30% above the atrial flutter rate. Pacing for up to 1 minute may be required.

   d. The pacer should be turned off abruptly. Sinus rhythm, a pause followed by sinus rhythm, atrial fibrillation, or recurrent flutter may be noted (Figure 11.18). If severe bradycardia develops, the pacemaker may be turned on at a rate around 60 until the sinus mechanism recovers.

F. **Atrioventricular pacing**

   1. Atrioventricular (AV) pacing is achieved by connecting both atrial wires to the atrial inlets and both ventricular wires to the ventricular inlets of an AV pacer (Figure 11.19). If two ventricular wires are not available or functioning, an atrial or skin lead can be used as a ground (the positive electrode) for ventricular pacing. The atrial and ventricular outputs are both set at 10–20 mA with a PR interval of 150 ms. Cardiac output can often be improved by increasing or decreasing the PR interval to alter ventricular filling time. The ECG will demonstrate both pacing spikes, although the atrial spike is often difficult to detect.

   2. Current external pacemakers, such as the Medtronic 5388, can pace in a variety of modes. The DDD mode senses atrial activity, following which the ventricle contracts at a preset time interval after the atrial contraction. This mode reduces the risk of triggering atrial, junctional, and pacemaker-induced arrhythmias. Careful monitoring is necessary in the event that the pacemaker tracks the atrial

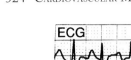

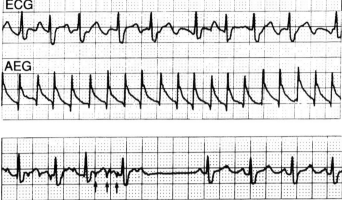

Figure 11.18 • Rapid atrial bipolar pacing of atrial flutter in sequential ECG tracings. The upper tracings confirm the rhythm as type I atrial flutter (rate 300/min) with variable AV block. In the lower tracing, rapid atrial pacing at a slightly faster rate entrains the atrium; the pacer is turned off and sinus rhythm resumes after a brief pause. The arrows indicate the atrial pacing stimulus artifact.

signal in atrial fibrillation/flutter, resulting in a very fast ventricular response. However, setting an appropriate upper rate limit on these pacemakers usually prevents this complication. Occasionally, a pacemaker-mediated tachycardia can develop from repetitive retrograde conduction from premature ventricular complexes, producing atrial deflections that are sensed and tracked.

3. If atrial activity is absent, either the DDD or DVI mode can be used. The DVI mode senses only the ventricle, so if a ventricular beat does not occur, both chambers are paced. This may lead to competitive atrial activity if the atrium is beating at a faster rate.

4. **Indications**
   a. Complete heart block
   b. Second-degree heart block to achieve 1:1 conduction
   c. First-degree heart block if 1:1 conduction cannot be achieved at a faster rate because of a long PR interval

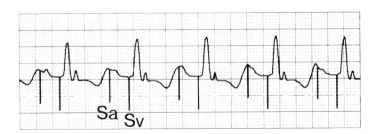

Figure 11.19 • Atrioventricular (AV) pacing at a rate of 75 bpm with a PR interval of about 220 ms. The P wave is often very poorly seen between the pacing stimulus artifacts (Sa, atrial; Sv, ventricular).

5. Additional comments

    a. Sequential AV pacing is ineffective during atrial fibrillation/flutter.

    b. AV pacing is always preferable to ventricular pacing because of the atrial contribution to ventricular filling. This is especially important in noncompliant ventricles, for which atrial contraction contributes up to 20–30% of the cardiac output. Atrial pacing alone in patients with normal conduction is superior to AV pacing by ensuring virtually simultaneous biventricular activation. Biventricular pacing provides superior hemodynamics to RA-RV pacing in patients with impaired LV function, especially with a prolonged QRS interval.[26–28]

    c. If sudden hemodynamic deterioration occurs during AV pacing, consider the possibility that atrial fibrillation has occurred with loss of atrial contraction. If AV conduction is slow, the ECG will demonstrate two pacing spikes with a QRS complex suggesting AV sequential pacing, although only ventricular pacing is occurring. This may be noted in the DDD mode with undersensing of AF or in the DVI mode in which the atrium is not sensed.

G. Ventricular pacing

    1. Ventricular pacing is achieved by connecting the two ventricular wires to the pulse generator for bipolar pacing or connecting one ventricular wire to the negative pole and an indifferent electrode (skin wire or an atrial wire) to the positive pole for unipolar pacing.

    2. The pacemaker is used in the VVI mode. The ventricular output is set at 10–20 mA in the synchronous (demand) mode. The rate selected depends on whether the pacemaker is being used for bradycardia backup, pacing at a therapeutic rate, or for overdrive pacing (Figure 11.20). Ventricular pacing in the VOO or VVI mode with undersensing of native R waves may result in the delivery of an inappropriate spike on the T wave at a time when the ventricle is vulnerable, inducing ventricular tachyarrhythmias.

    3. Indications

        a. A slow ventricular response to atrial fibrillation or flutter

        b. Failure of atrial pacing to maintain heart rate

        c. Ventricular tachycardia (overdrive pacing)

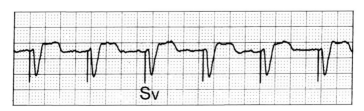

Figure 11.20 • Ventricular pacing at a rate of 80 bpm, demonstrating the wide ventricular complex. Since the patient's own mechanism is slower, the pacemaker produces all of the ventricular complexes. Sv, ventricular pacing stimulus artifact.

4. If a patient is dependent on AV or ventricular pacing, the pacing threshold must be tested. Gradually lower the mA until there is no capture. If the current necessary to generate electrical activity is rising or exceeds 10 mA, consideration should be given to placement of a transvenous pacing system (temporary or permanent).

5. If the pacemaker is in the demand mode, the sensing threshold should be checked. This determines the amplitude of the signal being measured in the chamber being sensed. Demand pacing relies on the native rhythm to determine when to pace. Undersensing results in inappropriate pacing, while oversensing inhibits pacing. To determine the sensing threshold, decrease the pacing rate to below the native rate and slowly decrease the sensitivity of the channel by increasing the sensing threshold (i.e., the amplitude below which the channel will not respond to a native signal). When an inappropriate pacing spike appears on the monitor or the "pacing" light begins to flash on the pacemaker when pacing should not be occurring, the sensing threshold will have been reached. **Ventricular tachycardia can be triggered by inappropriately sensing ventricular pacing wires.**

H. **Potential problems with epicardial pacing wire electrodes**

1. **Failure to function** may result from:

   a. Faulty connections of the connecting cord to the pacing wires or to the pulse generator

   b. A defective pacing cord

   c. Faulty pulse generator function (low battery)

   d. Electrodes located in areas of poor electrical contact and high threshold

   e. Undetected detachment of the wire electrode from the atrial or ventricular epicardium

   f. Undetected development of atrial fibrillation causing failure of atrial capture

2. **Options** to restore pacemaker function and reestablish a rhythm include:

   a. Checking all connections; changing the connecting cord

   b. Increasing the output of the pulse generator to maximal current (20 mA)

   c. Using a different wire electrode as the negative (conducting) electrode (reversing polarity)

   d. Unipolarizing the pacemaker by attaching the positive lead to a surface ECG electrode or skin pacing wire

   e. Converting to ventricular pacing if the atrial stimulus fails to produce capture

   f. Using a chronotrope (any of the catecholamines) to increase the intrinsic rate or possibly increase atrial sensitivity to the pacing stimulus

   g. Placing a transvenous pacing wire if the patient has heart block or severe bradycardia and is pacer-dependent

3. **Change in threshold.** The pacing threshold rises from the time of implantation because of edema, inflammation, thrombus, or the formation of scar tissue near the electrodes. If an advanced degree of heart block persists for more than a few days, consideration should be given to the placement of a permanent transvenous pacemaker system.

4. **Oversensing problems.** If the atrial activity of atrial fibrillation/flutter is sensed during DDD pacing, a very fast ventricular response will be noted. The upper rate

limit should be programmed (i.e., lowered) to prevent this. If this is not possible, the pacemaker should be converted to the VVI mode. Oversensing of T waves may lead to inhibition of VVI pacing.

5. **Competition with the patient's own rhythm.** When atrial or ventricular ectopy occurs during asynchronous pacing, suspect that the pacemaker is set at a rate similar to the patient's intrinsic mechanism. Turning off the pacemaker will eliminate the problem.

6. **Inadvertent triggering of VT or VF.** Use of ventricular pacing in the asynchronous mode can potentially trigger ventricular ectopy by competing with the patient's own mechanism. Appropriate sensing should always be confirmed if the pacemaker generator is left attached to the patient and is turned on. Ventricular pacing must always be accomplished in a demand mode (DVI, VVI, DDD). Pacing wires that are not being used should be electrically isolated to prevent stray AC or DC current near the wires from triggering VF. Wires should be placed in needle caps and left in accessible locations.

7. **Mediastinal bleeding** can occur if a pacing wire or the plastic carrier wire beyond the electrode (on Medtronic 6500 pacing wires) is placed close to bypass grafts, shearing them by intermittent contact during ventricular contractions. Bleeding from atrial or ventricular surfaces can occur if the wires are sewn too securely to the heart and excessive traction is used for their removal. If ventricular pacing wires are placed adjacent to small vessels on the surface of the heart, injury with bleeding may ensue during removal. Bleeding is unlikely to occur when the atrial wires are placed in a plastic sleeve producing superficial contact with the atrial wall. Pacing wires should generally be removed with the patient off heparin and before a therapeutic INR has been achieved in patients receiving warfarin. The patient should be observed carefully for signs of tamponade with frequent vital signs for several hours after removal of epicardial wires.

8. **Inability to remove the wire electrodes from the heart.** The wire can be caught beneath a tight suture on the heart or, more likely, under a sternal wire or subcutaneous suture. Constant gentle traction, allowing the heart to "beat the wire loose", should be applied. A lateral chest x-ray may reveal where the wires are entrapped. If the wires cannot be removed, they should be pulled out as far as possible, cut off at the skin level, and allowed to retract. Infection can occur in pacing wire tracts, but it is unusual.

I. Other temporary pacing modalities

1. Current monitor/defibrillators can provide transcutaneous pacing through gel pads attached to the patient's chest and back. This is most useful in emergency situations when epicardial pacing wires fail to function. This should not be relied on for more than a few hours because ventricular capture frequently deteriorates over time.

2. Placement of a 4–5 Fr temporary transvenous ventricular pacing wire is indicated if the patient is pacemaker-dependent and the threshold of the epicardial wires is high or the wires fail to function. These wires are usually placed through an introducer in the internal jugular or subclavian vein. These wires have balloon tips that assist in floating the pacing wire into the apex of the right ventricle, although fluoroscopy may occasionally be required.

3. Some Swan-Ganz catheters have extra channels that open into the right atrium and ventricle ("paceport catheters") through which pacing catheters can be placed. This

is convenient during and following minimally invasive cardiac operations. It is also helpful in emergency situations since central venous access has already been achieved. These pacing leads should not be relied upon for chronic pacing in the pacemaker-dependent patient.

4. Transesophageal atrial pacing is valuable during minimally invasive procedures and can be used in the intensive care unit on a temporary basis if AV conduction is preserved.[256]

J. Indications for permanent pacemakers

1. Although the temporary use of epicardial pacing is not uncommon after surgery, most patients with preoperative sinus rhythm will achieve a satisfactory sinus rate within a few days and can receive β-blockers for prevention of atrial fibrillation. Conduction abnormalities such as first-degree block and bundle branch blocks (BBBs) may be persistent, but are usually of little consequence and have not been shown to significantly affect clinical outcome following CABG. However, development of a LBBB does compromise the prognosis after an aortic valve replacement (AVR).[257,258]

2. Placement of a permanent pacemaker system is more likely to be indicated in elderly patients, in those with preoperative BBBs, and following valve surgery, mitral annular reconstructions, mitral valve operations performed through the superior transseptal approach,[259] reoperations, and generally more complex surgery with a longer ischemic time. It is also more common following surgery that can cause potential trauma to the conduction system (aortic valve replacement, operations for endocarditis, ablative arrhythmia surgery).[260–262] It is estimated that about 5% of patients undergoing AVR will require a pacemaker, more commonly in those with preoperative conduction problems or aortic regurgitation.[263]

3. If a permanent pacemaker is being considered, oral anticoagulation should be withheld, with use of heparin for atrial fibrillation or valve thromboprophylaxis, if indicated.

4. Postoperative pacemaker placement is indicated for the following conditions:

   a. Complete heart block

   b. Symptomatic or significant sinus node dysfunction

   c. Slow ventricular response to atrial fibrillation (usually at rates less than 50 bpm). The rate must remain slow after all potentially contributory medications are stopped. These include β-blockers, sotalol, amiodarone, CCBs, amiodarone, and digoxin.

   d. Tachycardia–bradycardia syndrome: when medications used to control a fast response to AF produce a very slow sinus mechanism upon conversion

   e. Advanced second-degree heart block with a slow ventricular response

5. The optimal timing for placement of a permanent pacemaker system has not been determined. In some patients, the indication may be a transient phenomenon, and waiting a few extra days may obviate its need. However, it often seems more cost-effective to implant a pacemaker after 3–4 days to expedite the patient's discharge from the hospital. A study from the Mayo Clinic showed that 40% of patients were not pacer-dependent at follow-up, although about 85% of patients requiring implantation for complete heart block had become pacer-dependent.[262]

XII. Cardiac Arrhythmias

The development of cardiac arrhythmias following open-heart surgery is fairly common. Supraventricular arrhythmias, especially atrial fibrillation (AF), are noted in about 25% of patients. Ventricular arrhythmias are less common and usually reflect some degree of myocardial injury. Whereas AF is usually benign, ventricular arrhythmias may warrant further evaluation and treatment because of their potentially life-threatening nature.

The mechanisms underlying the development of most arrhythmias are those of altered automaticity (impulse formation) and conductivity (impulse conduction). An understanding of these mechanisms and the electrophysiologic effects of the antiarrhythmic drugs has provided a rational basis for their use. The treatment of arrhythmias commonly noted after open-heart surgery is summarized in Table 11.14.

A. **Etiology.** Although the factors that contribute to the development of various cardiac arrhythmias may differ, there are several common causes that should be considered.

1. Cardiac problems
   a. Underlying heart disease
   b. Preexisting arrhythmias
   c. Myocardial ischemia or infarction
   d. Poor intraoperative myocardial protection
   e. Pericardial inflammation
2. Respiratory problems
   a. Endotracheal tube irritation or misplacement
   b. Hypoxia, hypercarbia, acidosis
   c. Pneumothorax
3. Electrolyte imbalance (hypo- or hyperkalemia, hypomagnesemia)
4. Intracardiac monitoring lines (PA catheter)
5. Surgical trauma (atriotomy, ventriculotomy, dissection near the conduction system)
6. Drugs (vasoactive drugs, proarrhythmic effects of antiarrhythmic medications)
7. Hypothermia
8. Fever, anxiety, pain
9. Gastric dilatation

B. **Assessment**
1. Check the arterial blood gases, ventilator function, position of the endotracheal tube, and chest x-ray for mechanical problems.
2. Check serum electrolytes (especially potassium).
3. Review a 12-lead ECG for ischemia and a more detailed examination of the arrhythmia. If the diagnosis is not clear-cut, obtain an atrial electrogram (AEG). This is frequently beneficial in differentiating among some of the more common arrhythmias by providing an amplified tracing of atrial activity.

C. **Sinus bradycardia**
1. Sinus bradycardia is present when the sinus rate is less than 60 bpm. It is frequently caused by persistent β-blockade and the use of narcotics, and may result in atrial, junctional, or ventricular escape rhythms.

Table 11.14 • Treatment of Common Arrhythmias

Arrhythmia	Treatment
1. Sinus bradycardia	Pacing: atrial or AV > ventricular Catecholamine infusion
2. Third-degree heart block	Pacing: AV > ventricular Catecholamine infusion
3. Sinus tachycardia	Address cause β-blocker
4. Premature atrial complexes	No treatment Atrial pacing (preferably dual-site) Magnesium sulfate β-blocker Amiodarone Calcium channel blockers

5. Atrial fibrillation	Cardioversion if hemodynamically compromised
	Rate control:
	    β-blocker
	    Diltiazem
	    Amiodarone
	    Digoxin
	Convert:
	    Amiodarone
	    Propafenone/ibutilide
	    Electrical cardioversion
	V-pace if slow response

6. Atrial flutter	Cardioversion if compromised Rapid atrial pacing See atrial fibrillation
7. Paroxysmal supraventricular tachycardia (PAT or AVNRT)	Atrial overdrive pacing Cardioversion Adenosine Verapamil/diltiazem β-blocker Digoxin
8. Slow junctional rhythm	Pacing: atrial > AV > ventricular Chronotropic medication

9. Nonparoxysmal AV junctional tachycardia	On digoxin: stop digoxin
	            potassium
	            phenytoin
	Not on digoxin: digoxin

10. Premature ventricular complexes	Treat hypokalemia Atrial overdrive pacing Lidocaine Amiodarone
11. Ventricular tachycardia/ fibrillation	Defibrillation Amiodarone Lidocaine

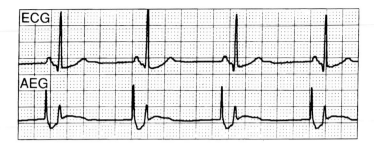

Figure 11.21 • Sinus bradycardia at a rate of 54 bpm recorded simultaneously in lead I and a unipolar AEG. The AEG demonstrates the larger atrial complex, a PR interval of 0.18 s, and the smaller ventricular complex.

2. Because sinus bradycardia reduces cardiac output, the heart rate should be maintained around 90 bpm following the termination of CPB to optimize hemodynamics. An increase in heart rate can improve myocardial contractility and cardiac output.

3. **Diagnosis**. See Figure 11.21.

4. **Treatment**

   a. Atrial pacing should be used to take advantage of the 20–30% increase in stroke volume that results from the contribution of atrial filling. This is particularly helpful in the early postoperative period when reperfusion and myocardial edema impair ventricular compliance and cause diastolic dysfunction. Atrial contraction is especially important in patients with left ventricular hypertrophy (LVH), such as those with aortic valve disease or systemic hypertension, in whom loss of atrial "kick" reduces stroke volume by 25–30%.

   b. AV pacing should be used if abnormal AV conduction is present with a slow ventricular rate (second- or third-degree AV block).

   c. If atrial pacing wires were not placed at the conclusion of surgery or if they fail to function, one of the catecholamines can be used to stimulate the sinus mechanism. Epinephrine 1–2 μg/min, dopamine 5–10 μg/kg/min, or isoproterenol 1–2 μg/min may be useful. However, these medications not only increase the heart rate, but have other hemodynamic effects as well. Atropine 0.01 mg/kg IV (usually 0.5–1 mg IV) can be used for severe symptomatic bradycardia on an emergency basis.

   d. Ventricular pacing can be used if the atrium fails to capture or there is little response to pharmacologic management. It will nearly always produce less effective hemodynamics than a supraventricular mechanism. If the ventricular pacing wires fail to function, the other pacing modes listed on pages 527–528 can be considered.

   e. If sinus bradycardia is induced by medications used to either prevent or treat atrial fibrillation, lower doses or cessation of those medications should be considered if the heart rate remains <60 bpm. Patients with known sick sinus or tachy-brady syndrome often have problems with slow heart rates postoperatively when medications are required to slow the response to AF, and may require placement of a permanent pacemaker.

D. **Conduction abnormalities and heart block**

1. Transient disturbances of conduction at the AV node are noted in about 25% of patients following coronary bypass surgery. They are more frequent when cold cardioplegic arrest is used for myocardial protection.

   a. Conduction abnormalities are more common in patients with compromised LV function, hypertension, severe coronary disease (especially involving the right coronary artery in a right-dominant system), long aortic cross-clamp periods, and extremely low myocardial temperatures. These findings suggest that ischemic or cold injury to the conduction system may be responsible for these problems. Although most will resolve within 24–48 hours, the persistence of a new left bundle branch block (LBBB) suggests the possible occurrence of a perioperative infarction.

   b. Conduction abnormalities occurring after aortic valve replacement (AVR) may be caused by hemorrhage, edema, suturing, or debridement near the AV node and His bundle. Although persistent conduction abnormalities do not appear to influence the long-term prognosis after CABG, LBBB is an ominous prognostic sign after AVR.[257,258]

   c. Exposure of the mitral valve by the biatrial transseptal approach involves division of the sinus node artery and anterior internodal pathways. Although some studies have not documented a higher incidence of postoperative rhythm disturbances, others have shown a high incidence of sinus node dysfunction with ectopic atrial rhythms, junctional rhythms, and varying degrees of heart block. About 10% of patients may require a permanent pacemaker for bradycardia or complete heart block when this approach is used.[259]

2. **Diagnosis.** See Figures 11.22–11.26.

3. **Treatment**

   a. Conduction abnormalies are best treated if both atrial and ventricular pacing wires are placed at the conclusion of surgery.

   b. **First-degree AV block** is characterized by prolongation of the PR interval to greater than 200 ms and usually does not require treatment. If the PR interval is markedly prolonged, attempts to achieve faster atrial pacing will not achieve 1:1 conduction because the AV node will remain refractory when the next impulse arrives. This will produce functional second-degree heart block. AV

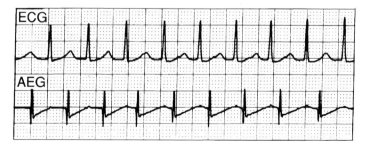

Figure 11.22 • First-degree AV block recorded simultaneously in lead II and a bipolar AEG. The PR interval is approximately 0.26s.

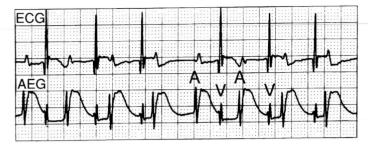

Figure 11.23 • Mobitz type I (Wenckebach) second-degree block. The unipolar AEG demonstrates a constant atrial rate of 120 bpm with progressive lengthening of the A–V (PR) intervals until the ventricular complex is dropped. In the AEG, the atrial activity is represented by the larger of the two complexes (A, atrial complex; V, ventricular complex).

pacing in the DDD or DVI mode can be used in this situation. Shortening a prolonged AV interval can significantly improve hemodynamics, especially in patients with impaired LV function.[255]

  c. **Second-degree AV** block is caused by intermittent failure of AV conduction.

   i. Mobitz type I (Wenckebach) is characterized by progressive PR interval prolongation culminating in a nonconducted P wave with no QRS complex (Figure 11.23). This usually does not require treatment unless the ventricular rate is slow. In this situation, it can be treated by AV pacing (DVI) at a slightly faster rate. If the atrial rate is too fast to overdrive, it can be treated by DDD pacing.

   ii. Mobitz type II is characterized by constant PR intervals and intermittent dropped QRS complexes. The P–P and R–R intervals remained unchanged. This reflects block in the His–Purkinje system and therefore is associated with a wide QRS complex. If the ventricular rate is too slow, AV pacing in the DVI or DDD mode should be used. If this rhythm persists, a permanent pacemaker should usually be implanted because it is likely to progress to complete heart block.

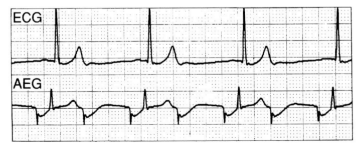

Figure 11.24 • Second-degree block. Atrial activity is present at a rate of 100/min with 2:1 block, producing a ventricular rate of 50/min.

iii. 2:1 AV block entails a constant PR interval with a dropped QRS complex every other beat (Figure 11.24). It is treated in a similar fashion to Mobitz type II block with AV pacing.

iv. High-grade second-degree heart block is evident when there is a constant PR interval but two or more consecutive atrial impulses do not conduct to the ventricle. It is treated by AV pacing and may require permanent pacing if persistent.

d. Third-degree (complete) heart block is characterized by failure of AV conduction of any atrial activity. Thus, there will usually be variable rates for the P waves and QRS complexes, which may be absent or represent escape rhythms at various rates (Figures 11.25 and 11.26). This usually requires AV pacing in either the DDD or DVI mode. If the atrial rate is acceptable, the DDD mode should be used to track the atrial rate and then provide a sequential ventricular contraction. If there is atrial inactivity or a slow atrial rate, either DDD or DVI pacing can be used. Ventricular pacing should be used if atrial fibrillation/flutter is present. Pacing is usually not necessary when there is an adequate junctional or idioventricular rate. However, AV pacing can be accomplished in the DVI mode or the DDD mode if the atrial rate is not too fast to take advantage of the atrial contribution to filling.

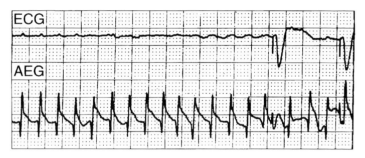

Figure 11.25 • Complete AV block. The AEG demonstrates type I atrial flutter, but the monitor ECG shows no ventricular complex until ventricular pacing is initiated.

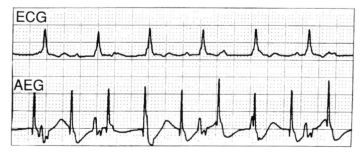

Figure 11.26 • Complete AV block with AV dissociation. The unipolar AEG demonstrates an atrial rate of 140/min (large spikes) with no clear-cut relationship to the QRS complex, which represents a junctional mechanism at a rate of 100/min.

e. If the patient is dependent on AV or ventricular pacing, the pacing threshold must be tested. Gradually lower the mA until there is no capture. If the current necessary to generate electrical activity is rising or exceeds 10 mA, consideration should be given to placement of a transvenous pacing system (temporary or permanent).

f. If advanced degrees of heart block persists, the patient's medications should be reviewed. Those that might accentuate AV block (β-blockers, amiodarone, calcium channel blockers, or digoxin) should be withheld to assess the patient's intrinsic rate and conduction. If complete heart block persists for more than a few days with the patient off these medications, a permanent pacemaker system should be placed. The most significant predictor of pacemaker dependency is its insertion for complete heart block.[262]

E. Sinus tachycardia

1. Sinus tachycardia is present when the sinus rate exceeds 100 bpm. It generally occurs at rates less than 130. A faster and regular ventricular rate suggests atrial flutter with 2:1 block or paroxysmal supraventricular (atrial or junctional) tachycardia.

2. Fast heart rates are detrimental to myocardial metabolism. They can exacerbate myocardial ischemia by increasing oxygen demand and decreasing the time for diastolic coronary perfusion. They also reduce the time for ventricular filling and can reduce stroke volume, especially in patients with LVH and diastolic dysfunction.

3. **Etiology**

   a. Benign hyperdynamic reflex response related to sympathetic overactivity:
   - Pain, anxiety, fever
   - Adrenergic rebound (patient on β-blockers preoperatively)
   - Drugs (catecholamines, pancuronium)
   - Gastric dilatation
   - Anemia
   - Hypermetabolic states (sepsis)

   b. Compensatory response to myocardial injury or impaired cardiorespiratory status:
   - Hypoxia, hypercarbia, acidosis
   - Hypovolemia or low stroke volumes noted with small, stiff left ventricles with LVH and diastolic dysfunction
   - Myocardial ischemia or infarction
   - Cardiac tamponade
   - Tension pneumothorax

   c. Once a patient is transferred from the ICU and is clinically stable, sinus tachycardia is usually caused by pain, anemia, hypovolemia, or respiratory issues. Some patients have higher sympathetic activity and a higher baseline heart rate with no other identifiable cause.

4. **Diagnosis**. See Figure 11.27.

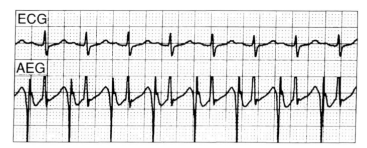

Figure 11.27 • Sinus tachycardia at a rate of 130 bpm on simultaneous recordings of monitor lead II and a unipolar AEG. Note the larger atrial and smaller ventricular complex in the unipolar AEG tracing, which demonstrates the 1:1 AV conduction.

5. **Treatment**

   a. Correction of the underlying cause

   b. Sedation and analgesia in the ICU setting; adequate analgesia subsequently on the postoperative floor

   c. β-blockers can be used if the heart is hyperdynamic with an excellent cardiac output. They must be used cautiously, however, when cardiac function is marginal. Tachycardia is a compensatory mechanism to maintain cardiac output when the stroke volume is low, and attempts to slow the heart rate may prove detrimental. Even when the cardiac output is satisfactory, β-blockers often lower the blood pressure significantly more than they reduce the heart rate.

      i. Esmolol 0.25–0.5 mg/kg IV over 1 minute followed by a continuous infusion of 50–200 μg/kg/min. A trial bolus of 0.125 mg/kg is recommended to determine whether the patient can tolerate esmolol.

      ii. Metoprolol 5 mg IV increments every 5 minutes for three doses

      iii. Increasing doses of oral metoprolol (25–100 mg bid) are usually used to control a postoperative sinus tachycardia on the floor. Some patients are refractory to its effects and respond better to atenolol (25–100 mg qd).

   d. Calcium channel blockers have mild negative chronotropic effects on the SA node, but they do not play a major role in the treatment of sinus tachycardia.

   e. **Note:** Both β-blockers and calcium channel blockers individually are safe to administer intravenously, but their simultaneous use should only be considered if functional pacing wires are present.

F. **Premature atrial complexes (PACs)**

   1. PACs are premature beats arising in the atrium that generally have a different configuration than the normal P wave and produce a PR interval that exceeds 120 ms. Although benign, they often herald the development of atrial fibrillation or flutter, and this occurrence can be very difficult to prevent.

   2. Magnesium sulfate may be beneficial in reducing the incidence of PACs in the immediate postoperative period. The dose is 2 g in 100 mL solution.

   3. **Diagnosis**. See Figure 11.28.

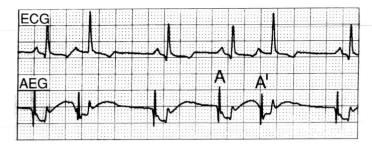

Figure 11.28 • Premature atrial complexes (PACs) in monitor lead II and a unipolar AEG. Note the slightly different morphology of the normal (A) and premature (A') atrial complexes and the slightly shorter PR interval following the PACs that indicates a focus different from the sinus node. The PR interval exceeds 120 ms, thus differentiating these beats from premature junctional complexes.

4. Treatment

    a. PACs generally do not need to be treated, but because they frequently precede the development of atrial fibrillation, medications that can alter atrial automaticity and conduction or slow the ventricular response to AF can be considered. These include β-blockers, calcium channel blockers, and amiodarone.

    b. Digoxin is useful in decreasing the frequency of PACs and slows conduction through the AV node if AF does develop. However, by increasing conduction velocity in the atrium, digoxin can theoretically increase the risk of developing AF if PACs are present.

    c. Temporary right atrial pacing at a faster rate ("overdrive pacing") may suppress PACs, but it may also trigger atrial arrhythmias and induce AF. This may occur even in the AAI mode when there is difficulty sensing atrial activity leading to inappropriate pacing. This problem generally does not occur with permanent dual-chamber pacemakers. If PACs occur during atrial pacing, one should suspect competition with the patient's own rhythm. Dual-site atrial pacing may suppress PACs and also prevent AF.

G. Atrial fibrillation or flutter

    1. Atrial fibrillation (atrial rate >380) and atrial flutter (atrial rate generally <380) are the most common arrhythmias noted after open-heart surgery. Despite various prophylactic measures to decrease their incidence, they still occur in about 25–30% of patients. There is probably a reversible trigger that causes AF in postoperative patients in whom there is an underlying substrate for its development, such as increased dispersion of atrial refractoriness with nonuniform atrial conduction. Age-related changes in the atrial myocardium are also contributory, since AF is more likely to occur in older patients. Inflammation may also play a major role.[264]

    2. Among the factors that increase the risk of AF are: older age, a history of atrial arrhythmias, obesity, COPD, LVH, right coronary artery disease, valve surgery, increased preoperative BNP levels, and increased P-wave duration. Operative considerations include redo surgery, inadequate myocardial protection, prolonged cross-clamp times, atrial trauma, and use of lower systemic temperatures.[265,266] The efficacy of off-pump coronary surgery in reducing the incidence of AF is controversial.[267,268] Postoperative pericardial effusions may also increase the risk of AF.[269]

3. Atrial fibrillation or flutter can compromise cardiac hemodynamics and also increase the risk of systemic thromboembolism and stroke from left atrial thrombus. AF tends to prolong hospital length of stay and increase hospital costs.

4. These arrhythmias occur most commonly on the second and third postoperative day. By that time, myocardial function has recovered to baseline and few adverse hemodynamic effects are noted. However, when atrial tachyarrhythmias occur during the first 24 hours, when the patient is hemodynamically unstable, or in patients with noncompliant hypertrophied ventricles, a rapid ventricular response can precipitate ischemia and lower cardiac output by eliminating the atrial contribution to ventricular filling.

5. After the initial 24 hours, AF is frequently an incidental finding on the ECG monitor. Symptoms such as palpitations, nausea, fatigue, or lightheadedness may be noted, especially in patients with LVH or poor ventricular function.

6. **Etiology**
   a. Enhanced sympathetic activity ("hyperadrenergic state") or adrenergic rebound in patients taking β-blockers preoperatively
   b. Atrial ischemia from poor myocardial preservation during aortic cross-clamping
   c. Atrial distention from fluid shifts
   d. Surgical trauma or inflammation (pericarditis)
   e. Metabolic derangements (hypoxia, hypokalemia, hypomagnesemia)

7. **Diagnosis**. See Figures 11.29 and 11.30.

8. **Prevention.**[270–273] Prophylactic therapy can reduce the risk of AF by approximately 50%, but cannot eliminate its occurrence.
   a. Initiation of low-dose **β-blockers** starting within 12–24 hours of surgery is the most effective pharmacologic intervention to lower the incidence of AF. Metoprolol 25–50 mg bid or atenolol 25 mg qd is most commonly used. β-blockers are beneficial whether or not the patient was taking them prior to surgery. One meta-analysis found a 65% reduction in the incidence of AF.[272] Several randomized trials have demonstrated the superiority of carvedilol, an α- and β-blocker commonly used in patients with depressed LV function, over metoprolol in reducing the incidence of AF.[274,275] This is being further evaluated in the COMPACT trial which was ongoing in 2010.[276]

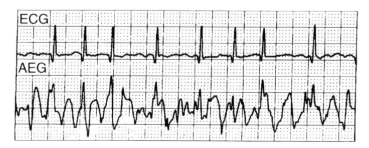

Figure 11.29 • Atrial fibrillation with a ventricular response of 130 bpm. The AEG demonstrates the chaotic atrial activity that is characteristic of atrial fibrillation.

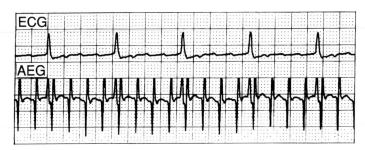

Figure 11.30 • Atrial flutter with 4:1 AV block. The unipolar AEG demonstrates an atrial rate of about 300 bpm with a ventricular response of about 75 bpm.

b. **Amiodarone** is a class III antiarrhythmic with some class I, II, and IV properties that is effective in reducing the incidence of AF, either when given alone or in conjunction with β-blockers. It is unclear if there is additive benefit to using both drugs. In several meta-analyses, it reduced the incidence of AF by about 45–50%.[271,272,277]

   i. The timing (pre-, intra-, or postoperative), route (IV vs. PO), and dosage of amiodarone which provides the best prophylaxis are unknown because different protocols have been used in virtually every study. Optimal benefit requires adequate dosing to achieve electrophysiologic effects at the time of highest risk for AF. Thus, regimens of preoperative oral loading must be long enough or use high enough doses to be effective since it takes several days to achieve effect. In the large PAPABEAR trial, a 50% reduction in postoperative AF was noted using a 6-day preoperative load of 10 mg/kg daily and a 13-day total course.[278] Other recommended dosing regimens for patients undergoing elective surgery include:[279]

   • 200 mg tid × 5 days, then 400 mg bid × 4–6 days postoperatively if surgery is scheduled in more than 5 days

   • 400 mg qid × 1 day, then 600 mg bid on day of surgery, then 400 mg bid × 4–6 days after surgery (if surgery scheduled within 1–5 days)

   ii. Logistic considerations in patients requiring more urgent surgery suggest that an alternative approach should be used that loads amiodarone intravenously during surgery and continues it for several days postoperatively. This can achieve effect within a few hours. An acceptable dosing regimen is a 150 mg IV load over 15 minutes, followed by a 60 mg/h infusion × 8 hours, then 30 mg/h × 16 hours with conversion to oral dosing starting at 400 mg bid. The efficacy of this approach is inferential, but there is at least one study of patients undergoing valve surgery, who could be considered at higher risk for the development of AF, which did not confirm any benefit to a perioperative 48-hour IV infusion of amiodarone in reducing the incidence of AF.[280]

   iii. Whether amiodarone should be used for all patients or only in those at higher risk has yet to be defined. Risk factors include age >60, history of AF, LV dysfunction, valvular heart disease or valve surgery, and a baseline heart rate >100 bpm.[279] Amiodarone may be particularly beneficial in patients with COPD, in whom the incidence and morbidity of AF are greater.[281] However, the potential for acute amiodarone toxicity that can produce hypoxemia must be kept in mind.[282]

iv. The benefits of continuing amiodarone after hospital discharge are uncertain. Amiodarone can probably be stopped at the time of discharge if effective for prophylaxis since it will have persistent electrophysiologic effects for weeks. If the patient does develop intermittent AF and converts, it is usually continued for about 1 month, with the dosage being weaned down to 200 mg qd. Some have argued that 1 week of therapy with any drug is adequate if the patient is discharged home in sinus rhythm.[283]

c. **Dronedarone** has similar electrophysiologic properties to amiodarone, but has a different chemical structure that avoids the risk of thyroid toxicity. It is effective in maintaining sinus rhythm after conversion from AF. It is given in a dose of 400 mg PO bid without a loading dose and has a much shorter half-life than amiodarone (1-2 days vs. nearly 2 months). Although there were no trials as of late-2010 that evaluated the use of dronedarone for the prophylaxis or treatment of AF in cardiac surgery patients, it is anticipated that studies will demonstrate the same clinical benefits as amiodarone.[284]

d. **Sotalol** is a β-blocker with class III antiarrhythmic properties that is arguably more effective than standard β-blockers and as effective as amiodarone in preventing supraventricular tachyarrhythmias when used at a dose of 80 mg bid.[285] However, it is a negative inotrope and is not tolerated in about 20% of patients, in whom hypotension, bradycardia, or AV block may develop. Sotalol may also cause QT prolongation and polymorphic ventricular arrhythmias, including torsades de pointes. It is excreted by the kidneys and should be avoided in patients with renal dysfunction. It is available in IV form (75 mg IV = 80 mg oral) if the patient cannot take the oral dose.

e. **Magnesium sulfate** (2 g in 100 mL) is often effective in decreasing the occurrence and number of episodes of postoperative AF. It appears to be most effective when given with a β-blocker (studies have evaluated combinations with sotalol and bisoprolol), and when the serum magnesium level is low.[286–289] Since its administration is benign and of potential benefit, it is worthwhile administering to all patients during surgery and on the first postoperative day in addition to β-blockers.

f. Although atrial pacing may increase atrial ectopy and does not reduce the incidence of AF, **dual-site atrial pacing** has been shown in numerous studies to reduce the incidence of AF, especially when given with β-blockers. It is theorized that intra-atrial conduction delays may contribute to AF. Dual-site pacing alters the atrial activation sequence and may achieve more uniform electrical activation of the atria. It may also overdrive-suppress PACs, eliminate compensatory pauses after PACs, and reduce the dispersion of refractoriness that may contribute to AF.[290–292]

g. Studies have identified other medications and substances which might reduce the incidence of AF:

  i. Dofetilide is effective in reducing the incidence of AF (by 50% in one study), but other medications are preferable due to its cost and risk of causing QT prolongation.[293] **Propafenone** 300 mg PO bid is also effective and was found comparable to atenolol in one study.[294] Other antiarrrhythmic drugs, including digoxin, verapamil, and diltiazem, have not been uniformly efficacious in preventing AF.

  ii. Steroids may reduce inflammation and the risk of AF, but commonly cause hyperglycemia and may increase the risk of infection. Study protocols include use of hydrocortisone 100 mg prior to surgery followed by 100 mg q8h × 3 days[295] or methylprednisolone 1 g before surgery with additional doses of dexamethasone 4 mg q6h × 24 hours[296]

 iii. Statins at high dose (atorvastatin 40 mg)[297,298]

 iv. ACE inhibitors[266]

  v. Ascorbic acid (vitamin C) given with β-blockers (2 g before surgery and 1 g daily for 5 days)[299]

 vi. N-3 fatty acids (fish oils) 2 g/day started preoperatively; this is not recommended because of the increased risk of perioperative bleeding from the antiplatelet effect.[300]

 vii. Triiodothyronine 0.8 µg/kg (about 50–80 µg) at the time of removal of the cross-clamp with a 6-hour infusion of 0.113 µg/kg/h (8–11 µg/h) has been shown to halve the rate of AF, but it is very expensive and rarely used.[102]

9. **Management** of the unstable patient developing atrial fibrillation initially involves cardioversion, whereas the strategy for the stable patient involves rate control, anticoagulation if AF persists, and attempts to achieve conversion to sinus rhythm (Table 11.15 and Figure 11.31). Presumably based on the placebo arm of trials, it is estimated that spontaneous conversion to sinus rhythm will occur in about 50% of patients. Nonetheless, following cardiac surgery, it is recommended that pharmacologic intervention be used to achieve conversion if AF persists for more than 24 hours to avoid the requirement for anticoagulation. Once the early hyperadrenergic effects of surgery have dissipated, most patients who develop AF will convert to sinus rhythm spontaneously or with medications, and invariably will remain in sinus rhythm subsequently without the long-term use of medications. This approach is in contradistinction to that often used for patients not undergoing cardiac surgery, in whom a rate-controlled strategy has similar survival results but potentially fewer adverse effects than pharmacologic attempts to achieve rhythm control.[301] However, even in these nonsurgical studies, patients in AF had a worse functional outcome.[302]

 a. Electric **cardioversion** with 50–100 joules can be used in a variety of circumstances.

  i. Cardioversion should always be considered first if there is evidence of significant hemodynamic compromise. This is more common in the early postoperative period when a very rapid ventricular response may be present and myocardial function is moderately depressed from surgery. It is also more likely to have adverse effects in patients with significant LVH.

  ii. If a patient fails to convert to normal sinus rhythm with medications within 48 hours, one strategy is to perform cardioversion to avoid the necessity for

Table 11.15 • *Management Protocols for Atrial Fibrillation/Flutter*

1. Prophylaxis

    a. Magnesium sulfate 2 g IV after CPB and on first postoperative morning

    b. β-blocker

       • Metoprolol 25–50 mg PO (per NG tube) bid starting 8 hours after surgery

       • Carvedilol 3.125–12.5 mg PO bid

    c. Alternatives

       • Amiodarone started either PO preoperatively or IV the day of surgery

       • Sotalol 80 mg bid

       • Dual-site atrial pacing

2. Treatment

    a. Cardioversion with 50–100 joules if unstable

    b. Rapid atrial pace if atrial flutter

    c. Increase prophylactic β-blocker dose if hemodynamically stable (heart rate < 100)

    d. Rate control if heart rate >100

       • IV **diltiazem** 0.25 mg/kg IV over 2 minutes, followed 15 minutes later by 0.35 mg/kg over 2 minutes, followed by a continuous infusion of 10–15 mg/h, if necessary

       • IV **metoprolol** 5 mg IV q5 min × 3 doses

    e. Conversion to sinus rhythm and anticoagulation

       • Magnesium sulfate 2 g IV

       • Option #1: **amiodarone** 150 mg over 30 minutes, followed by an infusion of 1 mg/min × 6 h, then 0.5 mg/min × 12 h, then 400 mg orally bid

          ⟶ If successful, continue amiodarone for 1–4 weeks

          ⟶ If unsuccessful, consider cardioversion at 36–48 hours without heparin or subsequently on heparin; consider TEE to rule out left atrial thrombus

          ⟶ If unsuccessful, continue anticoagulation and β-blockers, but stop amiodarone

       • Option #2: heparin/warfarin after 48 hours; await spontaneous conversion on β-blockers and discharge home in either SR or AF

       • Option #3: Consider alternative pharmacologic management with or without cardioversion if unsuccessful; anticoagulation after 48 hours

          ∗ **Sotalol** 80 mg q4h × 4 doses, then 80 mg bid and stop other β-blockers

          ∗ **Propafenone** 1 mg/kg IV over 2 minutes, followed 10 minutes later by another 1 mg/kg dose; if IV not available, give one oral dose of 600 mg

          ∗ **Ibutilide** 1 mg infusion over 10 minutes (0.01 mg/kg if <60 kg) with a second infusion 10 minutes later

          ∗ **Dofetilide** 500 µg PO bid

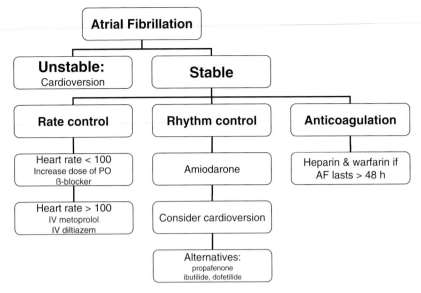

Figure 11.31 • Simplified algorithm for management of atrial fibrillation.

anticoagulation.[303] If AF has been present or recurrent for more than 48 hours and the patient has not been anticoagulated, a preliminary TEE must be performed to rule out left atrial thrombus before performing cardioversion.[304,305] The decision to continue warfarin for 1 month after delayed cardioversion must be considered, because de novo thrombus may form due to mechanical atrial inactivity after electrical cardioversion.[306]

 iii. If the patient cannot be converted pharmacologically or electrically, warfarin should be given for 3 weeks and then elective cardioversion attempted. If successful, warfarin is continued for an additional 4 weeks.

 b. **Rapid atrial overdrive pacing** should be attempted to convert atrial flutter (see Figure 11.18 and page 523 for technique of rapid atrial pacing). It is usually successful in converting only type I flutter (atrial rate less than 350/min). Several medications, such as propafenone and ibutilide, increase the efficacy of rapid atrial pacing by prolonging the atrial flutter cycle length.[307,308]

 c. **Rate control** can be achieved most readily with one of the rapid-acting intravenous medications and more chronically by use of digoxin. Once the rate has been controlled, the IV medications can be converted to oral ones. One study showed that 80% of patients receiving only "rate control" drugs, such as β-blockers and CCBs, converted to sinus rhythm within 24 hours, suggesting it was a spontaneous conversion, rather than the effects of the medications.[309]

  i. **β-blockers** are very effective in achieving rate control and have the advantage of converting about 50% of patients to sinus rhythm (whether considered spontaneous or not). If an oral β-blocker has already been given, it can be supplemented by an IV dose if the ventricular response is fast. If the patient has a relatively slow heart rate (whether already receiving a β-blocker or not) and then develops AF, diltiazem is a better selection to avoid the bradycardia that may occur after conversion.

- **Metoprolol** is the preferred β-blocker in that it can be given in the ICU or on the postoperative floor. It is a negative inotrope, so it must be used cautiously in patients with significantly compromised LV function or hypotension. For fairly rapid rates (>100 bpm), it is given in 5 mg IV increments q5 min up to a total dose of 15 mg. The onset of action is 2–3 minutes with a peak effect noted at 20 minutes. The duration of action is approximately 5 hours. Slower rates (<100 bpm) can be managed with increasing doses of oral metoprolol.[273]

- **Esmolol** can be used in the operating room or ICU setting with arterial line monitoring, but it is a very dangerous drug due to its tendency to produce hypotension. It has a rapid onset of action of 2 minutes with rapid reversal of effect in 10–20 minutes. Thus, it may be safer to use than longer-acting drugs in the immediate perioperative period in case adverse effects develop, such as bronchospasm, conduction disturbances, excessive bradycardia, or LV dysfunction. The dose is 0.125–0.5 mg/kg IV over 1 minute, followed by an infusion of 50–200 μg/kg/min.

ii. **Diltiazem** is an excellent alternative for patients with rapid AF and mildly to moderately compromised LV function in that it is a fairly weak negative inotrope. It must be used cautiously in hypotensive patients because of its mild vasodilatory effects, but blood pressure commonly improves with rate control. Concomitant use of an α-agent may be helpful if the blood pressure remains marginal. Diltiazem is also preferable in patients with a slow sinus mechanism prior to the development of AF. It is very effective in slowing the ventricular response but less effective in converting the patient to sinus rhythm. It is more effective in slowing the ventricular response to AF than atrial flutter.

- **Dosage.** It is given in a dose of 0.25 mg/kg IV over 2 minutes, followed 15 minutes later by 0.35 mg/kg over 2 minutes, followed by a continuous infusion of 10–15 mg/h, if necessary. Heart rate response is noted in about 3 minutes with a peak effect within 7 minutes. The reduction in heart rate lasts 1–3 hours after a bolus dose. The median duration of action is 7 hours after a 24-hour continuous infusion.

- **Note:** Extreme caution must be used when administering any IV calcium channel blocker concomitantly with an IV β-blocker because of the risk of inducing complete AV block. Availability of functional pacing wires is essential.

iii. **Amiodarone** is effective in reducing the ventricular response to AF due to its multiple mechanisms of action (β-blockade, class III effects), but the rapidity and degree of slowing is less than with the β-blockers and CCBs. It is especially useful in the patient with borderline hemodynamics and more compromised LV function because it has no negative inotropic effects. Thus, it can be recommended as first-line therapy if the ventricular response is not rapid or β-blockers and CCBs are contraindicated; otherwise, it should be added after rate control has been achieved, primarily in an attempt to achieve conversion to sinus rhythm.[273]

iv. **Digoxin** is ineffective in controlling heart rate in the acute postoperative setting which is associated with increased sympathetic tone. It may be combined with other medications to obtain better chronic rate control if AF persists.

- The initial dose is 0.5 mg IV, followed by 0.25 mg IV q4–6h × 3 doses (up to a total dose of 1.25 mg within 24 hours – less in elderly patients), and then 0.125–0.25 mg qd. The serum potassium level should be >4.0 mEqL when digoxin is given because hypokalemia can precipitate digoxin-toxic rhythms.
- The onset of action of IV digoxin is about 30 minutes with a peak effect in 2–3 hours.

d. **Anticoagulation.** Heparinization should be considered for patients with recurrent or persistent atrial fibrillation to minimize the risk of stroke from embolization of left atrial thrombus.[310] In one study, it was noted that 14% of patients developed thrombus and 39% had spontaneous echo contrast in the left atrium within 3 days of the development of AF.[311]

i. Due to lack of adequate data, guidelines are ambivalent on the timing of initiation of heparin and whether it is even necessary. The 2006 ACC/AHA guidelines state that anticoagulation with heparin or oral anticoagulation is appropriate when AF persists for over 48 hours,[267] but the 2008 ACCP guidelines only recommend starting warfarin after 48 hours of AF.[312] Use of warfarin alone will not provide adequate thromboprophylaxis against stroke for several days. Therefore heparin can be recommended after 48 hours of AF, but its use must always be tempered by the potential for bleeding. Thus, an aggressive anticoagulant strategy for AF that develops immediately after surgery must be individualized.

ii. A strategy of early cardioversion may avert the need for anticoagulation. However, anticoagulation is essential before later cardioversion to reduce the risk of thromboembolism. Alternatively, a TEE can be performed to rule out left atrial appendage thrombus prior to attempting cardioversion.

iii. If the patient remains in AF and is to be discharged on warfarin, bridging with low-molecular-weight heparin should be considered in patients at high risk (older patients, low ejection fraction, any valve patient).

e. **Conversion to sinus rhythm.** Conversion to sinus rhythm is fairly common with the use of β-blockers, amiodarone, or calcium channel blockers. As noted above, one study found that 80% of patients converted to normal sinus rhythm within 24 hours without use of class I or III medications, and this was more likely in patients receiving β-blockers postoperatively, especially in the absence of severe LV dysfunction and diabetes.[309] The conversion rate noted in this study seems quite high when compared with most studies of cardiac surgery patients, which have shown conversion rates of 50–60% with most medications. If a patient cannot be converted pharmacologically, a strategy of anticoagulation, rate control, and subsequent cardioversion is a viable and cost-effective alternative strategy.

i. **Magnesium sulfate** 2 gm IV over 15 minutes is a benign and relatively effective means of converting patients back to sinus rhythm, with a conversion rate of 60% within 4 hours in one study.[313]

ii. **β-blockers**, in addition to being used for prophylaxis, are effective for both rate control and conversion, more so than diltiazem.[314] The dosage of the prophylactic dose can be increased if the patient's blood pressure and heart rate are acceptable. Substitution of sotalol (80 mg bid) for the selective β-blockers may be considered, because it is slightly more successful in producing conversion. Many patients cannot tolerate sotalol because of bradycardia or hypotension.

iii. **Amiodarone** is probably the most effective drug for conversion of AF and produces adequate rate control, although not as promptly or effectively as β-blockers. Because it lacks other significant cardiac effects, it has an excellent safety profile. Hypotension is usually seen only with rapid IV infusion, and QTc prolongation, although common, is usually not accompanied by a proarrhythmic effect. (Note that the QT interval adjusted for heart rate (QTc) is normally <450−470 ms). For rapid effect, it is given with the standard IV load (150 mg IV load over 15−30 minutes, followed by a 60 mg/h infusion × 6 hours, then 30 mg/h × 18 hours), followed by an oral taper (400 mg bid for 1 week, 400 mg qd × 1 week, 200 mg qd × 2 weeks). If AF develops despite the use of prophylactic amiodarone, an additional 150 mg bolus given over 30 minutes can be used. Alternatively, it may be given to treat AF as an oral load of 400 mg tid × 1 week, followed by the same wean.

iv. The type IC and other type III antiarrhythmics have been successful in converting 50−70% of patients with recent-onset AF back to sinus rhythm. They generally cause less hypotension than amiodarone and produce more rapid conversion.

- **Propafenone** (class IC) is effective in slowing the ventricular response and in rapidly converting patients to sinus rhythm within a few hours. Studies have demonstrated similar efficacy of conversion with intravenous and oral dosing, although conversion takes longer with oral dosing.[315] The IV dose is 1−2 mg/kg IV over 15 minutes, followed 10 minutes later by another 1 mg/kg dose. The oral dose is 600 mg given once. IV propafenone is not available in the USA.

- **Ibutilide** (class III) is an effective medication for conversion of AF and especially atrial flutter.[316] It is given as a 1 mg infusion over 10 minutes (0.01 mg/kg if <60 kg) with a second infusion 10 minutes later, if necessary. Most patients will convert within 1 hour. Because of the proarrhythmic risk (VT and torsades), careful monitoring is required, and the infusion should be stopped as soon as the arrhythmia has terminated, VT occurs, or there is marked prolongation of the QT interval. Ibutilide is particularly useful in patients with poor ventricular function or chronic lung disease. In comparative studies, ibutilide was found to be just as effective as amiodarone in converting atrial fibrillation/flutter to sinus rhythm.[317]

- **Dofetilide** (class III) has no negative inotropic effects and is beneficial when there are contraindications to class I drugs (LV dysfunction) or β-blockers (bradycardia, COPD). It is usually given in a dose of 500 μg PO bid. One study using IV dofetilide (up to 8 μg/kg over 15 minutes) found that it was more successful in converting atrial flutter (70%) than fibrillation (30%) within 1 hour.[318] It also causes QT prolongation and is proarrhythmic. The dosage must be adjusted by creatinine clearance and the baseline QTc. One study showed that the addition of magnesium did not affect dofetilide conversion of AF, but did double the efficacy of electrical cardioversion.[319]

   v. **Vernakalant** is an atrial-selective potassium- and sodium-channel blocking agent which has been shown to convert about 50% of patients with new-onset postoperative AF to sinus rhythm at a median time of just over 10 minutes. The dosage is 3 mg/kg infused over 10 minutes with a subsequent 2 mg/kg infusion over 10 minutes if AF is still present after 15 minutes. The drug received approval by the European Union in September 2010, but was still awaiting FDA approval in late-2010.[320]

   vi. **Low-energy internal cardioversion** using epicardial defibrillation wires sewn to the left and right atria at the time of surgery is 90% successful in restoring sinus rhythm.[321]

H. **Other supraventricular tachycardias (SVTs)**

   1. This designation refers to a tachycardia of sudden onset that arises either in the atrium (paroxysmal atrial tachycardia, PAT) or in the AV nodal region (AV nodal reentrant tachycardia, AVNRT), or uses the AV node as an integral part of the reentrant circuit (AV reentrant tachycardia, AVRT). These rhythms usually occur at a rate of 150–250/min and are uncommon after cardiac surgery. PAT with AV block may be associated with ischemic heart disease and commonly results from digoxin toxicity. As with any arrhythmia causing a rapid ventricular response, immediate treatment is indicated because of potential adverse effects on myocardial metabolism and function.

   2. **Diagnosis.** Differentiation among sinus tachycardia, PAT, AVNRT, AVRT, and atrial flutter with 2:1 block may require examination of an AEG (Figure 11.32). Carotid sinus massage is often recommended as a diagnostic modality to differentiate among various arrhythmias by slowing the ventricular response to atrial tachyarrhythmias. However, it must be used cautiously in patients with coronary artery disease, not only because it may precipitate asystole, but because it may produce an embolic stroke in patients with coexistent carotid artery disease.

   3. **Treatment**

   a. Rapid atrial overdrive pacing may capture the atrium and cause reversion to sinus rhythm.

   b. Cardioversion should be considered if there is evidence of hemodynamic compromise.

   c. Vagal stimulation will often break a reentrant rhythm involving the AV node. Carotid sinus massage must be used cautiously as noted above.

   d. Adenosine produces transient high-grade AV block and is successful in terminating SVT caused by AVNRT.[322] It is given as a 6 mg rapid IV injection via a central line followed by a saline flush. A repeat dose of 12 mg may be given 2 minutes later. The half-life of adenosine is only 10 seconds. Adenosine can help distinguish AVRT and AVNRT, in which it terminates the circuit, from atrial flutter or fibrillation, in which it transiently slows AV conduction and the ventricular rate.

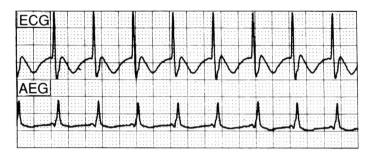

Figure 11.32 • AV junctional tachycardia at a rate of about 140 bpm recorded in simultaneous monitor and bipolar AEGs. Note the nearly simultaneous occurrence of retrograde atrial activation in the AEG and the antegrade ventricular activation in the monitor lead.

    e. Diltiazem given in standard doses (0.25 mg/kg IV over 2 minutes, followed 15 minutes later by 0.35 mg/kg, if necessary) is effective in converting AVNRT to sinus rhythm in about 90% of patients.[323]

    f. Additional measures that can be used for AVNRT if the above fail include:

      i. Digoxin 0.5 mg IV in a patient not previously on digoxin

      ii. Metoprolol 5 mg q5 min to a total dose of 15 mg

      iii. Edrophonium 5 mg slow IV push, followed by a 10 mg dose

    g. PAT with block is usually associated with digoxin toxicity and treatment should be provided accordingly:

      i. Digoxin should be withheld and a digoxin level obtained

      ii. Administration of potassium chloride (KCl)

      iii. Digibind (digoxin immune Fab [ovine]) starting at a dose of 400 mg (10 vials) over 30 minutes if severe digoxin toxicity

      iv. Phenytoin (Dilantin) 250 mg IV over 5 minutes

I. AV junctional rhythm and nonparoxysmal AV junctional tachycardia

    1. An AV junctional rhythm occurs when junctional tissue has a faster intrinsic rate than the sinus node. This generally occurs at a rate less than 60 bpm and is termed a junctional escape rhythm.

    2. Nonparoxysmal AV junctional tachycardia occurs at a rate of 70–130/min and usually results from enhanced automacity in the bundle of His. In the postoperative patient, this rhythm may reflect digitalis toxicity, pericarditis, or an inferior infarction. Its presence may be suggested by a regularized ventricular rate in a patient with underlying atrial fibrillation and can be confirmed with an atrial electrogram.

    3. As with any non-atrial rhythm, cardiac output is diminished by lack of synchronous atrial and ventricular contractions.

    4. Diagnosis. See Figures 11.32 and 11.33. The focus may be localized by the relationship of the P wave to the QRS on a surface ECG (short PR interval if high-nodal, invisible P wave if mid-nodal, and P wave following the QRS if low-nodal). The P-QRS relationship is more evident on an atrial electrogram.

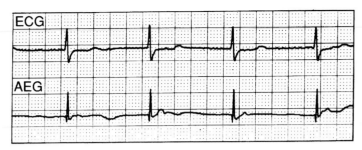

Figure 11.33 • Slow junctional rhythm at a rate of 54 bpm. Note the simultaneous occurrence of atrial and ventricular activation.

5. **Treatment**
   a. Slow junctional rhythm (junctional escape rhythm)
      i. Atrial pacing if AV conduction is normal.
      ii. AV pacing if AV conduction is depressed.
      iii. Use of a vasoactive drug with chronotropic β_1 action to stimulate the sinus mechanism; any drug the patient is receiving that might slow the sinus mechanism should be stopped.
   b. Nonparoxysmal junctional tachycardia
      i. If the patient is receiving digoxin, it should be stopped. Severe digoxin toxicity may be treated with digibind. Use of potassium, lidocaine, phenytoin, or a β-blocker may be helpful.
      ii. Overdrive pacing at a faster rate may establish AV synchrony.
      iii. If the patient is not on digoxin, it should be started. If the rhythm is not well tolerated, use of a β-blocker or calcium channel blocker can be considered to slow the junctional focus, with use of atrial or AV pacing to establish AV synchrony.

J. **Premature ventricular complexes (PVCs)**
   1. PVCs are fairly uncommon when complete revascularization has been accomplished with good myocardial protection. When they develop de novo, they may reflect transient perioperative phenomena, such as augmented sympathetic tone or increased levels of catecholamines (endogenous or exogenous), irritation from a Swan-Ganz catheter or endotracheal tube, abnormal acid–base status, hypoxemia, etc. Thus, most PVCs are self-limited, benign, and not predictive of more serious or life-threatening arrhythmias. Ventricular ectopy is also fairly common preoperatively in the postinfarction patient and may persist after surgery, although ischemia-induced ectopy may be improved.
   2. Nonetheless, PVCs developing de novo may also reflect poor intraoperative myocardial protection or myocardial ischemia or infarction, and may herald malignant ventricular arrhythmias. Therefore, some surgical groups believe that even occasional PVCs should never be ignored in the early postoperative period. During the first 24 hours after surgery, when a multitude of cardiac and noncardiac precipitating factors may be present, it is of potential benefit and little risk to treat any ventricular

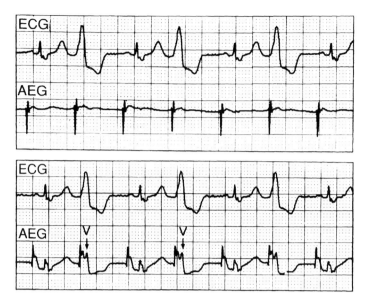

Figure 11.34 • Premature ventricular complexes (ventricular bigeminy) recorded simultaneously from monitor lead II and bipolar (upper) and unipolar (lower) AEGs. Note the wide QRS complex of unifocal morphology representing the PVC on the ECG. The bipolar AEG shows that the interval between atrial complexes is maintained despite the PVCs. The unipolar tracing shows that the PVC directly follows the sinus beat but leaves the ventricle refractory to the following beat, producing a full compensatory pause. V, premature ventricular complex.

ectopy. Persistent complex ventricular ectopy in patients with depressed left ventricular function (ejection fraction <35%) may require further evaluation and treatment.

3. **Diagnosis.** See Figure 11.34.

4. **Treatment**

   a. Correct the serum potassium with an intravenous KCl infusion at a rate up to 10–20 mEq/h through a central line. Some patients require potassium levels between 4.5 and 5.0 mEq/L to eliminate ventricular ectopy.

   b. Atrial pace at a rate exceeding the current sinus rate (overdrive pacing) unless tachycardia is present.

   c. Magnesium sulfate (2 g in 100 mL IV) administered at the termination of bypass has been shown to reduce the incidence of ventricular ectopy.[324]

   d. In patients with impaired LV function, recent infarction, ongoing ischemia, symptomatic PVCs, and perhaps in the immediate perioperative period as the heart recovers from surgery, use of drugs to control PVCs might be warranted. Commonly used drugs include:

      i. Lidocaine 1 mg/kg with 1–2 repeat doses of 0.5 mg/kg 10 minutes apart. A continuous infusion of 1–2 mg/min of a 1 g/250 mL mix should be started. Do not exceed 4 mg/min to avoid seizure activity. Consider the patient's weight, hepatic function, and any underlying congestive heart failure when calculating a maximum dose. Although a strategy of prophylactic lidocaine may reduce PVCs and the incidence of nonsustained VT after CABG, there is little evidence that this influences outcomes.[325]

ii. Amiodarone 150 mg IV load over 15 minutes, followed by a 60 mg/h infusion × 6 hours, then 30 mg/h × 18 hours. Control of ventricular ectopy is an added benefit when amiodarone is used prophylactically to prevent AF.

K. **Ventricular tachycardia (VT) and ventricular fibrillation (VF)**

1. **Etiology**

a. VT/VF occur postoperatively in about 1–3% of patients undergoing open-heart surgery and carry a mortality rate of 20–30%.[326–328]

b. Ventricular tachyarrhythmias result from disorders of impulse formation or propagation. When they are present preoperatively on the basis of ischemia, resolution may be anticipated with revascularization of the ischemic zones. However, if they occur preoperatively as a consequence of a prior infarction, they may be exacerbated by reperfusion.

c. Reperfusion of zones of ischemia or infarction can trigger de novo malignant ventricular arrhythmias. They are more common in patients with prior infarction, unstable angina, an ejection fraction <40%, NYHA class III–IV CHF, pulmonary and systemic hypertension, long pump times, low cardiac output syndromes, and when bypass grafts are placed to infarct zones or noncollateralized occluded vessels, especially the left anterior descending artery. Potential triggers include residual ischemia or development of a perioperative myocardial infarction secondary to incomplete revascularization, anastomotic problems, or acute graft closure. Elevated levels of catecholamines and autonomic imbalance early in the postoperative periods may be contributory.

i. Nonsustained VT (NSVT) (VT lasting less than 30 seconds) may be encountered for reasons similar to those of PVCs and may occur in patients with normal or abnormal ventricular function.

ii. Sustained monomorphic VT (VT lasting over 30 seconds) is usually noted in patients with a previous myocardial infarction and depressed LV function, often with formation of a left ventricular aneurysm. The border zone between scar and viable tissue provides the electrophysiologic substrate for a reentry mechanism that passes through myocyte bands surviving within the infarct.[329,330]

iii. Sustained polymorphic VT with a normal QT interval is usually caused by increased dispersion of repolarization in areas of reperfused ischemia or infarction. Triggered activity in the form of delayed afterdepolarizations and occasionally enhanced automaticity are the mechanisms involved. Polymorphic VT may be facilitated by perioperative phenomena such as ischemia, hemodynamic instability, use of catecholamines or intrinsic sympathetic activity, withdrawal of β-blockers, and other metabolic problems. Ventricular fibrillation may be triggered by an acute ischemic insult.[329,330]

iv. Polymorphic VT with QT prolongation is called **torsades de pointes.** The mechanism involves early afterdepolarizations, which is a form of triggered activity. It may complicate the use of type IA and III antiarrhythmic agents,

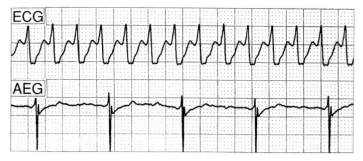

Figure 11.35 • Ventricular tachycardia recorded simultaneously in lead II and a bipolar AEG. There is dissociation between the sinus tachycardia at a rate of 72 bpm noted in the AEG and the wide complex ventricular tachycardia occurring at a rate of 210 bpm noted in the monitor lead.

especially if hypokalemia is present. Other medications that can contribute to torsades are metoclopramide, droperidol (for nausea), and high-dose haloperidol (>35 mg/day) used for agitation in the ICU.[331]

    d. If the patient has a VVI or DDD pacemaker, the use of electrocautery during surgery can inactivate the sensing circuit, converting it to the VOO mode. This may result in bizarre-appearing arrhythmias and may trigger ventricular fibrillation. These pacemakers must be evaluated upon arrival in the ICU and reprogrammed if necessary.[332]

2. Diagnosis. See Figures 11.35–11.38. An arrhythmia commonly confused with VT is atrial fibrillation with a rate-dependent conduction block (aberrancy) that produces a wide QRS complex. This should be distinguished by its irregularity, although it may be difficult to detect at fast heart rates.

3. Evaluation and treatment depend on the status of LV function, the nature of the arrhythmia (nonsustained vs. sustained, monomorphic vs. polymorphic VT), and whether the VT is inducible.

    a. Any potential triggering factors should be identified and managed. These include acid–base and electrolyte abnormalities, intracardiac catheters, myocardial ischemia or infarction, CHF, and potentially proarrhythmic medications.

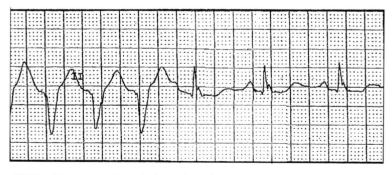

Figure 11.36 • Nonsustained ventricular tachycardia at a rate exceeding 130 bpm that spontaneously reverted to a sinus mechanism at a rate of 75 bpm.

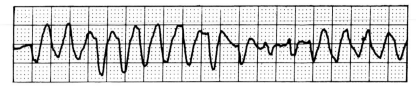

Figure 11.37 • Ventricular fibrillation on monitor lead.

    b. Nonsustained VT (NSVT) with preserved LV function has a favorable prognosis. Although lidocaine or amiodarone may be considered when this rhythm develops, β-blockers alone should suffice if evaluation reveals an ejection fraction >35%.[333]

    c. NSVT in patients with depressed LV function may be associated with a poor prognosis without treatment. Extrapolating from the MADIT I and MUSTT trials, an electrophysiology study and ICD placement should be considered if NSVT develops after surgery in these patients.[333]

    d. Sustained VT occurring without hemodynamic compromise can be managed by:

        i. Ventricular overdrive pacing to terminate the reentry circuit

        ii. Cardioversion if VT persists or hemodynamic compromise develops

        iii. Amiodarone 150 mg over 15 minutes, then 1 mg/min (60 mg/h) × 6 hours, then 0.5 mg/min (30 mg/h) × 18 hours

    e. Any patient developing **VF or sustained VT that is pulseless or associated with hemodynamic instability** requires immediate defibrillation per ACLS protocol (see pages 506–512). If unsuccessful, emergency resternotomy and open-chest massage are indicated.

    f. Electrophysiologic evaluation is essential for patients with sustained VT and impaired ventricular function to improve the long-term prognosis. In general, ICD placement can be justified in any patient with an ejection fraction <35% (see pages 58–59).[334,335]

        i. Monomorphic VT is inducible in 80% of patients with spontaneous VT and is usually associated with a remote infarct and an arrhythmogenic substrate causing a reentry mechanism. This usually requires antiarrhythmic therapy (usually amiodarone) as well as the placement of an ICD.

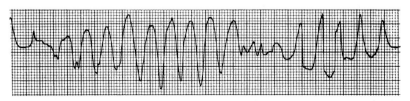

Figure 11.38 • Torsades de pointes on monitor lead. Note how the QRS complex appears to "twist" arouind the isoelectric baseline. Torsades usually has a pause-dependent onset initiated by a premature ventricular complex discharging at the end of a T wave, usually associated with a long QT interval.

  ii. Polymorphic VT is usually associated with myocardial infarction, ischemia, or reperfusion, and should prompt further evaluation for ongoing ischemia. This may involve coronary arteriography to identify potential graft occlusion or an anastomotic stenosis, which may a correctable problem. It is often transient and therapy must be individualized.

 g. Torsades de pointes[336]

  i. Cardiovert immediately for hemodynamic compromise or prolonged episodes (usually because VF is suspected to be present).

  ii. Administer potassium chloride, unless hyperkalemia is present, to shorten the QT interval.

  iii. Ventricular pace at 90–100 beats/min or start an isoproterenol infusion at 1–4 µg/min.[337] This will shorten the action potential to prevent early afterdepolarizations and triggered activity.

  iv. Magnesium 1–2 g and β-blockers may eliminate triggered activity to prevent recurrence, but do not shorten the QT interval.

XIII. Antiarrhythmic Medications

A variety of medications are available for the control of supraventricular and ventricular arrhythmias. A basic understanding of their mechanism of action is critical to the appropriate selection of these drugs for the treatment of various arrhythmias as noted in the preceding sections. In this section, drugs that may be used in patients undergoing cardiac surgery are presented. The reader is referred to any of the major cardiology textbooks or websites for more detailed information.

 A. Vaughan-Williams classification of antiarrhythmic medications

Class I	**Sodium channel blockers**	
	Class IA	Quinidine
		Procainamide
		Disopyramide
	Class IB	Lidocaine
		Mexiletine
		Phenytoin
	Class IC	Propafenone
		Flecainide
Class II	**β-adrenergic blockers**	
Class III	**Potassium channel blockers**	
	Amiodarone	
	Dofetilide	
	Dronedarone	
	Ibutilide	
	Sotalol	
Class IV	**Calcium channel blockers**	

Table 11.16 • Electrophysiologic Properties of Antiarrhythmic Drugs

Property		Class IA	Class IB	Class IC	Class II	Class III	Class IV
Automaticity							
SA node		—	—	—	↓	—	↓
Vent ectopic foci (Purkinje)		↓	↓	↓	↓	—	—
Delayed afterdepolarizations[a]		—	↓	↓	↓	—	↓
Conduction							
Atria	CV	↓	—	↓	—	—	—
	ERP	↑	—	↑	—	—	—
AV node	CV	—	—	↓	↓	—	↓
	ERP	—	—	↑	↑	—	↑
His-Purkinje	CV	↓	↓	↓	—	—	—
	ERP	↓	↑	↑	↑	—	—
Ventricle	CV	↓	↓	↓	—	—	—
	ERP	↑	↓	↑	—	↑	—

[a] Mechanism of digoxin-induced ventricular ectopy.
CV = conduction velocity; ERP = effective refractory period.

B. Table 11.16 shows the effects of the various classes of antiarrhythmic drugs on automaticity, conduction velocity (CV), and the effective refractory period (ERP). Some medications have multiple properties (such as amiodarone and sotalol), so they may have additional electrophysiologic effects. The appropriate classes of antiarrhythmic drug that can be selected for the management of the common arrhythmias are as follows:

1. Alterations in automaticity
   a. Sinus tachycardia (sinus node): class II, IV
   b. Ventricular ectopy (Purkinje and ventricular fibers): class IA, IB, IC, II, III
   c. Digoxin-toxic ectopy (delayed afterdepolarizations: class IB (phenytoin)
2. Alterations in conduction velocity and ERP
   a. Conversion of atrial fibrillation (atrium): class IA, IC, II, III

    b. To slow the response to atrial fibrillation (AV node): class II, III, IV, digoxin

    c. Conversion of AVNRT or AVRT: class II, IV, digoxin

    d. Ventricular tachycardia (interrupt reentrant circuits in His−Purkinje fibers or ventricle): class IA, IB, III

C. **Note:** The clinical indications listed below for each of the antiarrhythmic medications are those for which there is documented efficacy. US Food and Drug Administration (FDA) approval has not necessarily been provided for each of these indications.

D. Drugs that may be used in cardiac surgery patients are listed below in order from class I to class IV drugs.

E. **Procainamide** − Type IA

    1. Clinical indications (used infrequently due to the superiority of amiodarone)

      a. Prevention/conversion of atrial fibrillation

      b. Suppression of premature atrial and ventricular complexes and sustained ventricular tachyarrhythmias

      c. WPW syndrome (slows conduction over accessory pathways)

    2. Doses

      a. IV: 100 mg q5 min up to 1000 mg (never more than 50 mg/min), then a 2−4 mg/min drip (1 g/250 mL mix)

      b. PO procainamide was no longer available as of mid-2010

    3. Metabolism: hepatic to active metabolite *N*-acetylprocainamide (NAPA) and then excreted by the kidneys

    4. Therapeutic level: 4−10 μg/mL of procainamide and 2−8 μg/mL of NAPA

    5. Hemodynamic effects: decreases SVR, negative inotrope in high doses

    6. Electrophysiologic effects

      a. Slows conduction and decreases automaticity and excitability of the atrium and ventricle

      b. Slows the atrial rate in atrial flutter, but vagolytic effects on AV conduction may increase the ventricular response to atrial fibrillation/flutter. Medications that prevent accelerated AV conduction must be given first.

      c. Evidence of toxicity

        i. QT prolongation and polymorphic VT

       ii. Myocardial depression

      iii. NAPA may accumulate in patients with heart and renal failure. It has a longer half-life than procainamide (7 h vs. 4 h) and can lead to cardiac toxicity, including early afterdepolarizations, triggered activity, and ventricular arrhythmias, including torsades de pointes.

    7. Noncardiac side effects: GI (nausea, anorexia), CNS (insomnia, hallucinations, psychosis, depression), rash, drug fever, agranulocytosis, lupus-like syndrome with long-term use

F. **Disopyramide** − Type IA

    1. Clinical indications

      a. Suppression of ventricular and supraventricular arrhythmias

      b. Termination and prevention of recurrence of AVNRT

      c. Prevention/conversion of atrial fibrillation

      d. WPW syndrome (slows conduction over accessory pathways)

  2. Dose: 100–200 mg PO q6h

  3. Metabolism: 65% renal, 35% hepatic

  4. Therapeutic level: 2–5 µg/mL

  5. Hemodynamic effects: strong negative inotrope (thus useful in patients with hypertrophic obstructive cardiomyopathy)

  6. Electrophysiologic effects

      a. Reduces ventricular automaticity, slows conduction in the AV node, and prolongs the action potential

      b. May cause torsades de pointes or other ventricular tachyarrhythmias associated with QT prolongation

  7. Noncardiac side effects: anticholinergic (urinary retention, constipation, blurred vision), nausea, dizziness, insomnia

G. Lidocaine – Type IB

  1. Clinical indications: premature ventricular complexes and ventricular tachyarrhythmias

  2. Doses

      a. 1 mg/kg IV followed by a continuous infusion of 2–4 mg/min (1 g/250 mL mix); a dose of 0.5 mg/kg may be given 15 minutes later to achieve a stable plasma concentration.

      b. A rebolus of 0.5 mg/kg should be given to increase plasma levels if the infusion rate is increased.

  3. Metabolism: hepatic; half-life is 15 minutes after one dose and 2 hours with constant infusion (often longer with hepatic impairment)

  4. Therapeutic level: 1–5 µg/mL

  5. Hemodynamic effects: none in the absence of severe LV dysfunction

  6. Electrophysiologic effects: benefits are derived from suppression of abnormal automaticity in ventricular fibers

  7. Noncardiac side effects: CNS (dizziness, delirium, tremors, seizures), GI (nausea)

H. Propafenone – Type IC

  1. Clinical indication: conversion of atrial fibrillation

  2. Doses

      a. PO: 600 mg load, then 150–300 mg q8h

      b. IV: 1 mg/kg IV over 2 minutes, followed 10 minutes later by another 1 mg/kg dose (used for conversion of AF) (not available in the USA in 2010)

  3. Metabolism: hepatic

  4. Therapeutic level: 0.2–3.0 µg/mL

  5. Hemodynamic effects: negative inotrope in patients with compromised ventricular function

  6. Electrophysiologic effects

      a. Slows conduction in the atria, AV node, His–Purkinje system, and ventricle, and prolongs atrial refractoriness

      b. Has some β-blocker activity and can produce AV block and sinus node depression

      c. Proarrhythmic effects are noted in 5% of patients

      d. Doubles the digoxin level

  7. Noncardiac side effects are noted in 15% of patients: CNS (dizziness, diplopia), GI upset

I. β-adrenergic blockers – Type II

  1. Clinical indications

      a. Prevention/treatment of postoperative atrial fibrillation/flutter

      b. Sinus tachycardia

      c. Ventricular arrhythmias associated with digoxin toxicity, myocardial ischemia, or QT prolongation

      d. AVNRT and reciprocating tachycardias in WPW syndrome

  2. Doses

      a. Metoprolol (relative potency is 2.5:1 for IV:PO)

        i. IV: 5 mg q5 minutes for three doses

        ii. PO: 25–100 mg q12h

      b. Atenolol: 25–100 mg PO qd

      c. Esmolol: IV: 500 μg/kg load, then 50–200 μg/kg/min drip

  3. Metabolism: hepatic (metoprolol), renal (atenolol), blood (esmolol)

  4. Hemodynamic effects: negative inotropes (worsening of CHF), hypotension

  5. Electrophysiologic effects

      a. Reduce automaticity at all levels, slowing the heart rate

      b. Decrease AV conduction and can cause heart block

  6. Noncardiac side effects: bronchospasm (less with the cardioselective β-blockers atenolol and metoprolol), fatigue, diarrhea, impotence, depression, claudication

J. Amiodarone – Type III

  1. Clinical indications

      a. Prevention/conversion of postoperative atrial fibrillation

      b. Pulseless VT/VF (first choice to facilitate defibrillation success)

      c. Sustained ventricular tachyarrhythmias

  2. Doses

      a. PO: 400 mg tid, weaned down to 200 mg qd over several weeks (onset of action takes several days)

      b. IV: 150 mg over 15–30 min (300 mg during cardiac arrest), then 1 mg/min × 6 h, 0.5 mg/min × 18 h, then 1 g/day. Onset of action occurs within several hours, but serum levels fall within 30 minutes after infusion is stopped. Repeat bolus doses of 150 mg can be given over 30 minutes for recurrent AF.

  3. Metabolism: hepatic (half-life of 50 days); it may take several months for blood levels to reach equilibrium and clinical effect dissipates after 3 months.

4. Therapeutic level: 1.0–2.5 μg/mL
5. Hemodynamic effects: β-blocker (class II); coronary and peripheral vasodilator
6. Electrophysiologic effects
   a. Has class I, II, and IV activities as well
   b. Initial effects of IV infusion are prolongation of AV conduction and refractoriness, to some degree related to class II (β-blocking) and class IV (calcium channel blocking effects). This accounts for its early benefit in slowing the ventricular response to AF. With the initial infusion, there is less effective prolongation of repolarization in the atria and ventricles.
   c. May produce bradycardia and heart block
   d. Prolongs the QT interval but rarely causes ventricular arrhythmias; lengthens the PR interval, and may increase the QRS duration
7. Reduces clearance (and therefore increases serum levels) of drugs metabolized by the liver. These include **digoxin and warfarin**. Doses of these medications should be reduced by about one-half. Due to the increased risk of rhabdomyolysis, no more than 20 mg of **simvastatin** can be given to patients on amiodarone.
8. Noncardiac side effects are noted in more than 50% of patients, especially during chronic therapy. Minor problems include corneal microdeposits, elevated liver function tests (LFTs), photosensitivity, and alteration in thyroid function.[338] Baseline and follow-up LFTs and thyroid function tests should be performed. Peripheral neuropathy and myopathy may produce an unstable gait. The most serious complication is pulmonary toxicity, which is more common in patients on high-dose chronic amiodarone therapy, especially with abnormal chest x-rays or pulmonary function tests prior to surgery. Acute pulmonary toxicity, which probably represents a hypersensitivity reaction, can also occur, but is rare.[282] Baseline pulmonary function tests (PFTs) are also recommended for any patient in whom amiodarone will be used for more than 1 month.

K. **Dronedarone** – Type III
   1. Clinical indication – prevention of hospitalization in patients with paroxysmal AF; potential benefit in prophylaxis and treatment of AF[284]
   2. Dose: 400 mg PO bid
   3. Metabolism: hepatic (CYP 3A) with half-life of 1–2 days
   4. Therapeutic level: unknown, but levels are increased by substances that reduce CYP 3A activity, including grapefruit juice
   5. Hemodynamic effects: bradycardia and hypotension; can worsen CHF
   6. Electrophysiologic effects:
      a. Has class I (sodium-channel blocker), class II (β-blocker), class III (potassium-channel blocker), and class IV (calcium channel blocker) properties
      b. Can produce bradycardia and heart block
      c. Prolongs the QT interval and is contraindicated in patients with QT prolongation or in patients taking drugs that prolong the QT interval, including some antipsychotic and antidepressant medications and clarithromycin
   7. It inhibits CYP 3A and other hepatic metabolic pathways and raises serum levels of β-blockers, CCBs, digoxin and statins (especially simvastatin), which must be used in lower doses. Dronedarone does not influence INR levels.

8. Noncardiac side effects: GI (diarrhea, nausea, abdominal pain); hypokalemia and hypomagnesemia may occur in patients on potassium-depleting diuretics.

L. Dofetilide – Type III

1. Clinical indications: conversion of atrial fibrillation/flutter
2. Dose: 500 μg PO bid (based on renal function and QT prolongation)
3. Metabolism: 50% renal, 50% hepatic
4. Therapeutic level: unknown
5. Hemodynamic effects: no negative inotropic effects
6. Electrophysiologic effects
   a. Slightly decreases the sinus rate, but no effect on AV conduction
   b. Proarrhythmic effect from QT prolongation, so contraindicated if QT interval >440 ms (or if creatinine clearance <20 mL/min); torsades occurs in 4%
   c. Has drug interaction with verapamil, which contraindicates its use
   d. All class I or III antiarrhythmic medications should be stopped for 3 half-lives before it is given.
   e. Amiodarone must be stopped for 3 months (or a level <0.3 mg/L) before it is given.

M. Sotalol – Type III

1. Clinical indications
   a. Prevention/treatment of postoperative atrial fibrillation
   b. Suppression of ventricular tachyarrhythmias
2. Doses
   a. 80–160 mg PO bid
   b. 75–150 mg IV bid (administered over 5 hours)
3. Metabolism: excreted unchanged in the urine
4. Hemodynamic effects: causes bradycardia; negative inotropic effect can cause hypotension, fatigue, and CHF
5. Electrophysiologic effects
   a. Prolongs atrial and ventricular action potential and refractory periods
   b. Exhibits β-blocking and class III effects
   c. Produces torsades de pointes or proarrhythmic effects in about 4% of patients. Torsades de pointes is dose-related and predictable from the QT interval (avoid if QT >500 ms).
6. Noncardiac side effects: fatigue, dyspnea, dizziness, heart failure, nausea and vomiting

N. Ibutilide – Type III

1. Clinical indication: conversion of recent-onset atrial fibrillation and flutter
2. Dose: 1 mg IV over 10 minutes (0.01 mg/kg if <60 kg) with a second dose if no response.
3. Metabolism: hepatic
4. Therapeutic level: unknown
5. Hemodynamic effects: no significant hemodynamic effects

6. Electrophysiologic effects
   a. Increases refractoriness of atrium, AV node, and ventricle
   b. Dose-related prolongation of the QT interval (avoid if the QT interval exceeds 440 ms). QT prolongation may contribute to torsades de pointes, but sustained polymorphic VT may occur even in the absence of a prolonged QT interval.
   c. Monomorphic or polymorphic VT (sustained or nonsustained) is noted in about 10% of patients; careful monitoring in the ICU is essential for 4 hours after an administered dose (half-life is 6 hours) or until the QT interval has returned to baseline.
7. Noncardiac side effects: headache, nausea

O. **Calcium channel blockers** (verapamil and diltiazem) – Type IV
   1. Clinical indications
      a. Control rapid ventricular response to atrial fibrillation/flutter
      b. Treat supraventricular tachycardias including AVNRT, reciprocating tachycardias of WPW syndrome (AVRT), and multifocal atrial tachycardia – contraindicated for atrial fibrillation in WPW syndrome
      c. Ischemic ventricular ectopy
   2. Doses
      a. Diltiazem
         i. IV: 0.25 mg/kg IV bolus over 2 minutes, with a repeat bolus of 0.35 mg/kg 15 minutes later; then a continuous infusion of 10–15 mg/h (250 mg/250 mL mix).
         ii. PO: 30–90 mg q8h (or 180–360 mg qd of long-acting preparation)
      b. Verapamil
         i. IV: 2.5–10 mg bolus over 1 minute with repeat dose in 30 minutes; then a continuous infusion of 2–5 µg/kg/min (120 mg/250 mL mix).
         ii. PO: 80–160 mg q8h
   3. Metabolism: hepatic
   4. Therapeutic level: 0.1–0.15 µg/mL (verapamil)
   5. Hemodynamic effects: negative inotropes and vasodilators (verapamil more than diltiazem); cause hypotension and can worsen CHF
   6. Electrophysiologic effects
      a. Slow calcium channel action potentials in sinus and AV nodes. Can precipitate bradycardia, asystole, or heart block when used concomitantly with IV β-blockers.
      b. Verapamil reduces clearance of digoxin and increases the digoxin level by about 35%.
   7. Noncardiac side effects: GI (constipation, nausea), headache, dizziness, elevation in liver function tests

P. **Adenosine**
   1. Clinical indication: paroxysmal supraventricular tachycardias with AV nodal reentry (AVNRT or AVRT).

2. Dose: 6 mg rapid IV injection through a peripheral line followed by a saline flush; a second dose of 12 mg may be given 2 minutes later if necessary.
3. Metabolism: rapidly degraded in blood, with a half-life of less than 10 seconds.
4. Electrophysiologic effects: negative effects on SA and AV nodes; can produce asystole and transient high-grade AV block; the latter effect can unmask atrial activity to differentiate the causes of narrow and wide complex tachycardias.
5. Side effects: flushing, dyspnea, or chest pressure of very brief duration

Q. Digoxin

1. Clinical indications
   a. Rapid ventricular response to atrial fibrillation/flutter (less effective than calcium channel blockers or β-blockers due to the mechanism of early postoperative AF)
   b. Prevention of AVNRT
2. Doses
   a. IV: 0.5 mg, then 0.25 mg q4–6h to total dose of 1.0–1.25 mg, then 0.125 mg qd
   b. PO: 0.5 mg, then 0.25 mg q4–6h to total dose of 1.25 mg, then 0.25 mg qd (dosing without a load will take 7–10 days to reach a steady-state level)
      i. Maintenance dose depends on serum level and therapeutic effect
      ii. Dose is 0.125 mg qod for patients in renal failure
      iii. IV dose is two-thirds of the PO dose
3. Metabolism: hepatic (but renal failure prolongs its half-life and decreases its distribution)
4. Therapeutic level: 1–2 ng/mL (drawn not less than 6 hours after an oral dose or 4 hours after an IV dose)
   a. Serum levels are increased by medications that reduce its clearance or volume of distribution – thus digoxin dosing should be reduced accordingly.
   b. **Levels are increased by amiodarone** (by 70–100%) and verapamil (by 35%).
5. Hemodynamic effects: slight inotropic effect, peripheral vasodilation
6. Electrophysiologic effects: enhances vagolytic activity which reduces sinus node automaticity (slows the heart rate) and prolongs AV conduction and refractoriness (controls ventricular response to AF)
7. Noncardiac side effects: GI (anorexia, nausea, vomiting), CNS (headache, fatigue, confusion, seizures), visual symptoms

R. Comments on digoxin toxicity[339]

1. Digoxin is used primarily to slow the ventricular response to atrial fibrillation/flutter by virtue of its vagotonic effect (at low dose) and a direct effect (high dose) on the AV node. It is less effective than other medications in slowing the ventricular response to atrial fibrillation in the early postoperative period when a high adrenergic state is present. Thus, it is not the drug of choice for acute rate control. However, it can provide additional rate control, especially when AF is persistent.
2. Aggressive digitalization for rapid AF is usually not successful in achieving rate control and can lead to digoxin toxicity for a number of reasons in the early postoperative period.

a. There is increased sensitivity to digoxin related to augmented sympathetic tone, myocardial ischemia, electrolyte imbalance (hyper- or hypokalemia, hypercalcemia, hypomagnesemia), acid–base imbalance, or use of vasoactive or antiarrhythmic drugs (verapamil).

b. Large doses need to be given to achieve effect because digoxin's vagotonic effects are offset by increased sympathetic tone. IV doses are usually given to provide 1.25 mg within the first 24 hours but subsequent IV doses should be two-thirds of the oral doses to avoid toxicity.

c. The volume of distribution is less in many elderly patients with decreased lean body mass.

d. Hypokalemia from postoperative diuresis and hypomagnesemia predispose to digoxin toxicity.

e. Renal excretion may be impaired in patients with chronic kidney disease. Elderly patients have reduced glomerular filtration rates and excrete digoxin less efficiently.

3. Digoxin toxicity should be considered in any patient receiving digoxin who develops a change in rhythm. These include, in decreasing order of frequency:

a. Premature ventricular complexes (multiform and bigeminy)

b. Nonparoxysmal AV junctional tachycardia

c. AV block: first-degree or Wenckebach second-degree block

d. Paroxysmal atrial tachycardia with 2:1 block

e. Ventricular tachycardia (especially bidirectional VT at a rate of 140–180 bpm)

f. Sinus bradycardia or SA block

4. Digoxin toxicity in a patient with atrial fibrillation is usually manifested by:

a. Slow ventricular response (<50 bpm)

b. AV dissociation with AV junctional escape or accelerated junctional rhythm. Regularization of the ventricular rate in the presence of atrial fibrillation should always raise concern about the development of complete heart block with a junctional escape rhythm.

5. Treatment

a. Bradyarrhythmias are treated by atrial, AV, or ventricular pacing, depending on the underlying atrial rhythm and the status of AV conduction. Atropine can be used, but isoproterenol should be avoided because it may induce malignant ventricular arrhythmias.

b. Tachyarrhythmias

    i. Potassium chloride, except in the presence of high-grade AV block, because hyperkalemia can potentiate the depressant effect of digoxin on AV conduction.

    ii. Lidocaine at usual doses

    iii. Phenytoin (Dilantin), 100 mg IV every 5 minutes to a maximum of 1 g, then 100–200 mg PO q8h

c. Digibind (digoxin immune Fab [Ovine]) 400 mg (10 vials) IV, which may be repeated after several hours, can be used for life-threatening digoxin toxicity.

6. Special concerns

    a. Digoxin toxicity decreases the threshold for postcardioversion malignant arrhythmias. This may be exacerbated when hypokalemia or hypercalcemia is present. Use of lidocaine, phenytoin, or lower energy levels should be considered.

    b. Dialysis is ineffective in removing digoxin. Its half-life is 36–48 hours.

References

1. Douglas PS, Edmunds LH, Sutton MSJ, Geer R, Harken AH, Reichek N. Unreliability of hemodynamic indexes of left ventricular size during cardiac surgery. *Ann Thorac Surg* 1987;44:31–4.

2. Hansen RM, Viquerat CE, Matthay MA, et al. Poor correlation between pulmonary arterial wedge pressure and left ventricular end-diastolic volume after coronary artery bypass surgery. *Anesthesiology* 1986;64:764–70.

3. St. André AC, DelRossi A. Hemodynamic management of patients in the first 24 hours after cardiac surgery. *Crit Care Med* 2005;33:2082–93.

4. Schwann TA, Zacharias A, Riordan CJ, Durham SJ, Engoren M, Habib RH. Safe, highly selective use of pulmonary artery catheters in coronary artery bypass grafting: an objective patient selection method. *Ann Thorac Surg* 2002;73:1394–402.

5. Zimmermann A, Kufner C, Hofbauer S, et al. The accuracy of the Vigileo/FloTrac continuous cardiac output monitor. *J Cardiothorac Vasc Anesth* 2008;22:388–93.

6. Johnson RG, Thurer RL, Kruskall MS, et al. Comparison of two transfusion strategies after elective operations for myocardial revascularization. *J Thorac Cardiovasc Surg* 1992;104:307–14.

7. Spiess BD, Ley C, Body SC, et al. Hematocrit value on intensive care unit entry influences the frequency of Q-wave myocardial infarction after coronary artery bypass grafting. The Institutions of the Multicenter Study of Perioperative Ischemia (McSPI) Research Group. *J Thorac Cardiovasc Surg* 1998;116:460–7.

8. Ferraris VA, Ferraris SP, Saha SP, et al. Perioperative blood transfusion and blood conservation in cardiac surgery: the Society of Thoracic Surgeons and the Society of Cardiovascular Anesthesiologists clinical practice guidelines. *Ann Thorac Surg* 2007;83(5 suppl):S27–86.

9. Spiess BD. Choose one: damned if you do/damned if you don't! *Crit Care Med* 2005;33:1871–4.

10. Scott BH, Seifert FC, Grimson R. Blood transfusion is associated with increased resource utilisation, morbidity and mortality in cardiac surgery. *Ann Card Anaesth* 2008;11:15–9.

11. Sommers MS, Stevenson JS, Hamlin RL, Ivey TD, Russell AC. Mixed venous oxygen saturation and oxygen partial pressure as predictors of cardiac index after coronary artery bypass grafting. *Heart Lung* 1993;22:112–20.

12. Balik M, Pachl J, Hendl J, Martin B, Jan P, Jan H. Effect of the degree of tricuspid regurgitation on cardiac output measurements by thermodilution. *Intensive Care Med* 2002;28:1117–21.

13. Ardehali A, Ports TA. Myocardial oxygen supply and demand. *Chest* 1990;98:699–705.

14. Griffin MJ, Hines RL. Management of perioperative ventricular dysfunction. *J Cardiothorac Vasc Anesth* 2001;15:90–106.

15. Royster RL, Butterworth JF IV, Prough DS, et al. Preoperative and intraoperative predictors of inotropic support and long-term outcome in patients having coronary artery bypass grafting. *Anesth Analg* 1991;72:729–36.

16. Maganti MD, Rao V, Borger MA, Ivanov J, David TE. Predictors of low cardiac output syndrome after isolated aortic valve surgery. *Circulation* 2005;112(9 Suppl):I-448–52.

17. Ahmed I, House CM, Nelson WB. Predictors of inotrope use in patients undergoing concomitant coronary artery bypass graft (CABG) and aortic valve replacement (AVR) surgeries at separation from cardiopulmonary bypass (CPB). *J Cardiothorac Surg* 2009;4:24.

18. McKinlay KH, Schinderle DB, Swaminathan M, et al. Predictors of inotrope use during separation from cardiopulmonary bypass. *J Cardiothorac Vasc Anesth* 2004;18:404–8.

19. Bernard F, Denault A, Babin D, et al. Diastolic dysfunction is predictive of difficult weaning from cardiopulmonary bypass. *Anesth Analg* 2001;92:291–8.

20. Rao V, Ivanov J, Weisel RD, Cohen G, Borger MA, Mickle DA. Lactate release during reperfusion predicts low cardiac output syndrome after coronary bypass surgery. *Ann Thorac Surg* 2001;71:1925–30.

21. Breisblatt WM, Stein KL, Wolfe CJ, et al. Acute myocardial dysfunction and recovery: a common occurrence after coronary bypass surgery. *J Am Coll Cardiol* 1990;15:1261–9.

22. Smith RC, Leung JM, Mangano DT. Postoperative myocardial ischemia in patients undergoing coronary artery bypass surgery. *Anesthesiology* 1991;74:464–73.

23. Casthely PA, Shah C, Mekhjian H, et al. Left ventricular diastolic function after coronary artery bypass grafting: a correlative study with three different myocardial protection techniques. *J Thorac Cardiovasc Sug* 1997;114:254–60.

24. Imren Y, Tasoglu I, Oktar GL, et al. The importance of transesophageal echocardiography in diagnosis of pericardial tamponade after cardiac surgery. *J Cardiac Surg* 2008;23:450–3.

25. Weisel RD, Burns RJ, Baird RJ, et al. A comparison of volume loading and atrial pacing following aortocoronary bypass. *Ann Thorac Surg* 1983;36:332–44.

26. Muehlschlegel JD, Peng YG, Lobato EB, Hess PJ Jr, Martin TD, Klodell CT Jr. Temporary biventricular pacing postcardiopulmonary bypass in patients with reduced ejection fraction. *J Card Surg* 2008;23:324–30.

27. Berberian G, Quinin TA, Kanter JP, et al. Optimized biventricular pacing in atrioventricular block after cardiac surgery. *Ann Thorac Surg* 2005;80:870–5.

28. Vaughan P, Bhatti F, Hunter S, Dunning J. Does biventricular pacing provide a superior cardiac output compared to univentricular pacing wires after cardiac surgery? *Interact Cardiovasc Thorac Surg* 2009;8:673–8.

29. Eberhardt F, Heringlake M, Massalme MS, et al. The effect of biventricular pacing after coronary artery bypass grafting: a prospective randomized trial of different pacing modes in patients with reduced left ventricular function. *J Thorac Cardiovasc Surg* 2009;137:1461–7.

30. Richer M, Robert S, Lebel M. Renal hemodynamics during norepinephrine and low-dose dopamine infusions in man. *Crit Care Med* 1996;24:1150–6.

31. Morimatsu H, Uchino S, Chung J, Bellomo R, Raman J, Buxton B. Norepinephrine for hypotensive vasodilatation after cardiac surgery: impact on renal function. *Intensive Care Med* 2003;29:1106–12.

32. Albanese J, Leone M, Garnier F, Bourgoin A, Antonini F, Martin C. Renal effects of norepinephrine in septic and nonseptic patients. *Chest* 2004;126:534–9.

33. Nygren A, Thoren A, Ricksten SE. Norepinephrine and intestinal musocal perfusion in vasodilatory shock after cardiac surgery. *Shock* 2007;28:536–43.

34. Bragadottir G, Redfors B, Nygren A, Sellgren J, Ricksten SE. Low-dose vasopressin increases glomerular filtration rate, but impairs renal oxygenation in post-cardiac surgery patients. *Acta Anaesthesiol Scand* 2009;53:1052–9.

35. Nygren A, Thorén A, Ricksten SE. Vasopressin decreases intestinal mucosal perfusion: a clinical study on cardiac surgery patients in vasodilatory shock. *Acta Anaesthesiol Scand* 2009;53:581–8.

36. Tayama E, Ueda T, Shojima T, et al. Arginine vasopressin is an ideal drug after cardiac surgery for the management of low systemic vascular resistant hypotension concomitant with pulmonary hypertension. *Interact Cardiovasc Thorac Surrg* 2007;6:715–9.

37. Novella S, Martinez AC, Pagán RM, et al. Plasma levels and vascular effects of vasopressin in patients undergoing coronary artery bypass grafting. *Eur J Cardiothorac Surg* 2007;32:69–76.

38. Levin RL, Degrange MA, Bruno GF, et al. Methylene blue reduces mortality and morbidity in vasoplegic patients after cardiac surgery. *Ann Thorac Surg* 2004;77:496–9.

39. Leyh RG, Kofidis T, Strüber M, et al. Methylene blue: the drug of choice for catecholamine-refractory vasoplegia after cardiopulmonary bypass? *J Thorac Cardiovasc Surg* 2003;125:1426–31.

40. Shanmugam G. Vasoplegic syndrome – the role of methylene blue. *Eur J Cardiothorac Surg* 2005;28:705–10.

41. Boeken U, Feindt P, Limathe J, Kurt M, Gams E. Intraaortic balloon pumping in patients with right ventricular insufficiency after cardiac surgery: parameters to predict failure of IABP support. *Thorac Cardiovasc Surg* 2009;57:324–8.

42. Forrest P. Anaesthesia and right ventricular failure. *Anaesth Intensive Care* 2009;37:370–85.

43. Kerbaul F, Rondelet B, Demester JP, et al. Effects of levosimendan versus dobutamine on pressure-load induced right ventricular failure. *Crit Care Med* 2006;34:2814–9.

44. Salzberg SP, Filsoufi F, Anyanwu A, et al. High-risk mitral valve surgery: perioperative hemodynamic optimization with nesiritide (BNP). *Ann Thorac Surg* 2005;80:502–6.

45. Benharash P, Omari B. Administration of nesiritide in patients after coronary artery bypass surgery induces brisk diuresis. *Am Surg* 2005;71:794–6.

46. Ichinose F, Robert JD Jr, Zapol WM. Inhaled nitric oside. A selective pulmonary vasodilator. Current uses and therapeutic potential. *Circulation* 2004;109:3106–11.

47. George I, Xydas S, Topkara VK, et al. Clinical indication for use and outcomes after inhaled nitric oxide therapy. *Ann Thorac Surg* 2006;82:2161–9.

48. Frostell CG, Blomqvist H, Hedenstierna G, Lundberg J, Zapol WM. Inhaled nitric oxide selectively reverses human hypoxic pulmonary vasoconstriction without causing systemic vasodilation. *Anesthesiology* 1995;78:427–35.

49. Fullerton DA, Jaggers J, Piedalue F, Grover FL, McIntyre RC Jr. Effective control of refractory pulmonary hypertension after cardiac operations. *J Thorac Cardiovasc Surg* 1997;113:363–70.

50. Pearl JM, Nelson DP, Raake JL, et al. Inhaled nitric oxide increases endothelin-1 levels: a potential cause of rebound pulmonary hypertension. *Crit Care Med* 2002;30:89–93.

51. Solina A, Papp D, Ginsberg S, et al. A comparison of inhaled nitric oxide and milrinone for the treatment of pulmonary hypertension in adult cardiac surgery patients. *J Cardiothorac Vasc Anesth* 2000;14:12–7.

52. Winterhalter M, Simon A, Fischer S, et al. Comparison of inhaled iloprost and nitric oxide in patients with pulmonary hypertension during weaning from cardiopulmonary bypass in cardiac surgery: a prospective randomized trial. *J Cardiothorac Vasc Anesth* 2008;22:406–13.

53. Fattouch K, Sbraga F, Bianco G, et al. Inhaled prostacyclin, nitric oxide, and nitroprusside in pulmonary hypertension after mitral valve replacement. *J Card Surg* 2005;20:171–6.

54. Haché M, Denault A, Belisle S, et al. Inhaled epoprostenol (prostacyclin) and pulmonary hypertension before cardiac surgery. *J Thorac Cardiovasc Surg* 2003;125:642–9.

55. Lowson SM, Doctor A, Walsh BK, Doorley PA. Inhaled prostacyclin for the treatment of pulmonary hypertension after cardiac surgery. *Crit Care Med* 2002;30:2762–4.

56. De Wet CJ, Affleck DG, Jacobsohn E, et al. Inhaled prostacyclin is safe, effective, and affordable in patients with pulmonary hypertension, right heart dysfunction, and refractory hypoxemia after cardiothoracic surgery. *J Thorac Cardiovasc Surg* 2004;127:1058–67.

57. Rex S, Schaelte G, Metzelder S, et al. Inhaled iloprost to control pulmonary artery hypertension in patients undergoing mitral valve surgery: a prospective, randomized-controlled trial. *Acta Anaesthesiol Scand* 2008;52:65–72.

58. Yurtseven N, Karaca P, Uysal G, et al. A comparison of the acute hemodynamic effects of inhaled nitroglycerin and iloprost in patients with pulmonary hypertension undergoing mitral valve surgery. *Ann Thorac Cardiovasc Surg* 2006;12:319–23.

59. Baysal A, Bilsel S, Bulbul OG, Kayiacioglu I, Idiz M, Yekeler I. Comparison of the usage of intravenous iloprost and nitroglycerin for pulmonary hypertension during valvular heart surgery. *Heart Surg Forum* 2006;9:E536–42.

60. Aral A, Oğuz M, Özberrak H, et al. Hemodynamic advantages of left atrial epinephrine administration in open heart operations. *Ann Thorac Surg* 1997;64:1046–9.

61. Tritapepe L, Voci P, Cogliati AA, Pasotti E, Papalia U, Menichetti A. Successful weaning from cardiopulmonary bypass with central venous prostaglandin E1 and left atrial epinephrine infusion in patients with acute pulmonary hypertension. *Crit Care Med* 1999;27:2180–3.

62. Schmid ER, Bürki C, Engel MH, Schmidlin D, Tornic M, Seifert B. Inhaled nitric oxide versus intravenous vasodilators in severe pulmonary hypertension after cardiac surgery. *Anesth Analg* 1999;89:1108–15.

63. Trachte AL, Lobato EB, Urdaneta F, et al. Oral sildenafil reduces pulmonary hypertension after cardiac surgery. *Ann Thorac Surg* 2005;79:194–7.

64. Raja SG, Nayak SH. Sildenafil: emerging cardiovascular indications. *Ann Thorac Surg* 2004;78:1496–506.

65. Brutsaert DL, Sys SU, Gillebert TC. Diastolic dysfunction in post-cardiac surgical management. *J Cardiothorac Vasc Anesth* 1993;7(Suppl 1):18–20.

66. Butterworth JF IV, Prielipp RC, Royster RL, et al. Dobutamine increases heart rate more than epinephrine in patients recovering from aortocoronary bypass surgery. *J Cardiothorac Vasc Anesth* 1992;6:535–41.

67. Gatot I, Abramov D, Tsodikov V, et al. Should we give prophylactic renal-dose dopamine after coronary artery bypass surgery? *J Card Surg* 2004;19:128–33.

68. Lassnigg A, Donner E, Grubhofer G, Presterl E, Druml W, Hiesmayr M. Lack of renoprotective effects of dopamine and furosemide during cardiac surgery. *J Am Soc Nephrol* 2000;11:97–104.

69. Woo EB, Tang AT, el-Gamel A, et al. Dopamine therapy for patients at risk of renal dysfunction following cardiac surgery: fact or fiction? *Eur J Cardiothorac Surg* 2002;22:106–11.

70. Gelfman DM, Ornato JP, Gonzalez ER. Dopamine-induced increase in atrioventricular conduction in atrial fibrillation-flutter. *Clin Cardiol* 1987;10:671–3.

71. Romson JL, Leung JM, Bellows WH, et al. Effects of dobutamine on hemodynamics and left ventricular performance after cardiopulmonary bypass in cardiac surgical patients. *Anesthesiology* 1999;91:1318–28.

72. Fowler MB, Alderman EL, Oesterle SN, et al. Dobutamine and dopamine after cardiac surgery: greater augmentation of myocardial blood flow with dobutamine. *Circulation* 1984;70(suppl I): I-103–I-11.

73. Van Trigt P, Spray TL, Pasque MK, Peyton RB, Pellom GL, Wechsler AS. The comparative effects of dopamine and dobutamine on ventricular mechanics after coronary artery bypass grafting: a pressure-dimension analysis. *Circulation* 1984;70(suppl I):I-112–7.

74. DiSesa VJ, Brown E, Mudge GH Jr, Collins JJ Jr, Cohn LH. Hemodynamic comparison of dopamine and dobutamine in the postoperative volume-loaded, pressure-loaded, and normal ventricle. *J Thorac Cardiovasc Surg* 1982;83:256–63.

75. Feneck RO, Sherry KM, Withington PS, Oduro-Dominah A, and the European Milrinone multicenter trial group. Comparison of the hemodynamic effects of milrinone with dobutamine in patients after cardiac surgery. *J Cardiothorac Vasc Anesth* 2001;15:306–15.

76. Levy JH, Bailey JM, Deeb GM. Intravenous milrinone in cardiac surgery. *Ann Thorac Surg* 2002;73:325–30.

77. Liu JJ, Doolan LA, Xie B, Chen JR, Buxton BF. Direct vasodilator effect of milrinone, an inotropic drug, on arterial coronary bypass grafts. *J Thorac Cardiovasc Surg* 1997;113:108–13.

78. Lobato EB, Janelle GM, Urdaneta F, Martin TD. Comparison of milrinone versus nitroglycerin, alone and in combination, on grafted internal mammary artery flow after cardiopulmonary bypass: effects of α-adrenergic stimulation. *J Cardiothorac Vasc Anesth* 2001;15:723–7.

79. Lobato EB, Gravenstein N, Martin TD. Milrinone, not epinephrine, improves left ventricular compliance after cardiopulmonary bypass. *J Cardiothorac Vasc Anesth* 2000;14:374–7.

80. Lobato EB, Willert JL, Looke TD, Thomas J, Urdaneta F. Effects of milrinone versus epinephrine on left ventricular relaxation after cardiopulmonary bypass following myocardial revascularization: assessment by color M-mode and tissue Doppler. *J Cardiothorac Vasc Anesth* 2005;19:334–9.

81. Couture P, Denault AY, Pellerin M Tardif JC. Milrinone enhances systolic, but not diastolic function during coronary artery bypass grafting surgery. *Can J Anaesth* 2007;54:509–22.

82. Alhashemi JA, Hooper J. Treatment of milrinone-associated tachycardia with beta-blockers. *Can J Anaesth* 1998;45:67–70.

83. Kikura M, Sato S. The efficacy of preemptive milrinone or amrinone therapy in patients undergoing coronary artery bypass grafting. *Anesth Anal* 2002;94:22–30.

84. Kikura M, Lee MK, Safon RA, Bailey JM, Levy JH. The effects of milrinone on platelets in patients undergoing cardiac surgery. *Anesth Analg* 1995;81:44–8.

85. Duranteau J, Sitbon P, Teboul JL, et al. Effects of epinephrine, norepinephrine, or the combination of norepinephrine and dobutamine on gastric mucosa in septic shock. *Crit Care Med* 1999;27:893–900.

86. Shapira N, Schaff HV, White RD, Pluth JR. Hemodynamic effects of calcium chloride injection following cardiopulmonary bypass: response to bolus injection and continuous infusion. *Ann Thorac Surg* 1984;37:133–40.

87. DeHert SG, Ten Broecke PW, De Mulder PA, et al. The effects of calcium on left ventricular function early after cardiopulmonary bypass. *J Cardiothorac Vasc Anesth* 1997;11:864–9.

88. Drop LJ, Scheidegger D. Plasma ionized concentration: important determinant of the hemodynamic response to calcium infusion. *J Thorac Cardiovasc Surg* 1980;79:425–31.

89. Royster RL, Butterworth JF 4th, Prielipp RC, et al. A randomized, blinded, placebo-controlled evaluation of calcium chloride and epinephrine for inotropic support after emergence from cardiopulmonary bypass. *Anesth Analg* 1992;74:3–13.

90. Butterworth JF 4th, Zaloga GP, Prielipp RC, Tucker WY Jr, Royster RL. Calcium inhibits the cardiac stimulating properties of dobutamine but not of amrinone. *Chest* 1992;101:174–80.

91. Walker JD, Crawford FA Jr, Mukherjee R, Spinale FG. The direct effects of 3,5,3'-triodo-L-thyronine (T3) on myocyte contractile processes. Insights into mechanisms of action. *J Thorac Cardiovasc Surg* 1995;110:1369–80.

92. Batra YK, Singh B, Chavan S, Chari P, Dhaliwal RS, Ramprabu K. Effects of cardiopulmonary bypass on thyroid function. *Ann Card Anaesth* 2000;3:3–6.

93. Reinhardt W, Mocker V, Jockenhovel F, et al. Influence of coronary artery bypass surgery on thyroid hormone parameters. *Horm Res* 1997;47:1–8.

94. Ranasinghe AM, Quinn DW, Pagano D, et al. Glucose-insulin-potassium and tri-iodothyronine individually improve hemodynamic performance and are associated with reduce troponin I release after on-pump coronary artery bypass grafting. *Circulation* 2006;114(1 Suppl):I-245–50.

95. Spratt DI, Frohnauer M, Cyr-Alves H, et al. Physiological effects of nonthyroidal illness syndrome in patients after cardiac surgery. *Am J Physiol Endocrinol Metab* 2007;293:E310–5.

96. Bennett-Guerrero E, Jimenez JL, White WD, D'Amico EB, Baldwin BI, Schwinn DA; for the Duke T3 Study Group. Cardiovascular effects of intravenous triiodothyronine in patients undergoing coronary artery bypass surgery. A randomized, double-blind, placebo-controlled trial. *JAMA* 1996;275:687–92.

97. Klemperer JD. Thyroid hormone and cardiac surgery. *Thyroid* 2002;12:517–21.

98. Vohra HA, Bapu D, Bahrami T, Gaer JA, Satur CM. Does perioperative administration of thyroid hormone improve outcome following coronary artery bypass grafting? *J Card Surg* 2008;23:92–6.

99. Mullis-Jansson S, Argenziano M, Corwin S, et al. A randomized double-blind study of the effect of triiodothyronine on cardiac function and morbidity after coronary bypass surgery. *J Thorac Cardiovasc Surg* 1999;117:1128–35.

100. Park YJ, Yoon JW, Kim KI, et al. Subclinical hypothyroidism might increase the risk of transient atrial fibrillation after coronary artery bypass grafting. *Ann Thorac Surg* 2009;87:1846–52.

101. Kokonen L, Majahalme S, Koobi T, et al. Atrial fibrillation in elderly patients after cardiac surgery: postoperative hemodynamics and low postoperative serum triiodothyronine. *J Cardiothorac Vasc Anesth* 2005;19:182–7.

102. Klemperer JD, Klein IL, Ojamaa K, et al. Triiodothyronine therapy lowers the incidence of atrial fibrillation after cardiac operations. *Ann Thorac Surg* 1996;61:1323–9.

103. Mentzer RM Jr, Oz MC, Sladen RN, et al. Effects of perioperative nesiritide in patients with left ventricular dysfunction undergoing cardiac surgery: the NAPA trial. *J Am Coll Cardiol* 2007;49:716–26.

104. Brackbill ML, Stam MD, Schuller-Williams RV, Dhavle AA. Perioperative nesiritide versus milrinone in high-risk coronary artery bypass graft patients. *Ann Pharmacother* 2007;41:427–32.

105. Gordon GR, Schumann R, Rastegar H, Khabbaz K, England MR. Nesiritide for treatment of perioperative low cardiac output syndromes in cardiac surgical patients: an initial experience. *J Anesth* 2006;20:307–11.

106. Chen HH, Sundt TM, Cook DJ, Heublein CM, Burnett JC Jr. Low dose nesiritide and the preservation of renal function in patients with renal dysfunction undergoing cardiopulmonary-bypass surgery: a double-blind placebo controlled pilot study. *Circulation* 2007;116(11 Suppl):I-134–8.

107. Dyke CM, Bhatia D, Aronson S, Moazami N, Mentzer RM Jr. Perioperative nesiritide and possible renal protection in patients with moderate to severe kidney dysfunction. *J Thorac Cardiovasc Surg* 2008;136:1369–70.

108. Bothe W, Olschewski M, Beyersdorf F, Doenst T. Glucose-insulin-potassium in cardiac surgery: a meta-analysis. *Ann Thorac Surg* 2004;78:1650–8.

109. Raja SG, Rayen BS. Levosimendan in cardiac surgery: current best available evidence. *Ann Thorac Surg* 2006;81:1536–46.

110. Eriksson HI, Jalonen JR, Heikkinen LO, et al. Levosimendan facilitates weaning from cardiopulmonary bypass in patients undergoing coronary artery bypass grafting with impaired left ventricular function. *Ann Thorac Surg* 2009;87:448–54.

111. Kerbaul F, Rondelet B, Demester JP, et al. Effects of levosimendan versus dobutamine on pressure load-induced right ventricular failure. *Crit Care Med* 2006;34:2814–9.

112. Zangrillo A, Biondi-Zoccai G, Mizzi A, et al. Levosimendan reduces cardiac troponin release after cardiac surgery: a meta-analysis of randomized controlled studies. *J Cardiothorac Vasc Anesth* 2009;23:474–8.

113. Landoni G, Mizzi A, Biondi-Zoccai G, et al. Reducing mortality in cardiac surgery with levosimendan: a meta-analysis of randomized controlled trials. *J Cardiothorac Vasc Anesth* 2010;24:51–7.

114. Brezina A, Riha H, Pirk J. Prophylactic application of levosimendan in cardiac surgical patients with severe left ventricle dysfunction. *Exp Clin Cardiol* 2009;14:e31–4.

115. Tritapepe L, De Santis V, Vitale D, et al. Levosimendan pre-treatment improves outcomes in patients undergoing coronary artery bypass graft surgery. *Br J Anaesth* 2009;102:198–204.

116. De Hert SG, Lorsomradee S, Cromheecke S, Van der Linden PJ. The effects of levosimendan in cardiac surgery patients with poor left ventricular function. *Anesth Analg* 2007;104:766–73.

117. Flynn MJ, Winter DC, Breen P, et al. Dopexamine increases internal mammary artery blood flow following coronary artery bypass grafting. *Eur J Cardiothorac Surg* 2003;24:547–51.

118. Rosseel PM, Santman FW, Bouter H, Dott CS. Postcardiac surgery low cardiac output syndrome: dopexamine or dopamine? *Intensive Care Med* 1997;23:962–8.

119. El Mokhtari NE, Arlt A, Meissner A, Lins M. Inotropic therapy for cardiac low output syndrome: comparison of hemodynamic effects of dopamine/dobutamine versus dopamine/dopexamine. *Eur J Med Res* 2008;13:459–63.

120. MacGregor DA, Butterworth JF 4th, Zaloga CP, Prielipp RC, James R, Royster RL. Hemodynamic and renal effects of dopexamine and dobutamine in patients with reduced cardiac output following coronary artery bypass grafting. *Chest* 1994;106:835–41.

121. Onorati F, Renzulli A, De Feo M, et al. Perioperative enoximone infusion improves enzyme release after CABG. *J Cardiothorac Vasc Anesth* 2004;18:409–14.

122. Boldt J, Brosch C, Lehmann A, Suttner S, Isgro F. The prophylactic use of the beta-blocker esmolol in combination with phosphodiesterase III inhibitor enoximone in elderly cardiac surgery patients. *Anesth Analg* 2004;99:1009–17.

123. Feldman AM, Oren RM, Abraham WT, et al. Low-dose oral enoximone enhances the ability to wean patients wtih ultra-advanced heart failure from intravenous inotropic support: results of the oral enoximone in intravenous inotrope-dependent subjects trial. *Am Heart J* 2007;154:861–9.

124. Papaioannou TG, Stefanadis C. Basic principles of the intraaortic balloon pump and mechanisms affecting its performance. *ASAIO J* 2005;51:296–300.

125. Santa-Cruz RA, Cohen MG, Ohman EM. Aortic counterpulsation: a review of the hemodynamic effects and indications for use. *Catheter Cardiovasc Interv* 2006;67:68–77.

126. Tremper RS. Intra-aortic balloon pump therapy – a primer for perioperative nurses. *AORN J* 2006;84:34–44.

127. Field ML, Rengarajan A, Khan O, Spyt T, Richens D. Preoperative intra aortic balloon pumps in patients undergoing coronary artery bypass grafting. *Cochrane Database Syst Rev* 2007;1:CD004472.

128. Dyub AM, Whitlock RP, Abouzahr LL, Cinà CS. Preoperative intra-aortic balloon pump in patients undergoing coronary bypass surgery: a systematic review and meta-analysis. *J Card Surg* 2008;23:79–86.

129. Santarpino G, Onorati F, Rubino AS, et al. Preoperative intraaortic balloon pumping improves outcomes for high-risk patients in routine coronary artery bypass graft surgery. *Ann Thorac Surg* 2009;87:481–8.

130. Etienne PY, Papadatos S, Glineur D, et al. Reduced mortality in high-risk coronary patients operated off pump with preoperative intraaortic balloon counterpulsation. *Ann Thorac Surg* 2007;84:498–502.

131. Takami Y, Masumoto H. Effects of intra-aortic balloon pumping on graft flow in coronary surgery: an intraoperative transit-time flowmetric study. *Ann Thorac Surg* 2008;86:823–7.

132. Khir AW, Price S, Henein MY, Parker KH, Pepper JR. Intra-aortic balloon pumping: effects on left ventricular diastolic function. *Eur J Cardiothorac Surg* 2003;24:277–82.

133. Erdogan HB, Goksedef D, Erentug V, et al. In which patients should sheathless IABP be used? An analysis of vascular complications in 1211 cases. *J Card Surg* 2006;21:342–6.

134. Onorati F, Impiombato B, Ferraro A, et al. Transbrachial intraaortic balloon pumping in severe peripheral atherosclerosis. *Ann Thorac Surg* 2007;84:264–6.

135. Marcu CB, Donohue TJ, Ferneini A, Ghantous AE. Intraaortic balloon pump insertion through the subclavian artery. Subclavian artery insertion of IABP. *Heart Lung Circ* 2006;15:148–50.

136. Schreuder JJ, Maisano F, Donelli A, et al. Beat-to-beat effects of intraaortic balloon pump timing on left ventricular performance in patients with low ejection fraction. *Ann Thorac Surg* 2005;79:872–80.

137. Hurlé A, Llamas P, Meseguer J, Casillas JA. Paraplegia complicating intraaortic balloon pumping. *Ann Thorac Surg* 1997;63:1217–8.

138. Arafa OE, Pedersen TH, Svennevig JL, Fosse E, Geiran OR. Vascular complications of the intraaortic balloon pump in patients undergoing open heart operations: a 15-year experience. *Ann Thorac Surg* 1999;67:645–51.

139. Boffa DJ, Tak V, Jansson SL, Ko W, Krishnasastry KV. Atheroemboli to superior mesenteric artery following cardiopulmonary bypass. *Ann Vasc Surg* 2002;16:228–30.

140. Venkateswaran RV, Charman SC, Goddard M, Large SR. Lethal mesenteric ischaemia after cardiopulmonary bypass: a common complication? *Eur J Cardiothorac Surg* 2002;22:534–8.

141. Shimamoto H, Kawazoe K, Kito H, Fujita T, Shimamoto Y. Does juxtamesenteric placement of intra-aortic balloon interrupt superior mesenteric flow? *Clin Cardiol* 1992;15:285–90.

142. Ho AC, Hong CL, Yang MW, Lu PP, Lin PJ. Stroke after intraaortic balloon counterpulsation associated with mobile atheroma in thoracic aorta diagnosed using transesophageal echocardiography. *Chang Gung Med J* 2002;25:612–6.

143. Swartz MT, Sakamoto T, Arai H, et al. Effects of intraaortic balloon position on renal artery blood flow. *Ann Thorac Surg* 1992;53:604–10.

144. Christenson JT, Sierra J, Romand JA, Licker M, Kalangos A. Long intraaortic balloon treatment time leads to more vascular complications. *Asian Cardiovasc Thorac Ann* 2007;15:408–12.

145. Baskett RJF, Ghali WA, Maitland A, Hirsch GM. The intraaortic balloon pump in cardiac surgery. *Ann Thorac Surg* 2002;74:1276–87.

146. Davies AR, Bellomo R, Raman JS, Gutteridge GA, Buxton BF. High lactate predicts the failure of intraaortic balloon pumping after cardiac surgery. *Ann Thorac Surg* 2001;71:1415–20.

147. Stone ME. Current status of mechanical circulatory assistance. *Semin Cardiothorac Vasc Anesth* 2007;11:185–204.

148. Seyfarth M, Sibbing D, Bauer I, et al. A randomized clinical trial to evaluate the safety and efficacy of a percutaneous left ventricular assist device versus intra-aortic balloon pumping for treatment of cardiogenic shock caused by myocardial infarction. *J Am Coll Cardiol* 2008;52:1584–8.

149. Windecker S. Percutaneous left ventricular assist devices for treatment of patients with cardiogenic shock. *Curr Opin Crit Care* 2007;13:521–7.

150. Idelchik GM, Loyalka P, Kar B. Percutaneous ventricular assist device placement during active cardiopulmonary resuscitation for severe refractory cardiogenic shock afer acute myocardial infarction. *Tex Heart Inst J* 2007;34:204–8.

151. Klotz S, Deng MC, Stypmann J, et al. Left ventricular pressure and volume unloading during pulsatile versus nonpulsatile left ventricular assist device support. *Ann Thorac Surg* 2004;77:143–9.

152. Garcia S, Kandar F, Boyle A, et al. Effects of pulsatile- and continuous-flow left ventricular assist devices on left ventricular unloading. *J Heart Lung Transplant* 2008;27:261–7.

153. Samuels LE, Kaufman MS, Thomas MP, Holmes EC, Brockman SK, Wechsler AS. Pharmacological criteria for ventricular assist device insertion following cardiogenic shock: experience witih the Abiomed BVS system. *J Card Surg* 1999;14:288–93.

154. Rao V, Oz MC, Flannery MA, Catanese KA, Argenziano M, Naka Y. Revised screening scale to predict survival after insertion of a left ventricular assist device. *J Thorac Cardiovasc Surg* 2003;125:855–62.

155. Morales DL, Gregg D, Helman DN, et al. Arginine vasopressin in the treatment of 50 patients with postcardiotomy vasodilatory shock. *Ann Thorac Surg* 2002;69:102–6.

156. De Robertis F, Birks EJ, Rogers P, Dreyfus G, Pepper JR, Khaghani A. Clinical performance with the Levitronix Centrimag short-term ventricular assist device. *J Heart Lung Transplant* 2006;25:181–6.

157. Potapov EV, Loforte A, Weng Y, et al. Experience with over 1000 implanted ventricular assist devices. *J Card Surg* 2008;23:185–94.

158. Pal JD, Piacentino V, Cuevas AD, et al. Impact of left ventricular assist device bridging on posttransplant outcomes. *Ann Thorac Surg* 2009;88:1457–61.

159. Marquez TT, D'Cunha J, John R, Liao K, Joyce L. Mechanical support for acute right ventricular failure: evolving survival paradigms. *J Thorac Cardiovasc Surg* 2009;137:e39–40.

160. Klodell CT Jr, Morey TE, Lobato EB, et al. Effect of sildenafil on pulmonary artery pressure, systemic pressure, and nitric oxide utilization in patients with left ventricular assist devices. *Ann Thorac Surg* 2007;83:68–71.

161. Patel ND, Weiss ES, Schaffer J, et al. Right heart dysfunction after left ventricular assist device implantation: a comparison of the pulsatile HeartMate I and axial-flow HeartMate II devices. *Ann Thorac Surg* 2008;86:832–40.

162. Maeder MT, Leet A, Ross A, Esmore D, Kaye DM. Changes in right ventricular function during continuous-flow left ventricular assist device support. *J Heart Lung Transplant* 2009;28:360–6.

163. Kormos RL, Teuteberg JJ, Pagani FD, et al. Right ventricular failure in patients with the HeartMate II continuous-flow left ventricular assist device: incidence, risk factors, and effect on outcomes. *J Thorac Cardiovasc Surg* 2010;139:1316–24.

164. Matthews JC, Koelling TM, Pagani FD, Aaronson KD. The right ventricular failure risk score. A pre-operative tool for assessing the risk of right ventricular failure in left ventricular assist device candidates. *J Am Coll Cardiol* 2008;51:2163–72.

165. Fitzpatrick JR 3rd, Frederick JR, Hsu VM, et al. Risk score derived from pre-operative data analysis predicts the need for biventricular mechanical circulatory support. *J Heart Lung Transplant* 2008;27:1286–92.

166. Zahr F, Ootaki Y, Starling RC, et al. Preoperative risk factors for mortality after biventricular assist device implantation. *J Card Fail* 2008;14:844–9.

167. Schuerer DJE, Kolovos NS, Boyd KV, Coopersmith CM. Extracorporeal membrane oxygenation. Current clinical practice, coding, and reimbursement. *Chest* 2008;134:179–84.

168. Pagani FD, Aaronson KD, Swaniker F, Bartlett RH. The use of extracorporeal life support in adult patients with primary cardiac failure as a bridge to implantable left ventricular assist device. *Ann Thorac Surg* 2001;71(3 suppl):S77–81.

169. Smedira NG, Moazami N, Golding CM, et al. Clinical experience with 202 adult patients receiving extracorporeal membrane oxygenation for cardiac failure: survival at five years. *J Thorac Cardiovasc Surg* 2001;122:92–102.

170. Chen YS, Chao A, Yu HY, et al. Analysis and results of prolonged resuscitation in cardiac arrest patients by extracorporeal membrane oxygenation. *J Am Coll Cardiol* 2003;41:197–203.

171. Bartlett RH. Extracorporeal life support in the management for severe respiratory failure. *Clin Chest Med* 2000;21:555–61.

172. Yap HJ, Chen YC, Fang JT, Huang CC. Combination of continuous renal replacement therapies (CRRT) and extracorporeal membrane oxygenation (ECMO) for advanced cardiac patients. *Ren Fail* 2003;25:183–93.

173. Doll N, Kiaii B, Borger M, et al. Five-year results of 219 consecutive patients treated with extracorporeal membrane oxygenation for refractory postoperative cardiogenic shock. *Ann Thorac Surg* 2004;77:151–7.

174. Bakhtiary G, Keller H, Dogan S, et al. Venoarterial extracorporeal membrane oxygenation for treatment of cardiogenic shock: clinical experiences in 45 adult patients. *J Thorac Cardiovasc Surg* 2008;135:382–8.

175. Luo X, Wang W, Hu SS, et al. Extracorporeal membrane oxygenation for treatment of cardiac failure in adult patients. *Interact Cardiovasc Thorac Surg* 2009;9:296–300.

176. Wang J, Han J, Jia Y, et al. Early and intermediate results of rescue extracorporeal membrane oxygenation in adult cardiogenic shock. *Ann Thorac Surg* 2009;88:1897–904.

177. John R, Liao K, Lietz K, et al. Experience with the Levitronix CentriMag circulatory support system as a bridge to decision in patients with refractory cardiogenic shock and multisystem organ failure. *J Thorac Cardiovasc Surg* 2007;134:351–8.

178. Kamdar F, Boyle A, Liao K, Colvin-Adams M, Joyce L, John R. Effects of centrifugal, axial, and pulsatile left ventricular assist device support on end-organ function in heart failure patients. *J Heart Lung Transplant* 2009;28:352–9.

179. Pagani FD, Miller LW, Russell SD, et al. Extended mechanical circulatory support with a continuous-flow rotary left ventricular assist device. *J Am Coll Cardiol* 2009;54:312–21.

180. Lee MS, Makkar RR. Percutaneous left ventricular support devices. *Cardiol Clin* 2006;24:265–75.

181. Pitsis AA, Visouli AN, Burkhoff D, et al. Feasibility study of a temporary percutaneous left ventricular assist device in cardiac surgery. *Ann Thorac Surg* 2007;84:1993–9.

182. Prutkin JM, Strote JA, Stout KK. Percutaneous right ventricular assist device as support for cardiogenic shock due to right ventricular infarction. *J Invasive Cardiol* 2008;20:E215–6.

183. Gregoric ID, Jacob LP, La Francesca S, et al. The TandemHeart as a bridge to a long-term axial-flow left ventricular assist device (bridge to bridge). *Tex Heart Inst J* 2008;35:125–9.

184. Curtis JJ, McKenney-Knox CA, Wagner-Mann CC. Postcardiotomy centrifugal assist: a single surgeon's experience. *Artif Organs* 2002;26:994–7.

185. Haj-Yahia S, Birks EJ, Amrani M, et al. Bridging patients after salvage from bridge to decision directly to transplant by means of prolonged support with the CentriMag short-term centrifugal pump. *J Thorac Cardiovasc Surg* 2009;138:227–330.

186. Gazzoli F, Alloni A, Pagani F, et al. Arrow CorAide left ventricular assist system: initial experience of the cardio-thoracic surgery center in Pavia. *Ann Thorac Surg* 2007;83:279–82.

187. Samuels LE, Holmes EC, Thomas MP, et al. Management of acute cardiac failure with mechanical assist: experience with the Abiomed BVS 5000. *Ann Thorac Surg* 2001;71(3 suppl):S67–72.

188. Samoukovic G, Rosu C, Gianetti N, Cecere R. The Impella LP 5.0 as a bridge to long-term circulatory support. *Interact Cardiovasc Thorac Surg* 2009;8:682–3.

189. Sassard T, Scalabre A, Bonnefoy E, Sanchez I, Farhat F, Jegaden O. The right axillary artery approach for the Impella Recover LP 5.0 microaxial pump. *Ann Thorac Surg* 2008;85:1468–70.

190. John R, Kamdar F, Liao K, Colvin-Adams M, Boyle A, Joyce L. Improved survival and decreasing incidence of adverse events with the HeartMate II left ventricular assist device as bridge-to-transplant therapy. *Ann Thorac Surg* 2008;86:1227–34.

191. John R. Current axial-flow devices: the HeartMate II and Jarvik 2000 left ventricular assist devices. *Semin Thorac Cardiovasc Surg* 2008;20:264–72.

192. Haj-Yahia S, Birks EJ, Rogers P, et al. Midterm experience with the Jarvik 2000 axial flow left ventricular assist device. *J Thorac Cardiovasc Surg* 2007;134:199–203.

193. Vitali E, Lanfranconi M, Ribera E, et al. Successful experience in bridging patients to heart transplantation with the MicroMed DeBakey ventricular assist device. *Ann Thorac Surg* 2003;75:1200–4.

194. Garatti A, Bruschi G, Colombo T, et al. Clinical outcome and bridge to transplant rate of left ventricular assist device recipient patients: comparison between continuous-flow and pulsatile-flow devices. *Eur J Cardiothorac Surg* 2008;34:275–80.

195. Lietz K, Long JW, Kfoury AG, et al. Outcomes of left ventricular assist device implantation as destination therapy in the post-REMATCH era: implications for patient selection. *Circulation* 2007;116:497–505.

196. Dowling RD, Gray LA Jr, Etoch SW, et al. Initial experience with the AbioCor implantable replacement heart system. *J Thorac Cardiovasc Surg* 2004;127:131–41.

197. Roussel JC, Sénage T, Baron O, et al. CardioWest (Jarvik) total artificial heart: a single-center experience with 42 patients. *Ann Thorac Surg* 2009;87:124–30.

198. Goldstein DJ, Beauford RB. Left ventricular assist devices and bleeding: adding insult to injury. *Ann Thorac Surg* 2003;75(6 suppl):S42–7.

199. Steinlechner B, Dworschak M, Birkenberg B, et al. Platelet dysfunction in outpatients with left ventricular assist devices. *Ann Thorac Surg* 2009;87:131–8.

200. Malani PN, Dyke DB, Pagani FD, Chenoweth CE. Nosocomial infections in left ventricular assist device recipients. *Clin Infect Dis* 2002;34:1295–300.

201. Zierer A, Melby SJ, Voeller RK, et al. Late-onset driveline infections: the Achilles' heel of prolonged left ventricular assist device support. *Ann Thorac Surg* 2007;84:515–21.

202. Morgan JA, Park Y, Oz MC, Naka Y. Device related infections while on left ventricular assist device support do not adversely impact bridging to transplant or posttransplant survival. *ASAIO J* 2003;49:748–50.

203. Oz MC, Rose EA, Slater J, Kuiper JJ, Catanese KA, Levin HR. Malignant ventricular arrhythmias are well tolerated in patients receiving long-term left ventricular assist devices. *J Am Coll Cardiol* 1994;24:1688–91.

204. Shroder JN, Danesthman MA, Villamizar NR, et al. Heparin-induced thrombocytopenia in left ventricular assist device bridge-to-transplant patients. *Ann Thorac Surg* 2007;84:841–6.

205. Koster A, Huebler S, Potapov E, et al. Impact of heparin-induced thrombocytopenia on outcome in patients with ventricular assist device support: single-institution experience in 358 consecutive patients. *Ann Thorac Surg* 2007;83:72–6.

206. John R, Lietz K, Schuster M, et al. Immunologic sensitization in recipients of left ventricular assist devices. *J Thorac Cardiovasc Surg* 2003;125:578–91.

207. Levy J. Management of systemic and pulmonary hypertension. *Tex Heart Inst J* 2005;32:467–71.

208. Cheung AT, Cruz-Shiavone GE, Meng QC, et al. Cardiopulmonary bypass, hemolysis, and nitroprusside-induced cyanide production. *Anesth Analg* 2007;105:29–33.

209. Fremes SE, Weisel RD, Mickle DAG, et al. A comparison of nitroglycerin and nitroprusside: I. Treatment of postoperative hypertension. *Ann Thorac Surg* 1985;39:53–60.

210. Bojar RM, Rastegar H, Payne DD, et al. Methemoglobinemia from intravenous nitroglycerin: a word of caution. *Ann Thorac Surg* 1987;43:332–4.

211. Wijeysundera DN, Beattie WS, Rao V, Karski J. Calcium antagonists reduce cardiovascular complications after cardiac surgery: a meta-analysis. *J Am Coll Cardiol* 2003;41:1496–505.

212. Singla N, Warltier DC, Gandhi SD, et al. Treatment of acute postoperative hypertension in cardiac surgery patients: an efficacy study of clevidipine assessing its postoperative antihypertensive effect in cardiac surgery-2 (ESCAPE-2), a randomized, double-blind, placebo-controlled trial. *Anesth Analg* 2008;107:59–67.

213. Aronson S, Dyke CM, Stierer KA, et al. The ECLIPSE trials: comparative studies of clevidipine to nitroglycerin, sodium nitroprusside, and nicardipine for acute hypertension treatment in cardiac surgery patients. *Anesth Analg* 2008;107:1110–21.

214. Grigore AM, Castro JL, Swistel D, Thys DM. Nicardipine infusion for the prevention of radial artery spasm during myocardial revascularization. *J Cardiothorac Vasc Anesth* 1998;12:556–7.

215. Chanda J, Brichkov I, Canver CC. Prevention of radial artery graft vasospasm after coronary bypass. *Ann Thorac Surg* 2000;70:2070–4.

216. Chanda J, Canver CC. Reversal of preexisting vasospasm in coronary artery conduits. *Ann Thorac Surg* 2001;72:476–80.

217. Apostolidou IA, Despotis GJ, Hogue CW Jr. Antiischemic effects of nicardipine and nitroglycerin after coronary artery bypass grafting. *Ann Thorac Surg* 1999;67:417–22.

218. Sladen RN, Klamerus KJ, Swafford MW, et al. Labetalol for the control of elevated blood pressure following coronary artery bypass grafting. *J Cardiothorac Anesth* 1990;4:210–21.

219. Boldt J, Schindler E, Wollbruck M, Gorlach G, Hempelmann G. Cardiorespiratory response of intravenous angiotensin-converting enzyme inhibitor enalaprilat in hypertensive cardiac surgery patients. *J Cardiothorac Vasc Anesth* 1995;9:44–9.

220. Wagner F, Yeter R, Bisson S, Siniawski H, Hetzer R. Beneficial hemodynamic and renal effects of intravenous enalaprilat following coronary artery bypass surgery complicated by left ventricular dysfunction. *Crit Care Med* 2003;31:1421–8.

221. Gombotz H, Plaza J, Mahla E, Berger J, Metzler H. DA1-receptor stimulation by fenoldopam in the treatment of postcardiac surgical hypertension. *Acta Anaesthesiol Scand* 1998;42:834–40.

222. Yakazu Y, Iwasawa K, Narita H, Kindscher JD, Benson KT, Goto H. Hemodynamic and sympathetic effects of fenoldopam and sodium nitroprusside. *Acta Anaesthesiol Scand* 2001;45:1176–80.

223. Villacorta J, Oddoze C, Giorgi R, et al. Postoperative treatment with angiotensin-converting enzyme inhibitors in patients with preoperative reduced left ventricular systolic function. *J Cardiothorac Vasc Anesth* 2008;22:187–91.

224. Anthi A, Tzelepis GE, Alivizatos P, Michalis A, Palatianos GM, Geroulanos S. Unexpected cardiac arrest after cardiac surgery. Incidence, predisposing causes, and outcome of open chest cardiopulmonary resuscitation. *Chest* 1998;113:15–9.

225. Mackay JH, Powell SJ, Osgathorp J, Rozario CJ. Six-year prospective audit of chest reopening after cardiac arrest. *Eur J Cardiothorac Surg* 2002;22:421–5.

226. Ngaage DL, Cowen ME. Survival of cardiorespiratory arrest after coronary artery bypass grafting or aortic valve surgery. *Ann Thorac Surg* 2009;88:64–8.

227. 2005 American Heart Association guidelines for cardiopulmonary resuscitation and cardiovascular care. *Circulation* 2005;112(24 suppl):IV-1–IV-88. or at www.americanheart.org/cpr.

228. Dunning J, Fabbri A, Kolh PH, et al. Guideline for resuscitation in cardiac arrest after cardiac surgery. *Eur J Cardiothorac Surg* 2009;36:3–28.

229. Twomey D, Das M, Subramanian H, Dunning J. Is internal massage superior to external massage for patients suffering a cardiac arrest after cardiac surgery? *Interact Cardiovasc Thorac Surg* 2008;7:151–7.

230. Aung K, Htay T. Vasopressin for cardiac arrest: a systematic review and meta-analysis. *Arch Intern Med* 2005;165:17–24.

231. Jain U. Myocardial infarction during coronary artery bypass surgery. *J Cardiothorac Vasc Anesth* 1992;6:612–23.

232. Adabag AS, Rector T, Mithani S, et al. Prognostic significance of elevated troponin I after heart surgery. *Ann Thorac Surg* 2007;83:1744–50.

233. Paparella D, Cappabianca G, Visicchio G, et al. Cardiac troponin I release after coronary artery bypass grafting operation: effects on operative and midterm survival. *Ann Thorac Surg* 2005;80:1758–64.

234. Fellahi JL, Hedoire F, Le Manach Y, Monier E, Guillou L, Riou B. Determination of the threshold of cardiac troponin I associated with an adverse postoperative outcome after cardiac surgery: a comparative study between coronary artery bypass graft, valve surgery, and combined cardiac surgery. *Crit Care* 2007;11:R106.

235. Riedel BJ, Grattan A, Martin CB, Gal J, Shaw AD, Royston D. Long-term outcome of patients with perioperative myocardial infarction as diagnosed by troponin I after routine surgical coronary artery revascularization. *J Cardiothorac Vasc Anesth* 2006;20:781–7.

236. Croal BL, Hillis GS, Gibson PH, et al. Relationship between postoperative cardiac troponin I levels and outcome of cardiac surgery. *Circulation* 2006;114:1468–75.

237. Ramsay J, Shernan S, Fitch J, et al. Increased creatine kinase MB level predicts postoperative mortality after cardiac surgery independent of new Q waves. *J Thorac Cardiovasc Surg* 2005;129:300–6.

238. Engoren MC, Habib RH, Zacharias A, et al. The association of elevated creatinine kinase-myocardial band on mortality after coronary artery bypass grafting is time and magnitude limited. *Eur J Cardiothorac Surg* 2005;28:114–9.

239. Bignami E, Landoni G, Crescenzi G, et al. Role of cardiac biomarkers (troponin I and CK-MB) as predictors of quality of life and long-term outcome after cardiac surgery. *Ann Card Anaesth* 2009;12:22–6.

240. Petäjä L, Salmenperä M, Pulkki K, Pettilä V. Biochemical injury markers and mortality after coronary artery bypass grafting: a systematic review. *Ann Thorac Surg* 2009;87:1981–92.

241. Gavard JA, Chaitman BR, Sakai S, et al. Prognostic significance of elevated creatine kinase MB after coronary bypass surgery and after an acute coronary syndrome: results from the GUARDIAN trial. *J Thorac Cardiovasc Surg* 2003;126:807–13.

242. Svedjeholm R, Dahlin LG, Lundberg G, et al. Are electrocardiographic Q-wave criteria reliable for diagnosis of perioperative myocardial infarction after coronary surgery? *Eur J Cardiothorac Surg* 1998;13:655–61.

243. Chowdhury UK, Malik V, Yadav R, et al. Myocardial injury in coronary artery bypass grafting: on-pump versus off-pump comparison by measuring high-sensitivity C-reactive protein, cardiac troponin I, heart-type fatty acid-binding protein, creatine kinase-MB, and myoglobin release. *J Thorac Cardiovasc Surg* 2008;135:1110–9.

244. Alyanakian MA, Dehoux M, Chatel D, et al. Cardiac troponin I in diagnosis of perioperative myocardial infarction after cardiac surgery. *J Cardiothorac Vasc Anesth* 1998;12:288–94.

245. Vermes E, Mesguich M, Houel R, et al. Cardiac troponin I release after open heart surgery: a marker of myocardial protection? *Ann Thorac Surg* 2000;70:2087–90.

246. Thygesen K, Alpert JS, White HD on behalf of the Joint ESC/ACCF/AHA/AHF task force for the redefinition of myocardial infarction. *Circulation* 2007;116:2634–53 and *J Am Coll Cardiol* 2007;50:2173–95.

247. Steuer J, Horte LG, Lindahl B, Stahle E. Impact of perioperative myocardial injury on early and long-term outcome after coronary artery bypass grafting. *Eur Heart J* 2002;23:1219–27.

248. Force T, Hibberd P, Weeks G, et al. Perioperative myocardial infarction after coronary artery bypass surgery. Clinical significance and approach to risk stratification. *Circulation* 1990;82:903–12.

249. Guo LR, Myers ML, Kuntz EL. Coronary artery spasm: a rare but important cause of postoperative myocardial infarction. *Ann Thorac Surg* 2008;86:994–5.

250. Harskamp RE, McNeil JD, van Ginkel MW, Bastos RB, Baisden CE, Calhoon JH. Postoperative internal thoracic artery spasm after coronary artery bypass grafting. *Ann Thorac Surg* 2008;85:647–9.

251. Minato NM, Katayama Y, Sakaguchi M, Itoh M. Perioperative coronary artery spasm in off-pump coronary artery bypass grafting and its possible relationship with perioperative hypomagnesemia. *Ann Thorac Cardiovasc Surg* 2006;12:32–6.

252. Havrilla PL, Kane-Gill SL, Verrico MM, Seybert AL, Reis SE. Coronary vasospasm and atrial fibrillation associated with ondansetron therapy. *Ann Pharmacother* 2009;43:532–6.

253. Yasue H, Mizuno Y, Harada E, et al. Effects of a 3-hydroxy-3-methylglutaryl coenzyme A reductase inhibitor, fluvastatin, on coronary spasm after withdrawal of calcium-channel blockers. *J Am Coll Cardiol* 2008;51:1742–8.

254. Bethea BT, Salazar JD, Grega MA, et al. Determining the utility of temporary pacing wires after coronary artery bypass surgery. *Ann Thorac Surg* 2005;79:104–7.

255. Broka SM, Ducart AR, Collard EL, et al. Hemodynamic benefit of optimizing atrioventricular delay after cardiopulmonary bypass. *J Cardiothorac Vasc Anesth* 1997;11:723–8.

256. Atlee JL III, Pattison CZ, Mathews EL, Hedman AG. Transesophageal atrial pacing for intraoperative sinus bradycardia or AV junctional rhythm: feasibility as prophylaxis in 200 anesthetized adults and hemodynamic effects of treatment. *J Cardiothorac Vasc Anesth* 1993;7:436–41.

257. Cook DJ, Bailon JM, Douglas TT, et al. Changing incidence, type, and natural history of conduction defects after coronary artery bypass grafting. *Ann Thorac Surg* 2005;80:1732–7.

258. Thomas JL, Dickstein RA, Parker FB Jr, et al. Prognostic significance of the development of left bundle conduction defects following aortic valve replacement. *J Thorac Cardiovasc Surg* 1982;84:382–6.

259. Lukac P, Hjortdal VE, Pedersen AK, Mortensen PT, Jensen HK, Hansen PS. Superior transseptal approach to mitral valve is associated with a higher need for pacemaker implantation than the left atrial approach. *Ann Thorac Surg* 2007;83:77–82.

260. Elahi MM, Lee D, Dhannapuneni RRV. Predictors of permanent pacemaker implantation during the early postoperative period after valve surgery. *Tex Heart Inst J* 2006;33:455–7.

261. Gordon RS, Ivanov J, Cohen G, Ralph-Edwards AL. Permanent cardiac pacing after a cardiac operation: predicting the use of permanent pacemakers. *Ann Thorac Surg* 1998;66:1698–704.

262. Glikson M, Dearani JA, Hyberger LK, Schaff HV, Hammill SC, Hayes DL. Indications, effectiveness, and long-term dependency in permanent pacing after cardiac surgery. *Am J Cardiol* 1997;80:1309–13.

263. Dawkins S, Hobson AR, Kalra PR, Tang ATM, Monro JL, Dawkins KD. Permanent pacemaker implantation after isolated aortic valve replacement: incidence, indications, and predictors. *Ann Thorac Surg* 2008;85:108–12.

264. Anselmi A, Possati G, Gaudino M. Postoperative inflammatory reaction and atrial fibrillation: simple correlation or causation? *Ann Thorac Surg* 2009;88:326–33.

265. Mathew JP, Fontes ML, Tudor TC, et al. A multicenter risk index for atrial fibrillation after cardiac surgery. *JAMA* 2004;291:1720–9.

266. Fuster V, Rydén LE, Cannom DS, et al. ACC/AHA/ESC 2006 guidelines for the management of patients with atrial fibrillation: a report of the American College of Cardiology/American Heart Association Task Force on Practice Guidelines and the European Society of Cardiology Committee for Practice Guidelines (Writing committee to review the 2001 guidelines for the management of patients with atrial fibrillation) developed in collaboration with the European Heart Rhythm Association and the Heart Rhythm Society. *J Am Coll Cardiol* 2006;48:e149–246.

267. Salamon T, Michler RE, Knott KM, Brown DA. Off-pump coronary artery bypass grafting does not decrease the incidence of atrial fibrillation. *Ann Thorac Surg* 2003;75:505–7.

268. Wijeysundera DN, Beattie WS, Djaiani G, et al. Off-pump coronary artery surgery for reducing mortality and morbidity: meta-analysis of randomized and observational studies. *J Am Coll Cardiol* 2005;46:872–82.

269. Biancari F, Mahar MAA. Meta-analysis of randomized trials on the efficacy of posterior pericardiotomy in preventing atrial fibrillation after coronary artery bypass surgery. *J Thorac Cardiovasc Surg* 2010;139:1158–61.

270. Bradley D, Creswell LL, Hogue CW Jr, et al. Pharmacologic prophylaxis: American College of Chest Physicians guidelines for the prevention and management of postoperative atrial fibrillation after cardiac surgery. *Chest* 2005;128(2suppl):39S–47S.

271. Burgess DC, Kilborn MJ, Keech AC, et al. Interventions for prevention of post-operative atrial fibrillation and its complications after cardiac surgery: a meta-analysis. *Eur Heart J* 2006;27:2846–57.

272. Crystal E, Garfinkle MS, Connolly SS, et al. Interventions for preventing post-operative atrial fibrillation in patients undergoing heart surgery. *Cochrane Database Syst Rev* 2004;4:CD003611.

273. Khanderia U, Wagner D, Walker PC, Woodcock B, Prager R. Amiodarone for atrial fibrillation following cardiac surgery: development of clinical practice guidelines at a university hospital. *Clin Cardiol* 2008;31:6–10.

274. Haghjoo M, Saravi M, Hasemi MJ, et al. Optimal beta-blocker for prevention of atrial fibrillation after on-pump coronary artery bypass graft surgery: carvedilol versus metoprolol. *Heart Rhythm* 2007;4:1170–4.

275. Acikel S, Bozbas H, Gultekin B, et al. Comparison of the efficacy of metoprolol and carvedilol for preventing atrial fibrillation after coronary bypass surgery. *Int J Cardiol* 2008;126:108–13.

276. Kamei M, Morita S, Hayashi Y, Kanmura Y, Kuro M. Carvedilol versus metoprolol for the prevention of atrial fibrillation after off-pump coronary bypass surgery: rationale and design of the Carvedilol or Metoprolol Post-Revascularization Atrial Fibrillation Controlled Trial (COMPACT). *Cardiovasc Drugs Ther* 2006;20:219–27.

277. Aasbo JD, Lawrence AT, Krishnan K, Kim MH, Trohman RG. Amiodarone prophylaxis reduces major cardiovascular morbidity and length of stay after cardiac surgery: a meta-analysis. *Ann Intern Med* 2005;143:327–36.

278. Mitchell LB, Exner DV, Wyse G, et al. Prophylactic oral amiodarone for the prevention of arrhythmias that begin early after revascularization, valve replacement, or repair: PAPABEAR: a randomized controlled trial. *JAMA* 2005;294:3093–100.

279. DiDomenico RJ, Massad MG. Pharmacologic strategies for prevention of atrial fibrillation after open heart surgery. *Ann Thorac Surg* 2005;79:728–40.

280. Beaulieu Y, Denault AY, Couture P, et al. Perioperative intravenous amiodarone does not reduce the burden of atrial fibrillation in patients undergoing cardiac valvular surgery. *Anesthesiology* 2010;112:128–37.

281. Kuralay E, Cingöz F, Kiliç S, et al. Supraventricular tachyarrhythmia prophylaxis after coronary artery surgery in chronic obstructive pulmonary disease patients (early amiodarone prophylaxis trial). *Eur J Cardiothorac Surg* 2004;25:224–30.

282. Kaushik S, Hussain A, Clarke P, Lazar HL. Acute pulmonary toxicity after low-dose amiodarone therapy. *Ann Thorac Surg* 2001;72:1760–1.

283. Izhar U, Ad N, Rudis E, When should we discontinue antiarrhythmic therapy for atrial fibrillation after coronary artery bypass grafting? A prospective randomized study. *J Thorac Cardiovasc Surg* 2005;129:401–6.

284. Singh D, Cingolani E, Diamond GA, Kaul S. Dronedarone for atrial fibrillation. Have we expanded the antiarrhythmic armamentarium? *J Am Coll Cardiol* 2010;55:1569–76.

285. Wurdeman RL, Mooss AN, Mohiuddin SM, Lenz TL. Amiodarone vs. sotalol as prophylaxis against atrial fibrillation/flutter after heart surgery. A meta-analysis. *Chest* 2002;121:1203–10.

286. Shiga T, Wajima Z, Inoue T, Ogawa R. Magnesium prophylaxis for arrhythmias after cardiac surgery: a meta-analysis of randomized controlled trials. *Am J Med* 2004;117:325–33.

287. Shepherd J, Jones J, Frampton GK, Tanajewski L, Turner D, Price A. Intravenous magnesium sulphate and sotalol for prevention of atrial fibrillation after coronary artery bypass surgery: a systematic review and economic evaluation. *Health Technol Assess* 2008;12:iii–iv, ix–95.

288. Forlani S, De Paulis R, de Notaris S, et al. Combination of sotalol and magnesium prevents atrial fibrillation after coronary artery bypass grafting. *Ann Thorac Surg* 2002;74:720–6.

289. Behmanesh S, Tossios P, Homedan H, et al. Effect of prophylactic bisoprolol plus magnesium on the incidence of atrial fibrillation after coronary bypass surgery: results of a randomized controlled trial. *Curr Med Res Opin* 2006;22:1443–50.

290. Chung MK, Augostini RS, Asher CR, et al. Ineffectiveness and potential proarrhythmia of atrial pacing for atrial fibrillation prevention after coronary artery bypass grafting. *Ann Thorac Surg* 2000;69:1057–63.

291. Archbold RA, Schilling RJ. Atrial pacing for the prevention of atrial fibrillation after coronary artery bypass graft surgery: a review of the literature. *Heart* 2004;90:129–33.

292. Debrunner M, Naegeli B, Genoni M, Turina M, Bertel O. Prevention of atrial fibrillation after cardiac valvular surgery by epicardial, biatrial synchronous pacing. *Eur J Cardiothorac Surg* 2004;25:16–20.

293. Seraminovski N, Burke P, Khawaja O, Sekulic M, Machado C. Usefulness of dofetilide for the prevention of atrial tachyarrhythmias (atrial fibrillation or flutter) after coronary artery bypass grafting. *Am J Cardiol* 2008;101:1574–9.

294. Merrick AF, Odom NJ, Keenan DJ, Grotte GJ. Comparison of propafenone to atenolol for the prophylaxis of postcardiotomy supraventricular tachyarrhythmias: a prospective trial. *Eur J Cardiothorac Surg* 1995;9:146–9.

295. Halonen J, Halonon P, Järvinen O, et al. Corticosteroids for the prevention of atrial fibrillation after cardiac surgery. A randomized controlled trial. *JAMA* 2007;297:1562–7.

296. Prasongsukarn K, Abel JG, Jamieson WR, et al. The effects of steroids on the occurrence of postoperative atrial fibrillation after coronary artery bypass grafting surgery: a prospective randomized trial. *J Thorac Cardiovasc Surg* 2005;130:93–8.

297. Kouliouros A, De Souza A, Roberts N, et al. Dose-related effect of statins on atrial fibrillation after cardiac surgery. *Ann Thorac Surg* 2008;85:1515–2.

298. Liakokpoulos OJ, Choi YH, Kuhn EW, et al. Statins for prevention of atrial fibrillation after cardiac surgery: a systematic literature review. *J Thorac Cardiovasc Surg* 2009;138:678–86.

299. Eslami M, Badkoubeh RS, Mousavi M, et al. Oral ascorbic acid in combination with beta-blockers is more effective than beta-blockers alone in the prevention of atrial fibrillation after coronary artery bypass grafting. *Tex Heart Inst J* 2007;34:268–74.

300. Calò L, Bianconi L, Colivicchi F, et al. N-3 fatty acids for the prevention of atrial fibrillation after coronary bypass surgery: a randomized controlled trial. *J Am Coll Cardiol* 2005;45:1723–8.

301. The atrial fibrillation follow-up investigation of rhythm management (AFFIRM) investigators. A comparison of rate control and rhythm control in patients with atrial fibrillation. *N Engl J Med* 2003;347:1825–33.

302. Chung MK, Shemanski L, Sherman DG, et al. Functional status in rate- versus rhythm-control stategies for atrial fibrillation: results of the Atrial Fibrillation Follow-up Investigation of Rhythm Management (AFFIRM) functional status substudy. *J Am Coll Cardiol* 2005;46:1891–9.

303. Samuels LE, Holmes EC, Samuels FL. Selective use of amiodarone and early cardioversion for postoperative atrial fibrillation. *Ann Thorac Surg* 2005;79:113–6.

304. Klein AL, Grimm RA, Murray RD, et al. Use of transesophageal echocardiography to guide cardioversion in patients with atrial fibrillation. *N Engl J Med* 2001;344:1411–20.

305. Black IW, Fatkin D, Sagar KB, et al. Exclusion of atrial thrombus by transesophageal echocardiography does not preclude embolism after cardioversion of atrial fibrillation. A multicenter study. *Circulation* 1994;89:2509–13.

306. Harjai KJ, Mobarek SK, Cheirif J, Boulos LM, Murgo JP, Abi-Samra F. Clinical variables affecting recovery of left atrial mechanical function after cardioversion from atrial fibrillation. *J Am Coll Cardiol* 1997;30:481–6.

307. Stambler BS, Wood MA, Ellenbogen KA. Comparative efficacy of intravenous ibutilide versus procainamide for enhancing termination of atrial flutter by atrial overdrive pacing. *Am J Cardiol* 1996;77:960–6.

308. D'Este D, Bertaglia E, Mantovan R, Zanocco Z, Franceschi M, Pascotto P. Efficacy of intravenous propafenone in termination of atrial flutter by overdrive transesophageal pacing previously ineffective. *Am J Cardiol* 1997;79:500–2.

309. Soucier RJ, Mirza S, Abordo MG, et al. Predictors of conversion of atrial fibrillation after cardiac operations in the absence of class I or III antiarrhythmic medications. *Ann Thorac Surg* 2001;72:694–8.

310. Lahtinen J, Biancari F, Salmela E, et al. Postoperative atrial fibrillation is a major cause of stroke after on-pump coronary artery bypass surgery. *Ann Thorac Surg* 2004;77:1241–4.

311. Stoddard MF, Dawkins PR, Prince CR, Ammash NM. Left atrial appendage thrombus is not uncommon in patients with acute atrial fibrillation and a recent embolic event: a transesophageal echocardiographic study. *J Am Coll Cardiol* 1995;25:452–9.

312. Singer DE, Alerts GW, Dalen JE, et al. Antithrombotic therapy in atrial fibrillation: American College of Chest Physicians evidence-based clinical practice guidelines (8th edition). *Chest* 2008;133:546S–92S.

313. Gullestad L, Birkeland K, Molstad P, Hoyer MM, Vanberg P, Kjekshus J. The effect of magnesium versus verapamil on supraventricular arrhythmias. *Clin Cardiol* 1993;16:429–34.

314. Hilleman DE, Reyes AP, Mooss AN, Packard KA. Esmolol versus diltiazem in atrial fibrillation following coronary artery bypass graft surgery. *Curr Med Res Opin* 2003;19:376–82.

315. Boriani G, Capucci A, Lenzi T, Sanguinetti M, Magnani B. Propafenone for conversion of recent-onset atrial fibrillation. A controlled comparison between oral loading dose and intravenous administration. *Chest* 1995;108:355–8.

316. VanderLugt KT, Mattioni T, Denker S, et al. Efficacy and safety of ibutilide fumarate for the conversion of atrial arrhythmias after cardiac surgery. *Circulation* 1999;100:369–75.

317. Bernard EO, Schmid ER, Schmidlin D, Scharf C, Candinas R, Germann R. Ibutilide versus amiodarone in atrial fibrillation: a double-blinded, randomized study. *Crit Care Med* 2003;31:1031–4.

318. Lindeboom JE, Kingma JH, Crijns HJGM, Dunselman PHJM. Efficacy and safety of intravenous dofetilide for rapid termination of atrial fibrillation and flutter. *Am J Cardiol* 2000;85:1031–3.

319. Coleman CI, Sood N, Chawla D, et al. Intravenous magnesium sulfate enhances the ability of dofetilide to successfully cardiovert atrial fibrillation or flutter: results of the Dofetilide and Intravenous Magnesium Evaluation. *Europace* 2009;11:892–5.

320. Kowey PR, Dorian P, Mitchell LB, et al. Vernakalant hydrochloride for the rapid conversion of atrial fibrillation after cardiac surgery: a randomized, double-blind placebo-controlled trial. *Circ Arrhythm Electrophysiol* 2009;2:652–9.

321. Patel AN, Hamman BL, Patel AN, et al. Epicardial atrial defibrillation: successful treatment of postoperative atrial fibrillation. *Ann Thorac Surg* 2004;77:831–7.

322. Wilbur SL, Marchlinski FE. Adenosine as an antiarrhythmic agent. *Am J Cardiol* 1997;79(12A):30–7.

323. Dougherty AH, Jackman WM, Naccarelli GV, Friday KJ, Dias VC, for the IV Diltiazem Study group. Acute conversion of paroxysmal supraventricular tachycardia with intravenous diltiazem. *Am J Cardiol* 1992;70:587–92.

324. England MR, Gordon G, Salem M, Chernow B. Magnesium administration and dysrhythmias after cardiac surgery. A placebo-controlled, double-blind, randomized trial. *JAMA* 1992;268:2395–402.

325. Johnson RG, Goldberger AL, Thurer RL, Schwartz M, Sirois C, Weintraub RM. Lidocaine prophylaxis in coronary revascularization patients: a randomized, prospective trial. *Ann Thorac Surg* 1993;55:1180–4.

326. Steinberg JS, Gaur A, Sciacca R, Tan E. New-onset sustained ventricular tachycardia after cardiac surgery. *Circulation* 1999;99:903–8.

327. Ascione R, Reeves BC, Santo K, Khan N, Angelini GD. Predictors of new malignant ventricular arrhythmias after coronary surgery. A case-control study. *J Am Coll Cardiol* 2004;43:1630–8.

328. Yeung-Lai-Wah JA, Qi A, McNeill E, et al. New-onset sustained ventricular tachycardia and fibrillation early after cardiac operations. *Ann Thorac Surg* 2004;77:2083–8.

329. Azar RR, Berns E, Seecharran B, Veronneau J, Lippman N, Kluger J. De novo monomorphic and polymorphic ventricular tachycardia following coronary artery bypass grafting. *Am J Cardiol* 1997;80:76–8.

330. Saxon LA, Wiener I, Natterson PD, Laks H, Drinkwater D, Stevenson WG. Monomorphic versus polymorphic ventricular tachycardia after coronary artery bypass grafting. *Am J Cardiol* 1995;75:403–5.

331. Sharma ND, Rosman HS, Padhi ID, Tisdale JE. Torsades de pointes associated with intravenous haloperidol in critically ill patients. *Am J Cardiol* 1998;81:238–40.

332. Lamas GA, Antman EM, Gold JP, Braunwald NS, Collins JJ. Pacemaker backup-mode reversion and injury during cardiac surgery. *Ann Thorac Surg* 1986;41:155–7.

333. Pinto RP, Romerill DB, Nasser WK, Schier JJ, Surawicz B. Prognosis of patients with frequent premature ventricular complexes and nonsustained ventricular tachycardia after coronary artery bypass surgery. *Clin Cardiol* 1996;19:321–4.

334. Tung R, Zimetbaum P, Josephson ME. A critical appraisal of implantable cardioverter-defibrillator therapy for the prevention of sudden cardiac death. *J Am Coll Cardiol* 2008;52:111–21.

335. Epstein AE, DiMarco JP, Ellenbogen KA, et al. ACC/AHA/HRS 2008 guidelines for device-based therapy of cardiac rhythm abnormalities: executive summary. A report of the American College of Cardiology/American Heart Association task force on practice guidelines (Writing committee to revise the ACC/AHA/NASPE 2002 guideline update for implantation of cardiac pacemakers and antiarrhythmia devices). *J Am Coll Cardiol* 2008;51:2085–105. (available at acc.org)

336. Roden DM. A practical approach to torsade de pointes. *Clin Cardiol* 1997;20:285–90.

337. Laub GW, Muralidharan S, Janeira L, et al. Refractory postoperative torsades de pointes syndrome successfully treated with isoproterenol. *J Cardiothorac Vasc Anesth* 1993;7:210–2.

338. Piga M, Serra A, Boi F, Tanda ML, Martino E, Mariotti S. Amiodarone-induced thyrotoxicosis. A review. *Minerva Endocrinol* 2008;33:213–28.

339. Bhatia SJS, Smith TW. Digitalis toxicity: mechanisms, diagnosis, and management. *J Cardiac Surg* 1987;2:453–65.

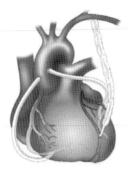

CHAPTER 12

Fluid Management, Renal, Metabolic, and Endocrine Problems

12 Fluid Management, Renal, Metabolic, and Endocrine Problems

Perioperative renal dysfunction is a major determinant of both operative and long-term mortality following cardiac surgery.[1-8] Even patients with mild renal dysfunction prior to surgery are more likely to experience acute kidney injury (AKI) afterwards with a compromised short- and long-term outcome.[9-14] Therefore, it is essential to identify patients at high risk for developing postoperative AKI who may benefit from specific interventions aimed at optimizing renal function. These must be considered during cardiac catheterization procedures, during surgery, and in the postoperative period, and include judicious fluid management, appropriate hemodynamic support, and use of adjunctive pharmacologic measures. Early aggressive use of renal replacement therapy may prove beneficial to patients with deteriorating renal function, and may reduce the high mortality associated with postoperative AKI.

A basic understanding of body water distribution, awareness of the factors that influence renal function and raise the risk of renal dysfunction, steps that can be taken to optimize renal perfusion, and early identification and treatment of incipient or established AKI are essential to optimize surgical outcomes.

I. Body Water Distribution

Approximately 60% of the body weight (50% in women) is water, with two-thirds of this residing in the intracellular space and one-third in the extracellular space. In the latter, two-thirds is in the interstitial space (the so-called "third space"), and one-third constitutes the intravascular volume.

  A. Water moves freely among all three compartments and shifts so as to normalize serum osmolality (which generally reflects the serum sodium concentration).

  B. Sodium moves freely between the intravascular and interstitial spaces but does not move passively into cells. Therefore, if a patient receives a hypotonic sodium load (e.g., 0.45% saline) which would lower the serum osmolality and sodium concentration, water will move from the extracellular space into the intracellular space to normalize these values. The presence of **a low serum sodium concentration in the postoperative patient usually indicates total body water overload.**

  C. Starling's law governs the influence of hydrostatic and oncotic pressures on fluid shifts. The primary determinant of oncotic pressure is serum protein, which remains within the intravascular space. Elevated hydrostatic pressure (e.g., increased pulmonary capillary wedge pressure, PCWP) or lower intravascular colloid oncotic pressure (e.g., low serum

Manual of Perioperative Care in Adult Cardiac Surgery, 5th Edition. By Robert M. Bojar.
Published 2011 by Blackwell Publishing Ltd.

albumin) will shift fluid from the intravascular space into the interstitial space, contributing to lung and tissue edema. Conversely, raising the intravascular oncotic pressure with colloid (e.g., 25% albumin) will tend to draw fluid from the lung interstitium back into the intravascular space.

D. It should be kept in mind that Starling's law describes fluid shifts in the absence of abnormalities in membrane integrity. However, extracorporeal circulation is associated with a "systemic inflammatory response", marked by increased membrane permeability and a transient capillary leak. When this leak is present, administered fluid will shift more readily into the interstitial space. Clinically, one may note impaired oxygenation and decreased pulmonary compliance (higher peak pressures on the ventilator) associated with increased extravascular lung water. This can produce the picture of noncardiogenic pulmonary edema. Expansion of the interstitial space and hyponatremia may also contribute to cerebral edema (mental obtundation), hepatic congestion (jaundice), and splanchnic congestion (ileus).

II. Effects of CPB and Off-Pump Surgery on Renal Function

A. Use of extracorporeal circulation (ECC) is associated with subtle effects on renal function with an increase in virtually all kidney-specific proteins that are markers for tubular damage.[15] Some of these, such as neutrophil gelatinase-associated lipocalin (NGAL), cystatin C, kidney injury molecule 1 (KIM-1), and interleukin-18 (IL-18), have been shown to be early biomarkers of AKI that correlate with the severity and duration of AKI.[15-18] However, very few centers routinely evaluate renal function other than by serum creatinine levels, and in the vast majority of cases, there is little significance to subtle changes in tubular function as long as the kidneys produce a satisfactory urine output with or without diuretics with minimal change in the serum creatinine.

B. The influence of extracorporeal circulation on renal function is multifactorial.[19] ECC involves nonpulsatile perfusion with hemodilution and variable degrees of hypothermia. It produces elevated levels of hormones that affect vascular tone, renal blood flow (RBF), glomerular filtration rate (GFR), filtration fraction, and electrolyte balance. It also evokes an inflammatory response with activation of complement and neutrophils, release of cytokines, and production of oxygen free radicals. Thus, there are a number of factors that influence renal function, including those that influence renal blood flow and trigger renal ischemia, and tubular insults associated with the inflammatory response. In general, ECC is accompanied by an increase in GFR and RBF with increased osmolar clearance and fractional excretion of sodium and potassium.[20]

1. Cardiopulmonary bypass (CPB) results in activation of the renin–aldosterone system (promoting sodium retention and potassium excretion), with elevation of angiotensin II levels (increasing renal vasoconstriction and sodium retention). It also activates the sympathoadrenal axis, elevating levels of epinephrine and norepinephrine (increasing systemic resistance), plasma free cortisol after bypass (promoting sodium retention and potassium excretion), and vasopressin levels (increasing renal vascular resistance). Release of vasodilatory mediators, including nitric oxide and prostacyclin, transiently impairs solute reabsorption. Other vasoactive substances released during CPB include complement, kallikrein, and bradykinin, which alter vascular tone and contribute to the generalized inflammatory response that increases capillary permeability.[21]

2. **Hypothermia** decreases renal cortical blood flow by producing vasoconstriction. It also decreases GFR slightly, decreases renal tubular function, and reduces free water and osmolar clearance. These effects are offset to some degree by hemodilution. During the phase of rewarming, vasodilation and hyperemia of tissue beds result in "third spacing" of fluid. Hypothermia may also cause hypokalemia due to a transcellular shift.

3. **Hemodilution** with a crystalloid prime reduces plasma oncotic pressure, promoting movement of fluid from the intravascular space into the interstitial space. A reduction in viscosity increases outer renal cortical blood flow, leading to an increase in urine output, free water clearance, and sodium and potassium excretion. However, a lower viscosity will reduce systemic blood pressure. A low hematocrit on pump (<21% in some studies and <24% in others) has been associated with an increased incidence of renal dysfunction, although this can be mitigated by increasing pump flow to increase oxygen delivery.[22-26]

4. **Medications.** Preoperative medications, including amiodarone, angiotensin-converting enzyme (ACE) inhibitors, angiotensin receptor blockers (ARBs), and calcium channel blockers, as well as drugs used during surgery, including nitroglycerin, inhalational anesthetics, narcotics, and anxiolytics, can produce significant vasodilation, which lowers the blood pressure and increases fluid requirements. It is generally recommended that ACE inhibitors and ARBs be withheld the day before and the morning of surgery to minimize their hypotensive effects during bypass, which could exacerbate kidney injury by lowering GFR. Furthermore, use of ACE inhibitors may attenuate the effects of norepinephrine.[21] However, studies have shown differing effects on the incidence of AKI, with evidence of both higher and lower risks of AKI in patients taking ACE inhibitors prior to surgery.[27,28]

C. The potential benefit of off-pump coronary bypass surgery (OPCAB) in reducing the risk of postoperative renal dysfunction by avoidance of CPB is controversial.

1. Although a few studies have shown benefits in patients with normal renal function,[29,30] and one showed benefits in diabetic patients with non-dialysis-dependent renal insufficiency,[31] most studies have been unable to demonstrate a benefit in patients with either normal or abnormal renal function.[32-35]

2. In theory, avoidance of CPB might preserve renal blood flow and glomerular function better by maintaining a higher systemic pressure. It may preserve tubular epithelial function because of decreased complement activation and a lessened inflammatory response. However, off-pump surgery is associated with significant fluid administration, use of comparable anesthetic and vasoactive medications, cytokine release that can damage proximal tubules, and alterations in perfusion pressure (lower systemic pressures with elevated venous pressures during exposure of the posterior heart and lower systemic pressures during construction of proximal anastomoses), all of which can adversely affect renal function.

3. Because postoperative renal dysfunction is related more to preexisting renal disease or significant hemodynamic alterations than to the inflammatory response, particular attention to fluid and hemodynamic management remains paramount no matter whether CPB is used or not.

III. Routine Fluid Management in the Early Postoperative Period

A. Hemodilution on CPB produces a state of total body sodium and water overload, expanding the body weight by about 5% (estimated at 800 mL/m²/h, but quite variable in amount). Cardiac filling pressures usually do not reflect this state of fluid overload because of a capillary leak from the systemic inflammatory response, decreased plasma colloid osmotic pressure, impaired myocardial relaxation (diastolic dysfunction) from ischemia/reperfusion after cardioplegic arrest, and vasodilation. Low filling pressures are consistent with hypovolemia despite the presence of body water overload, and additional fluid administration may be necessary to maintain satisfactory hemo-dynamics. High filling pressures may also be noted in the presence of hypovolemia, especially in patients with diastolic dysfunction, and additional fluid administration may be necessary in that situation as well.

B. This fluid requirement occurs at a time when urine output may be high or marginal (<1 mL/kg/h). During the first 4–6 hours after surgery, cardiac output is often depressed, and the achievement of satisfactory hemodynamics is dependent on both preload and inotropic support. Thus, fluid must invariably be administered to maintain intravascular volume and cardiac hemodynamics at the expense of expansion of the interstitial space. It should be noted that early extubation is helpful in reducing fluid requirements because it eliminates the adverse effects of positive-pressure ventilation on venous return and ventricular function.

C. It can be difficult to decide which fluid to administer to maintain filling pressures. Clearly, any fluid infused during a period of altered capillary membrane integrity will expand the interstitial space, but those that can more effectively expand the intravas-cular space while minimizing expansion of the interstitial space are preferable.

1. Blood and colloids are superior to hypotonic or even isotonic crystalloid solutions in expanding the intravascular volume. Although a rapid infusion of crystalloid is effective in increasing intravascular volume acutely, this benefit is transient.[36] For example, after a 5-minute infusion of 1 liter of lactated Ringer's, the intravascular volume expands approximately 630 mL. Yet due to rapid redistribution into the interstitial space, barely 20% of this volume is retained within the intravascular compartment after an hour. Similarly, only 25% (250 mL) of 1 liter of infused normal saline (NS) is retained in the intravascular compartment after 1 hour. In contrast, after a 5-minute infusion of 1 liter of 6% hetastarch, the intravascular volume expands by 1123 mL with more long-lasting effects. Five percent albumin can expand the plasma volume five times more than a comparable volume of normal saline.[37]

2. In general, it is reasonable to initially administer a moderate amount of inexpensive crystalloid (up to a liter) if the patient is oxygenating well.[38] Infusing greater amounts may contribute to tissue edema, commonly impairing oxygenation.

3. Colloids should be selected if additional volume is required. The selection of colloid should be based on the patient's pulmonary and renal function and the extent of mediastinal bleeding.[39–47]

a. **Albumin (5%)** provides excellent volume expansion (approximately 400 mL retained per 500 mL bottle administered) and has primarily dilutional effects on clotting parameters. Although it is a saline-based colloid, 5% albumin does preserve coagulation better than first-generation hydroxyethyl starchs in saline, and arguably better than colloids in balanced salt solutions (see Hextend, below). It has oxygen free-radical scavenging and anti-inflammatory properties, which may exert protective effects on the kidney.[45] Although albumin is effective in expanding the intravascular space, it does leak into the interstitial space due to the capillary leak and may cause movement of fluid out of the intracellular space. Albumin has a half-life of 16 hours and leaves the bloodstream at a rate of about 5–8 g/h.

b. Hydroxyethyl starch (HES) preparations are nonprotein colloid volume expanders. They are characterized in part by their molecular weight (MW) in kilodaltons (kDa) and their molar substitution (MS), which characterizes the rate at which they are broken down into smaller fragments. The first-generation HES are high MW solutions and include Hespan (6% hetastarch in saline) and Hextend (6% hetastarch in balanced electrolyte solution). Both are >600 kDa and 0.75 MS. They provide excellent volume expansion that decreases gradually over the ensuing 24–36 hours. They are retained in the intravascular space better than 5% albumin in conditions of capillary endothelial leakage. Concerns about use of HES preparations center around their effects on renal function and their potential to cause a coagulopathy. Although the high MW compounds are more likely to cause renal dysfunction than the lower MW ones,[44] none appear to be immune from this problem.[45] Furthermore, despite some claims that Hextend and the low MW HES solutions cause less of a coagulopathy than Hespan, all appear to be associated with postperative bleeding.[46]

  i. Hespan may contribute to a coagulopathy by binding to the von Willebrand/factor VIII complex causing platelet dysfunction and also contributing to fibrinolysis. Studies have shown that its use during CPB and even with off-pump surgery increases the risk of postoperative bleeding.[47,48] When used postoperatively for volume expansion, the dose should be limited to 20 mL/kg to minimize the risk of bleeding. Obviously, it is best avoided entirely if the patient is actively bleeding. These concerns about bleeding led to a US Food and Drug Administration (FDA) warning to avoid use of Hespan in cardiac surgery patients during surgery and the immediate postoperative period.[49]

  ii. Hextend provides similar volume expansion as Hespan. Although some studies suggest less of an impact on coagulation than Hespan,[50,51] other studies have demonstrated a similar decrease in clot tensile strength as Hespan with a comparable adverse effect on platelet function.[39,52,53] Hextend has been associated with increased blood loss after cardiac surgery, and thus the dosage should similarly be restricted to 20 mL/kg.[54]

  iii. Low MW compounds include pentastarch (6% HES 200/0.5 [Pentaspan]), available in Canada and Europe, and tetrastarch (6% HES 130/0.4 [Voluven]), available in the USA. It is recommended that daily doses of these two compounds be limited to 28 mL/kg and 50 mL/kg, respectively. These compounds produce volume expansion comparable to the first-generation compounds, although the volume effect is of shorter duration (estimated to be at least 6 hours for tetrastarch) because of more rapid elimination. Both are associated with less risk of renal dysfunction than the high MW compounds, and might have less impact on coagulation.[43,44] An increase in tissue oxygenation has also been demonstrated with HES 130/0.4 compared with lactated Ringer's, perhaps because of better microcirculatory flow.[55] Thus, the lowest MW HES, such as tetrastarch, may be the safest HES for volume expansion, although the duration of effect is less than with the higher MW HES.

iv. In Europe, gelatin solutions have been used effectively for volume expansion, but, because of the risk of life-threatening anaphylactic reactions and renal dysfunction, they are not available in the USA. Several comparative studies of 6% HES 130/0.4 (up to 50 mL/kg), 6% HES 200/0.5 (up to 33 mL/kg), 3% modified fluid gelatin, or 3% urea-linked gelatin demonstrated that all of these solutions were effective volume expanders.[56–58] However, there tended to be more bleeding noted with the HES 200/0.5 solution.

c. **Note:** There is concern that saline-based solutions (such as 5% albumin and Hespan) given in high dosage can induce renal dysfunction. They provide a chloride load that can produce progressive renal vasoconstriction, a decrease in GFR, and a hyperchloremic metabolic acidosis. Furthermore, patients receiving large amounts of normal saline can become hypernatremic, causing intracellular dehydration that may cause central nervous system changes and abdominal discomfort.[59] Thus, use of a balanced electrolyte vehicle may provide better acid–base and electrolyte balance and better organ perfusion. Notably, Hespan may contribute to a metabolic acidosis that might inappropriately raise the specter of poor tissue perfusion necessitating unnecessary intervention.[39]

d. Hypertonic solutions are effective in augmenting intravascular volume by extracting fluid from the interstitial and intracellular spaces. They may reduce the amount of fluid required to maintain intravascular volume when there is total body fluid overload. **25% albumin** can increase the intravascular volume by 450 mL for every 100 mL administered. **Hypertonic saline** (3%) can also be used, although it can produce neurologic problems with the development of acute hypernatremia. Studies from Europe have shown that hypertonic saline (7.5%) can produce renal vasodilation, increase GFR, and produce a diuresis.[60] It should be noted that use of these hypertonic colloids can produce hyper-oncotic renal failure in dehydrated patients because the glomerular filtration of hyperoncotic colloid molecules may cause hyperviscosity and stasis of tubular flow, resulting in tubular obstruction. This effect may also be one of the mechanisms of high MW HES-induced renal dysfunction.

e. An ideal solution for volume expansion would be a commercially available hemoglobin (Hb)-based oxygen carrier. Thromboelastographic studies of Oxyvita, a polymerized bovine-Hb-based oxygen carrier, have shown similar effects on the coagulation profile as Hespan at doses up to 23 mL/kg, but with minimal coagulopathic effects at the recommended dose of 2–3 mL/kg.[61]

D. It cannot be overemphasized that the objective of postoperative fluid management is to maintain **adequate** intravascular volume to ensure **satisfactory** cardiac output and tissue perfusion. Administration of excessive volume to maintain high filling pressures and the highest possible cardiac output will increase tissue edema, primarily manifest as increased extravascular lung water. This can be detrimental to pulmonary function and will often delay extubation. In addition, the hemodilution caused by intravascular volume expansion may decrease the hematocrit and also reduce the level of clotting factors, possibly precipitating bleeding and necessitating homologous blood or blood product transfusions.

E. When cardiac function is satisfactory, but there is an ongoing volume requirement to maintain filling pressures or blood pressure, often from a combination of the capillary leak, vasodilation, and an excellent urine output, "flooding" the patient with volume should be resisted. After 1.5–2 L of fluid is given, norepinephrine or vasopressin should be used to maintain filling pressures and improve the systemic blood pressure. Norepinephrine is the preferred drug in the vasodilated patient with good cardiac function since it will improve renal blood flow and actually lessen renal vascular resistance by lowering renal sympathetic tone.[62,63] Vasopressin (0.01–0.07 units/min) is very effective in the vasodilated "vasoplegic" patient with a good cardiac output in restoring blood pressure to within the renal autoregulatory range (generally >80 mm Hg).[63,64] In conditions of low cardiac output, however, it may increase the risk of splanchnic vasoconstriction and bowel ischemia. Phenylephrine should be utilized only when the cardiac output is satisfactory, because it provides a pure α effect on systemic vascular tone.

F. If both cardiac output and urine output remain marginal after adequate filling pressures have been achieved, inotropic support must be considered first, with use of vasoconstrictor drugs only if systemic resistance remains low. Use of α-agents at substantial doses is always of concern with a marginal cardiac output because they may produce renal vasoconstriction and compromise renal function.

G. Generally, diuretics are best avoided in the first 6 hours after surgery unless inexplicable oliguria, pulmonary edema, or borderline oxygenation is present. When the patient has achieved a stable core temperature and the capillary leak has ceased, usually after the first 6–12 hours, filling pressures will stabilize or rise with little fluid administration. By this time, myocardial function has usually recovered, inotropic support can be gradually withdrawn, and the patient can be extubated. Diuresis should then be initiated to excrete the excess salt and water administered during CPB and the early postoperative period. Patients who have undergone operations that require long periods of bypass (usually >3 hours) or who have persistent low output syndromes may experience a longer period of "capillary leak" that requires further fluid administration to maintain filling pressures.

H. **Diuresis** can be augmented most efficiently by the use of loop diuretics.[65]

1. Loop diuretics inhibit sodium reabsorption in the ascending limb of the loop of Henle and increase solute (sodium) presentation to the distal tubules. By inhibiting tubular water reabsorption, they increase natriuresis and diuresis and prevent tubular obstruction. To a lesser extent, they may also act as renal vasodilators, increasing RBF and GFR, and they may improve medullary oxygenation.

2. Most patients with preserved renal function respond to furosemide (Lasix) 10–20 mg IV. In the absence of renal insufficiency, furosemide has a half-life of 1.5–2 hours, and thus it can be repeated every 4 hours, if necessary. Not infrequently, the diuresis persists after one dose.

3. A gentle continuous diuresis may be obtained in patients with significant fluid overload and hemodynamic instability using a bolus dose of 40 mg followed by a continuous infusion of 0.1–0.5 mg/kg/h (usually 10–20 mg/h) of furosemide.[66]

This may decrease the total dosage requirements and usually improves the diuretic response, especially in patients who are diuretic "tolerant". This benefit is also seen in patients with chronic kidney disease.[67] The addition of a thiazide (chlorothiazide 500 mg IV) is beneficial in overcoming this problem of tolerance, which may be caused by compensatory hypertrophy of the distal nephron segments in response to increased exposure to solute from chronic use of loop diuretics.

4. Diuretics are continued in IV or oral form until the patient has achieved his/her preoperative weight. Despite the nearly universal use of routine diuretics to achieve an earlier diuresis, one study showed no clinical benefit to this practice in low-risk patients with normal renal function.[68]

5. Low-dose dopamine ($2-3\,\mu g/kg/min$) increases RBF and GFR, resulting in effective diuresis and natriuresis. This will lower filling pressures, reduce lung congestion, and improve oxygenation. It has been shown to be clinically beneficial while reducing the need for diuretics in postoperative patients with normal renal function.[69] However, one study found that low-dose dopamine was able to increase RBF only in patients with normal renal function. If moderate impairment was present, inotropic doses of dopamine were required to improve RBF.[70] Thus, in patients with normal renal function, dopamine may improve urine output and provide some clinical benefits, but there is no evidence that it improves outcomes or has any impact on preventing renal dysfunction. The same holds true for diuretics.

6. Guidelines for the hemodynamic and fluid management of typical postoperative scenarios are presented in Chapter 8.

IV. Prevention of Acute Kidney Injury[71-73]

A. The risk of developing postoperative acute kidney injury (AKI) is very low when a patient with normal renal function undergoes an uneventful operation and maintains satisfactory postoperative hemodynamics. In contrast, the presence of any degree of preoperative renal dysfunction increases the risk of postoperative AKI and mortality.[1-14] Therefore, it is important to identify patients with preoperative renal dysfunction and those with other risk factors for developing postoperative renal failure.

B. **Definition of preoperative renal dysfunction**   Renal dysfunction is commonly defined as a serum creatinine (Scr) >1.5 mg/dL or >130 μmol/L (1 mg/dL = 88 μmol/L). However, the Scr is not an ideal means of assessing kidney function because it may be normal with a greater than 50% reduction in GFR, which reflects the number of functioning nephrons. A more sensitive estimate of renal function can be obtained using the creatinine clearance (C_{Cr} in mL/min), which approximates the GFR.[74,75] This is more indicative of renal reserve and the ability of the kidneys to tolerate surgical stress. **A GFR $<60\,mL/min/1.73\,m^2$ is the best definition of renal dysfunction** and is the level below which there is an increased risk of worsening renal dysfunction and increased mortality.[2,3,5-7]

1. A 24-hour urine collection to precisely measure the C_{Cr} is considered to be no more reliable than an estimate using one of the following two predictive equations.

2. The Cockcroft and Gault equation can easily be calculated at the bedside and is generally indexed to the patient's weight. One study concluded that this

formula was better than the MDRD formula (below) in predicting in-hospital mortality.[76]

$$C_{Cr} = \frac{(140 - age) \times wt\,(kg) \times (0.85\,if\,female)}{72 \times Scr\,(mg/dL)}$$

3. The 2005 Modification of Diet in Renal Disease (MDRD) formula appears complex but is used in most laboratories to provide a GFR estimate. It is usually considered to be a more precise measure of abnormal renal function:[75]

$$GFR = 186 \times Scr^{-1.154} \times age^{-0.203} \times (0.742\,if\,female) \times (1.210\,if\,black)$$

where:

$GFR = mL/min/1.73\,m^2$

$Scr = mg/dL$

C. **The importance of preexisting renal dysfunction**

1. An elevated preoperative creatinine, or more specifically a reduction in C_{Cr} or GFR, is the most powerful predictor of AKI after surgery and is a major risk factor for operative mortality. An analysis of nearly 500,000 patients in the Society of Thoracic Surgeons (STS) database confirmed an increasing operative mortality with progressively lower GFRs of less than 60 mL/min/1.73 m^2.[2] Defining the degree of renal dysfunction (RD) by GFR, as recommended by the National Kidney Foundation (NKF) guidelines,[77] the mortality rates and requirements for dialysis in this representative analysis of patients undergoing CABG are shown in Table 12.1.

2. An assessment of GFR is very helpful in identifying patients with a milder degree of renal dysfunction, which is also associated with adverse renal outcomes and greater mortality.[9-14] Even patients with so-called "occult renal insufficiency" (Scr ≤1.1 mg/dL or ≤100 μmol/L with a GFR <60 mL/min), which is noted in about 13% of patients with a normal Scr, have significantly higher mortality and renal failure requiring renal replacement therapy (RRT) than those with normal renal function.[8,78]

Table 12.1 • Mortality Rates and Dialysis Requirements According to the Degree of Renal Dysfunction

Degree of Renal Dysfunction (RD)	GFR	Mortality	New Dialysis	NKF Stage
Normal	>90	1.3%	0.2%	stage 1 if albuminuria
Mild RD	60–90	1.8%	0.5%	stage 2 if albuminuria
Moderate RD	30–59	4.3%	1.8%	stage 3
Severe RD	<30	9.3%	10.9%	stages 4–5
Dialysis	–	9%	N/A	

3. Smaller studies correlating serum creatinine levels with mortality have shown somewhat higher mortality rates than those demonstrated in the STS study. Generally, the mortality risk for CABG patients is about 5% for patients with Scr 1.5–2.5 mg/dL, 15–30% in non-dialysis-dependent patients with Scr >2.5 mg/dL, and 10–15% for those on chronic dialysis.[2,79–81] One study found that the risk of AKI was increased 4.8-fold for each 1 mg/dL increment in Scr.[82] Another found that the risk of dialysis exceeded 30% if the pre-operative Scr was >2.5 mg/dL.[79] It is best to use the available risk models (Figures 12.1–12.4) to individualize the risks of AKI and RRT based upon an assessment of all contributing risk factors.

4. The operative mortality for patients who develop acute kidney injury that requires de novo dialysis ranges from 40% to 60% in several large series.[83–87] These alarming statistics emphasize the crucial importance of taking any steps possible to preserve renal function in the perioperative period, especially in patients at increased risk. The presence of any degree of preoperative renal insufficiency should therefore lead to a search for potentially treatable causes that might lower the risk of AKI postoperatively. Identifying and correcting these contributing factors before surgery and using prophylactic measures during and after surgery to optimize renal perfusion and tubular function may ameliorate the complications associated with the development of oliguric renal failure. These may include electrolyte abnormalities, pulmonary and cardiac dysfunction, bleeding, delayed return of gastrointestinal function affecting nutrition, and infection from immune dysfunction, not to mention the possibility of requiring dialysis and its attendant complications.

Risk Factor	Score
Age 70-74	1.5
Age 75-79	2.0
Age ≥ 80	2.5
Female	1.5
Diabetes	1.5
WBC > 12,000	1.5
Prior CABG	2.0
CHF	2.5
PVD	1.5
Hypertension	1.5
Preop IABP	3.0

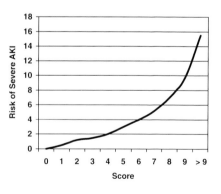

Figure 12.1 • Multivariate risk predictor for severe postoperative renal insufficiency in patients with normal or near normal preoperative renal function (GFR >60 mL/min/1.73 m^2). (Adapted with permission from Brown et al., *Circulation* 2007;116(Suppl I):I-139–43.)[89]

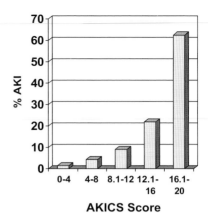

Risk factor	Points
Preop factors	
NYHA class III-IV	3.2
Scr > 1.2 mg/dL	3.1
Age > 65	2.3
Preop BS > 140 mg/dL	1.7
Intra- and postop factors	
Combined surgery	3.7
CPB time > 120 min	1.8
Low cardiac output	2.5
CVP > 14 cm H_2O	1.7

Figure 12.2 • Predictive model of acute kidney injury after cardiac surgery (AKICS score). Risk of developing postoperative AKI is defined as a serum creatinine (Scr) >2.0 mg/dL and a 50% increase in Scr (Adapted with permission from Palomba et al., *Kidney Int* 2007;72:624–31.)[90]

    D. **Predictive risk factors** for the development of postoperative AKI or the need for postoperative RRT have been elucidated in many studies and incorporated into risk stratification algorithms.[87–93] Figure 12.1 provides an estimate of the risk of developing severe AKI (GFR <30 mL/min/1.73 m^2) in patients with normal or near-normal renal function (GFR >60 mL/min/1.73 m^2) preoperatively.[89] Figure 12.2 provides a model to predict AKI (Scr >2.0 mg/dL and a 50% increase in Scr) based upon pre-, intra-, and postoperative parameters.[90] Figures 12.3 and 12.4 provides risk models for the prediction of RRT after cardiac surgery.[91,92] Most models include

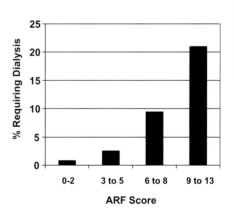

Risk Factor	Points
Female	1
CHF	1
EF < 35%	1
Preop IABP	2
COPD	1
Insulin-DM	1
Reoperation	1
Emergency surgery	2
Isolated valve surgery	1
CABG + Valve	2
Other non-CABG cardiac surgery	2
Preop Scr 1.2-2.0 mg/dL	2
Preop Scr > 2.0 mg/dL	5

Figure 12.3 • Cleveland Clinic model to predict the risk of acute renal failure requiring dialysis. The risk is divided into four quartiles depending on the risk score. (Adapted with permission from Thakar et al., *Am J Soc Nephrol* 2005;16:162–8.)[91]

Risk Factor	Points
Creatinine (mg/dL) x 10	5-40
Age: 1 point for each 5 yrs > 55	Up to 10
AVR	2
AVR-CABG	5
MV Surgery	4
MV-CABG	7
Diabetes – oral meds	2
Diabetes – insulin	5
MI < 3 weeks	3
Non-white race	2
COPD	3
Reoperation	3
NYHA class IV	3
Cardiogenic shock	7

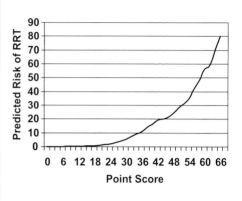

Figure 12.4 • Bedside model for predicting the risk of dialysis (STS model). (Adapted with permission from Mehta et al., *Circulation* 2006;114:2208–16.)[92]

preexisting renal dysfunction, older age (2.5-fold increase in risk for each 10-year increment in one study),[82] diabetes, hypertension, more tenuous hemodynamic status (shock, recent myocardial infarction, preoperative IABP, low ejection fraction), reoperations, and urgent or emergent surgery as risk factors. It is notable that several additional risk factors identified in other studies are not noted in all of these risk models. These include a long duration of CPB[94–96] and contrast studies within 5 days of surgery.[94]

E. **Classification and etiology of perioperative acute kidney injury (AKI).** AKI is usually categorized as prerenal (reduced renal perfusion), renal (intrinsic renal insults), or postrenal (obstructive uropathy). Mechanisms contributing to the first two categories in the perioperative period are noted in Table 12.2. When the kidneys have sustained an acute preoperative insult, either from the cardiac catheterization or more ominously from decompensated heart failure or cardiogenic shock from an acute ischemic event, they seem to be particularly sensitive to the nonpulsatile flow of CPB and to tenuous postcardiotomy hemodynamics. This is especially true in patients with "acute on chronic" renal dysfunction. The BUN and creatinine should therefore be allowed to return towards baseline, if possible, before proceeding with surgery.

F. Patients with **chronic kidney disease** are more susceptible to fluid overload, hyponatremia, hyperkalemia, and metabolic acidosis in the perioperative period. Patients on chronic dialysis should be dialyzed within the 24 hours before and after surgery. Intraoperative hemofiltration should also be performed to reduce the positive fluid balance. The overall mortality rate for patients on chronic dialysis undergoing open-heart surgery is approximately 10–15%, but even higher in those with advanced NYHA class and those undergoing urgent or emergent surgery.

Table 12.2 • Factors Contributing to Pre- and Postoperative Acute Kidney Injury

Preoperative factors	Low cardiac output states/hypotension (cardiogenic shock from acute MI, mechanical complications of MI) Medications that interfere with renal autoregulation (ACE inhibitors, NSAIDs) Nephrotoxins (contrast-induced ATN, especially in diabetic vasculopathy), medications (aminoglycosides, metformin) Renal atheroembolism (catheterization, IABP) Interstitial nephritis (antibiotics, NSAIDs, furosemide) Glomerulonephritis (endocarditis)
Intraoperative factors	Cardiopulmonary bypass (nonpulsatile, low flow, low pressure perfusion) Low cardiac output syndrome/hypotension after CPB Hemolysis and hemoglobinuria from prolonged duration of CPB
Postoperative factors	Low cardiac output states (decreased contractility, hypovolemia, absent AV synchrony in hypertrophied hearts) Hypotension Intense vasoconstriction (low flow states, α-agents) Atheroembolism (IABP) Sepsis Medications (cephalosporins, aminoglycosides, ACE inhibitors)

G. **Preoperative measures**

1. Prior to and during cardiac catheterization, consider the following interventions (Table 12.3):

   a. Avoid medications with adverse effects on renal function the day of the catheterization – especially metformin, which can cause lactic acidosis.

   b. Adequately hydrate with normal saline at 1 mL/kg/hour (usually about 75 mL/h) before, during, and after the study for up to 12 hours.

   c. Use low volumes of iso- or low-osmolar non-ionic contrast.

   d. Consider medications that may attenuate the nephrotoxic effects of contrast media in patients at increased risk of renal dysfunction.[97-99]

      i. **Sodium bicarbonate** 150 mEq (1 mEq/mL) added to 850 mL of D5W with an initial infusion of 3 mL/kg over 1 hour starting just prior to catheterization followed by a 1 mL/kg/h infusion for up to 12 hours. Bicarbonate infusion with hydration has been found to be superior to hydration alone in patients with mild precatheterization renal dysfunction.[100,101]

Table 12.3 • Preoperative and Intraoperative Measures to Reduce the Risk of Acute Kidney Injury

A. Preoperative measures
   1. Withhold metformin the day of catheterization
   2. Hydration during cardiac catheterization
   3. Use of sodium bicarbonate infusion
   4. Consider use of N-acetylcysteine
   5. Optimize hemodynamic status
   6. Repeat serum creatinine if preoperative renal dysfunction, especially in diabetics, and defer surgery, if possible, until creatinine has returned to baseline
   7. Correct all acid–base and metabolic problems
B. Intraoperative measures
   1. Perform off-pump surgery if possible
   2. Use antifibrinolytics (ε-aminocaproic [Amicar] or tranexamic acid) to minimize bleeding
   3. Pump considerations
      a. Maintain a high perfusion pressure (75–80 mm Hg) on bypass
      b. Keep the pump run as short as possible
      c. Consider use of a leukocyte-reducing filter
      d. Use hemofiltration to remove excess fluid
   4. Pharmacologic renoprotection
      a. Nesiritide (2 μg/kg bolus, then 0.01 μg/kg/min)
      b. Fenoldopam (0.1 μg/kg/min)
      c. Sodium bicarbonate (0.25 mEq/kg load, then 0.075 mEq/kg/h)
   5. Optimize postbypass hemodynamics

    ii. **N-acetylcysteine** (NAC) given in an oral dose of 600 mg bid beginning 12 hours before the procedure (if possible) and continuing q12h for a total of four doses. Alternatively, it may be given IV as 150 mg/kg in 500 mL NS over 30 minutes prior to contrast exposure followed by 50 mg/kg in 500 mL NS infused over the next 4 hours. The added effectiveness of NAC when used with adequate hydration is controversial.[98,99] Even though some studies suggest that the benefits of NAC are similar when combined with hydration or bicarbonate,[102] a meta-analysis suggested that the combination of NAC + bicarbonate was the best regimen to reduce the incidence of postcontrast AKI in patients at high risk.[103]

    iii. **Note:** Furosemide should be avoided during catheterization because it may increase the risk of AKI. Dopamine provides no advantage over hydration alone.[104]

2. Repeat the serum creatinine 12 hours after contrast studies and defer surgery, if possible, until the creatinine has returned to baseline.

3. Optimize hemodynamic status. Occasionally, emergency surgery is indicated in patients with marginal hemodynamics on inotropic support and an IABP, in which case one often has to accept the inevitable, but frequently transient, deterioration in renal function postoperatively.

4. Correct acid–base or metabolic abnormalities associated with renal insufficiency, such as hyponatremia, hyper- or hypokalemia, hypomagnesemia, hyperphosphatemia, metabolic acidosis (from chronic kidney disease) or alkalosis (from diuretics). Perform dialysis the day before surgery in patients on chronic dialysis.

5. Preoperative dialysis may be of benefit to patients with moderate renal dysfunction. One study showed that this approach to patients with a preoperative creatinine ≥2.5 mg/dL significantly reduced the need for postoperative dialysis, with less morbidity and significantly less mortality.[105] In patients with preoperative CHF and hypoxemia who require urgent surgery, ultrafiltration to remove fluid frequently proves beneficial as well.

H. **Intraoperative measures** should be taken to try to augment renal reserve by improving renal blood flow, enhancing the GFR, and preventing tubular damage in patients with known renal dysfunction or risk factors for its development (Table 12.3).[106,107]

1. Consider performing off-pump coronary surgery in diabetic patients with preoperative renal dysfunction.[31]

2. Maintain optimal hemodynamic performance before and after CPB.

3. Use antifibrinolytic drugs to minimize the bleeding diathesis that commonly accompanies renal dysfunction (uremic platelet dysfunction). ε-aminocaproic acid (Amicar) is commonly used and is generally safe, although it is associated with some degree of renal tubular dysfunction without a significant change in creatinine clearance.[108] Tranexamic acid is a good alternative. Aprotinin came under scrutiny in 2007 because of a report that it increased the risk of renal failure as well as other adverse outcomes.[109] However, numerous studies, including a previous analysis of the same database, have refuted this finding.[110–113] In fact, it was concluded that blood transfusions were associated with adverse renal outcomes, yet aprotinin was not an independent risk factor for AKI.[111,114] One study also showed a similar risk of renal dysfunction with EACA or aprotinin.[115] Nonetheless, aprotinin was withdrawn from the market in late 2007.

4. **Considerations during CPB**

a. Use heparin-coated circuits, if available, which may be beneficial in reducing the systemic inflammatory response.[116]

b. Use a miniaturized circuit, which may lower the incidence of postoperative AKI by reducing the systemic inflammatory response.[117]

c. Leukodepletion on pump using leukocyte-reducing filters may attenuate glomerular and tubular injury. This has been shown to lower the levels of microalbumin and retinol-binding protein indexed to creatinine.[118]

    d. Maintain a higher mean perfusion pressure on bypass (around 80 mm Hg) by increasing the systemic flow rate. If this does not raise the blood pressure to adequate levels, a vasopressor can be added. As long as an adequate systemic flow rate with satisfactory oxygen delivery is maintained (as evidenced by adequate venous oxygen saturations), a vasopressor, such as phenylephrine, norepinephrine, or vasopressin, can be used to increased systemic resistance. Autoregulation of renal flow occurs down to a pressure of about 80 mm Hg, but below that, flow is pressure-dependent. Nonetheless, one study did indicate that the incidence of postoperative AKI was no different whether mean pressures <60, 60–69, or >70 mm Hg were used during CPB, although urine output was less at lower pressures.[119]

    e. Keep the "pump run" as short as possible. Generally, the longer the duration of CPB, the greater the incidence of renal failure.[94–96]

    f. Avoid extreme hemodilution on CPB. Studies have suggested that there is a correlation between the lowest hematocrit on pump (usually <21%) and the incidence of AKI, especially in obese patients. However, the hematocrit is only one factor in oxygen delivery. Since AKI is more common below a critical level for oxygen delivery (272 mL/min/m^2), lower hematocrits may be acceptable as long as oxygen delivery is maintained above the critical level with increased pump flow rates.[22–26]

    g. Although moderate hypothermia may not be protective of renal function during surgery, rewarming up to $37\,^\circ$C may be harmful to the kidneys. One study showed that this produced a 40% greater chance of developing AKI than if the patient was only warmed to $34\,^\circ$C.[120] This may occur because the kidneys may rewarm more rapidly than other organs, including the brain, resulting in hyperthermia-related exacerbation of renal injury. However, rewarming to lower temperatures has its own problems, such as an increased risk of bleeding, shivering, delayed extubation, and infection.

    h. Prevent hyperglycemia during the pump run.[121]

    i. Hemofiltration can be performed to remove free water and solute during and at the conclusion of bypass. This is beneficial in removing excess fluid from patients with preoperative CHF and may improve pulmonary function. By removing potassium, it mitigates the concern about using high volumes of hyperkalemic cardioplegia solutions. Hemoconcentration can optimize the hematocrit and lower the requirement for transfusions. It may improve hemodynamics, hemostasis, and pulmonary function in higher-risk patients.[122,123]

    j. One study suggested that the use of sodium nitroprusside during rewarming on pump improved renal function in patients undergoing elective CABG, although this must not be allowed to occur at the expense of unacceptable hypotension.[124]

5. Nesiritide (B-type natriuretic peptide) has been demonstrated in several studies to provide a renoprotective benefit when used during surgery, primarily in patients with abnormal renal function, but also in patients with impaired left ventricular function and those undergoing high-risk surgery.[125–128] It dilates the renal afferent arterioles and, to a lesser extent, the efferent arterioles, leading to augmented glomerular filtration. During periods of neurohormonal activation, such as CPB, it inhibits the renin–angiotensin–aldosterone axis and has a direct tubular effect on sodium and water handling. Thus, it exhibits strong natriuretic and diuretic properties. Preliminary experience with human **atrial natriuretic peptide** (ANP) in patients with LV dysfunction undergoing CABG has shown that it provides a similar renoprotective benefit.[129]

   a. Indications: nesiritide should be considered in patients considered at medium-to-high risk for the development of postoperative renal failure using the risk algorithms noted in Figures 12.1–12.4. It is usually given to any patient with a Scr >1.4 mg/dL or a GFR <60 mL/min/1.73 m^2.

   b. Dosage: it is given in a bolus dose of 2 μg/kg over 1 minute prior to going on bypass followed by an infusion of 0.01–0.03 μg/kg/min. The infusion is usually continued for 18–24 hours after surgery, but may be given for a longer period if indicated. Occasionally the diuretic response is so dramatic that it needs to be stopped sooner. The dose of ANP is 0.02 μg/kg/min.

6. Fenoldopam is a selective agonist of the dopamine 1 (DA$_1$) receptor that produces a dose-dependent increase in renal plasma flow with a decrease in renal vascular resistance and maintenance of GFR. It increases blood flow to both the renal cortex and medulla and inhibits tubular reabsorption of sodium. Thus it produces diuresis, natriuresis, and kaliuresis. Studies have shown preservation of renal function, and in fact, some improvement in Scr and C$_{Cr}$ after CPB in patients with an elevated creatinine.[130–134] A reduction in mortality and the need for renal replacement therapy have also been documented.[132]

   a. Indications: fenoldopam is an alternative to nesiritide to provide renoprotection during surgery performed on CPB.

   b. Dosage: it is started as an infusion of 0.1 μg/kg/min before CPB and continued in the ICU for about 12–24 hours. A dose-dependent increase in renal blood flow is noted in doses up to 0.3 μg/kg/min, but doses greater than 0.1 μg/kg/min are associated with systemic vasodilation.[130]

7. Sodium bicarbonate may be an inexpensive means of preventing renal dysfunction after surgery. One report found the following dosing regimen reduced the risk of AKI after surgery: a bicarbonate load of 0.5 mmol/kg (0.25 mEq/kg) in 250 mL D5W after the induction of anesthesia followed by a 0.15 mmol/kg/h (0.075 mEq/kg/h) infusion over 24 hours for a total dose of approximately 4 mmol/kg (2 mEq/kg).[135]

8. Diltiazem has been evaluated as a means of preserving renal function, but its benefits are controversial. It reduces renal vascular resistance by dilating afferent arterioles, resulting in an increase in renal blood flow and GFR. It may limit calcium influx into renal tubular cells, preserving their integrity. It has been shown to increase sodium excretion and improve creatinine and free water clearance by a direct effect on tubular reabsorption.

   a. There have been concerns that diltiazem could adversely affect renal function because of its vasodilatory effect during pump. However, further investigation has shown that diltiazem is more likely to improve rather than reduce glomerular function in patients with mild-to-moderate renal dysfunction. This is a significant finding that should not dissuade the use of diltiazem for vasospasm prophylaxis when radial artery grafting is performed. Nonetheless, either nesiritide or fenoldopam should be used preferentially to provide renoprotection.[82,136,137]

  b. Dosage: 0.1 mg/kg bolus followed by an infusion of 2 µg/kg/min.

9. Medications often used during surgery with minimal renoprotective benefit:

  a. **Mannitol** is commonly added to the pump to increase tubular flow and produce a diuresis. It increases oncotic pressure, reduces tissue edema, and may reduce cell swelling after cardioplegic arrest. Usually 25–50 g is added to the pump prime. However, mannitol has not been demonstrated to provide any benefit to renal function in patients with normal or abnormal preoperative renal function.[138–140]

  b. **Furosemide** is often given during surgery to augment urine output and is beneficial in patients with significant volume overload, severe oliguria, or hyperkalemia. However, its use may be associated with an increased, rather than a decreased, risk of renal impairment, even in patients with normal preoperative function. Thus, although it will increase urine output, it is not renoprotective and should be used only for the indications listed.[141–143]

  c. **Dopamine** acts on DA_1 and DA_2 receptors as well as α_1-receptors in the kidney. Whereas DA_1 receptors reduce renal vascular resistance, the other receptors oppose this effect, potentially decreasing renal blood flow and GFR. Use of "renal-dose" dopamine (2–3 µg/kg/min) during surgery may improve urine output, but has been shown to produce early renal tubular damage equal to or worse than that noted in control patients. Numerous studies have failed to demonstrate any renoprotective effect of dopamine during surgery, in patients with both normal and abnormal renal function.[144–146] One study comparing fenoldopam (0.05 µg/kg/min) with dopamine found a comparable lack of benefit in preventing postoperative AKI.[147]

  d. Despite concerns over using either dopamine or diltiazem alone to provide renal protection, an infusion of dopamine (2 µg/kg/min) + diltiazem (2 µg/kg/min) has been shown to increase creatinine clearance, osmotic clearance, and free water clearance with no increase in markers of tubular damage.[148]

  e. Despite evidence of benefit in some trials, *N*-acetylcysteine given intra-operatively has generally not been shown to be effective in preventing renal dysfunction in patients at high risk.[149,150]

V. Postoperative Oliguria and Acute Kidney Injury

A. The use of hemodilution during CPB expands the extracellular volume and usually produces an excellent urine output in the immediate postoperative period. Oliguria is considered to be present in the postoperative cardiac surgical patient when the urine output is **less than 0.5 mL/kg/h**. Transient oliguria is commonly noted in the first 12 hours after surgery and usually responds to a volume infusion or low-dose inotropic support. However, the persistence of oliguria is usually a manifestation of an acute renal insult caused by prolonged hypotension or a low cardiac output state. The serum creatinine will frequently be lower immediately after bypass due to hemodilution, and may have a delayed rise despite a marked reduction in GFR as it takes time for creatinine to accumulate in the bloodstream. Thus, it is important to recognize that acute kidney injury may be associated with an abrupt and sustained decrease in urine output and/or a sustained decline in GFR, eventually evident by an increase in Scr. Measurement of biomarkers, as noted below, may be the most sensitive means of early detection of AKI.[18]

B. **Definition of acute kidney injury.** The incidence of postoperative renal dysfunction depends on its definition. A classification system (RIFLE) has been devised to identify progressively worsening degrees of renal dysfunction (Table 12.4). Since the function of the kidneys is both elimination of nitrogenous waste products and production of urine, either the creatinine level/GFR criteria or the urine output criteria can be used for classification in this model. It should be noted that urine output is determined by the difference between the GFR and the rate of tubular reabsorption. Therefore, if the GFR is low from chronic kidney disease in association with poor tubular absorption, the patient can have good urine output initially. With AKI, tubular absorption is initially normal with a low GFR and then falls.

1. In the RIFLE system, the first category of AKI ("risk") is defined by an increase in Scr × 1.5 or a decrease in GFR >25%. Approximately 20% of patients will develop this degree of AKI, with a 1% requirement for RRT and a 90-day mortality rate

---

Table 12.4 • *The RIFLE Criteria for Classification of Renal Failure*

	Scr/GFR Criteria	Urine Output	Overall Incidence
Risk	Increase in Scr × 1.5 *or* Decrease in GFR >25%	<0.5 mL/kg/h × 6 h	20–25%
Injury	Increase in Scr × 2 *or* Decrease in GFR >50%	<0.5 ml/kg/h × 12 h	5–7%
Failure	Increase in Scr × 3 *or* Decrease in GFR >75% *or* Scr >350 μmol/L (>4 mg/dL) *or* Acute Scr rise >44 μmol/L (>0.5 mg/dL)	<0.3 ml/kg/h × 24 h	1–3%
Loss	Persistent acute renal failure with complete loss of kidney function >4 weeks		
ESKD	End-stage kidney disease >3 months		

Adapted with permission from Bell et al. *Nephrol, Dial Transplant* 2005;20:354–60.

of 8%. The second level ("injury") is defined by a doubling of the Scr or a >50% decrease in GFR. This corresponds fairly well to the 2011 STS database specifications definition of AKI, which is an increase in Scr to ≥2.0 mg/dL and to twice the preoperative level. This occurs in about 5–7% of patients and is associated with a 7% need for RRT and a 21% 90-day mortality. Patients in the third category ("failure") require dialysis 55% of the time and have a 90-day mortality rate of 33%. However, once RRT is necessary, the mortality rate is usually about 50%.[151,152]

2. An elevation in many kidney-specific markers is common after open-heart surgery. A significant elevation in plasma and urinary levels of biomarkers, such as NGAL, cystatin C, kidney injury molecular 1 (KIM-2) and IL-18, may be noted within 2-6 hours of surgery and has been found to correlate with the extent and duration of AKI.[15–18,153] These are valuable early indicators of AKI that preceed elevation in Scr levels. Although cystatin concentration reflects baseline GFR more accurately than Scr, NGAL is rapidly induced in renal tubular cells in response to ischemic injury, and although its early appearance is independent of GFR, it is generally predictive of a subsequent decline in GFR. In patients developing early AKI, plasma NGAL levels >150 ng/mL and a 15-25 fold increase in urinary levels have been reported.[15–18] Because elevated NGAL levels may provide for earlier diagnosis and intervention of incipient AKI than elevations in Scr, some authors have recommended that all patients have baseline NGAL levels obtained for comparison with serial postoperative values.[17]

3. The Scr is influenced not just by glomerular function, but also by tubular function and the generation of creatinine. Thus, it tends to underestimate the degree of renal dysfunction, because as the GFR falls, creatinine secretion increases, minimizing the rise in Scr, upon which the GFR calculation is based. Although the Scr may not rise for several days after tubular injury has occurred, changes in Scr do reflect changes in GFR, and they are therefore valuable in making the diagnosis of AKI.[107] A fall in Scr is an indicator of renal recovery from AKI and correlates with long-term outcomes, whereas such a correlation with biomarkers is not clear but is being investigated.[154]

4. **Nonoliguric renal failure**, defined as a rise in creatinine with a urine output >400 mL/day, is the most common form of AKI and may occur after an uneventful operation in a patient with preexisting renal dysfunction or risk factors for its development, and occasionally without any precipitating factors. This condition usually reflects less renal damage and is associated with a mortality rate of about 5–10%. Most patients can be managed by judicious fluid administration, hemodynamic support as indicated, and high-dose diuretics to optimize urine output while awaiting spontaneous recovery of renal function.

5. **Oliguric renal failure** may occur in patients with varying degrees of reduction in GFR, but when the urine output is <0.3–0.5 mL/kg/h for 12–24 hours, the patient is in the second and third categories of the RIFLE system with a greater likelihood of requiring RRT. As noted, once this is necessary, the mortality rate approaches 50%.[83–88] This mortality rate has not changed much over the past 10–15 years despite the early institution of various forms of RRT and general improvements in postoperative care. This reflects the higher-risk population undergoing surgery and the morbidity of conditions frequently associated with renal failure, such as low cardiac output states, respiratory failure, infection, and stroke.

C. Etiology of postoperative acute kidney injury[155,156]

1. In patients with preexisting renal dysfunction, the complex effects of extracorporeal circulation will often induce some degree of AKI. Mechanisms include renal hypoperfusion from low-flow, low-pressure nonpulsatile perfusion with hemodilution and hypothermia, as well as an inflammatory response that may maintain afferent arteriolar constriction. Hopefully, utilization of the numerous steps delineated on pages 597–600 will be successful in minimizing the intraoperative insult. Most patients will recover back to their baseline renal function if no additional insult occurs. However, in the early postoperative period, the most common cause of a further renal result is a low cardiac output state. An additional contributing factor is intense peripheral vasoconstriction, often related to use of α-agents. Oliguria occurring as a consequence of reduced GFR is most clinically significant early after surgery when fluid overload and hyperkalemia can lead to pulmonary and myocardial complications and impair recovery from surgery.

2. The kidneys have a tremendous capacity to autoregulate and maintain RBF, GFR, filtration fraction, and tubular reabsorption in the face of reduced renal perfusion pressure. Intrinsic renal mechanisms that maintain autoregulation include a reduction in afferent arteriolar resistance and an increase in efferent arteriolar resistance. However, when a low cardiac output state or hypotension persists or potent vasopressor medications are used, these compensatory reserves gradually become exhausted, filtration reserve is exceeded, and endogenous and/or exogenous vasoconstrictors increase afferent arteriolar resistance, resulting in a fall in GFR. At this point of prerenal azotemia, oliguria may occur, but tubular function may still be intact. Aggressive management to optimize renal perfusion at this time is essential to try to avoid tubular damage.

3. However, a more protracted period of ischemia will eventually cause structural tubular injury with sloughing of cells that may obstruct the tubules with backleakage of fluid into the circulation. Impaired sodium absorption and increased sodium concentration in the distal tubules polymerizes proteins contributing to cast formation. There is also an oxidant injury and inflammatory phenomena that result in further hypoperfusion and damage to tubular cells. Some of this damage is reversible and some results in apoptotic cell death. The term "acute tubular necrosis" has commonly been applied to this condition, although it is a somewhat misleading term; therefore it is more commonly referred to as "acute kidney injury" (AKI).

4. It should be noted that an acute ischemic renal insult is a hypoperfusion injury that may be undetected in a normotensive patient.[157] If autoregulation is impaired, the kidney may be more susceptible to lesser degrees of hypoperfusion. Factors to consider are:

   a. Renal arteriolar disease, notably in elderly patients and those with hypertension, chronic kidney disease, or renal artery stenosis.

   b. Failure of afferent arterioles to dilate appropriately. NSAIDs and Cox-2 inhibitors decrease prostaglandin synthesis and allow endogenous vasoconstrictors to act unopposed; sepsis and liver failure increase afferent arteriole vasoconstriction.

   c. Use of vasoconstrictors during a low output state, which tend to reduce RBF despite achieving systemic normotension.

     d. Failure of efferent arterioles to constrict, noted with ACE inhibitors, ARBs, or renin inhibitors, such as aliskiren (Tekturna).

     e. Systemic venous hypertension, often as a result of right ventricular failure, tamponade, or an abdominal compartment syndrome which may reduce renal perfusion.[158]

  5. The acute development of oliguria and a rising Scr several days after surgery should always raise the specter of **cardiac tamponade**. The combination of systemic venous hypertension and a low output state can compromise renal perfusion even if hypotension is not evident. The patient may have nonspecific systemic symptoms, and a compensatory tachycardia may be absent with the use of β-blockers.

  6. Conditions of impaired oxygen delivery (profound anemia from bleeding, hypoxemia from respiratory failure) will contribute to renal ischemia in conditions of borderline hypoperfusion.

D. Three patterns of acute renal failure were described following open-heart surgery nearly 25 years ago and in principle still hold true today (Figure 12.5).[159] In the first, termed "**abbreviated ARF**", a transient intraoperative insult occurs that causes renal

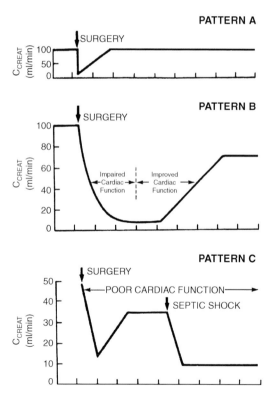

Figure 12.5 • Patterns of acute renal failure (ARF) observed after open-heart surgery. **(A)** Abbreviated ARF. **(B)** Overt ARF. **(C)** Protracted ARF. The reduction in creatinine clearance (C_{Cr}) noted here is paralleled by a rise in serum creatinine. (Reproduced with permission of the Massachusetts Medical Society from Myers et al., *N Engl J Med* 1986;314:97–105.)[157]

ischemia. The serum creatinine peaks on the fourth postoperative day and then returns to normal. In the second pattern, termed "**overt ARF**", the acute insult is followed by a more prolonged period of cardiac dysfunction. The creatinine usually rises to a higher level and gradually returns towards baseline over the course of 1–2 weeks once hemodynamics improve. The third pattern ("**protracted ARF**") is characterized by an initial insult followed by a period of cardiac dysfunction that resolves. Just as the creatinine begins to fall, another insult occurs, often from sepsis or a period of hypoperfusion/hypotension, that triggers a progressive, often irreversible rise in creatinine.

E. Assessment (Table 12.5)[160]

1. Assess cardiac hemodynamics (filling pressures, cardiac output). If the patient is no longer being intensively monitored, insertion of a Foley catheter is helpful in assessing urine output. Evidence of jugular venous distention or orthostatic vital signs raise the specter of tamponade. An echocardiogram may be considered to assess ventricular function and the presence of a significant hemopericardium.

2. Identify any drugs being prescribed with potential adverse effects on renal function (ACE inhibitors, ARBs, NSAIDs, nephrotoxic antibiotics).

3. Obtain a serum BUN, creatinine, electrolytes, and osmolality. **Note:** An elevation in creatinine with minimal or parallel rise in BUN is frequently noted with AKI. In contrast, a disproportionate rise in BUN with little rise in creatinine may reflect a prerenal process or increased protein intake, total parenteral nutrition (TPN), gastrointestinal (GI) bleeding, hypercatabolism, or steroid administration, which increase urea production.

4. Examine the urinary sediment. Tubular epithelial or granular ("muddy brown") casts are indicative of tubular injury, whereas hyaline casts are seen in low perfusion states. The sediment is important to examine because tests of tubular function, such as the urine sodium and osmolality, may be inaccurate with use of diuretics.

Table 12.5 • Evaluation of the Etiology of Oliguria

	Prerenal	Renal
BUN/Cr	>20:1	<10:1
U/P creatinine	>40	<20
U_{osm}	>500	<400
U/P osmolality	>1.3	<1.1
Urine specific gravity	>1.016	<1.010
U_{Na} (mEq/L)	<20	>40
FE_{Na}	<1%	>2%
Urinary sediment	Hyaline casts	Tubular epithelial cells Granular casts

5. Measure the urine sodium (U_{Na}) and creatinine (U_{Cr}) concentrations and the urine osmolality (U_{osm}). These tests can differentiate prerenal from renal causes, but their interpretation will be influenced by the use of diuretics. A U_{Na} <20 mEq/L and U_{osm} >500 mOsm/kg are strongly suggestive of prerenal disease. However, in oliguric patients, the U_{Na} will rise as the urine volume falls, leading to a higher U_{Na}, even in prerenal states.

a. In this situation, calculation of the fractional excretion of sodium (FE_{Na}) is helpful:

$$FE_{Na} = \frac{U_{Na} \times P_{Cr}}{P_{Na} \times U_{Cr}} \times 100$$

where U and P refer to the urinary and plasma concentrations, respectively, of sodium and creatinine.

b. In the oliguric patient, an FE_{Na} <1% reflects retained tubular function with absorption of sodium and water, consistent with a prerenal problem except in cases of contrast nephrotoxicity and hepatorenal syndrome. In contrast, an FE_{Na} >2% is usually caused by AKI. However, this may also be noted when a prerenal process is superimposed on chronic kidney disease, when the kidneys at baseline cannot conserve water and sodium appropriately. A rise in FE_{Na} may be noted during recovery of renal function due to sodium mobilization.

6. Monitor other electrolytes, blood glucose, and acid–base balance frequently.

7. Obtain a renal ultrasound to assess kidney size and rule out obstruction. A renal scan may be performed if a renal embolus is suspected.

F. **Management of oliguria and AKI** (Table 12.6).[156,160,161] Early aggressive intervention in patients with oliguria and early evidence of AKI may prevent progressive tubular injury and worsening of renal function. However, once AKI is established, very little can be done to promote recovery of renal function except to prevent additional insults. There is little evidence that strategies that increase renal blood flow or increase urine flow to reduce tubular obstruction have any impact on enhancing tubular epithelial cell proliferation and recovery of function.[162] Generally, attention should be directed towards maintaining urine output to reduce tissue edema and treating electrolyte or metabolic problems as they arise.

1. Ensure that the Foley catheter is within the bladder and is patent (this may rule out an obstructive uropathy). Irrigate with saline if necessary or consider changing the catheter empirically. If the Foley catheter has been removed, a bladder scan may indicate whether oliguria is real or spurious. A significant post-void residual may provide evidence of a post-obstructive uropathy as the cause of an elevated creatinine. Either way, replacement of the catheter may be helpful in further assessing the urine output.

2. Discontinue all potentially nephrotoxic drugs (ACE inhibitors, ARBs, NSAIDs, nephrotoxic antibiotics) and avoid any diagnostic studies requiring IV contrast.

3. Optimize hemodynamics. Although augmenting a good cardiac output may not be able to expedite recovery of renal function, it is clear that any additional insult that causes hypotension or hypoperfusion may contribute to a state of "protracted ARF". These insults include hypovolemia (often gastrointestinal bleeding), low cardiac output states (tamponade), arrhythmias (rapid atrial fibrillation, ventricular tachycardia), antihypertensive medications, or sepsis. Thus, there is little downside to optimizing hemodynamics to increase urine output even if the rate of renal recovery is not hastened.

Table 12.6 • Management of Low Urine Output

1. Ensure that Foley catheter is in the bladder and is patent

2. Optimize cardiac function
   - Treat hypovolemia
   - Control arrhythmias
   - Improve contractility
   - Reduce elevated afterload, but allow BP to drift up to 150 mm Hg

3. Diuretics or other medications
   - Give increasing doses of furosemide (up to 500 mg IV) or a continuous infusion of 10–20 mg/h
   - Add chlorothiazide 500 mg IV to the loop diuretic
   - Consider bumetanide 4–10 mg or 1 mg bolus, then 0.5–2 mg/h infusion
   - Give cocktail of furosemide + dopamine ± mannitol
   - Consider use of nesiritide 2 µg/kg over 1 minute followed by an infusion of 0.01–0.03 µg/kg/min if elevated filling pressures
   - Consider use of fenoldopam 0.1 µg/kg/min, especially if hypertensive

4. If above fail
   - Limit fluid to insensible losses
   - Readjust drug doses
   - Avoid potassium supplements
   - Nutrition: essential amino acid diet
     - → High nitrogen tube feeds if on dialysis
     - → Total parenteral nutrition with 4.25% amino acid/35% dextrose

5. Consider early renal replacement therapy

a. Optimize preload without being overzealous. Hemodynamic monitoring with a Swan-Ganz catheter may be indicated if a low cardiac output state is suspected. If the diagnosis is not clear, echocardiography can differentiate ventricular failure from tamponade from significant hypervolemia. Otherwise, assessment of fluid balance, central venous pressure monitoring, strict I & O's, and/or a careful physical examination may give an overall assessment of the patient's fluid balance and intravascular volume. Remember that in a state of capillary leak (often seen in sepsis, following surgery with a long duration of CPB, or with a persistent low output state) or with reduced oncotic pressure (as noted from hemodilution or poor nutritional condition), excessive fluid administration may produce noncardiogenic pulmonary edema.

b. Optimize heart rate and treat arrhythmias. Even though the patient may have a satisfactory heart rate, increasing the rate with pacing to augment the cardiac output might prove beneficial in improving renal perfusion and GFR.

    c. Improve contractility with inotropes if a low cardiac output state is present.

    d. Reduce afterload with vasodilators and try to eliminate drugs that cause renal vasoconstriction; avoid ACE inhibitors and ARBs.[163]

      i. Do not be overly aggressive in the reduction of systemic blood pressure in patients with preexisting hypertension and chronic kidney disease. They usually require a higher blood pressure (130–150 mm Hg systolic) to maintain renal perfusion.

      ii. If inotropic drugs with vasodilator properties are used, such as milrinone or dobutamine, an α-agent may be necessary to maintain systemic blood pressure. In this situation, norepinephrine is the preferred drug because it will also provide some inotropic support.[62–64] Use of a pure α-agent, such as phenylephrine, is more likely to cause renal vasoconstriction unless the cardiac output is excellent. Vasopressin should only be used in vasodilated states with good cardiac output.

    e. If the cardiac output remains marginal despite the use of multiple inotropes, consider the placement of an IABP. This may result in an abrupt and dramatic increase in urine output.

4. If oliguria persists despite optimization of hemodynamics, the next step is selection of a **diuretic**. Although a few studies suggest that loop diuretics may hasten a decline in creatinine and possibly shorten the duration of renal replacement therapy, the majority of studies have shown that loop diuretics do not have a direct effect on renal functional recovery or the natural history of AKI, and in fact may increase operative mortality and delay recovery of renal function.[164,165] However, loop diuretics have uniformly been shown to improve urine output and can often convert oliguric to nonoliguric renal failure if administered early after the onset of renal failure. This may minimize the adverse impact of fluid retention on pulmonary function. An improvement in urine output suggests that the extent of renal injury is less severe in patients with "diuretic-responsive" renal failure, and may portend an earlier decrease in Scr, contributing to an improvement in short- and long-term survival.[154]

    a. **Furosemide** is given in incremental doses starting at 10 mg IV. However, once acute renal failure is established, a dose of 100 mg IV is commonly required and should be given over 20–30 minutes to minimize ototoxicity. If urine output fails to increase within a few hours, the following steps can be taken:

      i. Increase the dose of furosemide up to 200 mg IV (limiting the cumulative daily dose to 1 g).

      ii. Use a continuous infusion of IV furosemide.[66] Give a loading dose of 40–100 mg, and then initiate an infusion of 10–20 mg/h. Rebolus before an increase in the infusion rate. This may be the best means of maintaining an adequate urine output.

      iii. Alternatively, bumetanide can be given either as a bolus dose of 4–10 mg IV or as a 1 mg load followed by a continuous infusion of 0.5–2 mg/h depending on the estimated creatinine clearance. There is little evidence, however, that one loop diuretic is better than any other.

    b. Various **combinations** of medications may be effective in improving diuresis.

      i. Add a **thiazide** diuretic to the loop diuretic. These include chlorothiazide 500 mg IV, metolazone (Zaroxolyn) 5–10 mg PO or via a nasogastric tube, or hydrochlorothiazide 50–200 mg PO qd. Thiazides block distal nephron sites and act synergistically with the loop diuretics to increase exposure of the distal tubules to solute. This combination is particularly effective in patients who tend to be diuretic-resistant.[166]

ii. The combination of dopamine and furosemide may be synergistic because the renal vasodilation and improved RBF produced by dopamine improve the delivery of furosemide to the loop diuretics to increase exposure.[167]

iii. The combination of mannitol (500 mL of 20% Osmitrol) + furosemide (1 g) + dopamine (2–3 μg/kg/min) started within the first 6 hours of oliguria has been shown to produce a significant diuresis with early restoration of renal function.[168]

5. **Nesiritide** is very effective in producing a diuresis and lowering pulmonary artery pressures in patients with heart failure and other states of neurohormonal activation (such as use of CPB). It acts primarily by dilating afferent arterioles and to a lesser extent efferent arterioles and improves renal blood flow. It can improve the delivery of diuretics to the tubules, thus producing a synergistic effect with the loop diuretics. It therefore may be of benefit to patients who are diuretic-resistant. It is given in a bolus dose of 2 μg/kg over 1 minute followed by an infusion of 0.01–0.03 μg/kg/min. There are limited data on use of nesiritide to treat postoperative AKI. One study found that nesiritide was very effective in improving diuresis and hemodynamics in patients whose oliguria did not respond to dopamine or diuretics.[169] Another report showed that patients with normal preoperative renal function who developed postoperative AKI had enhanced recovery of renal excretory function and a 50% reduction in the need for RRT when they received 50 ng/kg/min of recombinant human atrial natriuretic peptide.[170] It is likely that such a benefit may be demonstrated with nesiritide as well.

6. **Fenoldopam** has shown equivocal results in the treatment of established AKI after cardiac surgery. One study of patients receiving a 72-hour infusion for early acute AKI (a 50% rise in creatinine) showed a trend towards reduction in mortality and the need for dialysis in non-diabetic patients.[171] Another study using a 48-hour infusion of 0.1 μg/kg/min in similar patients found that it mitigated the progression of oliguria and increase in Scr and reduced the need for RRT.[172] A meta-analysis of fenoldopam studies in postoperative AKI confirmed the latter findings.[132] Another study comparing dopamine and fenoldopam in patients with early postoperative renal dysfunction found that fenoldopam was more effective in reversing renal hypoperfusion and improving creatinine levels, although urine output did not differ.[173]

7. Use of **"renal-dose" dopamine** (2–3 μg/kg/min) for postoperative oliguric renal failure has not been shown to influence the duration of AKI, the need for dialysis, or survival once AKI has developed.[174] Although it can produce a diuresis in patients with normal renal function, higher doses are required in patients with moderate renal dysfunction to improve RBF. Even if it does improve urine output, that may be its only benefit. Studies of dopamine use in critically ill patients have found it to be deleterious to recovery by worsening splanchnic oxygenation, impairing GI function, impairing endocrine and immunologic systems, and blunting the respiratory drive.[175] Comparisons of dopamine and dobutamine on renal function in critically ill patients have been evaluated in several studies. One showed that renal-dose dopamine

increased urine output without improving creatinine clearance, whereas dobutamine did just the opposite.[176] Another showed that dopamine produced a diuresis and improved creatinine clearance unrelated to any hemodynamic effects, whereas dobutamine had no effect on any renal variable.[177]

8. **Note: Mannitol** is an osmotic diuretic that is frequently used during surgery to increase serum osmolality during hemodilution to minimize tissue edema. It improves renal tubular flow, reduces tubular cell swelling, and also improves urine output. Nonetheless, it is best avoided in the postoperative period because its oncotic effect mobilizes fluid into the intravascular space. This could theoretically lead to pulmonary edema if fluid overload is present and urine output does not improve. In fact, a significant increase in serum osmolality can cause renal vasoconstriction and induce renal failure.

G. **Management of established renal failure**

1. Once oliguric renal failure is established, treatment should be directed towards optimizing hemodynamics while minimizing excessive fluid administration, providing appropriate nutrition, and initiating early renal replacement therapy to hopefully reduce morbidity and improve survival. The blood pressure should be maintained at a higher level than usual in hypertensive patients whose kidneys may require higher perfusion pressures.

2. Restrict fluids with mL/mL of fluid replacement (i.e., input = output) plus 500 mL D5W/0.2% normal saline/day (about 200 mL/m²/day). Daily weights are helpful in assessing changes in day-to-day fluid status, but must also take into consideration the influence of nutritional status on body mass.

3. Monitor electrolytes and blood glucose

   a. Avoid potassium supplements and medications that increase potassium levels (β-blockers, ACE inhibitors). Correct hyperkalemia as described on pages 616–617.

   b. Hyponatremia should be treated with fluid restriction.

   c. Metabolic acidosis should be corrected if serum bicarbonate falls below 15 mEq/L.

   d. Correct hyperglycemia and abnormalities of calcium, phosphate, or magnesium metabolism.

4. Medications

   a. Eliminate drugs that impair renal perfusion or are nephrotoxic (ACE inhibitors, ARBs, aminoglycosides, NSAIDs).

   b. Avoid or adjust doses of medications that are excreted or metabolized by the kidneys (particularly digoxin, low-molecular-weight heparin, and renally excreted antibiotics) (see Appendices 11 and 12).

   c. Give antacid medications (proton pump inhibitors) to minimize the risk of gastrointestinal bleeding, but avoid magnesium-containing antacids and laxatives.

5. Remove the Foley catheter and catheterize daily or prn depending on urine output. Culture the urine.

6. Improve the patient's nutritional state with enteral nutrition if possible.[178]

   a. If the patient is able to eat, an essential amino acid diet should be used. Protein should not be restricted if the patient is on hemodialysis, which can result in the loss of 3–5 g/h of protein. Patients on dialysis should receive approximately 1.5 g/kg/day of protein.

b. If the patient is unable to eat, but has a functional gastrointestinal tract, a high-nitrogen tube feeding can be used if the patient is on dialysis. For most patients with acute renal failure, there is no need to alter the amount of protein, and standard tube feedings can be used unless hyperkalemia is present. In patients with chronic kidney disease that does not require dialysis, a low-protein supplement can be used to provide 0.5–0.8 g/kg/day of protein.

c. If the patient is unable to tolerate enteral feedings, total parenteral nutrition using a 4.25% amino acid/35% dextrose solution that contains no potassium, magnesium, or phosphate is recommended.

7. Consider the prompt initiation of renal replacement therapy.

VI. Renal Replacement Therapy (Table 12.7)[179]

A. Various forms of renal replacement therapy (RRT) can be used to remove excessive fluid and solute to improve electrolyte balance and remove other nitrogenous waste products.

1. Indications. The most important indications for initiation of RRT are fluid overload, hyperkalemia, and metabolic acidosis. Other signs of uremia, such as a change in mental status, pericarditis, or GI bleeding, should also prompt initiation of RRT. However, a very important and sometimes difficult decision to make is whether RRT should be initiated at the first sign of persistent oliguria or a rising creatinine, especially since the latter tends to lag behind the extent of renal dysfunction. Studies suggest that early and aggressive dialysis, before the patient develops signs and symptoms of renal failure and before a marked elevation in

Table 12.7 • Techniques of Renal Replacement Therapy (Hemofiltration and Hemodialysis)

If the Patient Has:	HD	SCUF	CVVH	CVVHD
Unstable hemodynamics	–	+ + +	+ + +	+ + +
Contraindication to heparin	+ +	+	+	+
Vascular access problems	+ + +	+ + +	+ + +	+ + +
Volume overload	+ +	+ + +	+ + +	+ + +
Hyperkalemia	+ + +	0	+ +	+ + +
Severe uremia	+ + +	0	+	+ +
Respiratory compromise	+ +	+ + +	+ + +	+ + +

HD, hemodialysis; SCUF, slow continuous ultrafiltration; CVVH, continuous venovenous hemofiltration; CVVHD, continuous venovenous hemofiltration with dialysis.
– avoid; 0 minimal effect; + useful; + + better; + + + even better.

creatinine occurs, might improve outcomes.[180–184] Certainly, when marked oliguria is present early after surgery in a patient with significant fluid overload, a delay in initiating RRT may lead to respiratory compromise and prolonged ventilation with its attendant risks, as well as other complications commonplace to ventilated, sedated patients in the ICU. It is hopeful that an early aggressive approach will have some impact on the high mortality rate associated with postoperative RRT, which is even greater in patients with concomitant cardiac failure and when GI complications develop.[182]

2. An additional consideration in patients with moderate renal dysfunction (serum creatinine >2–2.5 mg/gL) is use of "prophylactic" preoperative dialysis. Several studies have demonstrated that this reduces the need for postoperative RRT, with a reduction in overall morbidity and mortality.[105,185]

3. The most common forms of RRT used in cardiac surgery patients are those of intermittent hemodialysis and continuous venovenous hemofiltration. Selection of a modality depends on the indications for it use (whether primarily for volume or solute removal), and the hemodynamic stability of the patient. Both modalities are associated with comparable outcomes, such as recovery of renal function and mortality.[186,187]

B. Intermittent hemodialysis (HD)

1. **Principle.** Solute passes by diffusion down a concentration gradient from the blood, across a hollow-fiber semipermeable membrane, and into a dialysate bath. Some solute is also transported by convection resulting from a difference in hydrostatic pressure (ultrafiltration).

2. **Indications.** HD is indicated for the management of hyperkalemia, acid-base imbalances, fluid overload, or a hypercatabolic state in the hemodynamically stable patient. It is the most efficient means of removing solute (urea, creatinine) and correcting severe acid-base abnormalities. It does not obligatorily remove fluid, but can be combined with ultrafiltration to achieve this goal.

3. **Access.** Standard intermittent HD is performed using a single 12 Fr double-lumen catheter (such as the Niagara Slim-Cath, Bard Access Systems, Inc.) placed in the internal jugular or subclavian vein, although the latter is more likely to be associated with venous thrombosis. Placement in the femoral vein may lead to lower-extremity venous thrombosis, but can be used for very short-term dialysis. To reduce the risk of infection in patients requiring more extended periods of dialysis, a double-lumen Permcath (Quinton Instrument Co.) or HemoGlide or HemoSplit long-term hemodialysis catheter (Bard Access Systems) can be placed into the internal jugular vein and brought through a subcutaneous tunnel. Subsequently, a fistula can be created for permanent dialysis. When recovery appears unlikely and a fistula is being considered, the arm vessels on one side should be protected from use as much as possible.

4. **Technique.** Intermittent HD is performed over a 3–4 hour period and usually provided at least three times per week until renal function recovers. The blood is pumped into the dialysis cartridge at a rate of 300–500 mL/min, while the dialysate solution is infused at a rate of 500 mL/min in a direction countercurrent to blood flow. Although heparin is commonly used, heparin-free HD is possible in patients with bleeding problems or heparin-induced thrombocytopenia.

5. Limitations

    a. Circulatory instability with hypotension from a blunted sympathetic reflex response to hypovolemia is the most common complication of HD, especially if large volumes are being removed in a short period of time. The rapid removal of solute will reduce plasma osmolality, prompting water movement into cells, exacerbating the depletion of extracellular volume. This problem has been mitigated to some degree by use of biocompatible membranes, bicarbonate baths, initial high dialysate sodium, cool temperatures, and volumetric control during dialysis. Colloid or blood transfusions and hemodynamic support (usually with α-agents or PO midodrine) are frequently necessary. Therefore, HD is best avoided in the hemodynamically unstable patient.

    b. Dialysis machines are complex and costly, and require special expertise.

C. Continuous venovenous systems can be used in a variety of ways, including slow continuous ultrafiltration (SCUF), continuous venovenous hemofiltration (CVVH), and continuous venovenous hemodiafiltration (CVVHD).

    1. Principle. An occlusive pump is included in a circuit that actively withdraws blood at a designated rate from the venous system, pumps it with hydrostatic pressure through the membrane of a hemofilter and then returns the blood to the venous system. This circuit achieves filtration or convection of plasma water. For CVVHD, dialysis fluid runs countercurrent to the direction of blood flow within the diafilter. Solute then passes by diffusion down a concentration gradient across a hemofilter into the dialysate solution.

    2. Indications. These systems are indicated for the management of fluid overload, especially in the hemodynamically unstable or hypotensive patient. Slow correction of electrolyte imbalance can be achieved with CVVH using a crystalloid solution of different composition for replacement fluid. Severe electrolyte imbalance or a hypercatabolic state is better managed with CVVHD.

    3. Access is obtained using a 12 Fr double-lumen catheter (12 gauge for each lumen) placed in the internal jugular, subclavian, or femoral vein.

    4. Technique (Figure 12.6)

        a. Most CVVH circuits are "integrated" systems that include the blood pump, pressure monitors, air detector with shut-off controls, and fluid balancing systems for ultrafiltrate control. A high-efficiency biocompatible hemodialysis cartridge is attached downstream to an occlusive pump and heparin is infused into the inflow portion of the circuit to maintain a dialyzer output (venous) PTT of 45–60 sec. Alternatively, regional citrate anticoagulation can be infused into the inflow limb instead of heparin, especially in patients with bleeding or heparin-induced thrombocytopenia.[188,189] When citrate is used, steps must be taken to avoid hypocalcemia and metabolic alkalosis. Calcium should be infused in the venous return line post-filter and alkaline buffers must be reduced in replacement fluids for CVVH or in the dialysate solution for CVVHD.

        b. For **CVVH**, the pump is usually set to deliver blood at a rate of 250 mL/min and the ultrafiltrate rate is usually set at a preselected rate around 16.7 mL/min or 1 L/h. This can provide a daily ultrafiltrate volume of 24 liters/day. The blood then passes through a bubble trap air detector and is returned to the patient.

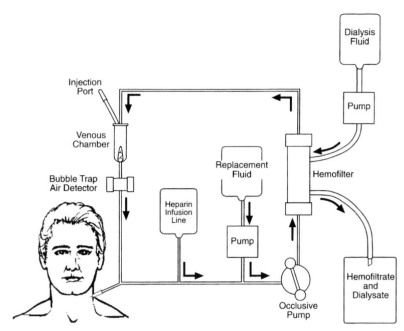

Figure 12.6 • Continuous venovenous hemofiltration (CVVH). An occlusive pump withdraws blood from the venous circuit, pumps it through a diafilter, and returns it to the venous system through a double-lumen catheter placed in the internal jugular vein.

Replacement fluid (alternating 1 L of 0.9% NS plus 1 ampoule (10 mL of a 10% solution) of calcium gluconate with 1 L of 0.45% NS plus 1 ampoule (50 mEq/ 50 mL) of 8.4% NaHCO$_3$) is infused into the outflow (return) circuit or into the venous chamber. The amount administered is dictated by the desired negative fluid balance per hour. This technique can achieve a moderate amount of solute removal. Clotting of the system is less likely because the dialyzer can be prediluted with a large volume of fluid.

c. For **SCUF**, the blood flow rate is set at 50–80 mL/min and the ultrafiltrate rate is set at the desired amount (about 5 mL/min) which can potentially achieve a net negative fluid balance of up to 7 L/day. The filter is more prone to clotting due to the slow flow and because the postfilter hematocrit is high. Since no replacement fluid is given and minimal solute is removed, SCUF is ineffective for uremia or hyperkalemia.

d. **CVVHD** combines the convective solute removal of CVVH with the diffusive solute removal of hemodialysis. The blood flow is set at 150–300 mL/min and the dialysate (Dianeal 1.5% with 4 mL of 23% NaCL per 2 L bag) is infused into the dialysis cartridge at a rate of 1–2 L/h or even higher. This technique is most useful in the highly catabolic patient for the removal of a large solute load. The effluent flow rate (hemofiltration rate + the dialysate flow rate) should be about 20 mL/kg.

5. **Advantages and limitations**

    a. Citrate anticoagulation eliminates concerns about use of heparin.

    b. High flow rates of CVVH/CVVHD reduce the potential for clotting of the filter noted with SCUF.

    c. Venous access eliminates vascular disease as an impediment to arterial access.

    d. Use of the blood pump enables CVVH to be performed when the patient is hypotensive or hemodynamically unstable.

    e. Because CVVH removes so much fluid, it is essential to carefully monitor electrolytes and modify the replacement solutions as necessary to maintain electrolyte balance.

    f. The pump adds some complexity and cost to the system compared with arteriovenous hemofiltration.

D. Continuous arteriovenous hemofiltration (CAVH) is used during surgery to remove excessive fluid before terminating CPB. It is beneficial in improving hemodynamics, hemostasis, and pulmonary function in higher-risk patients. Postoperatively, its use is limited by the need for arterial access, heparinization to minimize clotting of the hemofilter, and the requirement for satisfactory arterial pressure to provide the hydrostatic pressure to achieve hemofiltration. Because of these drawbacks, CAVH has been replaced by CVVH in most units.

E. Peritoneal dialysis (PD) is rarely used in cardiac surgical patients because it produces abdominal distention and glucose absorption that can compromise respiratory status, and it carries the risk of peritonitis. Its use is usually limited to patients on chronic peritoneal dialysis.

VII. Hyperkalemia[190,191]

A. Etiology

1. High-volume, high-potassium cardioplegia solutions used in the operating room. The potassium load is usually eliminated promptly by normally functioning kidneys, but hyperkalemia can be problematic in patients with intrinsic renal dysfunction or oliguria from other causes.

2. Low cardiac output states associated with oliguria. Potassium levels may rise with alarming and life-threatening rapidity.

3. Severe tissue ischemia, whether peripheral (from severe peripheral vascular disease or complication of an IABP) or intra-abdominal (mesenteric ischemia). Hyperkalemia is often the first clue to the existence of these problems.

4. Acute and chronic renal insufficiency

5. Medications that impair potassium excretion or increase potassium levels (ACE inhibitors, potassium-sparing diuretics, NSAIDs, ARBs, β-blockers)

Note: Remember that hyperkalemia is exacerbated by acidosis, which often accompanies low output or ischemic syndromes. A 0.2 unit change in pH produces about a 1 mEq/L change in serum potassium concentration. However, in conditions of organic acidosis, the potassium is more likely to rise from tissue breakdown and release of potassium from cells (lactic acidosis) or from insulin deficiency and hyperglycemia (ketoacidosis), than from a change in pH.

B. Manifestations are predominantly electrocardiographic due to depolarization of cardiac cell resting membrane potentials that decreases membrane excitability. An asystolic arrest may occur when the potassium rises rapidly to a level exceeding 6.5 mEq/L. The ECG changes of hyperkalemia do not always develop in classic progressive fashion and are more related to the rate of rise of serum potassium than to the absolute level. These changes include:

1. Peaked T waves
2. ST depression
3. Smaller R waves
4. Prolonged PR interval
5. Loss of P waves
6. QRS widening, bradycardia, asystole, ventricular fibrillation
   When the heart is being paced, hyperkalemia may result in failure to respond to the pacemaker stimulus.

C. **Treatment** entails stabilizing the cell membrane, shifting potassium into cells, and increasing its excretion from the body (Table 12.8).

1. It is essential to identify and remove any potential source of potassium intake or medications that may increase the potassium level (as above); use a low-potassium diet in patients with renal dysfunction and persistent hyperkalemia.

2. Optimize cardiac function:
   a. If there is evidence of advanced cardiac toxicity or ECG changes, usually when the potassium is >6.5 mEq/L, administer **calcium gluconate** 10 mL of a 10% solution (1 g) IV over 2−3 minutes to stabilize the cell membranes. Note that calcium should be avoided in patients on digoxin.
   b. Alternatively, calcium chloride 5−10 mL of a 10% solution (0.5−1 g) can be infused through a central line over several minutes.

Table 12.8 • Acute Treatment of Hyperkalemia

Medication	Dosage	Onset of Action	Duration of Action
Calcium gluconate	10 mL of 10% solution over 2–3 min	Immediate	30 min
Insulin	10 units regular insulin IV in 50 mL of 50% dextrose	15–30 min	2–6 hours
Sodium bicarbonate	1 amp 7.5% (44.6 mEq)	30 min	1–2 hours
Albuterol	10–20 mg by nebulizer	90 min (peak effect)	2–3 hours
Furosemide	20–40 mg IV	15–60 min	4 hours
Sodium polystyrene sulfonate (Kayexalate)	Oral: 30 g in 60–120 mL sorbitol PR: 50 g in retention enema	1–2 hours	4–6 hours

3. Shift potassium into cells:

    a. Regular insulin 10 units in 50 mL of a 50% dextrose solution IV. This should lower the potassium about 0.5–1.5 mEq/L within 15 minutes and last for several hours. This can be considered first if there is marked hyperkalemia but no ECG changes.

    b. Sodium bicarbonate ($NaHCO_3$) (1 ampoule of 50 mL of a 7.5% solution with 44.6 mEq or of an 8.4% solution with 50 mEq) should be given to raise the pH to 7.40–7.50 if the patient has a metabolic acidosis. This will lower the serum potassium in about 30 minutes with an effect that lasts for several hours. Bicarbonate also has a direct effect on hyperkalemia independent of a change in pH.[192] In hyponatremic patients, the sodium load may reverse some of the ECG changes of hyperkalemia.

    c. β_2-agonists activate the Na^+-K^+-ATPase system to drive potassium into cells and can lower the potassium level by 0.5–1.5 mEq/L. Recommended drugs include **albuterol** 10–20 mg in 4 mL NS by nebulizer, which has a peak effect in about 90 minutes, or an infusion of IV epinephrine 0.05 µg/kg/min, which achieves its peak effect in about 30 minutes.[193]

4. Enhance potassium excretion:

    a. Furosemide 20–40 mg IV is very effective in reducing serium potassium in patients with well-functioning kidneys. Higher doses may be required in patients with AKI or chronic kidney disease.

    b. Sodium polystyrene sulfonate (**Kayexalate**) enema 50 g in 150 mL of water can be given every 2–4 hours. **Note** that sorbitol should be avoided in an enema because of an association with colonic necrosis in early postoperative patients due to decreased colonic motility. Alternatively, 30 g in 60–120 mL of 20% sorbitol can be given orally up to three times daily. Each gram may bind up to 1 mEq of potassium. This is a reasonable first step in the stable postoperative patient with a slowly rising potassium >5.5 mEq/L despite withdrawal of contributing factors.

    c. Hemodialysis may be indicated if the above measures fail to lower the potassium to adequate levels. It can remove up to 50 mEq of potassium per hour.

VIII. Hypokalemia[194]

A. Etiology

1. Profound diuresis without adequate potassium replacement. Potassium excretion parallels the urine output after bypass, which tends to be copious because of hemodilution. The use of potent diuretics may produce a significant diuresis and kaliuresis in the early postoperative period.

2. Insulin to treat hyperglycemia

3. Alkalosis (metabolic or respiratory)

4. Significant nasogastric tube drainage

B. Manifestations. The primary concern with hypokalemia in the cardiac patient is the induction of cardiac reentrant arrhythmias due to enhanced cardiac automaticity and delayed ventricular repolarization. Hypokalemia may produce atrial, junctional, or ventricular ectopy (PACs, PVCs), paroxysmal atrial and junctional tachycardias, AV block and ventricular tachycardia/fibrillation. The ECG may demonstrate flattened ST segments, decreased T-wave amplitude and the presence of "u" waves. Factors that may promote the development of hypokalemic arrhythmias include myocardial ischemia, enhanced sympathetic tone (often from epinephrine or β_2-agonists), digoxin, and low magnesium levels (commonly seen after CPB). Hypokalemia can also result in weakness involving the respiratory muscles, the GI tract, producing an ileus, or the skeletal muscles.

C. **Treatment** is indicated for any potassium level below the normal range, although a level lower than 3.0 mEq/L is usually present before ECG changes become evident.

1. It is essential that renal function and urine output be evaluated before a potassium chloride (KCl) drip is started, because acute hyperkalemia can develop very rapidly when oliguria or renal dysfunction is present. A slower infusion rate is advisable in this situation, with frequent rechecking of the serum potassium level.

2. In the ICU setting, KCl is administered through a central line at a rate of 10–20 mEq/h (mix of 20 mEq/100 mL normal saline or 0.45% NS). A dextrose carrier should be avoided because it may lower the potassium level by stimulating secretion of insulin. The serum potassium rises approximately 0.1 mEq/L for each 2 mEq of KCl administered. Repeat potassium levels should guide therapy.

3. When a central line is not present, a concentrated potassium drip cannot be administered peripherally because it scleroses veins. The maximum concentration of KCl that can be administered peripherally is 60 mEq/L. Oral potassium (10–20 mEq tablets up to three to four times a day) will usually suffice for potassium levels of 3–4 mEq/L. However, doses of 40–60 mEq three to four times a day may be necessary to maintain normal potassium levels when the potassium is <3 mEq/L.

4. Particular attention should be paid to sources of urinary or GI loss of potassium that may require more aggressive replacement.

IX. Hypocalcemia

A. Calcium plays a complex role in myocardial energetics and reperfusion damage. Ionized calcium (normal = 1.1–1.3 mmol/L) should be measured, because total calcium levels, which are affected by protein binding, usually decrease during surgery because of hemodilution, hypothermia, shifts in pH, hypomagnesemia, and the use of citrated blood. Hypocalcemia is usually associated with prolongation of the QT interval on the ECG tracing. It reduces cardiac sensitivity to digoxin.

B. **Treatment**

1. It is common practice to empirically administer a 500 mg bolus of calcium chloride at the termination of bypass to support systemic vascular resistance and possibly increase myocardial contractility.[195] It is also commonly mixed with protamine to offset its vasodilatory effects.

2. It is questionable whether treatment of hypocalcemia identified in the ICU is of any value in improving cardiovascular function. In fact, calcium salts may attenuate the

cardiotonic effects of catecholamines, such as dobutamine or epinephrine, although they have little effect on the efficacy of milrinone.[196] Nonetheless, if the ionized calcium level is measured and found to be <1 mmol/L, calcium gluconate (10 mL of 10% solution in 50 mL D5W) may be given over 10–20 minutes, although there is no clear benefit to doing so. It may also be given as an infusion of 50 mL/h of a 10% solution (placing 100 mL in 1 L of D5W). Calcium chloride ($CaCl_2$) is best avoided for "asymptomatic" hypocalcemia to minimize any acute hemodynamic effects, but similar dosing is used. Because hypocalcemia can be difficult to correct if the serum magnesium levels is low, an infusion of magnesium sulfate 2 grams (16 mEq) of a 10% solution over 10–20 minutes may be given, with a subsequent infusion of 1 g (8 mEq) in 100 mL of fluid per hour.[197]

3. Calcium chloride (0.5–1 g IV) may be given in emergency situations to provide temporary circulatory support when a low cardiac output syndrome or profound hypotension develops suddenly. The transient improvement in hemodynamics allows time for analysis of causative factors and the institution of other pharmacologic support. $CaCl_2$ should not be given routinely during a cardiac arrest.

X. Hypomagnesemia

A. Magnesium plays a role in energy metabolism and cardiac impulse generation. Low levels have been associated with coronary spasm, low cardiac output syndromes, prolonged ventilatory support, a higher incidence of postoperative atrial and ventricular arrhythmias, perioperative infarction, and a higher mortality rate.[198,199]

B. Magnesium levels (normal = 1.5–2 mEq/L) are usually not measured during surgery, but are reduced in the majority of patients. This is usually the result of hemodilution during CPB as well as urinary excretion, but it is also very common in patients undergoing off-pump surgery.[200]

C. Administration of magnesium sulfate ($MgSO_4$) 2 g in 100 mL solution to raise the serum level to 2 mEq/L is effective in reducing the incidence of postoperative atrial fibrillation and ventricular arrhythmias after both on-pump and off-pump surgery.[201,202] Notably, magnesium has been found to inhibit the vasoconstrictive response to epinephrine, but not its cardiotonic effects.[203] Administering 1–2 g of $MgSO_4$ at the conclusion of bypass and on the first postoperative morning can be recommended.

XI. Metabolic Acidosis

A. Etiology

1. A low cardiac output state, which is often associated with peripheral vasoconstriction from hypothermia or use of vasoconstrictive drugs, is the primary cause of metabolic acidosis in the cardiac surgery patient.

2. Low-dose epinephrine occasionally causes a metabolic acidosis out of proportion to its α effects when the cardiac output is satisfactory. This may reflect a metabolic type B lactic acidosis (not associated with tissue hypoxia) caused by metabolic factors that increase lactic acid production, such as hyperglycemia and lipolysis.[204]

3. Intra-abdominal catastrophes, such as mesenteric ischemia from a low-flow state, should always be considered when progressive metabolic acidosis occurs.

4. Sepsis
5. High doses of sodium nitroprusside
6. Renal failure (which reduces acid excretion)
7. Acute hepatic dysfunction
8. Diabetic ketoacidosis

B. **Effects**

1. Adverse effects of metabolic acidosis usually do not occur until the pH is less than 7.20.[205] A pure metabolic acidosis (low serum bicarbonate with acidemic pH) may be noted in the heavily sedated patient in whom there is no respiratory compensation. However, compensatory hyperventilation to neutralize the acidosis will occur when the patient can breathe spontaneously, and for every 1 mEq/L fall in bicarbonate, the PCO_2 is generally reduced about 1.2 torr. However, it is not uncommon to see incomplete compensation with a mixed respiratory/metabolic acidosis. Notably, some of the deleterious effects of metabolic acidosis may be related to the metabolic products associated with the acidosis, rather than the absolute level of pH, although they may be reversed by administration of sodium bicarbonate.

2. The presence of a progressive or significant metabolic acidosis (as assessed by the serum bicarbonate level) is often an indication of a serious ongoing problem that must be corrected before adverse consequences occur. These include:

   a. Cardiovascular effects
      - Decreased contractility and cardiac output; reduction in hepatic and renal blood flow
      - Attenuation of the positive inotropic effects of catecholamines[206]
      - Venoconstriction and arteriolar dilatation which increase filling pressures and decrease systemic pressures
      - Increased pulmonary vascular resistance
      - Sensitization to reentrant arrhythmias and reduction in the threshold for ventricular fibrillation

   b. Respiratory effects
      - Dyspnea and tachypnea
      - Decreased respiratory muscle strength

   c. Metabolic changes
      - Increased metabolic demands
      - Hyperglycemia caused by tissue insulin resistance and inhibition of anaerobic glycolysis
      - Decreased hepatic update and increased hepatic production of lactate
      - Hyperkalemia
      - Increased protein catabolism

   d. Cerebral function
      - Inhibition of brain metabolism and cell volume regulation
      - Obtundation and coma

3. Type A lactic acidosis reflects impaired tissue oxygenation and anaerobic metabolism resulting from circulatory failure. The acidosis is self-perpetuating in that

excess lactate is being produced at a time when there is suppression of hepatic lactate utilization. The lactate ion, probably more than the acidosis, contributes to potential cardiovascular dysfunction. Elevated lactate levels (>3 mmol/L) upon arrival in the ICU are associated with a worse outcome. They are more commonly noted in patients with preexisting renal dysfunction, after long pump runs, and with use of intraoperative vasopressors. It is likely that this reflects inadequate oxygen delivery during bypass that can contribute to splanchnic and renal ischemia with the acidosis perpetuated by a low cardiac output syndrome.[25,204,207] Needless to say, the presence of elevated lactate levels during bypass or upon arrival in the ICU requires prompt attention. The development of a metabolic acidosis several days after surgery raises the specter of mesenteric ischemia, especially in patients requiring additional days of ICU care.

4. Type B lactic acidosis occurs in the absence of tissue hypoxia. It may be a catecholamine-induced metabolic effect (especially with epinephrine) caused by hyperglycemia and alterations in fatty acid metabolism that cause pyruvate accumulation and elevated levels of lactic acid. Acute hepatic failure may also be present with severe lactic acidosis due to failure to clear lactic acid. Metformin is associated with lactic acidosis in patients with renal insufficiency, low cardiac output states, and liver disease, and with use of contrast agents.

C. **Assessment**

1. Measurement of the anion gap (AG) is important is sorting out the etiology of acidosis (AG $= Na^+ - (Cl^- + HCO_3^-)$), with normal range being 3–13 mEq/L).

2. Although there are a number of factors that can influence the anion gap, an increase in AG generally reflects additional acid production, and high AG metabolic acidosis is what is most common after cardiac surgery. It may also be elevated in diabetic ketoacidosis due to production of hydroxybutyrate or in renal failure from retention of hydrogen ions.

3. A normal or low anion gap represents loss of bicarbonate (diarrhea, renal tubular acidosis).

D. **Treatment** should be directed primarily towards reversal of the underlying cause. This will allow for oxidation of lactate and regeneration of bicarbonate to correct the acidosis. Whether correction of a primary metabolic acidosis (not one that compensates for a primary respiratory alkalosis) should be considered when the serum bicarbonate is less than 15 mEq/L (base deficit greater than 8–10 mmol/L) is controversial.

1. Proponents of bicarbonate administration suggest that severe metabolic acidosis does have significant deleterious effects on cardiovascular function that can be corrected with a more normal pH. Furthermore, more responsiveness to catecholamines does seem to occur with a more normal pH. Thus, correction of the acidosis may be important when the etiology of the acidosis is unclear or not imminently remediable.[205]

2. Others argue that the use of bicarbonate can cause metabolic derangements with little evidence of hemodynamic improvement.[208,209] Sodium bicarbonate can cause fluid overload, hypernatremia, and hyperosmolarity, increased affinity of hemoglobin for oxygen (and thus less tissue release), and reduced ionized calcium, which may reduce cardiac contractility. It is proposed that bicarbonate may correct only

the blood pH, not the intracellular pH, and that the increased production of CO_2 that may not be eliminated in low output states may impair lactate utilization, perpetuating the elevated lactate levels.

3. If one elects to correct the pH, there are several compounds that can be used:

   a. **Sodium bicarbonate** is administered in a dose calculated from the following equation:

   $$0.5 \times \text{body weight in kg} \times \text{base deficit} = \text{mEq NaHCO}_3$$

   This should be administered over several hours in the patient with severe metabolic acidosis with careful monitoring of the serum sodium concentration. Because the bicarbonate is metabolized to CO_2, this can worsen a respiratory acidosis in a patient with compromised pulmonary function.

   b. **Carbicarb** (available in Canada) is an equimolar solution of sodium bicarbonate and sodium carbonate.[210] One of its advantages over $NaHCO_3$ alone is that it does not undergo significant breakdown into CO_2 and H_2O. However, it still runs the risk of producing hypernatremia and fluid overload. It may raise the intracellular pH more consistently than $NaHCO_3$. The recommended dose is:

   $$0.2 \times \text{kg} \times \text{base deficit} = \text{mEq sodium}$$

   c. **Tromethamine** 0.3 M (THAM or Tris buffer) is most beneficial in the patient with hypernatremia or a mixed metabolic/respiratory acidosis because it limits CO_2 generation and will not raise the serum sodium. In contrast to $NaHCO_3$, it does not lower serum potassium, but it can produce hypoglycemia and respiratory depression.[205] It is usually given as a continuous infusion and is contraindicated in renal failure.[211]

   $$\text{kg} \times \text{base deficit} = \text{mL of 0.3 M THAM}$$

4. In a mechanically ventilated patient, it is not unreasonable to hyperventilate the patient to lower the PCO_2; this will increase the intracellular and extracellular pH.

XII. Metabolic Alkalosis[212]

A. Etiology

1. Excessive diuresis, especially from the loop diuretics, which promotes hypovolemia and depletion of hydrogen ions and chloride
2. Nasogastric drainage and inadequate electrolyte replacement by IV solutions
3. Total parenteral nutrition with inappropriate solute composition
4. Secondary as compensation for respiratory acidosis

B. Pathophysiology

1. Hypovolemia stimulates aldosterone secretion, which causes sodium retention, which then prevents excretion of sodium bicarbonate. Aldosterone also increases hydrogen secretion into the tubules, increasing bicarbonate reabsorption.

2. Decreased available chloride delivered to the distal tubules results in less chloride–bicarbonate exchange and thus less bicarbonate excretion.

3. Potassium loss directly increases bicarbonate reabsorption. This shifts hydrogen into the cells in exchange for potassium, raising the plasma bicarbonate concentration, and the lower intracellular pH stimulates hydrogen secretion and bicarbonate reabsorption.

C. **Adverse effects**

1. Lowers the serum potassium level, potentially leading to atrial and ventricular arrhythmias (especially digoxin-induced arrhythmias) and to neuromuscular weakness.

2. Has an adverse effect on the cardiovascular response to catecholamines that is comparable to that of acidosis.[206]

3. Shifts the oxygen–hemoglobin dissociation curve to the left, impairing oxygen delivery to the tissues. This effect is offset in chronic metabolic alkalosis by an increase in 2,3-DPG in red cells.

4. Produces arteriolar constriction which can compromise cerebral and coronary perfusion. Neurologic abnormalities including headache, seizures, tetany, and lethargy may occur, probably because of the associated hypocalcemia induced by alkalosis. These effects are usually seen with a pH >7.60.

5. Decreases the central respiratory drive, leading to hypoventilation, CO_2 retention, and potentially hypoxemia.

D. **Treatment**

1. Metabolic alkalosis is sustained by volume depletion ("contraction alkalosis"), as well as by potassium and chloride depletion. Thus, therapy should be directed towards correction of these factors.

2. Potential contributors to alkalosis should be assessed.

   a. Reduce doses of loop diuretics or thiazides to avoid volume depletion. Use proton pump inhibitors to minimize loss of gastric acid through a nasogastric tube.

   b. Avoid lactated Ringer's solution and acetate (common in parenteral nutrition solutions) that are metabolized to bicarbonate.

3. The administration of chloride, usually as potassium (KCl) or sodium (NaCl), is the primary treatment for metabolic alkalosis. The appropriate solution depends on the patient's volume status and potassium level.

   a. In hypovolemic patients, 0.9% sodium chloride is the primary replacement fluid, and KCl may also be given for hypokalemia. Volume repletion removes the stimulus for sodium resorption, allowing for more bicarbonate excretion. Chloride repletion increases chloride delivery to the distal tubules and augments the chloride–bicarbonate exchange mechanism. Potassium moves into cells in exchange for hydrogen ions which buffer the bicarbonate. The reduction in intracellular pH in renal tubular cells reduces hydrogen secretion and bicarbonate reabsorption.

   b. In patients with total body water overload, typical in the postoperative state or with CHF, infusion of sodium chloride may exacerbate the edema. A KCl infusion is beneficial if the serum K^+ is not elevated, but it can only be given at a limited rate (20 mEq/L). During a profound diuresis with significant potassium loss, a faster infusion rate can be used. Alternative means of treating alkalosis in these states include the following:

i. **Acetazolamide** (Diamox) 250–500 mg IV can be given in conjunction with a loop diuretic to increase urine output. Acetazolamide is a carbonic an hydrase inhibitor that inhibits proximal bicarbonate reaborption by the kidneys, but it is a weak diuretic when used alone. It can lead to potassium depletion, so normokalemia should be present before it is started. One can also consider using a potassium-sparing diuretic, such as spironolactone 25 mg PO qd, amiloride 5 mg PO qd, or eplerenone 50 mg PO qd, an aldosterone antagonist.

ii. **Hydrochloric acid** 0.1 N (100 mEq/L) may be administered through a central line at a rate of 10–20 mEq/h. It is rarely required in cardiac surgical patients. The total dose can be calculated based on a bicarbonate space of 50% body weight from either of the two following methods:

- Chloride-deficit method:

$$\text{mEq HCl} = 0.5 \times \text{kg (IBW)} \times (103 - \text{measured chloride})$$

where IBW is ideal body weight.

- Base-excess method:

$$\text{mEq HCl} = 0.5 \times \text{kg (IBW)} \times (\text{serum HCO}_3^- - 24)$$

where (serum $HCO_3^- - 24$)) represents the base excess. If a profound alkalosis is present, these doses should be given over 12 hours with intermittent reevaluation.

XIII. Hyperglycemia

A. **Etiology**

1. The hormonal stress response to surgery, which induces insulin resistance in both diabetics (who also have impaired insulin production) and non-diabetics.[213] This is associated with elevated levels of the counterregulatory hormones, including cortisol, epinephrine, and growth hormone.[214]

2. Total parenteral nutrition with inadequate insulin response

3. Sepsis (often the first manifestation of an occult sternal wound infection or an intra-abdominal process)

B. **Manifestations.** Intraoperative and postoperative hyperglycemia are associated with an increase in morbidity and mortality in both diabetic and non-diabetic patients.[214–220]

1. Increased urine output from an osmotic diuresis. Although the hypotonic fluid loss may cause hypernatremia, the glucose-induced shift of water from cells into the extracellular fluid compartment may cause hyponatremia. In this situation, the plasma osmolality is elevated despite the low serum sodium, a condition treated by fluid administration, rather than restriction.

2. Impaired wound healing and increased risk of sternal wound infection. This is noted in diabetics and non-diabetics with hyperglycemia, indicating that the blood glucose level itself is an independent risk factor.[219]

3. Increased risk of atrial fibrillation, cardiac, respiratory, renal, neurologic, and infectious complications.[217-220]

4. Worsened cognitive function has arguably been noted in non-diabetics with intraoperative hyperglycemia, but not in diabetics.[221,222]

C. **Treatment**

1. Prevention of intraoperative hyperglycemia might result in less neurologic morbidity and possibly less renal dysfunction, and it should be considered an integral component of perioperative glucose management.[121] Therefore, IV insulin should be given to keep the blood glucose less than 180 mg/dL. Several studies have shown little difference in outcome when comparing a stringent intraoperative blood glucose control protocol (maintaining a blood glucose between 80 and 100 mg/dL) to one using insulin only if the glucose was >200 mg/dL.[223,224]

2. In the intensive care unit, maintaining a blood glucose <180 mg/dL during the first 48 hours after surgery has been shown to reduce the risk of wound infection and mortality, primarily in diabetic patients, with some evidence of benefits in non-diabetics as well.[225-228] Therefore, a hyperglycemia protocol should be followed with careful monitoring of blood glucose (Appendix 6). Novolin R is the usual preparation used for IV boluses and infusions. An intravenous bolus of insulin is rapidly cleared from the blood and may lower the potassium level without affecting the blood glucose. Therefore, a bolus followed by an infusion (using a mix of 100 units of regular insulin/100 mL normal saline) is recommended. Excessively stringent control (keeping glucose <120 mg/dL) is potentially dangerous and probably not necessary.

3. All diabetic patients should have a fingerstick blood glucose drawn before meals and at bedtime once they are started on an oral diet. The glucose level may be higher than suspected from the patient's oral intake because of the residual elevation of counterregulatory hormones from the operation. On the other hand, the blood glucose may remain acceptable without medications in some patients with poor oral intake.

4. Patients with type I diabetes mellitus should have their insulin doses gradually increased back to preoperative levels depending on blood glucose levels and early postoperative insulin requirements.[228] It is preferable to use a lower dose of intermediate or long-acting insulin initially (usually one-half of the usual dose) and supplement it with regular insulin as necessary (Table 12.9). Insulin doses may be increased when the patient becomes more active and has an improved caloric intake.

5. In type II diabetics, oral hypoglycemic medications should be restarted once the patient is taking a normal diet, with frequent checking of fingersticks to assess the adequacy of blood glucose control. Additional coverage may be given with regular insulin (Novolin R). If blood glucose is not well controlled postoperatively, or in patients with preoperative HbA1c levels >7, an endocrine consultation should be considered to initiate the patient on insulin therapy.

Table 12.9 • Commonly Used Insulin Products in Postoperative Patients

Preparation	Brand	Onset	Peak	Average Duration
Very fast–acting (give 15 minutes prior to meals)				
Insulin lispro	Humalog	< 15 min	30–90 min	2–4 h
Insulin aspart	Novolog	5–10 min	1–3 h	3–5 h
Short (fast)–acting				
Regular insulin	Humulin R	30–60 min	2–3 h	5–8 h
Regular insulin	Novolin R	30–60 min	2.5–5 h	5–8 h
Intermediate–acting				
NPH insulin	Humulin N	60–90 min	6–12 h	16–24 h
NPH insulin	Novolin N	60–90 min	4–12 h	16–24 h
Long–acting				
Insulin glargine	Lantus	60 min	none	24 h

1. Combinations of insulin lispro protamine/insulin lispro (Humalog 75/25), insulin aspart protamine/insulin aspart (Novolog mix 70/30), NPH/regular (Humulin 70/30, Novolin 70/30, Humulin 50/50) provide rapid onset of action with two peaks (the first at 1–3 hours and the second at 4–10 hours) with durations of effect of 10–16 hours for each preparation.

2. Onset, peak, and duration may vary depending in part on dose and patient activity.

Humulin products made by Lilly; Novolin products made by Novo Nordisk; Lantus made by Sanofi Aventis.

D. **Hyperosmolar, hyperglycemic, nonketotic coma** has been reported in type II diabetics following surgery. It commonly develops 4–7 days after surgery and is manifested by polyuria in association with a rising BUN or serum sodium. The resultant dehydration, often exacerbated by GI bleeding or use of high-nitrogen, hyperosmolar tube feedings, results in the hyperosmolar state.[229] Gradual correction of hypovolemia, hyperglycemia, hypokalemia, and hypernatremia is indicated. Consultation with an endocrinologist is important in the assessment and management of these patients.

E. **Diabetic ketoacidosis** is rarely seen following cardiac surgery, but may be noted in type I diabetics. An endocrine consultation and standard management with saline infusions, an insulin drip, and correction of potassium and acid–base abnormalities should be followed.

F. **Note: Hypoglycemia** is extremely uncommon after open-heart surgery. Possible causes include:

1. Administration of excessive doses of insulin (either SC or as a continuous infusion); repeating a blood glucose level every 2 hours is essential in patients on a continuous infusion, especially at high rates.

2. Premature resumption of preoperative insulin or oral hypoglycemic drug doses in patients with poor oral food intake.

3. Residual effects of oral hypoglycemic agents in patients with renal dysfunction.

4. A severe hepatic insult with impaired glucose production.

XIV. Hypothyroidism

A. Hypothyroidism is difficult to treat preoperatively in the patient with ischemic heart disease because thyroid replacement may precipitate ischemic symptoms. It may be present more often than realized in patients taking thyroid hormone replacement. One study showed a significantly greater operative mortality in patients taking thyroxine preoperatively, perhaps for this reason.[230] Nonetheless, cardiac surgery is well tolerated in most patients with mild-to-moderate hypothyroidism.

B. Serum total and free triiodothyronine (T_3 and free T_3) are significantly reduced after both on- and off-pump surgery and remain low for up to 6 days, whereas thyroxine (T_4) is low immediately after surgery, but returns to normal within 24 hours.[231,232] There is some evidence that patients with low T_3 levels preoperatively are more prone to the "nonthyroidal illness syndrome" (NTIS) and to a low cardiac output state after surgery.[233] Furthermore, a prolonged reduction in the conversion of T_4 to T_3 may account for the slower recovery of some patients after surgery.[231] Patients with NTIS may not feel that well, but there is generally little physiologic impact on cardiac function.[234,235]

C. Patients with true hypothyroidism may be somewhat lethargic and hypotensive from decreased myocardial contractility and bradycardia. They may occasionally have difficult weaning from the ventilator.[236]

D. **Treatment**

1. Should postcardiotomy ventricular dysfunction occur, triiodothyronine (T_3) in a dose of $10-20\,\mu g$ can be given in conjunction with an inotrope, such as milrinone or inamrinone, which do not depend on β-receptors for their action.[237]

2. For the hypothyroid patient who has tolerated surgery uneventfully, treatment is initiated postoperatively with levothyroxine (Synthroid) $50\,\mu g$ PO qd and subsequently increased depending on TSH and T_4 levels. If the patient is unable to take oral medications, one-half of the oral dose can be given intravenously.

3. If the patient is severely hypothyroid, consultation with an endocrinologist is imperative. Doses of T_4 that have been recommended include an initial IV dose of 0.4 mg, followed by three days of $0.1-0.2$ mg IV daily, and then a maintenance dose of $50\,\mu g$ PO qd.

XV. Adrenal Insufficiency

A. Adrenal insufficiency is a rare complication of cardiac surgery that may result from adrenal hemorrhage associated with heparinization (or other anticoagulation) and the hormonal stress response in an elderly patient.

B. Manifestations include flank pain, nonspecific GI complaints (anorexia, nausea, vomiting, ileus, abdominal pain or distention), fever, and delirium. Late signs include hyperkalemia, hyponatremia, and hypotension with poor response to vasopressors. The clinical scenario can be confused with sepsis.

C. Diagnosis is confirmed by a low serum cortisol level and failure of cortisol levels to rise one hour after a 0.25 mg IV dose of cosyntropin (a synthetic ACTH analog). The level should rise fourfold or to a level greater than 20 µg/mL.

D. Treatment is with 100 mg of hydrocortisone IV every 8 hours along with administration of glucose and normal saline. If an additional mineralocorticoid is needed, fludrocortisone 0.05–0.2 mg qd can be given.

XVI. Pituitary Abnormalities

A. **Pituitary apoplexy**[238–241]

1. **Etiology.** This rare phenomenon results from infarction of a pituitary tumor due to ischemia, edema, or hemorrhage. The risk is exacerbated by use of CPB with heparinization and reduced cerebral blood flow. If the patient has a pituitary adenoma, off-pump surgery should be considered.[237]

2. **Presentation.** Compression of the optic chiasm and parasellar structures results in ophthalmoplegia, a third nerve palsy, visual loss, and headache. An Addisonian crisis may be precipitated by the hypopituitarism.[239]

3. **Treatment**

   a. Decrease intracerebral edema with hyperventilation, mannitol, and steroids (dexamethasone 10 mg q6h)

   b. Urgent hypophysectomy if no improvement.

B. **Diabetes insipidus** (DI) is a rare complication of cardiac surgery caused by diminished production of antidiuretic hormone (ADH). It has been noted in patients taking lithium preoperatively for depression.[242] The presence of polyuria, a urine osmolarity of 50–100 mOsm/L, and hypernatremia should raise suspicion of the diagnosis. Treatment of central DI involves use of desmopressin, administered either intranasally (1–2 sprays = 10–20 µg) at bedtime, or 0.05–0.4 mg PO bid. This is not effective in nephrogenic DI, which is usually treated with nonhormonal therapy.

References

1. Mehta RH, Hafley GE, Gibson CM, et al. Influence of preoperative renal dysfunction on one-year bypass graft patency and two-year outcomes in patients undergoing coronary artery bypass surgery. *J Thorac Cardiovasc Surg* 2008;136:1149–55.

2. Cooper WA, O'Brien SM, Thourani VH, et al. Impact of renal dysfunction on outcomes of coronary artery bypass surgery: results from the Society of Thoracic Surgeons National Adult Cardiac Database. *Circulation* 2006;113:1063–70.

3. Hillis GS, Croal BL, Buchan KG, et al. Renal function and outcome from coronary artery bypass grafting: impact on mortality after a 2.3 year follow-up. *Circulation* 2006;113:1056–62.

4. Devbhandari MP, Duncan AJ, Grayson AD, et al. Effect of risk-adjusted, non-dialysis-dependent renal dysfunction on mortality and morbidity following coronary artery bypass surgery: a multi-centre study. *Eur J Cardiothorac Surg* 2006;29:964–70.

5. Brown JR, Cochran RP, MacKenzie TA, et al. Long-term survival after cardiac surgery is predicted by estimated glomerular filtration rate. *Ann Thorac Surg* 2008;86:4–11.

6. Kangasniemi OK, Mahar MAA, Rasinaho E, et al. Impact of estimated glomerular filtration rate on the 15-year outcome after coronary artery bypass surgery. *Eur J Cardiothorac Surg* 2008;33:198–202.

7. Gibson PH, Croal BL, Cuthbertson BH, et al. The relationship between renal function and outcome from heart valve surgery. *Am Heart J* 2008;156:893–9.

8. Najafi M, Goodarzynejad H, Karimi A, et al. Is preoperative creatinine a reliable indicator of outcome in patients undergoing coronary artery bypass surgery? *J Thorac Cardiovasc Surg* 2009;137:304–8.

9. Howell NJ, Keogh BE, Bonser RS, et al. Mild renal dysfunction predicts in-hospital and post-discharge survival following cardiac surgery. *Eur J Cardiothorac Surg* 2008;34:390–5.

10. Zakeri R, Freemantle N, Barnett V, et al. Relation between mild renal dysfunction and outcomes after coronary artery bypass grafting. *Circulation* 2005;112(suppl I):I-270–5.

11. Kilo J, Margreiter JE, Ruttmann E, Laufer G, Bonatti JO. Slightly elevated serum creatinine predicts renal failure requiring hemofiltration after cardiac surgery. *Heart Surg Forum* 2005;8:E34–8.

12. Ibáñez J, Riera M, Saez de Ibarra JI, et al. Effect of preoperative mild renal dysfunction on mortality and morbidity following valve cardiac surgery. *Interact Cardiovasc Thorac Surg* 2007;6:748–52.

13. van de Wal RMA, van Brussel BL, Voors AA, et al. Mild preoperative renal dysfunction as a predictor of long-term clinical outcome after coronary bypass surgery. *J Thorac Cardiovasc Surg* 2005;129:330–5.

14. Weerasinghe A, Hornick P, Smith P, Taylor K, Ratnatunga C. Coronary artery bypass grafting in non-dialysis-dependent mild-to-moderate renal dysfunction. *J Thorac Cardiovasc Surg* 2001;121:1083–9.

15. Boldt J, Wolf M. Identification of renal injury in cardiac surgery: the role of kidney-specific proteins. *J Cardiothorac Vasc Anesth* 2008;22:122–32.

16. Bennett M, Dent CL, Ma Q, et al. Urine NGAL predicts severity of acute kidney injury after cardiac surgery: a prospective study. *Clin J Am Soc Nephrol* 2008;3:665–73.

17. Cruz DN, Ronco C, Katz N. Neutrophil-gelatinase-associated lipocalin: a promising biomarker for detecting cardiac surgery-associated acute kidney injury. *J Thorac Cardiovasc Surg* 2010;139:1101–6.

18. Haase M, Bellomo R, Devarajan P, et al. Novel biomarkers early predict the severity of acute kidney injury after cardiac surgery in adults. *Ann Thorac Surg* 2009;88:124–30.

19. Lema G, Meneses G, Urzua J, et al. Effects of extracorporeal circulation on renal function in coronary surgical patients. *Anesth Analg* 1995;81:446–51.

20. Licker M, Schweizer A, Höhn L, Morel DR. Chronic angiotensin converting inhibition does not influence renal hemodynamic and function during cardiac surgery. *Can J Anaesth* 1999;46:626–34.

21. Licker M, Neidhart P, Lustenberger S, et al. Long-term angiotensin-converting enzyme inhibitor treatment attenuates adrenergic responsiveness without altering hemodynamic control in patients undergoing cardiac surgery. *Anesthesiology* 1996;84:789–800.

22. Karkouti K, Beattie WS, Wijeysundera DN, et al. Hemodilution during cardiopulmonary bypass is an independent risk factor for acute renal failure in adult cardiac surgery. *J Thorac Cardiovasc Surg* 2005;129:391–400.

23. Habib RH, Zacharias A, Schwann TA, et al. Role of hemodilutional anemia and transfusion during cardiopulmonary bypass in renal injury after coronary revascularization: implications on operative outcome. *Crit Care Med* 2005;33:1749–56.

24. Habib RH, Zacharias A, Schwann TA, Riordan DJ, Durham SJ, Shah A. Adverse effects of low hematocrit during cardiopulmonary bypass in the adult: should current practice be changed? *J Thorac Cardiovasc Surg* 2003;125:1438–50.

25. Ranucci M, Romitti F, Isgrò G, et al. Oxygen delivery during cardiopulmonary bypass and acute renal failure after coronary operations. *Ann Thorac Surg* 2005;80:2213–20.

26. Ranucci M. Perioperative renal failure: hypoperfusion during cardiopulmonary bypass? *Semin Cardiothorac Vasc Anesth* 2007;11:265–8.

27. Arora P, Rajagopalam S, Ranjan R, et al. Preoperative use of angiotensin-converting enzyme inhibitors/angiotensin receptor blockers is associated with increased risk for acute kidney injury after cardiovascular surgery. *Clin J Am Soc Nephrol* 2008;3:1266–73.

28. Benedetto U, Sciarretta S, Roscitano A, et al. Preoperative angiotensin-converting enzyme inhibitors and acute kidney injury after coronary artery bypass grafting. *Ann Thorac Surg* 2008;86:1160–5.

29. Di Mauro M, Gagliardi M, Iacò, AL, et al. Does off-pump coronary surgery reduce postoperative renal failure? The importance of preoperative renal function. *Ann Thorac Surg* 2007;84:1496–503.

30. Weerasinghe A, Athanasiou T, Al-Ruzzeh S, et al. Functional renal outcome in on-pump and off-pump coronary revascularization: a propensity-based analysis. *Ann Thorac Surg* 2005;79:1577–83.

31. Sajja LR, Mannam G, Chakravarthi RM, et al. Coronary artery bypass grafting with or without cardiopulmonary bypass in patients with preoperative non-dialysis dependent renal insufficiency: a randomized study. *J Thorac Cardiovasc Surg* 2007;133:378–88.

32. Chukwuemeka A, Weisel A, Maganti M, et al. Renal dysfunction in high-risk patients after on-pump and off-pump coronary artery bypass surgery: a propensity score analysis. *Ann Thorac Surg* 2005;80:2148–54.

33. Gamoso MG, Phillips-Bute B, Landolfo KP, Newman MF, Stafford-Smith M. Off-pump versus on-pump coronary artery bypass surgery and postoperative renal dysfunction *Anesth Analg* 2000;91:1080–4.

34. Cheng DC, Bainbridge D, Martin JE, Novick RJ. Does off-pump coronary artery bypass reduce mortality, morbidity, and resource utilization when compared with conventional coronary artery bypass? A meta-analysis of randomized trials. *Anesthesiology* 2005;102:188–203.

35. Asimakopoulos G, Karagounis AP, Valencia O, et al. Renal function after cardiac surgery off- versus on-pump coronary artery bypass: analysis using the Cockroft-Gault formula for estimating creatinine clearance. *Ann Thorac Surg* 2005;79:2024–31.

36. McIlroy DR, Kharasch ED. Acute intravascular volume expansion with rapidly administered crystalloid or colloid in the setting of moderate hypovolemia. *Anesth Analg* 2003;96:1572–7.

37. Ernest D, Belzberg AS, Dodek PM. Distribution of normal saline and 5% albumin infusions in cardiac surgical patients. *Crit Care Med* 2001;29:2299–302.

38. Gallagher JD, Moore RA, Kerns D, et al. Effects of colloid or crystalloid administration on pulmonary extravascular water in the postoperative period after coronary artery bypass grafting. *Anesth Analg* 1985;64:753–8.

39. Boldt J. Saline versus balanced hydroxethyl starch: does it matter? *Curr Opin Anaesthesiol* 2008;21:679–83.

40. Boldt J. Modern rapidly degradable hydroxyethyl starches: current concepts. *Anesth Analg* 2009;108:1574–82.

41. James MFM. Pro: hydroxyethyl starch is preferable to albumin in the perioperative management of cardiac patients. *J Cardiothorac Vasc Anesth* 2008;22:482–4.

42. Green RS, Hall RI. Con: starches are not preferable to albumin during cardiac surgery: a contrary opinion. *J Cardiothorac Vasc Anesth* 2008;22:485–91.

43. Boldt J. Pro: use of colloids in cardiac surgery. *J Cardiothorac Vasc Anesth* 2007;21:453–6.

44. Boldt J, Brosch C, Ducke M, Papsdorf M, Lehmann A. Influence of volume therapy with a modern hydroxyethylstarch preparation on kidney function in cardiac surgery patients with compromised renal function: a comparison with human albumin. *Crit Care Med* 2007;35:2740–6.

45. Davidson IJ. Renal impact of fluid management with colloids: a comparative review. *Eur J Anaesthesiol* 2006;23:721–38.

46. Haynes GR. Fluid management in cardiac surgery: is one hydroxyethyl starch solution safer than another? *J Cardiothorac Vasc Anesth* 2006;20:916–7.

47. Wilkes MM, Navickis RJ, Sibbald WJ. Albumin versus hydroxyethylstarch in cardiopulmonary bypass surgery: a meta-analysis of postoperative bleeding. *Ann Thorac Surg* 2001;72:527–33.

48. Hecht-Dolnik M, Barkan H, Taharka A, Loftus J. Hetastarch increases the risk of bleeding complications in patients after off-pump coronary bypass surgery: a randomized clinical trial. *J Thorac Cardiovasc Surg* 2009;138:703–11.

49. Haynes GR, Havidich JE, Payne KJ. Why the Food and Drug Administration changed the warning label for hetastarch. *Anesthesiology* 2004;101:560–1.

50. Martin G, Bennett-Guerrero E, Wakeling H, et al. A prospective, randomized comparison of thromboelastographic coagulation profile in patients receiving lactated Ringer's solution, 6% hetastarch in balanced-saline vehicle, or 6% hetastarch in saline during major surgery. *J Cardiothorac Vasc Anesth* 2002;16:441–6.

51. Weeks DL, Jahr JS, Lim JC, Butch AW, Driessen B. Does Hextend impair coagulation compared to 6% hetastarch? An ex vivo thromboelastography study. *Am J Ther* 2008;15:225–30.

52. Dailey SE, Dysart CB, Langan DR, et al. An in vitro study comparing the effects of Hextend, Hespan, normal saline, and lactated Ringer's solution on thromboelastography and the activated partial thromboplastin time. *J Cardiothorac Vasc Anesth* 2005;19:358–61.

53. Roche AM, James MF, Bennett-Guerrero E, Mythen MG. A head-to-head comparison of the in vitro coagulation effects of saline-based and balanced electrolyte crystalloid and colloid intravenous fluids. *Anesth Analg* 2006;102:1274–9.

54. Moskowitz DM, Shander A, Javidroozi M, et al. Postoperative blood loss and transfusion associated with use of Hextend in cardiac surgery patients at a blood conservation center. *Transfusion* 2008;48:768–75.

55. Lang K, Boldt J, Suttner S, Haisch G. Colloids versus crystalloids and tissue oxygen tension in patients undergoing major abdominal surgery. *Anesth Analg* 2001;93:405–9.

56. Boldt J, Brosch Ch, Röhm K, Papsdorf M, Mengistu A. Comparison of the effects of gelatin and a modern hydroxyethyl starch solution on renal function and inflammatory response in elderly cardiac surgery patients. *Br J Anaesth* 2008;100:457–64.

57. Van der Linden PJ, De Hert SG, Deraedt D, et al. Hydoxyethyl starch 130/0.4 versus modified fluid gelatin for volume expansion in cardiac surgery patients: the effects on perioperative bleeding and transfusion needs. *Anesth Analg* 2005;101:629–34.

58. Van der Linden PJ, De Hert SG, Daper A, et al. 3.5% urea-linked gelatin is as effective as 6% HES 200/0.5 for volume management in cardiac surgery patients. *Can J Anaesth* 2004;51:236–41.

59. Williams EL, Hildebrand KL, McCormick SA, Bedel MJ. The effect of intravenous lactated Ringer's solution versus 0.9% sodium chloride solution on serum osmolality in human volunteers. *Anesth Analg* 1999;88:999–1003.

60. Järvelä K, Koskinen M, Kaukinen S, Kööbi T. Effects of hypertonic saline (7.5%) on extracellular fluid volumes compared with normal saline (0.9%) and 6% hydroxyethylstarch after aortocoronary bypass graft surgery. *J Cardiothorac Vasc Anesth* 2001;15:210–5.

61. Jahr JS, Weeks DL, Desai P, et al. Does Oxyvita, a new-generation hemoglobin-based oxygen carrier, or oxyglobin acutely interfere with coagulation compared with normal saline or 6% hetastarch? An ex vivo thromboelastography study. *J Cardiothorac Vasc Anesth* 2008;22:34–9.

62. Morimatsu H, Uchino S, Chung J, Bellomo R, Raman J, Buxton B. Norepinephrine for hypotensive vasodilatation after cardiac surgery: impact on renal function. *Intensive Care Med* 2003;29:1106–12.

63. Bellomo R, Wan L, May C. Vasoactive drugs and acute kidney injury. *Crit Care Med* 2008;36(Suppl):S179–86.

64. Egi M, Bellomo R, Langenberg C, et al. Selecting a vasopressor drug for vasoplegic shock after adult cardiac surgery: a systematic literature review. *Ann Thorac Surg* 2007;83:715–23.

65. Brater DC. Diuretic therapy. *N Engl J Med* 1998;339:387–95.

66. Yelton SL, Gaylor MA, Murray KM. The role of continuous infusion loop diuretics. *Ann Pharmacother* 1995;29:1010–4.

67. Sanjay S, Annigeri RA, Seshadri R, Rao BS, Prakash KC, Mani MK. The comparison of the diuretic and natriuretic efficacy of continuous and bolus intravenous furosemide in patients with chronic kidney disease. *Nephrology (Carlton)* 2008;13:247–50.

68. Lim E, Ali ZA, Attaran R, Cooper G. Evaluating routine diuretics after coronary surgery: a prospective randomized controlled trial. *Ann Thorac Surg* 2002;73:153–5.

69. Gatot I, Abramov D, Tsodikov V, et al. Should we give prophylactic renal-dose dopamine after coronary artery bypass surgery? *J Card Surg* 2004;19:128–33.

70. Drieghe B, Manoharan G, Heyndrickx GR, et al. Dopamine-induced changes in renal blood flow in normals and in patients with renal dysfunction. *Catheter Cardiovasc Interv* 2008;72:725–30.

71. Schetz M, Bove T, Morelli A, Mankad S, Ronco C, Kellum JA. Prevention of cardiac surgery-associated acute kidney injury. *Int J Artif Organs* 2008;31:179–89.

72. Stafford-Smith M. Evidence-based renal protection in cardiac surgery. *Semin Cardiothorac Vasc Anesth* 2005;9:65–76.

73. Venkataraman R. Can we prevent acute kidney injury? *Crit Care Med* 2008;36:S166–71.

74. Stevens LA, Coresh J, Greene, T, Levey AS. Assessing kidney function – measured and estimated glomerular filtration rate *N Engl J Med* 2006;354:2473–83.

75. Walter J, Mortasawi A, Arnrich B, et al. Creatinine clearance versus serum creatinine as a risk factor in cardiac surgery. *BMC Surg* 2003;3:4–12.

76. Lin Y, Zheng Z, Li Y, et al. Impact of renal dysfunction on long-term survival after isolated coronary artery bypass surgery. *Ann Thorac Surg* 2009;87:1079–84.

77. Levey AS, Coresh J, Balk E, et al. National Kidney Foundation practice guidelines for chronic kidney disease: evaluation, classification, and stratification. *Ann Int Med* 2003;139:137–47.

78. Wijeysundera DN, Karkouti K, Beattie WS, Rao V, Ivanov J. Improving the identification of patients at risk of postoperative renal failure after cardiac surgery. *Anesthesiology* 2006;104:65–72.

79. Durmaz I, Buket S, Atay Y, et al. Cardiac surgery with cardiopulmonary bypass in patients with chronic renal failure. *J Thorac Cardiovasc Surg* 1999;118:306–15.

80. Bechtel JFM, Detter C, Fischlein T, et al. Cardiac surgery in patients on dialysis: decreased 30-day mortality, unchanged overall survival. *Ann Thorac Surg* 2008;85:147–53.

81. Rahmanian PB, Adams DH, Castillo JG, Vassalotti J, Filsoufi F. Early and late outcome of cardiac surgery in dialysis-dependent patients: single-center experience with 245 consecutive patients. *J Thorac Cardiovasc Surg* 2008;135:915–22.

82. Young EW, Diab A, Kirsh MM. Intravenous diltiazem and acute renal failure after cardiac operations. *Ann Thorac Surg* 1998;65:1316–9.

83. Filsoufi F, Rahmanian PB, Castillo JG, Silvay G, Carpentier A, Adams DH. Predictors and early and late outcomes of dialysis-dependent patients in contemporary cardiac surgery. *J Cardiothorac Vasc Anesth* 2008;22:522–9.

84. Leacche M, Winkelmayer WC, Paul S, et al. Predicting survival in patients requiring replacement therapy after cardiac surgery. *Ann Thorac Surg* 2006;81:1385–92.

85. Thakar CV, Worley S, Arrigain S, Yared JP, Paganini EP. Improved survival in acute kidney injury after cardiac surgery. *Am J Kidney Dis* 2007;50:703–11.

86. Bove T, Calabrò MG, Landoni G, et al. The incidence and risk of acute renal failure after cardiac surgery. *J Cardiothorac Vasc Anesth* 2004;18:442–5.

87. Chertow GM, Lazarus JM. Christensen CL, et al. Preoperative renal risk stratification. *Circulation* 1997;95:878–84.

88. Fortescue EB, Bates DW, Chertow GM. Predicting renal failure after coronary bypass surgery: cross-validation of two risk-stratification algorithms. *Kidney Int* 2000;57:2594–602.

89. Brown JR, Cochran RP, Leavitt BJ, et al. Multivariable prediction of renal insufficiency developing after cardiac surgery. *Circulation* 2007;116(Suppl I):I-239–43.

90. Palomba H, de Castro I, Neto AL, Lage S, Yu L. Acute kidney injury prediction following elective cardiac surgery: AKICS score. *Kidney Int* 2007;72:624–31.

91. Thakar CV, Arrigain S, Worley S, Yared JP, Paganin EP. A clinical score to predict acute renal failure after cardiac surgery. *Am J Soc Nephrol* 2005;16:162–8.

92. Mehta RH, Grab JD, O'Brien SM, et al. Bedside tool for predicting the risk of postoperative dialysis in patients undergoing cardiac surgery. *Circulation* 2006;114:2208–16.

93. Wijeysundera DN, Karkouti K, Dupuis JY, et al. Derivation and validation of a simplified predictive index for renal replacement therapy after cardiac surgery. *JAMA* 2007;297:1801–9.

94. Del Duca D, Iqbal S, Rahme E, Goldberg P, de Varennes B. Renal failure after cardiac surgery: timing of cardiac catheterization and other perioperative risk factors. *Ann Thorac Surg* 2007;84:1264–71.

95. Boldt J, Brenner T, Lehmann A, Suttner SW, Kumle B, Isgro F. Is kidney function altered by the duration of cardiopulmonary bypass? *Ann Thorac Surg* 2003;75:906–12.

96. Rahmanian RB, Filsoufi F, Castillo JG, et al. Predicting postoperative renal failure requiring dialysis, and an analysis of long-term outcome in patients undergoing valve surgery. *J Heart Valve Dis* 2008;17:657–65.

97. Sterling KA, Tehrani T, Rudnick MR. Clinical significance and preventive strategies for contrast-induced nephropathy. *Curr Opin Nephrol Hypertens* 2008;17:616–23.

98. Pannu N, Wiebe N, Tonelli M, Alberta Kidney Disease Network. Prophylaxis strategies for contrast-induced nephropathy. *JAMA* 2006;295:2765–79.

99. Kelly AM, Dwamena B, Cronin P, Bernstein SJ, Carlos RC. Meta-analysis: effectiveness of drugs for preventing contrast-induced nephropathy. *Ann Intern Med* 2008;148:284–94.

100. Maioli M, Toso A, Leoncini M, et al. Sodium bicarbonate versus saline for the prevention of contrast-induced nephropathy in patients with renal dysfunction undergoing coronary angiography or intervention. *J Am Coll Cardiol* 2008;52:599–604.

101. Hogan SE, L'Allier P, Chetcuti S, et al. Current role of sodium bicarbonate-based preprocedural hydration for the prevention of contrast-induced acute kidney injury: a meta-analysis. *Am Heart J* 2008;156:414–21.

102. Ozcan EE, Guneri S, Akdeniz B, et al. Sodium bicarbonate, N-acetylcysteine, and saline for prevention of radiocontrast-induced nephropathy. A comparison of 3 regimens for protecting contrast-induced nephropathy in patients undergoing coronary procedures. A single-center prospective controlled trial. *Am Heart J* 2007;154:539–44.

103. Brown JR, Block CA, Malenka DJ, O'Connor GT, Schoolwerth AC, Thompson CA. Sodium bicarbonate plus N-acetylcysteine prophylaxis. A meta-analysis. *JACC Cardiovasc Interv* 2009;2:1116–24.

104. Gare M, Haviv YS, Ben-Yehuda A, et al. The renal effect of low-dose dopamine in high-risk patients undergoing coronary angiography. *J Am Coll Cardiol* 1999;34:1682–8.

105. Durmaz I, Yagdi T, Calkavur T, et al. Prophylactic dialysis in patients with renal dysfunction undergoing on-pump coronary artery bypass surgery. *Ann Thorac Surg* 2003;75:859–64.

106. Bellomo R, Auriemma S, Fabbri A, et al. The pathophysiology of cardiac surgery-associated acute kidney injury (CSA-AKI). *Int J Artif Organs* 2008;31:166–78.

107. Rosner MH, Portilla D, Okusa MD. Cardiac surgery as a cause of acute kidney injury: pathogenesis and potential therapies. *J Intensive Care Med* 2008;23:3–18.

108. Stafford-Smith M, Phillips-Bute B, Reddan DN, Black J, Newman MF. The association of epsilon-aminocaproic acid with postoperative decrease in creatinine clearance in 1502 coronary bypass patients. *Anesth Analg* 2000;91:1085–90.

109. Mangano DT, Tudor IC, Dietzel L; Multicenter Study of Perioperative Ischemia Research Group; Ischemia Research and Education Foundation. The risk associated with aprotinin in cardiac surgery. *N Engl J Med* 2006;354:353–65.

110. Furnary AP, Wu Y, Hirazka LF, Grunkemeier GL, Page US 3rd. Aprotinin does not increase the risk of renal failure in cardiac surgery patints. *Circulation* 2007;116(Suppl I):I-127–33.

111. Dietrich W, Busley R, Boulesteix AL. Effects of aprotinin dosage on renal function. An analysis of 8,548 cardiac surgical patients treated with different dosages of aprotinin. *Anesthesiology* 2008;108:189–98.

112. Mangano CM, Diamondstone LS, Ramsay JG, Aggarwal A. Hershkowitz A, Mangano DT. Renal dysfunction after myocardial revascularization: risk factors, adverse outcomes, and hospital resource utilization. *Ann Intern Med* 1998;128:194–203.

113. Westaby S. Aprotinin: twenty-five years of claim and counterclaim. *J Thorac Cardiovasc Surg* 2008;135:487–91.

114. Kulier A, Levin J, Moser R, et al. Impact of preoperative anemia on outcome in patients undergoing coronary artery bypass graft surgery. *Circulation* 2007;116:471–9.

115. Maslow AD, Chaudrey A, Bert A, Schwartz C, Singh A. Perioperative renal outcome in cardiac surgical patients with preoperative renal dysfunction: aprotinin versus epsilon aminocaproic acid. *J Cardiothorac Vasc Anesth* 2008;22:6–15.

116. Suehiro S, Shibata T, Sasaki Y, et al. Heparin-coated circuits prevent renal dysfunction after open heart surgery. *Osaka City Med J* 1999;45:149–57.

117. Benedetto U, Luciani R, Goraci M, et al. Miniaturized cardiopulmonary bypass and acute kidney injury in coronary artery bypass graft surgery. *Ann Thorac Surg* 2009;88:529–36.

118. Bolcal C, Akay HT, Bingol H, et al. Leukodepletion improves renal function in patients with renal dysfunction undergoing on-pump coronary bypass surgery: a prospective randomized study. *Thorac Cardiovasc Surg* 2007;55:89–93.

119. Sirvinskas E, Andrejaitiene J, Raliene L, et al. Cardiopulmonary bypass management and acute renal failure: risk factors and prognosis. *Perfusion* 2008;23:323–7.

120. Boodhwani M, Rubens FD, Wozny D, Nathan HJ. Effects of mild hypothermia and rewarming on renal function after coronary artery bypass grafting. *Ann Thorac Surg* 2009;87:48–95.

121. Lazar HL, McDonnell M, Chipkin SR, et al. The Society of Thoracic Surgeons practice guidelines series: blood glucose management during adult cardiac surgery. *Ann Thorac Surg* 2009;87:663–9.

122. Kamohara K, Yoshikai M, Yunoki J, et al. Safety of perioperative hemodialysis and continuous hemodiafiltration for dialysis patients with cardiac surgery. *Gen Thorac Cardiovasc Surg* 2007;55:43–9.

123. Luciani R, Goracci M. Simon C, et al. Reduction of early postoperative morbidity in cardiac surgery patients treated with continuous veno-venous hemofiltration during cardiopulmonary bypass. *Artif Organs* 2009;33:654–7.

124. Kaya K. Oğuz M, Akar AR, et al. The effect of sodium nitroprusside infusion on renal function during reperfusion period in patients undergoing coronary artery bypass grafting: a prospective randomized clinical trial. *Eur J Cardiothorac Surg* 2007;31:290–7.

125. Chen HH, Sundt TM, Cook DJ, Heublein CM, Burnett JC Jr. Low dose nesiritide and the preservation of renal function in patients with renal dysfunction undergoing cardiopulmonary-bypass surgery: a double-blind placebo-controlled pilot study. *Circulation* 2007;116(suppl I):I-134–8.

126. Mentzer RM Jr, Oz MC, Sladen RN, et al. Effects of perioperative nesiritide in patients with left ventricular dysfunction undergoing cardiac surgery: the NAPA trial. *J Am Coll Cardiol* 2007;49:716–26.

127. Dyke CM, Bhatia D, Aronson S, Moazami N, Mentzer RM Jr. Perioperative nesiritide and possible renal protection in patients with moderate to severe kidney dysfunction. *J Thorac Cardiovasc Surg* 2008;136:1369–70.

128. Beaver TM, Winterstein AG, Shuster JJ, et al. Effectiveness of nesiritide on dialysis or all-cause mortality in patients undergoing cardiothoracic surgery. *Clin Cardiol* 2006;29:18–24.

129. Sezai A, Hata M, Niino T, et al. Continuous low-dose infusion of human atrial natriuretic peptide in patients with left ventricular dysfunction undergoing coronary artery bypass grafting. *J Am Coll Cardiol* 2010;55:1844–51.

130. Meco M, Cirri S. The effect of various fenoldopam doses on renal perfusion in patients undergoing cardiac surgery. *Ann Thorac Surg* 2010;89:497–504.

131. Ranucci M, Soro G, Barzaghi N, et al. Fenoldopam prophylaxis of postoperative acute renal failure in high-risk cardiac surgery patients. *Ann Thorac Surg* 2004;78:1332–7.

132. Landoni G, Biondi-Zoccai GG, Marino G, et al. Fenoldopam reduces the need for renal replacement therapy and in-hospital death in cardiovascular surgery: a meta-analysis. *J Cardiothorac Vasc Anesth* 2008;22:27–33.

133. Cogliati AA, Vellutini R, Nardini A, et al. Fenoldopam infusion for renal protection in high-risk cardiac surgery: a randomized clinical study. *J Cardiothorac Vasc Anesth* 2007;21:847–50.

134. Barr LF, Kolodner K. N-acetylcysteine and fenoldopam protect the renal function of patients with chronic renal insufficiency undergoing cardiac surgery. *Crit Care Med* 2008;36:1427–35.

135. Haase M, Haase-Fielitz A, Bellomo R, et al. Sodium bicarbonate to prevent increases in serum creatinine after cardiac surgery: a pilot double-blind, randomized trial. *Crit Care Med* 2009;37:39–47.

136. Bergman AS, Odar-Cerderlöf I, Westman L, Bjellerup P, Höglund P, Ohqvist G. Diltiazem infusion for renal protection in cardiac surgical patients with preexisting renal dysfunction. *J Cardiothorac Vasc Anesth* 2002;16:294–9.

137. Manabe S, Tanaka H, Yoshizaki T, Tabuchi N, Arai H, Sunamori M. Effects of postoperative administration of diltiazem on renal function after coronary artery bypass grafting. *Ann Thorac Surg* 2005;79:831–6.

138. Poullis M. Mannitol and cardiac surgery. *Thorac Cardiovasc Surg* 1999;47:58–62.

139. Yallop KG, Sheppard SV, Smith DC. The effect of mannitol on renal function following cardio-pulmonary bypass in patients with normal pre-operative creatinine. *Anaesthesia* 2008;63:576–82.

140. Smith MN, Best D, Sheppard SV, Smith DC. The effect of mannitol on renal function after cardiopulmonary bypass in patients with established renal dysfunction. *Anaesthesia* 2008;63:701–4.

141. Lassnigg A, Donner E, Grubhofer G, Presterl E, Druml W, Hiesmayr M. Lack of renoprotective effects of dopamine and furosemide during cardiac surgery. *J Am Soc Nephrol* 2000;11:97–104.

142. Mahesh B, Yim B, Robson D, Pillai R, Ratnatunga C, Pigott D. Does furosemide prevent renal dysfunction in high-risk cardiac surgical patients? Results of a double-blinded prospective randomised trial. *Eur J Cardiothorac Surg* 2008;33:370–6.

143. Lombardi R, Ferreiro A, Servetto C. Renal function after cardiac surgery: adverse effects of furosemide. *Ren Fail* 2003;25:775–86.

144. Yavuz S, Ayabakan N, Dilek K, Ozdemir A. Renal dose dopamine in open heart surgery. Does it protect renal tubular function? *J Cardiovasc Surg (Torino)* 2002;43:25–30.

145. Woo EB, Tang AT, el-Gamel A, et al. Dopamine therapy for patients at risk of renal dysfunction following cardiac surgery: fact or fiction? *Eur J Cardiothorac Surg* 2002;22:106–11.

146. Carcoana OV, Mathew JP, Davis E, et al. Mannitol and dopamine in patients undergoing cardiopulmonary bypass: a randomized clinical trial. *Anesth Analg* 2003;97:1222–9.

147. Bove T, Landoni G, Calabrò MG, et al. Renoprotective action of fenoldopam in high-risk patients undergoing cardiac surgery. A prospective, double-blind, randomized clinical trial. *Circulation* 2005;111:3230–5.

148. Yavuz S, Ayabakan N, Goncu MT, Ozdemir IA. Effect of combined dopamine and diltiazem on renal function after cardiac surgery. *Med Sci Monit* 2002;8:PI45–50.

149. Adabag AS, Ishani A, Koneswaran S, et al. Utility of N-acetylcysteine to prevent acute kidney injury after cardiac surgery: a randomized controlled trial. *Am Heart J* 2008;155:1143–9.

150. Nigwekar SU, Kandula P. N-acetylcysteine in cardiovascular-surgery-associated renal failure: a meta-analysis. *Ann Thorac Surg* 2009;87:139–47.

151. Kuitunen A, Vento A, Suojaranta-Ylinen R, Pettilä V. Acute renal failure after cardiac surgery: evaluation of the RIFLE classification. *Ann Thorac Surg* 2006;81:542–6.

152. Karkouti K, Wijeysundera DN, Yu TM, et al. Acute kidney injury after cardiac surgery: focus on modifiable risk factors. *Circulation* 2009;119:495–502.

153. Ristikankare A, Pöyhiä R, Kuitunen A, et al. Serum cystatin C in elderly cardiac surgery patients. *Ann Thorac Surg* 2010;89:689–95.

154. Swaminathan M, Hudson CCC, Phillips-Bute BG, et al. Impact of early renal recovery on survival after cardiac surgery-associated acute kidney injury. *Ann Thorac Surg* 2010;89:1098–105.

155. Hudson C, Hudson J, Swaminathan M, Shaw A, Stafford-Smith M, Patel UD. Emerging concepts in acute kidney injury following cardiac surgery. *Sem Cardiothorac Vasc Anesth* 2008;12:320–30.

156. Lameire N, Biesen WV, Vanholder R. Acute kidney injury. *Lancet* 2008;372:1863–5.

157. Abuelo JG. Normotensive ischemic acute renal failure. *N Engl J Med* 2007;357:797–805.

158. Shear W, Rosner MH. Acute kidney dysfunction secondary to the abdominal compartment syndrome. *J Nephrol* 2006;19:556–65.

159. Myers BD, Moran SM. Hemodynamically mediated acute renal failure. *N Engl J Med* 1986;314:97–105.

160. Esson ML. Schrier RW. Diagnosis and treatment of acute tubular necrosis. *Ann Intern Med* 2002;137:744–52.

161. Tolwani A, Paganini E, Joannidis M, et al. Treatment of patients with cardiac surgery associated-acute kidney injury. *Int J Artif Organs* 2008;31:190–6.

162. Liu KD, Brakeman PR. Renal repair and recovery. *Crit Care Med* 2008;36(suppl):S187–92.

163. Manche A, Galea J, Busuttil W. Tolerance to ACE inhibitors after cardiac surgery. *Eur J Cardiothorac Surg* 1999;15:55–60.

164. Bagshaw SM, Delaney A, Haase M, Ghali WA, Bellomo R. Loop diuretics in the management of acute renal failure: a systematic review and meta-analysis. *Crit Care Resusc* 2007;9:60–8.

165. Bagshaw SM, Bellomo R, Kellum JA. Oliguria, volume overload, and loop diuretics. *Crit Care Med* 2008;36(Suppl):S172–8.

166. Vánky F, Broquist M, Svedjeholm R. Addition of a thiazide: an effective remedy for furosemide resistance after cardiac operations. *Ann Thorac Surg* 1997;63:993–7.

167. Lindner A. Synergism of dopamine and furosemide in diuretic-resistant, oliguric acute renal failure. *Nephron* 1983;33:121–6.

168. Sirivella S, Gielchinsky I, Parsonnet V. Mannitol, furosemide, and dopamine infusion in postoperative renal failure complicating cardiac surgery. *Ann Thorac Surg* 2000;69:501–6.

169. Benharash P, Omari B. Administration of nesiritide in patients after coronary artery bypass surgery induces brisk diuresis. *Am Surg* 2005;71:794–6.

170. Swärd K, Valsson G, Odencrants P, Samuelsson O, Ricksten SE. Recombinant human atrial natriuretic peptide in ischemic acute renal failure: a randomized placebo-controlled trial. *Crit Care Med* 2004;32:1310–5.

171. Tumlin LA, Finkel KW, Murray PT, Samuels J, Cotsonis G, Shaw AD. Fenoldopam mesylate in early acute tubular necrosis: a randomized, double-blind, placebo-controlled clinical trial. *Am J Kidney Dis* 2005;46:26–34.

172. Roasio A, Lobreglio R, Santin A, Landoni G, Verdecchia C. Fenoldopam reduces the incidence of renal replacement therapy after cardiac surgery. *J Cardiothorac Vasc Anesth* 2008;22:23–6.

173. Brienza N, Malcangi V, Dalfino L, et al. A comparison between fenoldopam and low-dose dopamine in early renal dysfunction of critically ill patients. *Crit Care Med* 2006;34:707–14.

174. Friedrich JO, Adhikari N, Herridge MS, Beyene J. Meta-analysis: low-dose dopamine increases urine output but does not prevent renal dysfunction or death. *Ann Intern Med* 2005;142:510–24.

175. Holmes CL, Walley KR. Bad medicine: low-dose dopamine in the ICU. *Chest* 2003;123:1266–75.

176. Duke GJ, Briedis JH, Weaver RA. Renal support in critically ill patients: low-dose dopamine or low-dose dobutamine? *Crit Care Med* 1994;22:1919–25.

177. Ichai C, Soubielle J, Carles M, Giunti C, Grimaud D. Comparison of the renal effects of low to high doses of dopamine and dobutamine in critically ill patients: a single-blind randomized study. *Crit Care Med* 2000;28:921–8.

178. Valencia E, Marin A, Hardy G. Nutrition therapy for acute renal failure: a new approach based on "risk, injury, failure, loss and end-stage kidney" classification (RIFLE). *Curr Opin Clin Nutr Metab Care* 2009;12:241–4.

179. John S, Eckardt KU. Renal replacement strategies in the ICU. *Chest* 2007;132:1379–88.

180. Palevsky PM. Indications and timing of renal replacement therapy in acute kidney injury. *Crit Care Med* 2008;36(suppl):S224–8.

181. Iyem H, Tavli M, Akcicek F, Büket S. Importance of early dialysis for acute renal failure after an open-heart surgery. *Hemodialy Int* 2009;13:55–61.

182. Demirkiliç U, Kuralay E, Yenicesu M, et al. Timing of replacement therapy for acute renal failure after cardiac surgery. *J Card Surg* 2004;19:17–20.

183. Elahi MM, Lim MY, Joseph RN, Dhannapuneni RR, Spyt TJ. Early hemofiltration improves survival in post-cardiotomy patients with acute renal failure. *Eur J Cardiothorac Surg* 2004;26:1027–31.

184. Bapat V, Sabetai M, Roxburgh J, Young C, Venn G. Early and intensive continuous veno-venous hemofiltration for acute renal failure after cardiac surgery. *Interact Cardiovasc Thorac Surg* 2004;3:426–30.

185. Bingol H, Akay HT, Iyem H, et al. Prophylactic dialysis in elderly patients undergoing coronary bypass surgery. *Ther Apher Dial* 2007;11:30–5.

186. Bagshaw SM, Berthiaume LR, Delaney A, Bellomo R. Continuous versus intermittent renal replacement therapy for critically ill patients with acute kidney injury: a meta-analysis. *Crit Care Med* 2008;36:610–7.

187. Bouchard J, Weidemann C, Mehta RL. Renal replacement therapy in acute kidney injury: intermittent versus continuous? How much is enough? *Adv Chronic Kidney Dis* 2008;15:235–47.

188. Kutsogiannis DJ, Gibney RT, Stollery D, Gao J. Regional citrate versus systemic heparin anticoagulation for continuous renal replacement in critically ill patients. *Kidney Int* 2005;67:2361–7.

189. Bihorac A, Ross EA. Continuous venovenous hemofiltration with citrate-based replacement fluid: efficacy, safety, and impact on nutrition. *Am J Kidney Dis* 2005;46:908–18.

190. Parham WA, Mehdirad AA, Biermann KM, Fredman CS. Hyperkalemia revisited. *Tex Heart Inst J* 2006;33:40–7.

191. Hollander-Rodriguez JC, Calvert JF Jr. Hyperkalemia. *Am Fam Physician* 2006;73:283–90.

192. Fraley DS, Adler S. Correction of hyperkalemia by bicarbonate despite constant blood pH. *Kidney Int* 1977;12:354–60.

193. Liou HH, Chiang SS, Wu SC, et al. Hypokalemic effects of intravenous infusion or nebulization of salbutamol in patients with chronic renal failure: comparative study. *Am J Kidney Dis* 1994;23:266–71.

194. Gennari FJ. Hypokalemia. *N Engl J Med* 1998;339:451–8.

195. Dinardo JA. Pro: calcium is routinely indicated during separation from cardiopulmonary bypass. *J Cardiothorac Vasc Anesth* 1997;11:905–7.

196. Butterworth JF, Zaloga GP, Prielipp RC, Tucker WY Jr, Royster RL. Calcium inhibits the cardiac stimulating properties of dobutamine but not of amrinone. *Chest* 1992;101:174–80.

197. Cooper MS, Gittoes NJ. Diagnosis and management of hypocalcaemia. *BMJ* 2008;36:1298–302.

198. Booth JV, Phillips-Bute B, McCants CB, et al. Low serum magnesium level predicts adverse cardiac events after coronary artery bypass graft surgery. *Am Heart J* 2003;145:1108–13.

199. Minato N, Katayama Y, Sakaguchi M, Itoh M. Perioperative coronary artery spasm in off-pump coronary artery bypass grafting and its possible relation with perioperative hypomagnesemia. *Ann Thorac Cardiovasc Surg* 2006;12:32–6.

200. Inoue S, Akazawa S, Nakaigawa Y, Shimizu R, Seo N. Changes in plasma total and ionized magnesium concentrations and factors affecting magnesium concentrations during cardiac surgery. *J Anesth* 2004;18:216–9.

201. Wilkes NJ, Mallett SV, Peachey T, Di Salvo C, Walesby R. Correction of ionized plasma magnesium reduces the risk of postoperative cardiac arrhythmia. *Anesth Analg* 2002;95:828–34.

202. Maslow AD, Regan MM, Heindle S, Panzica P, Cohn WE, Johnson RG. Postoperative atrial tachyarrhythmias in patients undergoing coronary artery bypass graft surgery without cardiopulmonary bypass: a role for intraoperative magnesium supplementation. *J Cardiothorac Vasc Anesth* 2000;14:524–30.

203. Prielipp RC, Zaloga GP, Butterworth JF IV, et al. Magnesium inhibits the hypertensive but not the cardiotonic actions of low-dose epinephrine. *Anesthesiology* 1991;74:973–9.

204. Maillet JM, Le Besnerais P, Cantoni M, et al. Frequency, risk factors, and outcome of hyperlactatemia after cardiac surgery. *Chest* 2003;123:1361–6.

205. Adrogué HJ, Madias NE. Management of life-threatening acid–base disorders. First of two parts. *N Engl J Med* 1998;338:26–34.

206. Kaplan JA, Guffin AV, Yin A. The effects of metabolic acidosis and alkalosis on the response to sympathomimetic drugs in dogs. *J Cardiothorac Anesth* 1988;2:481–7.

207. Ranucci M, De Toffol B, Isgrò G, Romitti F, Conti D, Vicentini M. Hyperlactatemia during cardiopulmonary bypass: determinants and impact on postoperative outcome. *Crit Care* 2006;10:R167.

208. Forsythe SM, Schmidt GA. Sodium bicarbonate for the treatment of lactic acidosis. *Chest* 2000;117:260–7.

209. Cooper DJ, Walley KR, Wiggs BR, Russell JA. Bicarbonate does not improve hemodynamics in critically ill patients who have lactic acidosis. A prospective, controlled clinical study. *Ann Intern Med* 1990;112:492–8.

210. Leung JM, Landow L, Franks M, et al. Safety and efficacy of intravenous Carbicarb® in patients undergoing surgery: comparison with sodium bicarbonate in the treatment of mild metabolic acidosis. *Crit Care Med* 1994;22:1540–9.

211. Hoste EA, Colpaert K, Vanholder RC, et al. Sodium bicarbonate versus THAM in ICU patients with mild metabolic acidosis. *J Nephrol* 2005;18:303–7.

212. Androgué HJ, Madias NE. Management of life-threatening acid–base disorders. Second of two parts. *N Engl J Med* 1998;338:107–11.

213. Liao P, DeSantis AJ, Schmeltz LR, et al. Insulin resistance following cardiothoracic surgery in patients with and without a preoperative diagnosis of type 2 diabetes during treatment with intravenous insulin therapy for postoperative hyperglycemia. *J Diabetes Complications* 2008;22:229–34.

214. Rassias AJ. Intraoperative management of hyperglycemia in the cardiac surgical patient. *Semin Thorac Cardiovasc Surg* 2006;18:330–8.

215. Doenst T, Wijeysundera D, Karkouti K, et al. Hyperglycemia during cardiopulmonary bypass is an independent risk factor for mortality in patients undergoing cardiac surgery. *J Thorac Cardiovasc Surg* 2005;130:1144–50.

216. Jones KW, Cain AS, Mitchell JH, et al. Hyperglycemia predicts mortality after CABG: postoperative hyperglycemia predicts dramatic increases in mortality after coronary artery bypass graft surgery. *J Diabetes Complications* 2008;22:365–70.

217. Ascione R, Rogers CA, Rajakaruna C, Angelini GD. Inadequate blood glucose control is associated with in-hospital mortality and morbidity in diabetic and nondiabetic patients undergoing cardiac surgery. *Circulation* 2008;118:113–23.

218. Ouattara A, Lecomte P, Le Manach Y, et al, Poor intraoperative blood glucose control is associated with worsened hospital outcome after cardiac surgery in diabetic patients. *Anesthesiology* 2005;103:687–94.

219. Swenne CL, Lindholm C, Borowiec J, Schnell AE, Carlsson M. Peri-operative glucose control and development of surgical wound infections in patients undergoing coronary artery bypass graft. *J Hosp Infect* 2005;61:201–12.

220. Gandhi GY, Nuttall GA, Abel MD, et al. Intraoperative hyperglycemia and perioperative outcomes in cardiac surgery patients. *Mayo Clin Proc* 2005;80:862–6.

221. Puskas F, Grocott HP, White WD, Mathew JP, Newman MF, Bar-Yosef S. Intraoperative hyperglycemia and cognitive decline after CABG. *Ann Thorac Surg* 2007;84:1467–73.

222. Butterworth J, Wagenknecht LE, Legault C, et al. Attempted control of hyperglycemia during cardiopulmonary bypass fails to improve neurologic or neurobehavioral outcomes in patients without diabetes mellitus undergoing coronary artery bypass grafting. *J Thorac Cardiovasc Surg* 2005;130:1319–25.

223. Gandhi GY, Nuttall GA, Abel MD, et al. Intensive intraoperative insulin therapy versus conventional glucose management during cardiac surgery: a randomized trial. *Ann Intern Med* 2007;146:233–43.

224. Chan RP, Galas FR, Hajjar LA, et al. Intensive perioperative glucose control does not improve outcomes of patients submitted to open-heart surgery: a randomized controlled trial. *Clinics* 2009;64:51–60.

225. Furnary AP, Gao G, Grunkemeier GL, et al. Continuous insulin infusion reduces mortality in patients with diabetes undergoing coronary artery bypass grafting. *J Thorac Cardiovasc Surg* 2003;125:1007–21.

226. Zerr KJ, Furnary AP, Grunkemeier GL, Bookin S, Kanhere V, Starr A. Glucose control lowers the risk of wound infection in diabetics after open heart operations. *Ann Thorac Surg* 1997;63:356–61.

227. Schmeltz LR, DeSantis AJ, Thiyagarajan V, et al. Reduction of surgical mortality and morbidity in diabetic patients undergoing cardiac surgery with a combined intravenous and subcutaneous insulin glucose management strategy. *Diabetes Care* 2007;30:823–8.

228. Carr JM, Sellke FW, Fey M, et al. Implementing tight glucose control after coronary artery bypass surgery. *Ann Thorac Surg* 2005;80:902–9.

229. Seki S. Clinical features of hyperosmolar hyperglycemic nonketotic diabetic coma associated with cardiac operations. *J Thorac Cardiovasc Surg* 1986;91:867–73.

230. Zindrou D, Taylor KM, Bagger JP. Excess coronary artery bypass graft mortality among women with hypothyroidism. *Ann Thorac Surg* 2002;74:2121–5.

231. Velissaris T, Tang AT, Wood PJ, Hett DA, Ohri SK. Thyroid function during coronary surgery with or without cardiopulmonary bypass. *Eur J Cardiothorac Surg* 2009;36:148–54.

232. Sabatino L, Cerillo AG, Ripoli A, Pilo A, Glauber M, Iervasi G. Is the low tri-iodothyronine state a crucial factor in determining the outcome of coronary artery bypass patients? Evidence from a clinical pilot study. *J Endocrinol* 2002;175:577–86.

233. Reinhardt W, Mocker V, Jockenhövel F, et al. Influence of coronary artery bypass surgery on thyroid hormone parameters. *Horm Res* 1997;47:1–8.

234. Cerillo AG, Storti S, Mariani M, et al. The non-thyroidal illness syndrome after coronary artery bypass grafting: a 6-month follow-up study. *Clin Chem Lab Med* 2005;43:289–93.

235. Spratt DI, Frohnauer M, Cyr-Alves H, et al. Physiological effects of nonthyroidal illness syndrome in patients after cardiac surgery. *Am J Physiol Endocrinol Metab* 2007;293:E310–5.

236. Sarma AK, Krisna M, Karunakaran J, Neema PK Neelakandham KS. Severe hypothyroidism after coronary artery bypass grafting. *Ann Thorac Surg* 2005;80:714–6.

237. Klemperer JD. Thyroid hormone and cardiac surgery. *Thyroid* 2002;12:517–21.

238. Levy E, Korach A, Merin G, Feinsod M, Glenville B. Pituitary apoplexy and CABG: should we change our strategy? *Ann Thorac Surg* 2007;84:1388–90.

239. Zayour DH, Azar ST. Silent pituitary infarction after coronary artery bypass grafting procedure: case report and review of the literature. *Endocr Pract* 2006;12:59–62.

240. Mattke AF, Vender JR, Anstadt MR. Pituitary apoplexy presenting as Addisonian crisis after coronary artery bypass grafting. *Tex Heart Inst J* 2002;29:193–9.

241. Hidiroglu M, Kucuker A, Ucaroglu E, Kucuker SA, Sener E. Pituitary apoplexy after cardiac surgery. *Ann Thorac Surg* 2010;89:1635–7.

242. Leeman MF, Vuylsteke A, Ritchie AJ. Lithium-induced nephrogenic diabetes insipidus after coronary artery bypass. *Ann Thorac Surg* 2007;84:656–7.

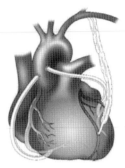

CHAPTER 13

Post-ICU Care and Other Complications

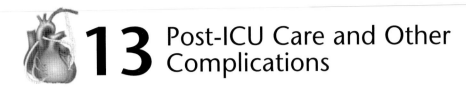

13 Post-ICU Care and Other Complications

I. General Comments

A. Following a brief stay in the intensive care unit, most patients undergoing cardiac surgical procedures follow a routine pattern of recovery. The use of fast-track protocols and critical care pathways ensures that the healthcare team and the patient have a clear understanding of what to expect at different junctures during recovery. Critical pathways are designed to standardize care and identify variances from the expected. However, they are not a substitute for careful patient examination that may identify problems that might otherwise be ignored by rigid adherence to protocols.

B. Most patients are transferred to an intermediate care unit or the postoperative cardiac surgical floor on the first postoperative day. Invasive monitoring is no longer utilized, although bedside telemetry should be considered for several days to identify arrhythmias. It should be remembered that patients are still in an early phase of recovery from surgery with many physiologic derangements still present. Restoring the patient to a normal physiologic state requires careful attention to the prevention, identification, and treatment of complications that may develop at any time during the hospital stay. A detailed daily examination of the patient must be performed with particular attention paid to each organ system. Orders must be thought out carefully and written on an individualized basis to ensure the best possible postoperative care.

C. Although postoperative complications are more common in elderly patients and those with comorbidities, they may still develop unpredictably in low-risk, healthy patients despite an uneventful surgical procedure and early postoperative course. Problems such as atrial arrhythmias are very common and quite benign, with little influence on the patient's hospital course or long-term prognosis. In contrast, less common complications, such as stroke, mediastinitis, tamponade, renal failure, or an acute abdomen, may be devastating, resulting in early death or prolonged hospitalization with multisystem organ failure.

II. Transfer from the ICU and Postoperative Routines

The patient recovering uneventfully from open-heart surgery is usually extubated within 6–12 hours and off all inotropic support by the first postoperative morning. The following interventions represent standardized steps in a critical care pathway which are applicable to most patients (Table 13.1). In more critically ill patients who require an additional period of

Manual of Perioperative Care in Adult Cardiac Surgery, 5th Edition. By Robert M. Bojar.
Published 2011 by Blackwell Publishing Ltd.

Table 13.1 • Critical Pathway for Coronary Artery Bypass Grafting

	Preop Day or Office Visit	Day of Surgery	POD #1	POD #2-3	POD #4-5
Cardiovascular	Bilateral BP Height & weight O_2 saturation	Monitor & treat: shivering bleeding arrhythmias hemodynamics Meds (start 8 h postop): aspirin metoprolol	VS q2h Telemetry D/C neck & arterial lines Meds: 2 g $MgSO_4$	VS q4-8h Telemetry	VS before D/C Remove pacing wires
Respiratory	RA O_2 saturation; ABGs if <90% PFTs if COPD	Wean to extubate within 12 hours IS when awake q1h	40% face mask or nasal cannula IS when awake q1h Splinted cough	Nasal cannula at 2-4 L/min for O_2 sat < 95% IS when awake q1h Splinted cough	Room air
Fluids and electrolytes		I & O q1h Keep u/o > 1 mL/kg/h	Weight I & O q2h Furosemide IV	Weight I & O qshift Furosemide IV	Weight Furosemide IV/PO until at preop weight
Wounds and drains	Hibiclens shower	OR dressing × 12 h unless Dermabond used Monitor/manage CT drainage	DSD with betadine wipe to wounds (unless Derma-bond used) & pacing wire sites D/C CT when total drainage <100 mL/last 8 hours	DSD with betadine wipe to wounds (unless Derma-bond used) & pacing wire sites	Wounds open to air

Pain control		Continuous or low dose IV MS bolus NSAID	IV → PCA MS IV ketorolac	Oxycodone or Tylenol #3	Oxycodone or Tylenol #3
Nutrition/GI	NPO after MN	NPO NG tube to low suction	D/C NG tube Clear liquids	Advance to hi cal, hi prot, NAS diet ADA for diabetics Metamucil/Colace	Progress on diet
Activity	Ambulatory	OOB to chair × 1 after extubation	OOB to chair q8h	Ambulate × 3 in room with assist, then in hallway × 4	Ambulate × 6 in hallway; stair climb 12 stairs × 1
Tests and labs	CXR, ECG, PT, PTT, CBC, plts, LBC, LFTs, urinalysis	On arrival: CXR, ECG, CBC, plts, K^+, ABG If bleeding: INR, PTT, repeat HCT & plts Obtain K^+ q4h × 3	CXR after CT removal LBC, CBC INR (on warfarin)	K^+ if on furosemide INR (on warfarin) PTT (on heparin)	CXR, ECG, CBC, LBC day before discharge Echo for valve patients
Anticoagulation	D/C warfarin 4 days before surgery		Warfarin (valve patients)	Warfarin (valve patients)	Start heparin if subtherapeutic INR for patients with mechanical valves

(continued)

Table 13.1 • *(Continued)*

	Preop Day or Office Visit	Day of Surgery	POD #1	POD #2–3	POD #4–5
Discharge planning	Home assessment	Reevaluate home situation		D/C planning status discussed by care team with discharge planners	Final review of meds; VNA follow-up, clinic or MD office follow-up
Teaching	Videos, critical pathway, NPO, shower instructions, incentive spirometry (IS)				Patient & family attend discharge class or view discharge video Nutrition instructions Medication instructions

ventilatory or pharmacologic support, the temptation to adhere to these time-related recommendations must be resisted, and withdrawal of "intensive care" must be carefully evaluated and not rushed. Typical orders for transfer to the postoperative floor are noted in Table 13.2 and Appendix 4.

A. Postoperative day and night
   1. Wean vasoactive medications
   2. Wean from ventilator and extubate
   3. Remove nasogastric tube
   4. Remove Swan-Ganz and arterial lines
   5. Get patient out of bed (OOB) in a chair
   6. Initiate β-blocker therapy and aspirin

B. POD #1
   1. Remove chest tubes if minimal drainage
   2. Transfer to floor; place on telemetry and pulse oximetry × 72 hours
   3. Get patient out of bed and ambulating
   4. Advance diet
   5. Remove Foley catheter
   6. Start warfarin for valve patients

C. POD #2–3
   1. Remove chest tubes if minimal drainage
   2. Stop antibiotics (after 48 hours maximum)
   3. Advance diet to achieve satisfactory nutrition
   4. Increase activity level
   5. Continue diuresis to preoperative weight
   6. Commence planning for home services or rehabilitation

D. POD #3–4
   1. Obtain predischarge laboratory data (hematocrit, electrolytes, BUN, creatinine, chest x-ray, ECG)
   2. Remove pacing wires
   3. Assess potential discharge location (home vs. rehab)
   4. Initiate discharge teaching

E. POD #4–5
   1. Consider heparin for patients receiving mechanical valves
   2. Carefully review discharge medications and instructions with patient and family
   3. Discharge home or to rehab facility

III. Differential Diagnosis of Common Postoperative Symptoms

The development of chest pain, shortness of breath, fever, or just feeling "plain lousy" with a poor appetite and fatigue during the early convalescent period is not unusual, especially in elderly patients. Although the cause of these signs and symptoms may be benign, they should

Table 13.2 • Typical Transfer Orders from the ICU

ALLERGIES: _____

1. Transfer to: _____

2. Procedure: _____

3. Condition: _____

4. NURSING

    ☐ Vital signs q4h × 2 days, then q shift

    ☐ ECG telemetry

    ☐ I & O q 8 hours

    ☐ Daily weights

    ☐ Foley catheter to gravity drainage; D/C on __/__ at __; due to void in 8 h

    ☐ Chest tubes to −20 cm H_2O suction

    ☐ Ambulate in hall with cardiac rehab

    ☐ T.E.D. stockings

    ☐ SpO_2 q8h and 1 time before and after ambulation

    ☐ Wire and wound care per protocol

    ☐ Wean oxygen via nasal prongs from 6 L/min to 2 L/min to keep $SpO_2 > 92\%$

    ☐ Incentive spirometry q1h when awake

    ☐ Glucose via fingerstick/glucometer AC and qHS in diabetics

    ☐ Notify housestaff for heart rate >110 or systolic blood pressure >150 mm Hg

    ☐ Saline lock, flush q8h and prn

5. Diet

    ☐ NPO

    ☐ Clear liquids/no added salt (NAS)

    ☐ Full liquids/NAS

    ☐ NAS, low fat, low cholesterol diet

    ☐ _____ cal ADA, NAS low cholesterol diet, if diabetic

    ☐ Fluid restriction ___ mL per 24 hours (IV + PO)

6. Temporary pacemaker settings

    ☐ Pacemaker on: Mode: ☐ Atrial ☐ VVI ☐ DVI ☐ DDD

                       Atrial output___mA   Ventricular output ___mA

                       Rate ___/min   AV interval ___msec

    ☐ Pacer attached but off

    ☐ Detach pacer but keep at bedside

7. Laboratory studies

    ☐ Chest x-ray after chest tube removal

    ☐ In AM after transfer: CBC, lytes, BUN, creatinine, blood glucose

    ☐ Daily PT/INR if on warfarin

    ☐ Daily PTT and platelet count if on heparin (see Appendix 7)

Table 13.2 • (Continued)

☐ Fingerstick blood glucose at 4 AM on POD #2 (___/___); if >150 mg/dL, treat per insulin sliding scale protocol and repeat fingerstick at 5:30 AM

☐ On day prior to discharge: chest x-ray, ECG, CBC, electrolytes, BUN, creatinine

8. Consults

☐ Cardiac rehabilitation

☐ Social services

☐ Physical therapy

☐ Occupational therapy

☐ Nutrition

9. Medications

a. Antibiotics

☐ Cefazolin 1 g IV q8h for ___ more doses (6 doses total); last dose on___/___ at _____ hours

☐ Vancomycin 1 g IV q12h for ___ more doses (4 doses total); last dose on___/___ at _____ hours

☐ Mupirocin 2% (Bactroban ointment) via Q-tip nasal swab the evening after surgery and bid × 3 days total

☐ Chlorhexidine 0.12% oral wash (Peridex) 15 mL with brushing q12 hr

b. Cardiovascular medications

☐ Metoprolol___ mg PO q12h. Hold for HR < 60 or SBP < 100

☐ Carvedilol ___ mg PO q12h. Hold for HR < 60 or SBP < 100

☐ Amiodarone ___ mg PO q12h

☐ Lisinopril ___ mg PO qd

☐ Diltiazem 30 mg PO q6h (radial artery grafts)

☐ Amlodipine 5 mg PO qd (radial artery grafts)

☐ Imdur (sustained release) 20 mg PO qd (radial artery grafts)

☐ Simvastatin ___ mg qd hs (no more than 20 mg if on amiodarone)

c. Anticoagulants/antiplatelet agents

☐ Enteric-coated aspirin ☐81 mg ☐325 mg PO qd (hold for platelet count <75,000)

☐ Clopidogrel 75 mg PO qd

☐ Low-molecular-weight heparin (Lovenox) ___ mg SC___

☐ Heparin 5000 units SC bid

☐ Heparin 25,000 units/500 mL D5W at ___units/h starting on _____ (per protocol – see Appendix 7)

☐ Warfarin ___mg PO qd starting on____; daily dose check with HO (per protocol – see page 672 and Appendix 8)

d. Pain medications

☐ Morphine sulfate via PCA pump or 10 mg IM q3h prn severe pain

☐ Ketorolac 15–30 mg IV q6h prn moderate-to-severe pain (4–10 on pain scale); D/C after 72 hours

(continued)

Table 13.2 • (Continued)

- ☐ Acetaminophen with oxycodone (Percocet) 1–2 tabs PO q4h prn pain (start with one tablet for moderate pain (4–6 pain scale); give additional tablet after 1 hour if no change in pain; give 2 tablets for severe pain (7–10 pain scale)
- ☐ Acetaminophen with codeine (Tylenol #3) 1–2 tabs PO q4h prn mild pain (1–3 pain scale)
- ☐ Acetaminophen 650 mg PO q4h prn mild pain (1–3 pain scale)

e. GI medications

- ☐ Pantoprazole (Protonix) 40 mg PO qd
- ☐ For nausea:
  - ☐ Metoclopramide 10 mg IV/PO q6h prn
  - ☐ Ondansetron 4–8 mg q4h IV/PO prn
  - ☐ Prochlorperazine 10 mg PO/IM/IV q6h prn
- ☐ Milk of magnesia 30 mL PO qhs prn
- ☐ Docusate (Colace) 100 mg PO bid
- ☐ Bisacodyl (Dulcolax) 10 mg suppository prn constipation

f. Diabetes medications

- ☐ Oral hypoglycemic: _____
- ☐ ___ units regular insulin (Novolin R or Humulin R) SC ___ qAM ___qPM
- ☐ ___ units NPH insulin (Novolin N or Humulin N) SC ___qAM ___qPM
- ☐ Sliding scale: treat fingerstick/glucometer glucose according to the following scale at 06:00, 11:00, 15:00, and 20:00:
  - ☐ 140–160, give 2 units regular insulin SC (Novolin R or Humulin R)
  - ☐ 161–200, give 4 units regular insulin SC
  - ☐ 201–250, give 6 units regular insulin SC
  - ☐ 251–300, give 8 units regular insulin SC
  - ☐ 301–350, give 10 units regular insulin SC
  - ☐ > 350, call house officer

g. Other medications

- ☐ Acetaminophen 650 mg PO q3h prn temp >38.5°C
- ☐ Chloral hydrate 0.5–1.0 g PO qhs prn sleep
- ☐ Furosemide ___ mg IV/PO q __ h
- ☐ Potassium chloride___ mEq PO bid (while on furosemide)
- ☐ Albuterol 2.5 mg/5 mL NS via nebulizer q4h prn
- ☐ Levalbuterol (Xopenex) 0.63 mg in 3 mL NS q8h via nebulizer or two inhalations q4–6h through a pressured MDI
- ☐ Duoneb inhaler q6h
- ☐ Other:_____

not be taken lightly because they may indicate the presence of potentially serious problems that warrant investigation. Careful questioning and examination of the patient on a daily or more frequent basis can prioritize diagnoses, direct the evaluation, and lead to prompt and appropriate treatment.

A. **Chest pain**

1. **Differential diagnosis**. The development of chest pain following cardiac surgery often raises the suspicion of myocardial ischemia, but the differential diagnosis must include several other potential causes. The greatest fear to a patient is that the recurrence of chest pain indicates a failed operation; the surgeon meanwhile may purposely try to provide alternative explanations. Although musculoskeletal pain is the most common cause of chest discomfort, significant problems that must be considered include:

   a. Myocardial ischemia

   b. Pericarditis

   c. Arrhythmias

   d. Pneumothorax

   e. Pneumonia

   f. Pulmonary embolism

   g. Sternal wound infection

   h. Aortic dissection

   i. Gastroesphageal reflux

2. **Evaluation**. Careful physical examination (breath sounds, pericardial rub, sternal wound), a chest x-ray, and 12-lead ECG will usually provide the appropriate diagnosis and direct additional testing. Differentiation of ST-segment elevation related to ischemia as opposed to pericarditis is important (Figure 8.2, page 321). Consultation with the cardiology service is essential in managing patients with a suspected cardiac origin to their chest pain. Stress imaging or even coronary angiography may be warranted. Other diagnostic modalities include echocardiography, computed tomography (CT) pulmonary angiography to rule out pulmonary embolism, and sternal wound aspiration.

B. **Shortness of breath**

1. **Differential diagnosis**. Shortness of breath is usually caused by splinting from chest wall discomfort and is not uncommon in the anemic patient with underlying lung disease. However, significant shortness of breath, its acute onset, or deterioration in pulmonary status should raise awareness of a significant problem. The source may be of a primary pulmonary nature, but it may also be the consequence of cardiac or renal dysfunction. Diagnoses to be considered include:

   a. Pleuropulmonary problems
   - Atelectasis and hypoxia from mucus plugging or poor inspiratory effort
   - Pneumothorax
   - Pneumonia (aspiration)
   - Bronchospasm
   - An enlarging pleural effusion
   - Pulmonary embolism

    b. Cardiopulmonary problems – low cardiac output states or acute pulmonary edema caused by:

- Acute myocardial ischemia or infarction
- Cardiac tamponade
- Residual or new-onset mitral regurgitation (ischemic, associated with systemic hypertension) or a recurrent ventricular septal defect
- Fluid overload (often associated with oliguric renal failure)
- Severe diastolic dysfunction
- Atrial or ventricular tachyarrhythmias

    c. Compensatory response to metabolic acidosis (low cardiac output state)

    d. Sepsis

  2. Evaluation. Careful lung examination may reveal absent breath sounds or diffuse rales/rhonchi suggesting a parenchymal process or pulmonary edema. Clinical evidence of cardiac tamponade (muffled heart sounds, orthostatic blood pressure changes, pulsus paradoxus) should be sought. An arterial blood gas (ABG), chest x-ray, and ECG should be obtained. An echocardiogram gives an assessment of ventricular function, detects valve dysfunction or recurrent shunting, and may also identify a large pleural or pericardial effusion or tamponade. A CT pulmonary angiogram should be performed if pulmonary embolism is suspected.

C. Fever

  1. Differential diagnosis. Fever is very common during the first 48–72 hours and is usually caused by atelectasis from poor inspiratory effort. Thorough evaluation of recurrent fevers is warranted after the first 72 hours. Potential causes of postoperative fever include:

    a. Atelectasis or pneumonia

    b. Urinary tract infection (UTI)

    c. Wound infections – sternum or leg

    d. *Clostridium difficile* colitis or other intra-abdominal process

    e. Sinusitis (usually in patients with indwelling endotracheal or nasogastric tubes)

    f. Catheter sepsis

    g. Endocarditis (especially on a prosthetic valve)

    h. Decubitus ulcer

    i. Drug fever

    j. Deep venous thrombosis (DVT) and pulmonary embolism

    k. Postpericardiotomy syndrome (PPS)

  2. Evaluation. The lungs, chest and leg incisions should be examined carefully. A CBC with differential, chest x-ray, urinalysis, and appropriate cultures should be performed. A stool sample for *C. difficile* should be obtained if the patient has abdominal pain or diarrhea. Indwelling central and arterial lines should be cultured and removed if in place for more than 5 days or if cultures return positive.[1] If the WBC is normal, a drug fever may be present. Occult sternal infections may be investigated with a chest CT scan, but results are usually nonspecific; needle aspiration should be performed if suspicion is high. Head CT scans can identify sinusitis. A transesophageal echocardiogram can evaluate the heart valves for vegetations consistent with endocarditis.

3. **Treatment**. It is ideally best to defer antibiotic therapy until an organism has been identified. However, a broad-spectrum antibiotic may be initiated based on the presumed source and organisms involved as soon as cultures have been obtained. This is especially important in patients who have received prosthetic material (valves, grafts). A more narrow-spectrum antibiotic may be substituted subsequently. Empiric metronidazole may be started for suspected *C. difficile* colitis. Occasionally a patient will have a fever and elevated WBC with no evident source, but will respond to a brief course of antibiotics. Further comments on nosocomial infections and sepsis are found on pages 674–676.

IV. Respiratory Care and Complications

A. Respiratory function is still impaired when the patient is transferred to the postoperative floor, with many patients exhibiting shortness of breath with some splinting from chest wall discomfort. Arterial desaturation is not uncommon, and all patients should have an arterial saturation measured daily by pulse oximetry until the SaO_2 remains above 90%. It is not uncommon to see significant desaturation when the patient becomes ambulatory. Most patients have some degree of fluid overload and require diuresis, and steps must be taken to overcome a poor inspiratory effort and atelectasis. Potential complications, such as pneumonia, bronchospasm, pleural effusions, or pneumothorax can be identified by examination and a chest x-ray. Standard orders should include:

1. Supplemental oxygen via nasal cannula at 2–6 L/min

2. Frequent use of incentive spirometry to encourage deep breathing

3. Progressive mobilization

4. Provision of adequate, but not excessive, analgesia. Patient-controlled analgesia (usually morphine) is particularly beneficial for 1 or 2 days following surgery, and may be supplemented with other pain medications, such as ketorolac (Toradol) 15–30 mg IV q6h for a few days. Most patients obtain adequate analgesia with oral medications 2–3 days after surgery and seem to do better with regular, rather than prn, pain medications.

5. Bronchodilators administered via nebulizers should be used if copious secretions or bronchospasm are present, (see page 428). These commonly include albuterol, levalbuterol (Xopenex), or a combination of albuterol and ipratropium (Duoneb). Chest physical therapy may benefit patients having difficulty raising secretions.

6. Measures to reduce the risk of venous thromboembolism (VTE) (antiembolism stockings, sequential compression devices [SCDs], subcutaneous heparin or low-molecular-weight heparin [LMWH]) should be considered depending on the patient's mobility and risk (see section on pulmonary embolism, page 655–656).

B. Patients with preexisting lung disease and a history of heavy smoking often have a tenuous respiratory status postoperatively, and acute decompensation can occur with little provocation, including ambulation. Mucus plugging, atelectasis from poor inspiratory effort, mobilization of "third space" fluid, or even a minor cardiac event can cause arterial desaturation and respiratory distress. In patients without significant underlying lung disease, acute decompensation usually indicates the presence of a significant process, such as a pleuropulmonary event (significant pneumothorax, pneumonia, pulmonary embolism), myocardial ischemia, worsening mitral regurgitation, cardiac tamponade, or acute fluid overload from acute kidney injury with oliguria.

C. The management of respiratory insufficiency, pneumothorax, pleural effusions, and bronchospasm was discussed in Chapter 10. Other complications, including diaphragmatic dysfunction from phrenic nerve paresis and pulmonary embolism, are discussed below.

D. **Diaphragmatic dysfunction** from phrenic nerve injury has been noted in 10–20% of patients following open-heart surgery in several studies.[2–4]

   1. **Etiology**

      a. Cold injury to the phrenic nerve from use of iced saline slush in the pericardial well is the primary cause of this problem. Systemic hypothermia may also be contributory.[5] Cooling pads to protect the phrenic nerve from cold solutions, minimizing systemic hypothermia, and avoiding iced slush reduce the incidence of phrenic nerve paresis.[2–4,6]

      b. The phrenic nerve may be injured directly during dissection of the internal thoracic artery (ITA) in the upper mediastinum, especially on the right side.[7] It may also be damaged when making a V-incision in the pericardium to allow for better lie of the ITA pedicle. Phrenic nerve devascularization with compromise of the pericardiophrenic artery may also be contributory. Although some studies suggest that a phrenic neuropathy is more common in diabetics, other studies could not identify this as a risk factor.[3,8,9]

   2. **Presentation**

      a. Most patients with unilateral phrenic nerve paresis have few respiratory symptoms and are extubated uneventfully. Difficulty weaning, shortness of breath, and the requirement for reintubation may be noted in patients with severe chronic obstructive pulmonary disease (COPD).

      b. Bilateral phrenic nerve palsy usually produces tachypnea, paradoxical abdominal breathing, and CO_2 retention during attempts to wean from mechanical ventilation.

   3. **Evaluation**

      a. A chest x-ray will demonstrate an elevated hemidiaphragm at end-expiration during spontaneous ventilation, most commonly on the left side. This will not be evident during mechanical ventilation. An elevated hemidiaphragm may be difficult to appreciate if basilar atelectasis or a pleural effusion is present. Therefore, when considering performing a thoracentesis or tube thoracostomy for a left pleural effusion, one must always consider the possibility of an obscured, elevated left hemidiaphragm. The position of the gastric bubble on chest x-ray should identify the position of the diaphragm. If the diaphragm is elevated, one might inadvertently insert a needle below the diaphragm, risking injury to intra-abdominal structures.

      b. Diaphragmatic fluoroscopy ("sniff test") will demonstate paradoxical upward motion of the diaphragm during spontaneous inspiration if unilateral paralysis is present.

   c. Ultrasonography will show a hypokinetic, immobile, or paradoxically moving diaphragm during respiration.

   d. Transcutaneous phrenic nerve stimulation in the neck with recording of diaphragmatic potentials over the seventh and eighth intercostal spaces can measure phrenic nerve conduction velocities and latency times.[10] This is helpful in assessing whether phrenic nerve dysfunction may be a contributing factor to a patient's respiratory problems.

   e. Transdiaphragmatic pressure measurements can be used to make the diagnosis in patients with bilateral phrenic nerve palsies.[9]

  4. Treatment is supportive until phrenic nerve function recovers, which may take up to 2 years. One study of patients with COPD found that nearly 25% of patients had persistent pulmonary problems with a decreased quality of life at midterm follow-up.[11] Diaphragmatic plication can provide significant symptomatic and objective improvement in patients with marked dyspnea from unilateral paralysis. This can be performed via a thoracotomy or laparoscopically.[12-14] Ventilatory support is usually necessary for patients with bilateral involvement. Some patients can be managed at home with a cuirass respirator or a rocking bed.

E. Pulmonary embolism (PE) is noted in about 1% of patients following surgery and is invariably linked to the development of deep venous thrombosis (DVT) of the lower extremities.[15,16] Although symptomatic DVT is also noted in about 1–2% of patients after cardiac surgery, screening noninvasive studies have documented an incidence of around 20%, with half being from the non-harvest leg.[16] In fact, an incidence of 13% was noted in a study in which patients were treated with enoxaparin and intermittent pneumatic calf compression per the 2008 American College of Chest Physicians (ACCP) guidelines.[17] Furthermore, PE can occur in the absence of symptomatic DVT. It has been presumed, perhaps inappropriately so, that the risk of venous thromboembolism (VTE) is low because of heparinization and hemodilution during surgery and the presence of thrombocytopenia and platelet dysfunction in the early postoperative period. However, other studies have shown that platelet activity may in fact be increased, rather than decreased, immediately after surgery.[18] Furthermore, there have been concerns that off-pump surgery may be associated with a prothrombotic state that may increase the risk of pulmonary embolism, although the risk of symptomatic VTE is still only 1%.[19]

  1. Risk factors for VTE in the perioperative period include older age, obesity (BMI >30), prolonged bed rest and immobility pre- and postoperatively, recent groin catheterization, COPD, hyperlipidemia, blood transfusions, prolonged mechanical ventilation and postoperative CHF. VTE occurring several weeks after surgery may be related to delayed-onset heparin-induced thrombocytopenia (HIT).

  2. Prevention. Although there are no clinical trials of VTE prophylaxis in cardiac surgery patients, several recommendations for mechanical or pharmacologic prophylaxis can be made.[15,20-22]

   a. Elastic graduated compression stockings (GCS), such as T.E.D. stockings, should be placed after the initial leg dressing and ace wrap are removed, and should be placed on both legs.

   b. Although a similar rate of VTE has been shown with the addition of sequential compression devices (SCDs) or intermittent pneumatic compression stockings

(PCS) (Venodyne) to GCS,[17] SCDs are commonly recommended for patients remaining in the ICU, especially those who remain sedated on mechanical ventilation. One study did show that the addition of SCDs to SC heparin reduced the incidence of PE by 60% (from 4% to 1.5%).[23]

    c. Heparin should be considered in many patients, taking into consideration the potential risk of hemopericardium and tamponade.[24,25] Several published guidelines recommend routine use of unfractionated heparin (UFH) 5000 units SC bid starting the day after surgery with use of a more intensive regimen (enoxaparin 40 mg qd or 30 mg bid) in patients at higher risk.[20,21] The 2008 ACCP guidelines state that the benefit of routine thromboprophylaxis for patients undergoing CABG is uncertain, yet it was recognized that many patients are at high risk for VTE and early mobilization is not always predictable. A general recommendation was made for use of *either* LMWH, low-dose UFH, *or* optimally used bilateral GCS or PCS.[22] Clearly, in patients at higher risk for bleeding, which may include elderly patients with fragile tissues and patients with early mediastinal bleeding, the risk of anticoagulation may exceed the benefits.

3. Manifestations. Pleuritic chest pain and shortness of breath are usually present. The acute onset of these symptoms distinguishes them from typical postoperative respiratory symptoms. The new onset of atrial fibrillation, sinus tachycardia, or fever of unknown origin may be clues to the diagnosis. Calf tenderness and edema are unreliable signs of DVT, especially in the leg from which the vein has been harvested. However, the new development of such findings several days to weeks after surgery should prompt further evaluation.

4. Assessment. Arterial blood gases, chest x-ray, ECG, and contrast-enhanced multislice CT pulmonary angiography (CTPA) should be obtained.[26] Although lung scintigraphy (V/Q scans) combined with a chest x-ray may be as sensitive as CTPA in detecting PE, the latter is usually selected in postoperative cardiac surgical patients unless there are reasons to avoid contrast (i.e., allergy or renal dysfunction).[27] The presence of a low arterial oxygenation saturation is nonspecific, but may be compared with values obtained earlier in the postoperative course. A positive venous noninvasive study of the lower extremities in association with respiratory symptoms and hypoxia is suggestive evidence of a pulmonary embolism and should prompt further evaluation. A low platelet count with VTE mandates evaluation for HIT, for which alternative anticoagulation should be initiated.

5. Treatment entails bedrest and anticoagulation with IV heparin for 1 week (unless HIT is present), followed by warfarin for 6 months. Thrombolytic therapy is contraindicated because of the recent sternotomy incision. An inferior vena cava filter is recommended because of the high risk of recurrence despite anticoagulation and should be performed if anticoagulation is contraindicated. Interventional methods, including suction embolectomy and fragmentation therapy, may be beneficial in patients with massive PE, reserving surgery for salvage situations to avoid a redo sternotomy and pump run.[28,29] However, some groups now recommend pulmonary embolectomy for hemodynamically stable patients with massive PE and right ventricular dysfunction, although few patients in these series have recently had open-heart surgery.[30]

V. Cardiac Care and Complications

A. Upon transfer to the postoperative floor, the patient should be attached to a telemetry system to continuously monitor the heart rate and rhythm for several days. Vital signs are obtained every shift if the patient is stable, but more frequently if the patient's heart rate, rhythm, or blood pressure is abnormal or marginal.

B. The evaluation and management of complications noted most frequently in the intensive care unit are presented in Chapter 11. These include low cardiac output states, perioperative infarction, cardiac arrest, coronary spasm, hypertension, and arrhythmias. This section will discuss several cardiac problems commonly noted during subsequent convalescence.

C. Arrhythmias and conduction problems

   1. Atrial arrhythmias are the most common complication of open-heart surgery and occur with a peak incidence on the second or third postoperative day. Although some patients become symptomatic with lightheadedness, fatigue, or palpitations, most have no symptoms and are noted to be in atrial fibrillation or flutter on the ECG monitor. Treatment entails rate control, attempted conversion to sinus rhythm, and anticoagulation if AF persists or recurs. Management protocols are discussed in detail on pages 537–547 and in Table 11.15 (page 542).

   2. Ventricular arrhythmias are always of concern because they may be attributable to myocardial ischemia or infarction and may herald cardiac arrest. Low-grade ectopy or nonsustained ventricular tachycardia (VT) with normal ventricular function does not require aggressive therapy. In contrast, VT with impaired LV function requires further evaluation and probable placement of an implantable cardioverter-defibrillator (ICD). These issues are discussed on pages 58–59.

   3. Temporary pacemaker wires are routinely removed on the third postoperative day if there is no evidence of symptomatic sinus bradycardia, lengthy sinus pauses, advanced degrees of heart block, or a slow ventricular response to atrial fibrillation. If these issues are present, medications that reduce atrial automaticity or reduce AV conduction (β-blockers, amiodarone, calcium channel blockers, digoxin) should be stopped. If they persist, permanent pacemaker implantation should be considered.

   a. Patients undergoing valve surgery are more prone to conduction disturbances and more frequently require implantation of a permanent pacemaker.[31] Patients with sick sinus or tachycardia/bradycardia syndrome may have a rapid ventricular response to AF intermixed with a slow sinus mechanism that limits use of β-blockers. A permanent pacemaker system should be considered if these problems persist beyond 3 days. Studies have shown, however, that pacemaker dependence usually resolves within a few months in patients in whom pacemakers are placed, unless the indication was complete heart block.[32]

   b. When pacemaker wires are removed, there is always the potential for bleeding and the development of tamponade. It is recommended that they be removed when the INR is less than 2, but this does not eliminate the possibility of bleeding. If the INR remains persistently elevated, the wires may be cut and left behind. After removal, vital signs should be taken every 15 minutes for the first hour and then hourly for a few hours to monitor for orthostatic changes. Tamponade can occur within minutes or hours and can prove fatal unless the possibility is entertained. If concern is raised because of hypotension or a complaint of chest pain, a STAT echocardiogram can be helpful. Emergency thoracotomy at the bedside may be lifesaving.

D. Hypertension. When the patient is transferred from the ICU, oral antihypertensive medications must be substituted for the potent intravenous drugs used in the ICU. Blood pressure tends to return to its preoperative level several days after surgery once myocardial function has returned to baseline, the patient has been mobilized, and chest wall pain improves with moderate analgesia. Aggressive patient-specific management is important to prevent blood pressure-related issues. For example, a patient with renal dysfunction may need a slightly higher blood pressure to ensure renal perfusion. In contrast, more strict control of blood pressure may be essential in an elderly patient with fragile tissues or in patients with perioperative bleeding. Not only can hypertension increase cardiac wall stress and increase any residual mitral regurgitation, but it can precipitate an aortic dissection from graft or cannulation sites.

1. A decrease in systolic blood pressure from preoperative levels may be noted in patients who are hypovolemic or anemic, or in those experiencing a perioperative infarction. In these patients, preoperative antihypertensive medications can be held and then restarted at lower doses when the blood pressure increases. In contrast, patients who have ongoing pain issues or have had AVR for aortic stenosis may develop significant systolic hypertension.

2. If the patient's blood pressure was well controlled before surgery, the same medications should usually be restarted in gradually increasing doses. Other considerations when selecting an antihypertensive medication include:

   a. Poor ventricular function: use one of the ACE inhibitors or angiotensin receptor blockers (ARBs).

   b. Sinus tachycardia with good LV function, evidence of residual myocardial ischemia: use a β-blocker.

   c. Coronary spasm or use of a radial artery graft: use a nitrate or calcium channel blocker (amlodipine, diltiazem, or nicardipine). These are excellent first-line medications to use in patients without significant ventricular dysfunction.

E. Hypotension may develop after transfer to the floor and should be evaluated using the differential diagnosis of shock or a low cardiac output state (see Chapter 11).

1. **Etiology.** The possibility of a significant clinical condition should always be considered in a patient with hypotension, although transient hypotension is usually of a benign etiology. Concerns must always include the possibility of hypoxemia, myocardial ischemia, and especially delayed **tamponade** (see section G, page 660). However, the more common causes of hypotension several days after surgery include:

   a. Hypovolemia, usually from aggressive diuresis

   b. Anemia

   c. β-blockers or amiodarone used prophylactically to prevent atrial fibrillation

   d. Significant bradycardia

   e. Arrhythmias (especially a rapid ventricular response to atrial fibrillation/flutter), and the medications used to treat them, which usually lower the blood pressure (β-blockers, calcium channel blockers, amiodarone)

   f. Initiating too high a dose of the patient's preoperative medications. Often the patient's initial postoperative hypertension is related to pain and sympathetic overactivity, and once these resolve, hypotension may result, necessitating fluid resuscitation and unnecessary transfusions.

2. **Assessment and management**

a. Review of the patient's medications, fluid status, orthostatic blood pressure measurements, heart rate and rhythm, pulse oximetry reading, 12-lead ECG, and hematocrit should be sufficient to delineate the mechanism for hypotension. If the patient appears warm and well perfused, administration of a moderate amount of volume and modification of the medical regimen should suffice.

b. Management of hypotension associated with atrial fibrillation can be problematic, in that medications that slow the rate tend to cause vasodilation and lower the blood pressure further (especially dilitiazem). However, in most patients, rate control improves left ventricular filling and the blood pressure. If the patient has refractory hypotension with a fast rate that is difficult to control pharmacologically, cardioversion may be indicated.

c. If the patient has refractory hypotension and does not appear well perfused, the likelihood of tamponade is increased and a STAT echocardiogram should be performed.

F. **Recurrent myocardial ischemia.** The development of recurrent angina or new ECG changes (ST segments) postoperatively always requires careful evaluation for evidence of ischemia or myocardial infarction. Manifestations may include a low output state, congestive heart failure and pulmonary edema, ventricular arrhythmias, or cardiac arrest.

1. **Etiology**

a. Acute thrombotic graft occlusion (usually from an anastomotic problem but occasionally from an incompletely endarterectomized vessel)

b. Hypoperfusion from anastomotic narrowing (technical issue) or inadequate flow (for example, using a small ITA graft or replacing a moderately diseased vein graft with a small ITA at reoperation)

c. Unbypassed, diseased coronary arteries (incomplete revascularization)

d. Coronary vasospasm

2. **Evaluation**

a. Empiric use of a nitrate and/or calcium channel blocker may be helpful for ischemia or spasm and can be diagnostic.

b. Urgent coronary arteriography should be considered when there are significant ECG changes. It may identify a technical problem with a graft or confirm the diagnosis of spasm.

c. In less urgent situations, a nuclear stress imaging study can be performed to identify the presence of myocardial ischemia and differentiate between ischemic and nonischemic causes of chest pain.

3. **Treatment**

a. Intensification of a medical regimen with nitrates and β-blockers is indicated.

b. Placement of an intra-aortic balloon pump (IABP) is beneficial for ongoing ischemia or evidence of hemodynamic compromise, especially in the immediate postoperative period. However, it should only be considered a supportive measure until the etiology of the problem is identified.

c. If a technical problem with a graft is identified by coronary angiography, percutaneous coronary intervention (PCI) is often the best treatment because it can be performed most expeditiously. If this is not feasible, but a major area of myocardium is in jeopardy and the patient has not suffered a significant perioperative myocardial infarction (PMI), reoperation should be considered. In contrast, medical management may be indicated if the coronary vessels supplying an ischemic zone are small and diffusely diseased, if they were bypassed but graft flow was limited by vessel runoff, or if they were not bypassable. PCI of larger more proximal stenotic segments may provide some benefit by improving inflow. Inability to address small vessels should only leave a minor area of the heart potentially ischemic.

  d. The long-term results of coronary bypass surgery are influenced by the development of atherosclerotic disease in bypass conduits, unbypassed native arteries, or native arteries beyond the bypass sites. Factors that can improve these results include use of ITA grafting, aggressive control of risk factors (abstinence from smoking, statins for hypercholesterolemia, optimal control of hypertension and diabetes), and indefinite use of aspirin (use for 1 year will improve vein graft patency).[20] On rare occasions, the late development of ischemia has been attributed to a coronary steal syndrome, either from a coronary-subclavian steal or an ITA-pulmonary artery fistula.[33]

G. Delayed tamponade. Pericardial effusions are noted in about 60% of patients following surgery but usually resolve completely.[34] A small percentage of patients will have effusions that gradually increase in size and produce a low cardiac output state and tamponade.[35] This may be noted within the first week of surgery or weeks later. Suspicion of this problem must remain high because symptoms may develop insidiously and can be difficult to differentiate from those noted in patients recovering slowly from surgery. **This is one of the most serious yet most potentially correctable of all postoperative problems**.

  1. Etiology

  a. Use of antiplatelet agents (aspirin, clopidogrel) or anticoagulation (heparin, warfarin) can cause slow intrapericardial bleeding from any source (soft tissues, raw pericardium, suture lines). This may occur even if the patient had minimal bleeding in the immediate postoperative period. This is of particular concern because of some recommendations to initiate heparin on the first postoperative day to prevent VTE.[20,21]

  b. Acute hemorrhage may result from laceration of a superficial artery or vein overlying the right ventricle or from the right ventricle itself during pacemaker wire removal. This usually occurs after the chest tubes have been removed. Bleeding during withdrawal of atrial pacing wires may occur if the wires are directly attached to the atrial wall rather than placed into a plastic sleeve that is sewn to the heart (the Medtronic model 6500 wires). Rarely, a patient may develop a delayed rupture of an infarct zone or LV rupture from a mitral valve prosthesis.

  c. Late serous or serosanguineous effusions may develop from postpericardiotomy syndrome (PPS), which is considered to be one type of the "postcardiac injury" syndromes.[36]

  2. Presentation. Acute hemorrhage will present with refractory hypotension and the clinical picture of acute cardiac tamponade. The classic picture of delayed tamponade is a low output state manifest by malaise, shortness of breath, chest discomfort, anorexia, nausea, or a low-grade fever. These symptoms are frequently ascribed to medications or simply a slow recovery from surgery. Jugular venous distention, a pericardial rub, progressive orthostatic hypotension, tachycardia (often masked by use of β-blockers), and a pulsus paradoxus are often noted. Occasionally, the first sign is a decrease in urine output with a rise in the BUN and creatinine caused by progressive renal dysfunction from the low output state and systemic venous hypertension.

3. **Evaluation.** A chest x-ray may reveal enlargement of the cardiac silhouette, but frequently is normal, depending on the site and rapidity of blood accumulation. Two-dimensional echocardiography can identify the pericardial effusion, confirm tamponade physiology, and also assess the status of ventricular function.[37] It is important to recognize that tamponade may be caused by selective compression of individual cardiac chambers, often by small effusions, and not necessarily by large circumferential effusions.[35,38] **A surface echo often has limitations in obtaining certain acoustic windows,** which may be related to the patient's body habitus. Thus, it will occasionally not identify an effusion. If the clinical suspicion remains high and transthoracic imaging is suboptimal, a **transesophageal echocardiogram** (TEE) should be performed as it is more sensitive in detecting posterior fluid collections (Figure 13.1).[39]

4. **Treatment**

   a. Emergency mediastinal exploration is indicated for active bleeding.

   b. Pericardiocentesis is the least invasive means of draining a large effusion that has produced cardiac tamponade. This is usually performed in the cardiac catheterization laboratory under ECG or two-dimensional echocardiographic guidance.

   c. Subxiphoid exploration should be considered when the echocardiogram suggests that the fluid collection cannot be successfully approached percutaneously (usually a posterior collection) or when it is loculated. If this approach is ineffective in draining the effusion, the entire sternal incision may need to be opened.

   d. A pericardial "window" or limited pericardiectomy through a left thoracotomy approach can be considered for loculated posterior effusions or recurrent effusions several weeks after surgery.

   e. Anti-inflammatory medications or steroids can be used for large effusions attributable to PPS that have not produced hemodynamic compromise. NSAIDs may reduce the inflammatory response and lower the incidence of pericardial effusions, and a trial of colchicine is under way to assess its prophylactic role in preventing PPS.[40]

   f. Several studies have demonstrated that performance of a small posterior pericardiotomy incision at the conclusion of surgery reduces the incidence of posterior pericardial effusions.[41] It is also possible that placement of one of the mediastinal tubes below the heart, rather than two tubes anteriorly, might improve drainage and reduce the incidence of residual effusions.

H. **Postpericardiotomy syndrome** (PPS) has been reported in 15−20% of patients following open-heart surgery and is considered to represent an autoimmune inflammatory response.[36,42] It is also a phenomenon that may occur after pacemaker

(A)

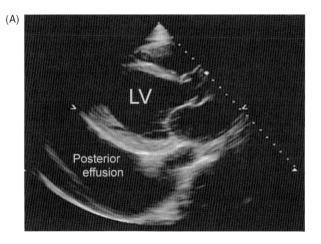

(B)

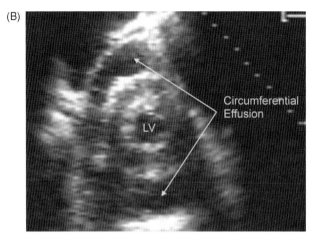

Figure 13.1 • Two-dimensional echocardiograms of significant postoperative pericardial effusions. (A) A transthoracic study in the parasternal long-axis view demonstrating a significant posterior effusion. (B) A transesophageal study in the transgastric short-axis view. Note the circumferential pericardial effusion that prevents adequate ventricular filling. Evidence of diastolic collapse will confirm the hemodynamic significance of the effusion.

implantation, PCI, transmural myocardial infarctions, or radiofrequency arrhythmia ablation, presumably as a response to cardiac injury. It may occur within the first week of surgery or several weeks to months later. PPS is more common in younger patients and those with a history of pericarditis or steroid usage. It must be aggressively treated because it may contribute to cardiac tamponade, early vein graft closure, or constrictive pericarditis. Use of prophylactic NSAIDs or colchicine (1.5 g/day) after surgery may reduce the incidence of PPS.[40,42]

1. **Presentation.** Fever, malaise, pleuritic chest pain, arthralgias, and a pericardial rub are the diagnostic criteria. A pleural or pericardial effusion is usually present.

2. **Evaluation.** Lymphocytosis, eosinophilia, and an elevated ESR are noted, but a fever work-up is negative. Effusions are usually demonstrable by chest x-ray and echocardiography. In one study, the presence of cardiac muscle antibodies correlated with PPS, but another suggested that this reflected an immune response to pericardial or myocardial injury, rather than being causally related. Other inflammatory markers of myocardial injury are not predictive of its occurrence.[43-45]

3. **Treatment**

   a. Diuretics and aspirin should be used as the initial treatment. If there is minimal symptomatic relief, a 1-week course of an NSAID, such as ibuprofen 400 mg qid, is 90% effective.[42] Aspirin should be stopped if an NSAID is used to minimize gastric irritation. Prednisone can be used if symptoms persist. It should be noted that regular use of NSAIDs (especially ibuprofen) may inhibit the cardioprotective antiplatelet effect of aspirin.[46]

   b. Pericardiocentesis may be necessary to drain a large symptomatic pericardial effusion.

   c. Pericardiectomy is recommended for recurrent large effusions.

I. **Constrictive pericarditis** is a late complication of cardiac surgery that is extremely uncommon despite the development of dense adhesions that form within the mediastinum following surgery. It has been noted in patients with undrained early postoperative hemopericardium, use of warfarin, early PPS, and previous mediastinal radiation.[47] Similar pathophysiology will be encountered in patients who develop constrictive epicarditis without thickening of the pericardium.[48]

1. **Presentation.** The patient will note the insidious onset of dyspnea on exertion, chest pain, and fatigue. Peripheral edema and jugular venous distention are common, but pulsus paradoxus is infrequent.

2. **Evaluation**

   a. The chest x-ray is frequently normal in the absence of a pericardial effusion.

   b. Two-dimensional echocardiography will demonstrate signs of constriction, such as septal bounce and diminished respiratory variation in the inferior vena cava.

   c. A CT scan usually documents a thickened pericardium and occasionally a small pericardial effusion. However, in cases of constrictive epicarditis, pericardial thickening may not be seen.

   d. Right-heart catheterization provides the most definitive information. It will document the equilibration of diastolic pressures and demonstrate a diastolic dip-and-plateau pattern ("square-root" sign) in the right ventricular pressure tracing (pages 63–64). On occasion, significant fluid overload will produce hemodynamics consistent with constriction, when in fact there is no pathoanatomic evidence of a thickened pericardium or epicarditis other than standard postoperative scarring.

3. **Treatment.** If there is no clinical response to diuretics and steroids, a pericardiectomy is indicated to decorticate the heart. This is best performed through a sternotomy incision, which allows for adequate decortication of the right atrium and

ventricle and much of the left ventricle. It also allows for the institution of cardiopulmonary bypass in the event of a difficult or bloody operation. Relief of epicardial constriction is difficult and may result in surgical damage to bypass grafts or significant bleeding. A "waffle" or "turtle shell" procedure is performed with crisscrossing incisions made in the epicardial scar to relieve the constriction.

VI. Renal, Metabolic, and Fluid Management and Complications

A. Routine care

1. Most patients are still substantially above their preoperative weight when transferred to the postoperative floor. Comparison of the patient's preoperative weight with daily weights obtained postoperatively is a guide to the use of diuretics to eliminate excess fluid. Achievement of dry body weight may require more aggressive diuresis if CHF was present before surgery. In the chronically ill patient, preoperative weight may be achieved despite fluid overload due to poor nutrition.

2. Dietary restriction (sodium and water) need not be overly strict in most cases. With the availability of potent diuretics to achieve negative fluid balance and the common problem of a poor appetite after surgery, it is more important to provide palatable food without restriction to improve the patient's caloric intake.

3. If a patient required diuretics before surgery (especially valve patients and those with poor myocardial function), it is advisable to continue them upon discharge from the hospital even if preoperative weight has been attained.

B. Transient renal failure (see also Chapter 12). Patients with preoperative renal insufficiency, severe hypertension, postoperative low cardiac output syndromes, or those requiring substantial doses of vasopressors may develop postoperative acute kidney injury (AKI). Although diuretics are useful in reducing the immediate postoperative fluid overload, they do not influence the course of AKI and can in fact exacerbate renal dysfunction by causing prerenal azotemia from intravascular volume depletion. Management can be very difficult on the postoperative floor when methods of monitoring intravascular volume are limited.

1. A common scenario is gradual elevation in the BUN and creatinine with low serum sodium, reflective of persistent total body water and salt overload. Medications must be adjusted to allow the normally hypertensive patient's blood pressure to rise to higher levels than normal. ACE inhibitors should be withheld, NSAIDs avoided, and diuretics must be used gently, if at all, to maintain adequate intravascular volume. If the patient was aggressively diuresed and has a poor appetite, additional hydration may be necessary. In most patients, the renal dysfunction is transient as long as the cardiac output remains satisfactory.

2. If fluid retention persists, contributing to respiratory compromise, and the BUN continues to rise, further evaluation and treatment are indicated. On occasion, medications (such as Bactrim) or an obstructive uropathy may be the cause of an unexplained rise in creatinine. If the patient is profoundly oliguric, return to the ICU for intravenous inotropic support, ultrafiltration, or dialysis may be indicated. **A rising BUN and creatinine of unclear etiology, especially when associated with new-onset oliguria, should always raise the suspicion of delayed tamponade.** An echocardiogram should be performed to assess myocardial function and look for possible cardiac tamponade.

C. **Hyperkalemia** usually occurs in association with renal dysfunction. Its manifestations and treatment are discussed on pages 615–617. Particular attention should be directed to stopping any exogenous potassium intake and ACE inhibitors, and reevaluating renal function.

D. **Hyperglycemia** in diabetics is a common postoperative problem. The blood glucose level may be elevated due to insulin resistance and residual elevation of the counter-regulatory hormones (glucagon, cortisol) after surgery.[49] Stringent control of blood glucose during the early postoperative period with an IV insulin protocol has been shown to reduce not only the incidence of wound infection, but also other morbidities and operative mortality (Appendix 6).[50–52] Once the patient is transferred to the floor, frequent fingersticks should be obtained (usually before meals and at bedtime) to assess the adequacy of blood glucose control.

1. Insulin resistance is commonly noted during the early postoperative period. Patients with type I diabetes should have their insulin doses gradually increased back to preoperative levels depending on oral intake and blood glucose levels. It is preferable to use a lower dose of intermediate-acting insulin initially and supplement it with regular insulin as necessary (see Table 12.9, page 626, for commonly used insulin preparations).

2. Oral hypoglycemics can be restarted once the patient has an adequate oral intake, usually starting at half the preoperative dose, and increasing the dose depending on oral intake and blood glucose.

E. Other electrolyte and endocrine complications are fairly unusual once the patient has been transferred to the postoperative floor. Chapter 12 discusses the evaluation and management of some of these problems.

VII. Hematologic Complications and Anticoagulation Regimens

A. **Anemia**

1. Despite the obligatory hemodilution associated with cardiopulmonary bypass (CPB), use of effective blood conservation strategies has reduced the requirements for perioperative blood transfusions. Furthermore, off-pump surgery is associated with a reduced transfusion requirement. Generally, the hematocrit should be maintained around 20% during CPB and then at least 22–24% postoperatively. However, transfusion to a higher hematocrit should be considered for elderly patients, those who feel significantly weak and fatigued, and those with ECG changes, hypotension, or significant tachycardia.

2. Although the hematocrit may rise gradually with postoperative diuresis, it frequently will not increase as the fluid is mobilized into the bloodstream from the extracellular tissues. Furthermore, the hematocrit may be influenced by the shortened red cell life span caused by extracorporeal circulation and the loss of 30% of transfused red cells within 24 hours of transfusion.

3. Any patient with a hematocrit below 30% should be placed on iron therapy (ferrous sulfate or gluconate 300 mg tid for 1 month) at the time of discharge. Exogenous iron may not be necessary if the patient has received multiple transfusions because of the storage of iron from hemolyzed cells.

    4. Consideration may also be given to use of recombinant erythropoietin (Epogen or Procrit) to stimulate red cell production (50–100 units/kg SC three times a week).

B. Thrombocytopenia is caused by platelet destruction and hemodilution during extracorporeal circulation, but platelet counts gradually return to normal within several days. Impaired hemostasis noted in the early postoperative period is caused more commonly by platelet dysfunction induced by CPB or use of antiplatelet medications, although it is attenuated somewhat by the use of the antifibrinolytic drugs. Documentation of a falling platelet count after the initial postoperative recovery of the platelet count raises the specter of heparin-induced thrombocytopenia (HIT).

    1. Etiology

        a. Platelet activation or dilution during CPB

        b. Excessive bleeding without platelet replacement therapy

        c. Use of an IABP

        d. Medications that may reduce the platelet count, such as heparin or inamrinone

        e. Sepsis

        f. Heparin-induced thrombocytopenia. **Note:** Platelet counts must be monitored on a daily basis in any patient receiving heparin. A falling platelet count or heparin resistance may be an indication for *in vitro* aggregation testing to identify HIT.

        g. Thrombotic thrombocytopenic purpura (TTP), which is usually associated with fever, altered mental status, renal insufficiency, thromboembolic events, and a microangiopathic hemolytic anemia with schistocytes on blood smear.[53]

    2. Treatment. Platelet transfusions are indicated:

        a. When platelet count is <20,000–30,000/μL (<20–30 × 10^9/L).

        b. For ongoing bleeding when the platelet count is <100,000/μL. Platelet administration may be considered when the platelet count is higher if platelet dysfunction is suspected.

        c. For a planned surgical procedure (such as percutaneous IABP removal) when the platelet count is <60,000/μL (<60 × 10^9/L).

C. **Heparin-induced thrombocytopenia** (HIT) is a very serious problem that may result in widespread arterial and venous thrombosis, and carries a mortality rate of about 20%. Because of its high risk and the necessity for treatment with direct thrombin inhibitors, early suspicion, identification, and management are essential.[53–55]

    1. HIT is an immune-mediated phenomenon caused by the formation of IgG antibodies that bind to the heparin–platelet factor 4 (PF4) complex, producing platelet activation. This results in release of procoagulant microparticles that lead to thrombin generation. This binding causes release of more PF4, promoting more platelet activation. Antibody binding to glycosaminoglycans on the surface of endothelial cells leads to endothelial cell damage and tissue factor expression. This procoagulant milieu promotes arterial and venous thrombosis in about 30% of patients, causing stroke, myocardial infarction, mesenteric thrombosis, and deep venous thrombosis.

2. The diagnosis of HIT requires the presence of heparin antibodies and thrombocytopenia. The suspicion of HIT is based on the degree of thrombocytopenia, the timing of its occurrence, and its relationship to thrombotic events.

   a. Thrombocytopenia is extremely common postoperatively and may be related to hemodilution, platelet damage on pump, clearance of transfused platelets, and sepsis. However, the platelet count generally begins to rebound by the 3rd–4th day after surgery. A subsequent fall in platelet count >50% is more consistent with HIT.

   b. HIT is more common with use of bovine heparin and is 8–10 times more likely to occur with UFH than LMWH.

   c. Although immediate-onset HIT (occurring within hours of giving heparin) may develop in patients who received heparin within 100 days due to residual circulating HIT antibodies, it is rare for a patient receiving short-term preoperative heparin to develop HIT within the first 4 days after surgery. The general pattern is for HIT to occur 5–14 days after surgery.

   d. Delayed-onset HIT (occurring after heparin has been discontinued due to residual heparin-PF4 platelet-activating antibodies) is often manifested by venous thromboembolism, and is commonly not diagnosed because platelet counts are rarely checked after heparin is stopped. If there is evidence of a thrombotic event, a low platelet count should raise suspicion of this entity.

   e. It is estimated that 30% to as high as 75% of patients who develop HIT will develop evidence of thrombosis, indicating the necessity for additional treatment beyond stopping heparin.[56,57] Disturbingly, it is estimated that 25% of patients may develop thrombosis before developing thrombocytopenia.[54] This is a very difficult management problem because of the tendency to administer heparin for a thrombotic event when it might be contraindicated. More commonly, however, patients will develop thrombosis as the platelet count is falling and reaching its nadir, but, as noted, it may occur even after the heparin has been stopped (delayed-onset HIT). Thus there are clinical scenarios when HIT may be present but the suspicion is low, leading to complications from delayed recognition and management.

3. **Diagnostic testing.** ELISA serologic testing for heparin-PF4 antibodies is positive in up to 19% of preoperative and 35–65% of postoperative cardiac surgical patients, yet only 2% of patients develop HIT. It is estimated that only 30–60% of patients with anti-PF4 antibodies by ELISA have heparin-dependent platelet-activating antibodies, indicating the nonspecificity of ELISA testing for HIT-causing antibodies.[56–58] More specific functional assays of washed platelet activation (serotonin release assay and to a lesser degree heparin-induced platelet aggregation studies) are able to more accurately identify antibodies that trigger platelet activation. The importance of identifying HIT-causing antibodies to avoid unnecessary treatment is borne out by multiple studies which have shown a high prevalence of non-HIT antibodies after catheterization or surgery with a very low incidence of thrombocytopenia or clinical thrombosis. Thus, preoperative testing for heparin antibodies is not recommended in the absence of thrombocytopenia or thrombosis.[54]

4. **Management**

   a. If HIT is identified preoperatively with positive testing and thrombocytopenia, an alternative method of anticoagulation must be used during surgery (see Chapter 4, pages 201–204). Antibodies generally clear within 3 months of the last heparin administration and heparinization can be performed safely if the HIT testing is negative.

b. With any suspicion of postoperative HIT, even before testing results become available, all heparin administration must be stopped. This includes cessation of heparin flushes and removal of heparin-coated pulmonary artery catheters. However, if the likelihood of HIT is low based upon clinical grounds, yet an anticoagulant is indicated for prophylaxis (such as for VTE), fondaparinux 2.5 mg qd SC can be given safely. As of late 2010, there had been only limited preliminary experience with use of fondaparinux to treat HIT-associated hypercoagulability.[59]

c. Platelets should not be administered because they may promote thrombosis.

d. Warfarin should ***not*** be started immediately, because tissue necrosis from microvascular thrombosis may occur due to depletion of the Vitamin K-dependent natural anticoagulant protein C. This has been noted in patients who rapidly develop a supratherapeutic INR. Warfarin may be started safely after the platelet count reaches 150×10^9/L and should overlap the non-heparin anticoagulant for 5 days, even when the INR is in therapeutic range.

e. Alternative anticoagulation is indicated to minimize the risk of thrombotic events and also to provide protection for the process for which the heparin was originally indicated. This is essential because the risk of symptomatic thrombosis remains greater than 25% if only the heparin is stopped.

   i. **Lepirudin** is a direct thrombin inhibitor that may be selected first, although it must be used cautiously in patients with renal dysfunction. It is given as a 0.2–0.4 mg/kg load, followed by a continuous infusion of 0.1 mg/kg/h. It is monitored by the PTT, aiming for 1.5–2.5 times baseline.

   ii. **Argatroban** is a synthetic direct thrombin inhibitor that is preferred in patients with renal dysfunction because it undergoes hepatic metabolism. It is given starting at a dose of 2 µg/kg/min once heparin effect has been eliminated (usually 4 hours for UFH and 12 hours after the last dose of LMWH), and maintained at a rate of 0.5–1.2 µg/kg/min. It is monitored by the PTT, aiming for 1.5–3 times baseline. Conversion from argatroban to warfarin can be somewhat problematic because both affect the INR. Generally, warfarin should be given in doses of 2.5–5 mg for 5 days of overlapping treatment. Once the platelet count exceeds 150×10^9/L and the INR is >4, the argatroban should be stopped. The INR should be rechecked in 4–6 hours. If the INR drops below 2.0, the argatroban should be restarted.

   iii. **Bivalirudin** is a direct thrombin inhibitor that produces reversible binding to thrombin and has a short half-life of only 25 minutes. It can be used off-label for the management of HIT with an initial infusion rate of 0.15–0.2 mg/kg/h with a target PTT of 1.5–2.5 times baseline. Advantages include 80% enzymatic metabolism (although some modification is indicated in patients with renal dysfunction), nonimmunogenicity, and no effect on the INR.

   iv. **Danaparoid** is a heparinoid that has a low degree of reactivity with heparin antibodies. It is given in a bolus dose of 2250 anti-Xa U, followed by 400 U/h × 4 h, then 300 U/h × 4 h, then a maintenance infusion of 200 U/h. It is monitored by anti-Xa levels, trying to achieve a level of 0.5–0.8 U/mL. It is not available in the United States.

D. **Coronary bypass surgery.** Postoperative aspirin should be utilized to increase saphenous vein graft patency, although there is no documented benefit in improving the patency of arterial conduits. It should be started within 24 hours of surgery, but ideally should being given down the nasogastric tube starting 6 hours postoperatively if the patient is not bleeding because of concerns that platelet reactivity may be enhanced immediately after surgery.[18]

1. The 2008 ACCP guidelines recommend use of aspirin 75–100 mg postoperatively.[60] The 2005 Society of Thoracic Surgeons (STS) and 2008 European guidelines suggest using a daily dose of 325 mg/day, although greater efficacy with the higher dose has not been proven.[20,61] Graft patency is not improved by use of preoperative aspirin or postoperative use of aspirin for longer than 1 year. However, due to the benefits of aspirin in the primary and secondary prevention of coronary artery disease, indefinite use of aspirin is recommended for all patients undergoing CABG independent of the types of grafts utilized.[60]

2. Clopidogrel 75 mg/day may be substituted for aspirin if the patient is allergic to aspirin and may be beneficial when used with aspirin in patients undergoing CABG following non-ST-elevation infarction (NSTEMI).[20,60] In other patients, it is not clear if there is any benefit to adding clopidogrel to aspirin. One study showed no benefit of adding aspirin to using clopidogrel alone,[62] but another showed that addition of clopidogrel to aspirin did reduce mortality after both on- and off-pump surgery, although there was no difference in the occurrence of ischemic or thrombotic events.[63] Platelet inhibition is more effectively achieved postoperatively with aspirin than with clopidogrel given without a loading dose.[64] Therefore, if the patient cannot take aspirin, a 300 mg load of clopidogrel is recommended. Potential benefits of warfarin in patients undergoing extensive coronary endarterectomy have not been defined, but if used, aspirin should also be given in low doses to achieve an antiplatelet effect.

E. **Prosthetic heart valves.** Heart valves are more susceptible to thromboembolic complications during the first 3 months after implantation, during which time a vitamin K antagonist (VKA) such as warfarin is recommended. Furthermore, some patients are considered at "higher risk" for thromboembolism, and more aggressive anticoagulation with VKAs is indicated. These include patients with atrial fibrillation, hypercoagulable states, previous systemic embolism, left atrial enlargement, and left ventricular dysfunction. The following recommendations (summarized in Table 13.3) are from the ACCP evidence-based clinical practice guidelines (8th edition) and the American College of Cardiology/American Heart Association (ACC/AHA) guidelines published in 2008.[65,66] Updates of the ACC/AHA guidelines may be found at www.cardiosource.com.

1. **Tissue valves**

a. **Aortic valves.** Aspirin 75–100 mg (usually 81 mg) is recommended indefinitely if the patient is in sinus rhythm and has none of the risk factors noted above. If risk factors are present, warfarin is recommended to achieve a target INR of 2.5 (2.0–3.0) and should be given along with aspirin 75–100 mg daily.

Table 13.3 • Recommended Anticoagulation Regimens for Prosthetic Heart Valves

	Warfarin	Antiplatelet Drugs
AVR – tissue	INR 2.0–3.0 for 3 months if risk factors (ACC/AHA)	Aspirin 75–100 mg alone if no risk factors
AVR – mechanical	INR 2.0–3.0 indefinitely	Aspirin 75–100 mg
Mitral valve repair	INR 2.0–3.0 for 3 months (use either warfarin or aspirin)	Aspirin 75–100 mg (use either warfarin or aspirin)
MVR – tissue	INR 2.0–3.0 for 3 months (ACCP) Continue indefinitely if risk factors	Aspirin 75–100 mg with warfarin if risk factors Aspirin 75–100 mg alone if no risk factors (ACC/AHA) Aspirin 75–100 mg after warfarin is stopped
MVR – mechanical	INR 2.5–3.5 indefinitely	Aspirin 75–100 mg
AVR-MVR – tissue	INR 2.0–3.0 for 3 months	Aspirin 325 mg after 3 months
AVR-MVR – mechanical	INR 3.0–4.5 indefinitely	Aspirin 75–100 mg
Atrial fibrillation with any of above	Continue warfarin indefinitely	

Risk factors: hypercoagulable state, history of systemic thromboembolism, ejection fraction <35%, history of anteroapical infarction, atrial fibrillation.

ACCP, American College of Chest Physicians recommendations 2008;[65] ACC/AHA, American College of Cardiology/American Heart Association recommendations 2008.[66]

b. **Mitral valves.** Warfarin should be started by the first postoperative day and given for 3 months to achieve a target INR of 2.5 (range 2.0–3.0). The initiation of heparin can be considered in the hospital (see below). The patient can then be discharged on LMWH until the INR reaches the therapeutic range. After 3 months, warfarin is stopped and aspirin 75–100 mg (usually 81 mg) is given if the patient is in sinus rhythm. However, warfarin should be continued indefinitely in patients at high risk and aspirin should be added to the regimen. In contrast to the ACCP recommendations, the 2008 ACC/AHA guidelines recommend use of aspirin alone following bioprosthetic MVR if there are no risk factors (class I recommendation), and the addition of aspirin to warfarin if there are risk factors.[66]

c. **Mitral rings.** Use of warfarin for 3 months following mitral valve repairs is recommended by the European Society of Cardiology (there is no ACCP recommendation for these patients). This conclusion is based primarily on evidence that about 30% of patients discharged in sinus rhythm will experience atrial fibrillation shortly thereafter, not based upon thromboembolic risk from the prosthetic rings.[66] However, small studies suggest that aspirin alone may be sufficient.[67,68]

2. **Mechanical valves**

    a. Aortic valves. Current-generation tilting-disc (Medtronic-Hall) or bileaflet valves (St. Jude) should receive warfarin indefinitely starting by the day after surgery to achieve a target INR of 2.5 (range 2.0–3.0). In patients at "high risk" for thromboembolism, those with Starr-Edwards or Bjork-Shiley valves, and probably those with double mechanical valves, the target INR should be 3.0 (range 2.5–3.5). The ACC/AHA guidelines give a class IIa recommendation to have a target INR of 3.0 for the first 3 months after surgery (but a class I recommendation for an INR of 2.5 if no risk factors are present). Aspirin 75–100 mg/day is also recommended for all mechanical valves (ACC/AHA recommendation).[66]

    b. Mitral valves. Patients should receive warfarin indefinitely starting by the day after surgery to achieve a target INR of 3.0 (range 2.5–3.5). The ACC/AHA recommends the addition of aspirin; the ACCP recommends addition of aspirin for patients at high risk for thromboembolism and in those with peripheral vascular disease.

3. In patients receiving mechanical valves or those with tissue mitral valves in atrial fibrillation, there is a potential increased risk of thromboembolism when the patient is not therapeutically anticoagulated. Therefore, use of heparin is recommended until the INR becomes therapeutic. However, the timing of initiation of heparin as a bridge is not well defined and must be individualized. Early initiation may increase the risk of bleeding, so a safe approach is to initiate UFH or LMWH on the 4th–5th postoperative day if the INR is less than 1.8.[25,69] Although the 2008 ACCP guidelines do not comment on the timing of initiation of heparin, they do recommend that IV UFH or SC LMWH be given until the INR is >2.0 for two consecutive days.[65] Several studies have documented the safety and efficacy of LMWH as a bridge, and a patient can usually be discharged home at any level of INR on LMWH.[70,71]

4. **Dosing and overanticoagulation.**[72] Warfarin is a dangerous drug that requires thoughtful administration and careful monitoring to avoid overanticoagulation. It results in the more rapid depletion of factors VII, IX, and X than factor II (prothrombin), which has a longer half-life. Thus, it exhibits an antihemostatic effect before it achieves an antithrombotic effect, which is attributable primarily to a reduction in factor II. Following cardiac surgery, it is essential that warfarin not be loaded and that doses be carefully individualized to avoid rapid overanticoagulation. An initial dose of 5 mg is given to most patients. However, 2.5 mg should be given to small elderly women, patients with hepatic dysfunction, chronic illness, and those receiving antibiotics or amiodarone (Table 13.4). The INR generally begins to rise in 2–3 days, but often takes 5–7 days to achieve a stable dosing level. Potential dangers of overanticoagulation include cardiac tamponade from intrapericardial bleeding, and gastrointestinal, intracranial, or retroperitoneal hemorrhage. Although there are antithrombotic benefits to the combined use of warfarin and aspirin, this combination increases the short-term risk of delayed tamponade as well as the long-term risk of bleeding.[73,74]

Table 13.4 • Protocol for Initiation of Warfarin Doses

Assess whether patient is at greater risk for sensitivity to warfarin – if so, use low-dose protocol

a. Small, elderly females
b. Over age 75
c. Renal (creatinine > 1.5 mg/dL) or hepatic dysfunction
d. Interacting medications (amiodarone, antibiotics)

Day	INR	Standard	Low-Dose
1	WNL	5 mg	2.5 mg
2	<1.5	5 mg	2.5 mg
	1.5–1.9	2.5 mg	1.25 mg
	≥2	HOLD*	HOLD*
3	<1.5	7.5 mg	5 mg
	1.5–1.9	5 mg	2.5 mg
	2–3	2.5 mg	HOLD*
	>3	HOLD*	HOLD*
4	<1.5	10 mg	7.5 mg
	1.5–1.9	7.5 mg	5 mg
	2–3	5 mg	HOLD*
	>3	HOLD*	HOLD*
5	<1.5	10 mg	10 mg
	1.5–1.9	10 mg	5 mg
	2–3	5 mg	HOLD*
	>3	HOLD*	HOLD*
6	<1.5	12.5 mg	10 mg
	1.5–1.9	10 mg	7.5 mg
	2–3	5 mg	2.5 mg
	>3	HOLD*	HOLD*

*Restart warfarin when INR is less than 3

A protocol for the management of overanticoagulation with warfarin is noted in Figure 13.2.

a. If the patient has significant bleeding with a significantly elevated INR, warfarin should be held, and fresh frozen plasma (up to 15 mL/kg) should be given. Vitamin K 10 mg IV in 50 mL NS over 30 minutes should be given and may be repeated every 12 hours for persistent INR elevation. In addition,

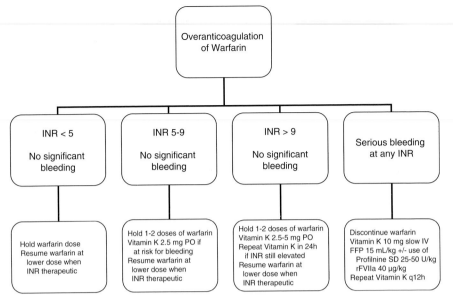

Figure 13.2 • Algorithm for overanticoagulation management.

use of prothrombin complex concentrate (PCC or Profilnine) 25−50 units/kg or recombinant factor VIIa 40 µg/kg may be considered.

b. If the patient has no evidence of bleeding, general recommendations for management of elevated INRs are as follows, although rapid elevation of the INR in the early postoperative period may warrant more aggressive therapy.

    i. INR ≥ 9: hold warfarin, give vitamin K 2.5−5 mg orally (INR should fall within 24−48 hours)

    ii. INR ≥ 5 and <9: hold warfarin for 1−2 days and restart when INR is <4; alternatively omit one dose of warfarin and give 1−2.5 mg of vitamin K orally

    iii. INR above therapeutic range but ≤5: lower or omit one dose until at therapeutic range

c. Vitamin K given in small oral doses can reduce the INR to a therapeutic level within a few days and is usually the best approach when withholding of warfarin does not reduce the INR. Use of large doses of IV vitamin K will produce more rapid reversal of the INR, but is associated with a small risk of anaphylaxis. It may also lead to warfarin resistance and generally should be avoided. If the INR becomes subtherapeutic (which is usually safer than a markedly elevated INR), heparin can be always be given until the INR rises back to the therapeutic range. In patients on long-term warfarin with variable INR responses, concomitant administration of vitamin K 100−200 µg/day orally helps stabilize the INR.[75,76]

VIII. Wound Care and Infectious Complications

A. General Comments

1. Prophylactic antibiotics are indicated to minimize the risk of postoperative mediastinitis. A cephalosporin is usually chosen (cefazolin or cefuroxime), although vancomycin is substituted if there is a penicillin allergy and is commonly selected for patients undergoing valve or graft placement because of its effectiveness against Gram-positive organisms. Some studies suggest it might be preferable in CABG patients as well.[77] The STS guidelines recommend that additional Gram-negative coverage be given when vancomycin is used, although this is not a common practice. Antibiotics are started within 1 hour (cephalosporins) or 2 hours (vancomycin) of surgery and continued for 24–48 hours. They should not be continued any longer even if invasive lines and catheters remain in place.[78,79]

2. Wounds closed with subcuticular sutures and covered with 2-octylcyanoacrylate adhesive (Dermabond) at the conclusion of surgery do not require dressing coverage. Otherwise, the wound should be cleansed and covered with a dressing every day for the first 3 postoperative days. Subsequent coverage is not necessary unless drainage is noted. All drainage should be cultured and sterile occlusive dressings applied.

B. Nosocomial infections develop in 5–10% of patients undergoing cardiac surgery using CPB. Most infections involve the respiratory tract, central line-associated bacteremias, the surgical site, and the urinary tract. Infections are less common in patients undergoing OPCAB, presumably because of a lower risk of blood transfusions and the absence of the immunomodulatory effects of extracorporeal circulation.[80] A nosocomial infection not only increases the length of stay, but significantly increases operative mortality (to about 20%) because of the frequent development of multisystem organ failure.[81–85] *Staphylococcus* is the most common organism noted in bacteremias and wound infections, whereas Gram-negative infections are more common in the respiratory tract. The high mortality rates of mediastinitis (about 20–25%) and septicemia (30–50%) do not differ much between patients with methicillin-resistant *Staphylococcus aureus* (MRSA) and other organisms.[86]

1. **Risk factors** have been identified in multiple studies, most of which are included in the STS risk model for major infection shown in Figure 13.3.[85]

   a. Comorbidities: older age, females, diabetes, obesity

   b. Nasal carriage of *Staphylococcus aureus*, which is associated with a significant incidence of postoperative MRSA infections (about 20%) with a mortality risk of 15–30%.[86–88]

   c. Operative factors: long complex operations, urgent/emergent surgery, reoperations; use of an IABP

   d. Postoperative factors (with specific relationships in parentheses)
   - Hyperglycemia (wound infections)
   - Prolonged duration of intubation or need for reintubation (pneumonia)
   - Prolonged duration of indwelling Foley catheter (UTI)
   - Prolonged duration of central venous catheter placement (bacteremia)
   - Multiple blood transfusions (usually over 4–5 units) (pneumonia)

Risk Factors	Preop	Combined
Age (for each 5 years > 5)	1	1
BMI 30–40 kg/m²	4	3
BMI 40⁺ kg/m²	9	8
Diabetes	3	3
Renal failure	4	4
CHF	3	3
PVD	2	2
Female	2	2
COPD	2	3
Cardiogenic shock	6	N/A
MI	2	N/A
Concomitant surgery	4	N/A
Perfusion time 100-200 min	N/A	3
Perfusion time 200-300 min	N/A	7
IABP	N/A	5

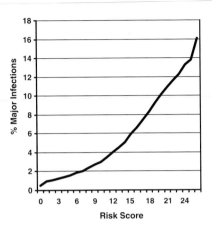

Figure 13.3 • Society of Thoracic Surgeons (STS) risk model for major infections after cardiac surgery (Adapted with permission from Fowler et al., *Circulation* 2005;112(9 Suppl):I-358–65.)[85]

- Reoperation for bleeding
- Empiric use of broad-spectrum antibiotics
- Low cardiac output syndromes
- Postoperative stroke
- Early development of postoperative renal failure

2. **Preventive measures** that may reduce the incidence of nosocomial infections include:

   a. Perioperative use of intranasal mupirocin to reduce staphylococcal nasal carriage. Although selective use limited to carriers is most appropriate and can be accomplished using polymerase chain reaction assessment, this is not always logistically possible, so it is easier to treat all patients as soon as possible before surgery and for 3–5 days postoperatively.[87–91]

   b. Chlorhexidine gluconate 0.12% (Peridex) oral rinse has been shown to reduce the rate of nosocomial respiratory infections, wound infections, and mortality.[92,93]

   c. Aggressive use of a hyperglycemia protocol to maintain early postoperative blood glucose <180 mg/dL.[49,52]

   d. Early removal of invasive catheters, especially central lines.

   e. Strict adherence to guidelines to avoid prolonged usage of prophylactic antibiotics. One study showed that early postoperative pneumonia was usually caused by organisms that colonized the respiratory tract prior to surgery. However, prolonged use of antibiotics was ineffective in reducing the incidence of pneumonia.[94]

f. Aggressive ventilatory weaning protocols to reduce the duration of mechanical ventilation and other steps to avoid ventilator-associated pneumonia (see page 417). Selective decontamination of the gut has arguably been effective in reducing this problem.

g. Raising the threshold for blood transfusions (transfuse only if hematocrit <25% unless clinically indicated).[95]

3. The **treatment** of a nosocomial infection requires appropriate antibiotic selection for the organism involved and recognition of the appropriate time course of treatment. Prolonged treatment is often unnecessary and may lead to the development of resistant strains or fungal infections, and not infrequently to hepatic or renal dysfunction. When a Gram-positive bacteremia occurs in a patient with a prosthetic heart valve, a 6-week course of treatment for presumed endocarditis may be indicated. In complex situations, infectious disease consultation is essential.

C. Sepsis

1. Clinical features. Sepsis resulting in hemodynamic compromise and multisystem organ failure is an uncommon, yet highly lethal, complication of cardiac surgery, with an estimated mortality rate of greater than 30%. It is usually noted in critically ill patients who remain in the ICU with multiple invasive monitoring lines, develop respiratory complications, and often have some element of renal dysfunction. It may be the first manifestation of an occult sternal wound infection.

2. Management. Aggressive ICU-directed, goal-oriented therapy may be able to reduce the high mortality associated with sepsis.[96–99] Important features of this approach include:

a. Optimization of hemodynamics with early aggressive fluid resuscitation, inotropic support, and selective use of vasoconstrictors (initially α-agents, and then vasopressin if necessary). This should be assessed by adequate hemodynamic monitoring (PA catheter and central or mixed venous oxygen saturations), aiming for an oxygen saturation >70%.

b. Initiation of broad-spectrum antibiotic coverage after panculturing with prompt modification to cover the specific organism isolated.

c. Low tidal volume ventilation if ARDS develops; minimizing sedation to promote early extubation.

d. Early aggressive use of renal replacement therapies (CVVH).

e. Tight control of blood glucose (<150 mg/dL).

f. Adequate nutrition, preferably by the enteral route.

g. VTE prophylaxis (pneumatic compression devices, possibly SC heparin).

h. Stress ulcer prophylaxis (sucralfate, proton pump inhibitors).

i. Low-dose stress steroids may be considered in patients with documented inadequate response to an ACTH challenge.

j. Recombinant activated protein C (drotrecogin alfa [Xigris]) has reduced mortality in patients with severe sepsis associated with organ system dysfunction by modulating the inflammatory and fibrinolytic responses to sepsis. It should only be considered in severely ill patients after consultation with an infectious disease expert.

D. Sternal wound infections (SWI) complicate about 1% of cardiac surgical procedures performed via a median sternotomy and are associated with significant hospital mortality (around 20%). Coagulase-negative staphylococcus and *S. aureus* are the most common pathogens encountered despite the use of prophylactic antibiotics specifically directed at these organisms. Sternal infections are a major source of physical, emotional, and economic stress, although advances in plastic surgical coverage techniques have improved results dramatically.

1. **Risk factors.** Numerous models have been devised to predict the risk of developing mediastinitis, including those from the Society of Thoracic Surgeons (available as part of the risk calculator at www.sts.org) and the Northern New England Cardiovascular Disease Study Group (page 160).[85,100,101] Among the risk factors identified in these and other studies are the following:[102–106]

   a. Comorbidities: obesity, diabetes, COPD, renal dysfunction, peripheral vascular disease (PVD), older age, impaired nutritional status (low serum albumin)

   b. Surgical considerations
      - Emergency surgery
      - Reoperations
      - Bilateral ITA usage in diabetics (controversial)[101,106–108]
      - Prolonged duration of CPB or surgery
      - Use of bone wax[109,110]

   c. Postoperative complications
      - Excessive mediastinal bleeding, reexploration for bleeding, multiple transfusions
      - Prolonged ventilatory support (usually in patients with COPD who are actively colonized)
      - Low cardiac output states
      - Refractory hyperglycemia in the ICU, independent of whether the patient has a history of diabetes[50,51,111]
      - Renal failure

2. **Prevention.** Several measures can be taken to reduce the risk of SWI.

   a. Preoperative measures
      - Identify and treat preexisting infections
      - Hibiclens wash several times the night before and the morning of surgery to reduce the bacterial skin count; positive cultures from the subcutaneous tissue have been obtained in 31% and 89% of patients prior to closure in two studies![112,113]
      - Intranasal mupirocin to reduce nasal carriage of staphylococcal organisms[90]
      - Hair clipping just prior to surgery
      - Appropriate timing and dosage of prophylactic antibiotics (within 1 hour of surgery for cephalosporins, 2 hours for vancomycin)[78]

   b. Intraoperative measures
      - Careful skin prep with chlorhexidine-alcohol rather than povidone-iodine and consideration of use of a microbial sealant that immobilizes bacteria (InteguSeal, Kimberly-Clark).[114]

- Ensure a midline sternotomy and provide a secure sternal closure.
- Be selective in use of bilateral ITAs in diabetic patients. Skeletoning the ITA may be helpful, but avoidance of bilateral usage in patients with other risk factors, such as severe obesity and COPD, is prudent.[115]
- Use meticulous surgical technique with respect for tissues and obtain adequate hemostasis to minimize mediastinal bleeding.
- Avoid bone wax.
- Use subcuticular sutures rather than skin staples and seal wound with a topical adhesive (Dermabond).
- Apply platelet gel to the sternal edges.[116]
- Consider use of a topical antibiotic to be applied to the sternum in patients at high risk. Vancomycin paste was shown decades ago to reduce the risk of infection, but more recent studies of its efficacy are lacking.[117] Use of "collagen/gentamicin sponges" placed within the sternotomy at the time of closure has been shown to reduce the incidence of infection.[118]

  c. Postoperative measures

- Maintain blood glucose <180−200 mg/dL during surgery and the early postoperative course.
- Raise the transfusion trigger for blood products during and after surgery.

3. Presentation of a mediastinal wound infection can be either overt or occult and often depends on the infectious agent. For example, *S. aureus* infections tend to be virulent and present within the first 10 days of surgery. In contrast, coagulase-negative staphylococcal infections tend to present late in an indolent fashion with an insidious onset.[119]

  a. The classification of sternal wound infections is somewhat controversial. The Centers for Disease Control (CDC) definitions differentiate between superficial incisional, deep incisional, and organ/space surgical site infections. However, the latter two definitions tend to overlap. This is particularly true since it is difficult to rule out sternal or retrosternal infection when the prepectoral fascia or sternal wires are involved in the infectious process.[120] A classification system for mediastinitis was proposed in 1996 to refine its management, but the eventual approach often depends on operative findings.[121]

  b. Minor/superficial infections usually present with local tenderness, erythema, serous drainage, or a localized area of wound breakdown with purulent drainage. The sternum is usually stable.

  c. Major/deep incisional infections (deep subcutaneous, osteomyelitis, mediastinitis) may have any of the above, but usually present with significant purulent drainage, often with an unstable sternum. The patient commonly has fever, chills, lethargy, and chest wall pain. Leukocytosis is invariably present. Sternal instability may be noted when mediastinitis is present, but, in the absence of other clinical evidence, may represent a sterile mechanical dehiscence.

  d. Inexplicable chest wall pain or tenderness, fever, Gram-positive bacteremia, or leukocytosis should raise suspicion of a sternal wound infection. Sternal wound infections account for more than 50% of postoperative Gram-positive bacteremias. Occult infections are particularly common in diabetic patients, who often mount a very poor inflammatory response and may present several weeks after surgery with extensive purulent mediastinitis but few systemic signs.

e. A chronic draining sinus tract or sternocutanous fistula is a common delayed presentation of chronic osteomyelitis, and often originates from the sternal wires.[110]

4. **Evaluation**

a. Assessment of the degree of sternal instability is important in deciding how to proceed. If the sternum is unstable, operative exploration is indicated. If it is stable, further diagnostic tests are warranted in an attempt to identify a deep infection.[120]

b. Culture of purulent drainage may identify the organisms and direct appropriate antibiotic therapy.

c. Wound aspiration may diagnose an infection when purulent drainage is not present.[122]

d. Chest CT scanning may be beneficial if the sternum is stable. It may help identify a deep infection if there is loss of the integrity of retrosternal soft tissue fat planes or an undrained retrosternal abscess with air. Although there are reports that CT scanning is quite sensitive and specific for diagnosing wound infections,[123] one must be cautious in its interpretation because hematoma formation and fibrin along the chest tube tracts are commonly present in the retrosternal area and may be interpreted as "consistent with infection". Clinical correlation and usually a wound aspirate are necessary before exploring a patient.

e. White cell scanning, using indium or technetium labeling, or ^{99m}Tc-labeled monoclonal granulocyte antibody scintigraphy, are among the radionuclide tests that have been helpful in identifying the presence and/or location of infections.[124,125]

f. Occasionally, the infection will have to "declare itself" by spontaneous drainage when diagnostic techniques are inconclusive but the clinical suspicion remains high.

5. **Treatment of minor infections**

a. Minor superficial site infections usually respond to oral antibiotics, opening of the wound, and local wound care. Persistence of a sinus tract or multiple areas of recurrent breakdown suggest a deeper-seated infection, often involving the sternal sutures. This usually requires surgical exploration rather than dressing changes *ad infinitum*. It may respond to simple wire removal and curetting of the involved bone with a 6-week course of antibiotics. The additional use of negative-pressure wound therapy may be helpful in cases of sternocutaneous fistulas.[110]

b. If the sternal wires or the bone are exposed at an early stage, a deeper infection must be ruled out and mediastinal exploration is indicated. This may introduce infection into the mediastinum from the superficial tissues, but may allow for primary reclosure over drains depending on the extent of infection.

6. **Treatment of major infections.** Major infections require mediastinal exploration for debridement of infected tissues, removal of foreign bodies, drainage, and elimination of dead space. Antibiotic therapy is generally recommended for 6 weeks.

  a. The closed method entails primary sternal reclosure with wires and placement of substernal drainage catheters for postoperative antibiotic irrigation (usually 0.5% povidone-iodine) or suction. This may be successful if performed within 2−3 weeks of surgery if there is a sterile dehiscence, minimal purulence, a healthy-appearing sternum, and mediastinal tissues that are pliable enough to eliminate dead space.[126] However, this technique is associated with a significant failure rate if not used in patients who satisfy these criteria. If there is a substantial amount of dead space behind the sternum, but minimal infection and a healthy bone, omental transposition beneath the bone (especially over prosthetic material or exposed grafts), can be considered.[127] Placement of redon catheters below and above the closed sternum which are attached to significant negative suction may be helpful.[128] If the sternum can be closed, but the subcutaneous tissue is infected and unhealthy, a vacuum-assisted closure (VAC) system dressing can expedite healing.

  b. The open method is used for more severe mediastinitis or when sternal osteomyelitis requires extensive debridement and the sternum cannot be reapproximated. This is preferential when there are concerns about the vascularity of the sternum, as in cases of bilateral ITA usage. Immediate coverage of the wound with muscle flaps (pectoralis major or rectus abdominis) may not be possible if extensive infection is present. Omentum can be placed over the heart, but this poses the risk of intra-abdominal contamination during mobilization. If immediate closure cannot be performed, it is imperative to mobilize the heart off the back of the sternum; otherwise, lateral distraction with patient movement or coughing may cause right ventricular rupture, which is usually fatal.[129] In addition, it is advisable to keep the patient intubated and sedated to minimize movement until the wound is covered. It is important to augment the patient's nutritional status to ensure a satisfactory result from flap coverage. Once the wound appears to be improving, muscle flap coverage can then be performed.[130,131]

  c. Vacuum-assisted closure (VAC) is extremely helpful in expediting the healing process, whether used as a bridge to muscle flap coverage, to subsequent sternal rewiring if an adequate amount of sternum remains, or in fact without additional coverage.[132,133] This system consists of a polyurethane ether foam with an evacuation tube that drains into an effluent canister connected to negative suction. The wound is covered with an adhesive drape to create a closed system. The VAC system produces arteriolar dilatation and improves microcirculatory flow, which encourages granulation tissue formation and accelerates wound healing. At the same time, it reduces wound edema and bacterial colonization. Equivalent sternal stabilization can be achieved with negative pressures of −50 to −100 mm Hg as with higher negative pressures.[134] It has also been suggested that by stabilizing the remaining sternal halves, it may help prevent right ventricular rupture, but this complication has been reported.[135] Although it has been recommended that several layers of paraffin or Vaseline gauze should be placed over the heart to prevent this from occurring, this coverage is not rigid and does not prevent displacement of the heart into the space between the sternal edges, which could result in RV injury and rupture.[136]

7. The **prognosis** of patients developing a deep SWI is very poor. The in-hospital mortality rate is around 20%, usually from multisystem organ failure, and the long-term survival of patients who are discharged is also compromised.[102] One of the most significant risk factors for mortality is ventilator-associated pneumonia, so earlier wound coverage or use of a VAC after appropriate mobilization of the heart should allow for earlier weaning from the ventilator.[137]

8. Preservation of the sternum should be the goal in patients who develop a sternal dehiscence in the absence of infection. Frequently, a sternum fragmented by wires which have pulled through the sternal halves can be difficult to reconstruct, requiring sternectomy and muscle flap coverage. Transverse titanium plates with rib-to-rib stabilization have been used successfully in these difficult situations.[138] This system can also be used prophylactically to reinforce standard wire closures in patients with narrow or osteoporotic sternums or very heavy patients who are at risk for dehiscence. It may be feasible to use these systems to stabilize the sternum in patients with infections, but one has to be cautious because of the large amount of hardware that will be placed in the chest.[139]

E. **Leg wound** complications are noted in 10–20% of patients having saphenous vein harvesting via the open technique.[140,141] Patients at higher risk include those with severe PVD and female patients with diabetes and obesity. Most complications are related to poor surgical technique with creation of flaps, failure to eliminate dead space, use of excessive suture material, or hematoma formation. Endoscopic vein harvesting using a single knee incision and "poke holes" to ligate the vein proximally and distally has reduced the incidence of complications to well under 5%. Nonetheless, the potential still exists for hematoma formation within the endoscopic tract and for infection to occur in the small incision near the knee. With the technique of multiple skip incisions, infections can also occur in a similar fashion to open incisions, especially since this technique may be accompanied by significant tissue trauma from retraction of the tissues for visualization.

1. **Presentation**
   a. Cellulitis
   b. Wound breakdown with purulent drainage
   c. Skin necrosis from thin flaps or a large subcutaneous hematoma; formation of eschar
   d. Warm, indurated wound overlying an endoscopic tract, often with accompanying hematoma or skin ecchymosis and significant leg edema

2. **Prevention**
   a. Use careful surgical technique: avoid tissue trauma, minimize flap formation, obtain meticulous hemostasis, and avoid excessive suture material and tissue strangulation, especially in the small knee incision for endoscopic harvesting.
   b. Use antibiotic wound irrigation prior to closure.

    c. Roll a sponge over the endoscopic tract prior to closure to evacuate any blood that may accumulate during heparinization. If there is concern about ongoing bleeding, reinspect the wound after protamine administration to ensure hemostasis and then close the wound. If there remains a concern about bleeding, place a suction drain to evacuate blood and eliminate dead space underneath a flap.

    d. Ace wrap the leg fairly tightly at the conclusion of surgery.

  3. **Treatment** of minor leg infections after endoscopic harvest requires oral antibiotics, removal of exposed foreign suture material, and drainage. Infections in endoscopic tunnels may require opening of the skin, but often can be managed by opening the skin incision and placing a Blake drain for antibiotic irrigation.[142] If a large hematoma or necrotic skin edges are present after open harvesting, early return to the operating room should be considered to evacuate the hematoma and close the leg primarily. Eschar formation from devitalized flaps may require more aggressive debridement.

F. **Radial artery harvesting.** Obtaining adequate hemostasis during open harvesting and before performing a layered closure that leaves the fascia open should prevent hematoma formation. Cellulitis is the most common manifestation of infection and will respond to antibiotics. Rarely, a purulent infection may occur that requires further drainage. Endoscopic harvesting is usually performed with a tourniquet in place, and blood accumulating in the endoscopic tract after the tourniquet is released should be manually evacuated. A drain is usually placed to evacuate blood and eliminate the dead space.

G. **Antibiotic prophylaxis** for dental procedures is mandatory for all patients with prosthetic valves and grafts. The ACC/AHA guidelines for endocarditis prophylaxis changed significantly in 2007 with the withdrawal of the recommendation to use antibiotics except for dental procedures and only in high-risk patients. These recommendations are available online at www.acc.org and are shown in Table 13.5.[143,144]

IX. Neurologic Complications

Neurologic complications following cardiac surgery may involve the central nervous system (CNS) or peripheral nerves. CNS injury has been subdivided into type 1 neurologic events (including focal stroke, encephalopathy, and coma) and type 2 neurocognitive deficits (which include impairment in memory or intellectual function). The risk of developing a type I deficit is more likely with use of CPB, following valvular surgery, and in older patients, who generally have more atherosclerosis. Although off-pump surgery is arguably associated with a reduction in the risk of stroke, the occurrence of neurocognitive dysfunction does not appear to be affected.[145–147]

A. **Central nervous system deficits**

  1. **Risk factors for stroke** have been identified in multiple studies, and risk models have been derived from the STS database and the Northern New England Cardiovascular Disease Study Group.[145,147–154]

    a. Preoperative factors

      • Prior stroke provides evidence of known cerebrovascular disease or risk factors for its development (such as atrial fibrillation). It is likely that CPB can

Table 13.5 • Antibiotic Prophylaxis to Prevent Endocarditis in Adult Patients

Dental Procedures	
Standard regimen	Amoxicillin 2.0 g PO 1 h before procedure
Unable to take PO medications	Ampicillin 2.0 g IV/IM within 30 minutes of procedure **or** Cefazolin or ceftriaxone 1 gm IV/IM
Penicillin-allergic	Cephalexin 2 g **or** Clindamycin 600 mg **or** Azithromycin or clarithromycin 500 mg PO
Penicillin-allergic and unable to take PO	Cefazolin or ceftriaxone 1 g IM/IV **or** Clindamycin 600 mg IM

GI/GU procedures do not require prophylaxis, even in patients at high risk

Dental prophylaxis is recommended for patients at high risk:

1. Prosthetic heart valves
2. Previous infectious endocarditis
3. Cardiac transplant recipients
4. Congenital heart disease: unrepaired, repaired with prosthetic material (within 6 months), or remaining defect near the site of prosthetic repair

Adapted with permission from Wilson et al., *Circulation* 2007;116:1736–54.[143]

exacerbate preexisting cerebral ischemia or cause cerebral edema in areas where prior damage has caused disruption of the blood–brain barrier. One study reported that 44% of patients with a history of stroke developed a focal neurologic deficit after surgery. Of these, 8.5% were new, 27% represented reappearance of the old deficit, and 8.5% were worsening of the old deficit.[155] Notably, about 5% of patients will have abnormal diffusion-weighted imaging (DWI) MRI scans prior to surgery in the absence of known clinical stroke, and these patients may be more likely to develop new neurologic deficits.[156]

- Cerebrovascular disease, whether intracranial or significant extracranial carotid disease
- Increasing age (risk of up to 10% in patients > age 75)
- Female gender
- Comorbidities, including diabetes, smoking, hypertension, PVD, and renal dysfunction

- Low ejection fraction or CHF
- Reoperative surgery
- Urgent/emergency surgery

b. Intraoperative/postoperative findings/events
- Ascending aortic and arch atherosclerosis and calcification
- Long duration of CPB (>2 hours)
- High transfusion requirement
- Left ventricular mural thrombus
- Opening of a cardiac chamber during surgery with possible air embolization
- Perioperative hypotension or cardiac arrest
- Postoperative atrial fibrillation

2. **Mechanisms**[145]

a. Thromboembolic strokes account for about two-thirds of strokes encountered after surgery, most commonly arising from the aorta. Some studies suggest that right hemispheric strokes are more common, while others suggest the left hemisphere is more commonly affected.[147,157] Nevertheless, aortic manipulation and/or arch disease commonly account for the development of stroke, and minimizing aortic manipulation can reduce the risk.[158,159] Transcranial Doppler studies have demonstrated an association between cerebral complications and the number of microemboli detected during surgery.[160] Although overt manifestations of stroke are not that common, radiographic evidence of cerebral embolization is quite common – in some studies, up to 45% of patients will have new abnormalities identified by DWI.[161,162] Embolic sources may be from:
- Atherosclerotic aorta (during cannulation, cross-clamping or unclamping, application of a side-clamp for proximal anastomoses)
- Solid (lipid) or gaseous microembolism debris from the extracorporeal circuit, which is more significant in patients in whom cardiotomy suction is utilized
- Air embolism from the left heart
- Left atrial or left ventricular thrombus (atrial fibrillation is the most common cause of "delayed" stroke)
- Platelet–fibrin debris from carotid ulcerations
- Multiple blood and blood component transfusions (especially platelets)[163]

b. Cerebral hypoperfusion may result from systemic hypotension or impaired cerebral flow from intra- or extracranial carotid disease.
- Systemic hypotension is common during CPB, although cerebral autoregulation can maintain cerebral blood flow down to a mean pressure of 40 mm Hg. This compensatory mechanism is usually inoperative in diabetic, hypertensive patients, and may be impaired by cerebral microembolization.[164] Blood pressure usually must be raised to provide adequate cerebral flow independent of the systemic flow rate. One study showed a fourfold greater incidence of watershed infarcts when there was a 10 mm decrease in intraoperative mean blood pressure compared with preoperative levels.[165]
- The blood pressure may be compromised during off-pump surgery during manipulation of the heart, and is usually reduced pharmacologically during

construction of proximal anastomoses when a side-clamp is placed on the ascending aorta.

- The potential exists for cerebral hypoperfusion during an episode of postoperative hypotension. This may result in a watershed infarct, especially in patients with uncorrected carotid disease.
- Cerebral hypoxemia from a low hematocrit during CPB may be associated with an increased risk of stroke. One study showed that the risk of stroke increased 10% for every percent decrease in hematocrit, but the risk rose primarily once the hematocrit was below 21%.[166]

3. **Presentation.** Several studies have suggested that "early stroke" (noted upon emergence from anesthesia) is noted in 50–67% of patients as a result of an intraoperative event.[147] However, other studies have suggested just the opposite – that 67% of strokes are "delayed strokes" that are noted after a period of normal neurologic recovery.[149,167,168] Either way, embolization is considered to be the most common mechanism. Consistent with this hypothesis is a study in which postoperative scanning revealed that 77% of patients had large territory embolic infarcts, 16% were watershed, and 7% had a mixed pattern.[151] For delayed strokes, it is not clear why intraoperative manipulation would be causative, but one study found that aortic atherosclerosis, diabetes, a prior neurological event, and the combination of low cardiac output and atrial fibrillation, but not AF alone, were associated with delayed strokes.[168] Another study showed that the early stroke risk was lower in patients undergoing on-pump CABG, but the risk of delayed stroke was similar for on- and off-pump CABGs.[149] The clinical presentation depends primarily on the site and extent of the cerebral insult. As noted, many patients will have subclinical infarcts noted by DWI.

   a. Focal deficits most commonly produce hemiparesis/hemiplegia, aphasia, or dysarthria. Visual deficits may occur as the result of retinal embolization, occipital lobe infarction, or anterior ischemic optic neuropathy.[169] The latter is more common in patients with long pump runs with extreme hemodilution. One study found that posterior strokes involving the posterior cerebral artery and cerebellum were the most common location, although embolization to the middle cerebral artery (MCA) was also encountered in about 50% of patients since multiple emboli were commonly noted.[170] Another found that the distributions of the MCA and anterior cerebral artery were the most common locations.[147]

   b. Transient ischemic attacks (TIAs) or reversible neurologic deficits (RNDs)

   c. Severe confusion or delirium

   d. Coma

4. **Prevention** of neurologic complications requires the identification and appropriate treatment of potential precipitating factors.

   a. Preoperative **evaluation for extracranial carotid disease** should be considered in any patient with current or remote neurologic symptoms or the presence of a carotid bruit. Noninvasive studies followed by magnetic resonance angiography, if indicated, may identify significant carotid disease. The approach to symptomatic carotid disease invariably involves a preliminary carotid endarterectomy (CEA) or carotid stenting or simultaneous CABG-CEA procedure.[171–174] The management of high-grade asymptomatic carotid disease at the time of cardiac surgery is controversial, and general recommendations are presented on pages 145–146.

b. Preoperative use of statins may lower not only the risk of stroke,[152] but also the risk of delirium.[175]

c. Intraoperative epiaortic echocardiography can be used to identify aortic atherosclerosis that might alter cannulation and clamping techniques to prevent manipulation of a diseased ascending aorta.[176,177] If not used routinely, it should be considered in patients with other markers for aortic atherosclerosis, such as hypertension, PVD, cerebrovascular disease, renal dysfunction, and COPD, or when increased thickness of the descending aorta is noted by TEE.[178]

d. Use of single aortic cross-clamping during on-pump bypass surgery.[159,179]

e. Use of membrane oxygenators for CPB with avoidance of cardiotomy suction.

f. Use of off-pump surgery with an aortic "no touch" technique. This may involve use of proximal anastomotic occluders, such as the HEARTSTRING device (Maquet Cardiovascular) to avoid aortic side-clamping, or use of the ITAs as inflow vessels.[159]

g. In patients with severe aortic calcification requiring CPB, circulatory arrest may be indicated to avoid aortic cross-clamping.

h. Flooding of the operative field with carbon dioxide to evacuate air, especially during valve cases, may reduce the incidence of neurologic impairment.[180]

i. Particulate emboli can be captured by use of the Embol-X intra-aortic filter (Edwards Lifesciences) at the time of unclamping.

j. Use of the Somanetics Invox cerebral oximeter may identify a significant decrease in cerebral oxygenation that can be improved by various maneuvers, such as maintaining a higher mean arterial pressure during CPB, raising the PCO_2 to increase cerebral blood flow, or transfusing for a profound anemia.[181] Theoretically these interventions should be able to reduce the incidence of neurologic impairment, especially watershed infarcts caused by low flow.[165]

k. Avoidance of hyperglycemia and systemic hyperthermia during rewarming may be helpful since they might contribute to worsening symptoms of type I deficits and possibly to neurocognitive deficits.[182]

l. Anticoagulation for postoperative atrial fibrillation (see page 545).

5. Evaluation requires an assessment of the degree of functional impairment by careful neurologic examination and identification of the anatomic extent of cerebral infarction by CT or DWI MRI scanning. Scanning is most important in assessing whether hemorrhage is present or not, since up to 30% of infarctions may develop hemorrhagic conversion that will contraindicate use of heparin.[151] It is common for an initial CT scan to not demonstrate an infarction consistent with the clinical scenario, although abnormalities will usually be evident on subsequent scans. Ideally, a DWI MRI should be obtained because it is more sensitive than CT scanning in identifying ischemic changes, watershed infarcts, or multiple embolic infarcts.[165] However, this procedure can be difficult to obtain in a critically ill patient on a ventilator and multiple infusion pumps. Furthermore, it is important to analyze whether the findings are consistent with an acute infarct, since many patients will have undiagnosed preoperative infarctions demonstrable by DWI. Evaluation should also be undertaken to search for a possible source of the stroke that might require additional attention (echocardiogram, carotid noninvasive studies).

6. **Treatment**

    a. The use of heparin in patients suffering an embolic stroke is controversial. It is recommended for patients with atrial fibrillation, possible valve thrombus, or other sources of intracardiac thrombus, but has unclear benefit in preventing further aortic atheroembolism. It might improve cerebral microcirculatory flow, but the possibility of subsequent hemorrhage into an infarct zone must always be taken into consideration. Some neurologists feel that heparin should be withheld for at least 72 hours to minimize the risk of hemorrhagic conversion.

    b. Standard measures to reduce intracranial pressure, including diuresis, mannitol, and steroids, may be indicated depending on the extent of cerebral infarction.

    c. A carotid endarterectomy may be considered in patients with severe carotid stenosis and postoperative transient neurologic deficits or small strokes.

    d. Early institution of physical therapy is important.

7. **Prognosis** is favorable for patients with small or temporary deficits, but the operative mortality rate for patients suffering permanent strokes is around 20%. The outlook for comatose patients is extremely poor, with over 50% dying or remaining in a vegetative state. Five-year survival following a postoperative stroke is only about 50–60%, with most patients continuing to manifest moderate-to-severe disability.[153,183,184] With such a dismal prognosis, any steps that can possibly be taken to reduce the incidence of stroke must be entertained.

B. **Encephalopathy and delirium** represent an acute change in a patient's mental status that is associated with a global impairment of cognitive function. These problems are fairly common after open-heart surgery requiring CPB, especially in elderly patients, with an incidence of upwards of 20%.[185] The etiology is frequently not clear, but in the early postoperative period, it may be related to metabolic/electrolyte disturbances superimposed on either microembolization from CPB or mild cerebral hypoperfusion. The contribution of CPB to the development of delirium is suggested by a lower incidence in patients undergoing off-pump surgery,[186] although many studies suggest that the incidence of neurocognitive changes is fairly comparable.[145] In patients requiring prolonged ICU stays, the incidence of delirium is very high. Delirium is associated with more respiratory complications, contributes to sternal instability problems, impairs mobilization, and increases operative mortality. Furthermore, patients with delirium are more prone to the development of dementia, perhaps reflecting its greater occurrence in patients with less cognitive reserve.[187] Although delirium is usually transient and has a fluctuating course, it can be very disturbing to the patient and his/her family.

1. **Risk factors**

    a. Older age

    b. Recent use of alcohol or opiates

    c. Preoperative organic brain disease (history of cognitive dysfunction, delirium, dementia, or functional impairment)

    d. Severe cardiac disease and high-risk status at the time of surgery (cardiogenic shock, urgent status, severe LV dysfunction)

    e. Multiple associated medical illnesses (especially diabetes, cerebrovascular disease, PVD) and poor nutritional status

  f. Atrial fibrillation

  g. Complex and prolonged surgical procedures on CPB, especially valve procedures

2. Common contributing causes

  a. Medication toxicity (including benzodiazepines and analgesics)

  b. Metabolic disturbances

  c. Alcohol withdrawal

  d. Low cardiac output syndromes; this may include periods of marginal cerebral blood flow during bypass that are just above the threshold for cerebral infarction

  e. Hypoxia

  f. Sepsis

  g. Recent/new stroke

3. Manifestations

  a. Disorientation, confusion, attention deficit, memory loss, disturbed sleep-wake cycle

  b. Lethargy or agitation

  c. Paranoia and hallucinations

4. Evaluation

  a. Review current medications and drug levels.

  b. Identify possible history of recent alcoholism or substance abuse.

  c. Neurologic examination, often with brain CT or MRI.

  d. ABGs, electrolytes, BUN, creatinine, CBC, magnesium, calcium, cultures.

5. Management[188]

  a. Use soft restraints and keep side rails up to prevent falls out of bed.

  b. Correct metabolic abnormalities.

  c. Stop inappropriate medications.

  d. Carefully select sedative medications in the ICU to minimize the risk of delirium. Dexmedetomidine is associated with less postoperative delirium than propofol or midazolam when used for immediate postoperative sedation.[189] It is also more effective than haloperidol in controlling the agitated, delirious, intubated patient, allowing for earlier extubation.[190]

  e. Select the appropriate medication to control agitation and the delirious state.

    i. Haloperidol 2.5–5.0 mg PO/IM/IV q6h is the most commonly prescribed medication for delirium.[191] One should always be aware of the risk of torsades de pointes in patients receiving IV haloperidol.[192]

    ii. Benzodiazepines (especially lorazepam [Ativan]) are best avoided for sedation of ventilated patients because they may cause delirium. If delirium is present, they can exacerbate confusion and produce agitation and stupor, especially in elderly patients. However, olanzepine (Zyprexa), a thieno-benzodiazepine, has been used successfully in delirious critically ill patients, and has been associated with fewer side effects than haloperidol.[193] It is given in a dose of 5–10 mg PO qd.

   iii. Ondansetron (Zofran), which is a $5-HT_3$-receptor antagonist that counteracts activation of the serotoninergic system, has been successful in treating postcardiotomy delirium without major side effects. It is given in a dose of 4–8 mg IV or PO.[194] A similar medication dolasetron (Anzemet) 12.5–25 mg IV can also be used. These medications are usually prescribed for control of postoperative nausea.

   iv. Other atypical antipsychotic medications including risperidone and quetiapine may have some benefit in managing delirium.[195]

  f. Treat suspected alcohol withdrawal[196]

   i. Benzodiazepines (lorazepam, diazepam, or chlordiazepoxide) are indicated in this situation for several days and should be gradually tapered. Patients often require a few additional days of ventilatory support during a period of sedation to avoid agitation and self-destructive behavior. Reintubation may be necessary when symptoms develop after early extubation has been accomplished.

   ii. Thiamine 50–100 mg IM/PO bid and folate 1 mg PO qd

   iii. Psychotherapy: reassurance and support

C. **Seizures** may accompany cerebral insults from hypoxia, or air and particulate emboli. However, they can also result from medication overdoses (e.g., lidocaine). Contributing factors should be addressed and the patient evaluated by a neurologist. A CT or MRI scan, EEG, or anticonvulsant therapy should be considered upon advice from a neurologist.

D. **Neurocognitive dysfunction** is a disturbing complication of cardiac surgery traditionally thought to be associated with the use of CPB. The prevalence in various studies is quite variable. In one study of CABG patients, significant cognitive dysfunction was virtually absent;[197] in another classic study, the incidence of type II deficits was 3%,[198] yet in another review the prevalence was estimated to be as high as 50%.[145] Clearly, the extent and variability of dysfunction depends on the definition of cognitive decline, the type of surgery performed, the timing of evaluation, and extent of the neuropsychologic tests performed.

  1. **Predisposing factors**

   a. Risk factors include older age, diabetes, and preexisting cerebrovascular disease. Aortic atherosclerosis may be a risk factor, with some studies indicating there is an association between aortic atheroma burden and cognitive dysfunction, while others have not.[199,200]

   b. Off-pump surgery was popularized with the assumption that avoidance of CPB would minimize the risk of neurologic deficits. However, OPCABs have not been shown to unequivocally reduce the incidence of neurocognitive deficits compared with on-pump surgery.[145,201–203]

   c. Numerous studies have addressed the relationship between preexisting cognitive abnormalities or abnormal MRI scans and the development of postoperative cognitive decline.

    i. Although neurocognitive dysfunction may occur in the absence of demonstrable ischemic lesions on DWI, the presence of pre- or postoperative cerebral infarction, whether symptomatic or not, is likely to be associated with neurocognitive decline. Many patients have preexisting asymptomatic cerebral infarcts, and up to 45% of patients develop MRI evidence of new cerebral infarction postoperatively.[161] In one study, virtually all patients with abnormal MRIs had cognitive decline;[204] in another, the presence of multiple infarctions was asymptomatic in two-thirds of patients but associated with cognitive decline in 25%.[205] An additional study suggested that the only correlate of late cognitive decline was early cognitive decline, not the presence of ischemic changes on MRI.[206]

    ii. Late neurocognitive decline is more common in patients with preexisting evidence of cognitive dysfunction or dementia, less cognitive reserve, or a history of anxiety/depression.[207,208]

    iii. Preoperative cognitive abnormalities are very common if tested for, with an incidence as high as 45%.[209,210] Patients with less cognitive reserve are inclined to experience more disabling cognitive dysfunction.

d. It is difficult to independently correlate the type of surgical procedure with the development of neurocognitive decline, and it is frequently associated with the use of general anesthesia in elderly patients. Furthermore, studies show that the rate of cognitive decline or impairment in memory after 6 years is no different in coronary artery disease patients managed medically or surgically or with on-pump vs. offpump surgery.[211,212]

2. **Mechanisms** for early and late postoperative cognitive decline appear to be different. Early decline may be related to cerebral microembolization, hypoperfusion, or the systemic inflammatory response to CPB and may be reversible.[145] Late decline is most likely related to preexisting cerebrovascular disease.

    a. Cerebral microembolization is believed to be the most likely source of cognitive decline, but the contribution of CPB is controversial. Studies of cell-saving devices to reduce lipid embolization have shown benefit.[213] However, the reduction in microembolization noted with off-pump surgery has not translated into a reduction in neurocognitive dysfunction.[214,215] As noted, the correlation between aortic atherosclerosis and neurocognitive decline is controversial, in contrast to the clear association of atherosclerosis with the occurrence of perioperative stroke.[199,200]

    b. Cerebral hypoperfusion is often considered the mechanism for encephalopathy, delirium, and neurocognitive dysfunction.

    c. One study proposed that early deficits may arise from either embolization or hypoperfusion; intermediate-term cognitive symptoms, particularly memory problems, are usually the results of multiple emboli, and late cognitive effects, usually pertaining to visuospatial abilities, may be related to hypoperfusion or the combination of hypoperfusion and microemboli.[216]

    d. The systemic inflammatory response syndrome (SIRS) may be a contributory factor to neurologic injury, although not a causative mechanism. The use of complement inhibitors to reduce SIRS has reduced the degree of neurocognitive decline.

    e. Intraoperative hyperglycemia and hyperthermia during rewarming have been associated with neurocognitive dysfunction.[182]

3. Presentation

a. Neurocognitive abnormalities include a deterioration in intellectual function and impaired memory. Forgetfulness, problems with word finding, altered attention span, reduction in psychomotor function, and impaired visual and verbal memory are among the abnormalities that may be present.

b. In some patients, the degree of cognitive dysfunction is immediately obvious; in others, it can only be detected by comparison of pre- and postoperative studies.

4. Prevention.

Steps mentioned above to reduce cerebral embolization and maintenance of a higher perfusion pressure during surgery are important in patients at high risk. Other recommended strategies include α-stat pH regulation during profound hypothermia cases (see page 245), control of intraoperative glucose levels, and avoidance of hyperthermia. Cerebral oximetry may be useful in identifying cerebral desaturation that has been associated with watershed infarcts, but it has not been shown conclusively to predict the occurrence of cognitive dysfunction.[165,217]

5. Evaluation.

MRI scanning often shows multiple infarctions, although such findings are also commonly seen in patients who are asymptomatic. Brain SPECT studies have shown worse cerebral perfusion at baseline and during surgery in patients with cognitive decline after surgery.

6. Natural history.

The duration of cognitive decline varies in numerous studies. One seminal study of CABG patients reported that 53% of patients had cognitive decline at hospital discharge, which decreased to 24% at 6 months but then increased to 42% at 5 years.[218] Most studies concur that cognitive function improves from the time of hospital discharge up to 1 year, only to worsen during subsequent follow-up. The fact that long-term cognitive function was similar in patients managed medically suggests that the late decline is most likely due to the presence of poorly-controlled risk factors for cerebrovascular disease, including hypertension and diabetes.

E. Psychiatric problems are fairly common in patients undergoing open-heart surgery. Anxiety and depression occur frequently in patients with known psychiatric disorders, but are also noted in patients who have lost family members due to coronary disease. The occurrence of these symptoms after surgery is associated with a more unfavorable outcome, including mortality.[219-221] Exacerbation of preexisting disorders, such as affective (bipolar) and personality disorders, is also not unusual. A psychiatrist with an interest in postoperative problems is invaluable in helping patients resolve distressing psychiatric symptoms and in providing advice on the appropriate use of psychotropic medications. Cognitive behavior therapy and support stress management are helpful in alleviating postoperative depression.[222]

F. Critical illness polyneuropathy is a syndrome of unknown etiology that complicates the course of sepsis and multisystem organ failure, especially respiratory and renal failure. Because of its association with critical illness, it is associated with a mortality rate greater than 50%. It usually presents as failure to wean from the ventilator due to weakness of the diaphragm and chest wall muscles. Axonal degeneration of motor and sensory fibers is the underlying pathologic process and is manifested by proximal muscle atrophy and paresis, decreased deep tendon reflexes, and, in some cases, by laryngeal and pharyngeal weakness, producing swallowing difficulties. It may produce motor and sensory deficits and can be diagnosed by electromyography and nerve conduction studies. The syndrome is self-limited and has no specific treatment other than supportive care (ventilatory support and physical therapy). It must be distinguished from other causes of postoperative muscle weakness, such as medications, nutritional deficiency, disuse atrophy, and other neuromuscular disorders.[223,224]

G. **Brachial plexus injuries**

1. **Etiology and prevention**. Stretch of the inferior cords of the brachial plexus by lateral sternal retraction or asymmetric elevation during ITA harvesting are the most likely causes of this injury. The incidence may be minimized by cautious and limited asymmetric retraction for ITA takedown, ensuring a midline sternotomy, caudad placement of the retractor, opening it only as much as necessary for adequate exposure, and maintaining a neutral head position.[9] The incidence may also be lessened by positioning the patient in the "hands up" position.[225]. Despite taking all of these precautions, a small number of patients will still develop a brachial plexus stretch injury, most probably related to their individual chest wall architecture. Routine electrophysiologic studies identify abnormalities in upwards of 20% of patients, although most patients are asymptomatic.[226] First rib fractures are often noted by bone scan, although they are frequently missed by routine chest x-rays.

2. **Presentation**. Sensory changes, including numbness, paresthesias, and occasionally sharp pains as well as weakness are common in the ulnar nerve distribution (T8–T1), which commonly affects the fourth and fifth fingers. Weakness of the interosseous muscles may also be noted. In more extreme forms, the median or radial nerve distribution may be involved. Radial nerve deficits are more likely to be caused by direct arm compression from retraction bars used for the ITA takedown or from positioning issues.

3. **Evaluation**. Electromyography, motor and sensory conduction velocities, and somatosensory evoked potentials can be used to assess changes in nerve function, but their significance is not clear. They may be useful in assessing the extent of the deficit and the return of function.

4. **Treatment**. Symptoms resolve in more than 95% of patients within a few months. Rarely, recovery may take up to a year, and some patients may have persistent, bothersome symptoms. Physical therapy is essential to maintain motor tone. If the patient has significant pain, amitriptyline (Elavil) 10–25 mg qhs, gabapentin (Neurontin) starting at 300 mg qd, or carbamazepine (Tegretol) 50–100 mg qid may be helpful.

H. **Paraplegia** is a very rare complication of open-heart surgery. It may occur as the result of an aortic dissection or as a complication of an IABP, presumably on the basis of atherosclerotic plaque shift or rupture, or from cholesterol embolism to the spinal cord. When it occurs after an isolated CABG, it is invariably associated with a period of hypotension in a patient with preexisting hypertension and severe vascular disease that compromises spinal cord perfusion.[227,228]

I. **Common peroneal or sciatic/tibial nerve palsies** are rare complications of surgery that usually have no identifiable contributing factor. Common peroneal nerve injuries cause weakness and sensory changes over the lateral lower leg and foot; tibial nerve problems affect the posterior calf and dorsum of the foot. Direct nerve injury is virtually impossible during vein harvesting, so the suspected mechanism is ischemia caused by direct pressure on the nerves with leg positioning. Older patients with diabetes, peripheral vascular disease, and subnormal body weight with atrophic tissues may be more predisposed to this problem, which is more likely to occur during longer operations involving CPB. However, in most cases, this complication is an unpredictable and unpreventable event. Fortunately, most patients recover satisfactory sensorimotor function and are not limited in their activities.[229]

J. **Compartment syndrome (CS)** may occur following periods of prolonged compromised blood flow to the lower extremities. It may rarely affect the thigh musculature.

1. **Mechanism.** A compartment syndrome develops when the interstitial tissue tension within a confined compartment exceeds the pressure in the microcirculation, resulting in tissue ischemia. A prolonged period of ischemia followed by reperfusion results in cell membrane damage with fluid leakage into the interstitial compartment, which initially compromises the blood supply to nerve tissue and eventually will compress major blood vessels causing loss of pulses. Thus, loss of pulses is one of the last manifestations of a compartment syndrome, at which time tissue loss has already occurred.

2. **Predisposing factors.** CS is rarely encountered with use of an IABP, most likely because of vigilant attention to leg edema and distal perfusion and the absence of a documented period of prolonged severe leg ischemia. However, CS has been noted in patients requiring prolonged groin cannulation (usually >4–6 hours) for CPB (aortic surgery, minimally invasive or robotic surgery). There are case reports of its occurrence after CABG, following both open and endoscopic vein harvesting (EVH).[230–232] With EVH, the proposed mechanism is retraction of venous branches which then bleed into the muscle.[232]

3. **Prevention.** CS can be prevented by using alternative methods of groin cannulation that allow for distal perfusion (sewing a graft to the femoral artery or proximal and distal cannulation).[233–235] However, these are rarely done because the duration of CPB is not always predictable – usually being lengthened when there are technical problems during the surgical procedure. Although placing a femoral arterial cannula via the Seldinger technique avoids the placement of a distal snare, distal flow is quite limited by the size of the cannula and vasoconstriction during periods of hypothermia. Obtaining adequate hemostasis during EVH should avoid development of a CS after CABG.

4. **Monitoring and treatment.** Any patient with a prolonged period of groin cannulation requires careful assessment for the development of a CS. Because patients are anesthetized and sedated for a number of hours, they are unable to complain of severe leg pain, which is one of the first manifestations of a compartment syndrome. Assessment of the calf diameter and palpation for tenseness and tenderness, if possible, are essential. Comparison with the contralateral leg may be beneficial, although less helpful if vein harvesting has been performed. If there is any doubt, obtaining a compartment pressure with a needle attached to a manometer is helpful. A pressure greater than 35 mm Hg or within 20 mm of the diastolic pressure is generally consistent with a compartment syndrome. If suspected, the patient should be returned to the operating room for a four-compartment fasciotomy. The wound can be closed several days later if muscle tissue is still viable once the edema resolves. The muscle becomes nonviable from inside to out, so the superficial muscle may bleed despite ongoing necrosis of deeper muscle, and careful reassessment is important.

K. Saphenous neuropathy is caused by damage to small branches of the saphenous nerve that lie adjacent to the saphenous vein in the lower leg.[9] It causes sensory changes along the medial side of the calf and foot to the level of the great toe and is fairly common after open vein harvesting. Vein dissection from the ankle up has been found to be more likely to cause this problem than dissection from the top down. It is proposed that the former is more likely to cause avulsion of the pretibial or infra-patellar branches of the nerve. Neuropathy is also more common when an open incision is closed in two layers, producing neuropraxia from too tight a closure. These symptoms are much less frequent when the vein is harvested endoscopically, but damage to the nerve in the lower leg can still occur.

L. Forearm neurologic symptoms following radial artery harvesting are not unusual. In one study comparing open vs. endoscopic harvesting, symptoms occurred in 42% and 64% of patients after open and endoscopic harvesting, respectively. Impaired sensation and paresthesias were more common in the superficial radial nerve distribution with open harvesting, but damage to the lateral antebrachial cutaneous nerve was only seen with open harvests.[236]

M. Vocal cord paralysis has been noted in 1–2% of patients after cardiovascular operations and is initially manifested by hoarseness. Eight different mechanisms have been elucidated, but most involve an indirect injury to the recurrent laryngeal nerve producing a reversible neuropraxia.[237] A major contributing factor is a longer operation, which is usually associated with a longer period of postoperative intubation. Direct injury may occur during ITA mobilization at the apex of the chest, during central line placement, or during aortic arch surgery. In addition to hoarseness, vocal cord paralysis leads to an ineffective cough, stridor, and the potential for aspiration pneumonia and respiratory failure.[237,238] Diagnosis can be made by laryngoscopy, which will distinguish it from laryngeal edema. Symptomatic improvement usually occurs within a few months, but if symptoms persist, it is more likely that the injury is permanent. In that situation, vocal cord medialization or thyroplasty may be indicated for unilateral paralysis.

N. Phrenic nerve palsy. See page 654.

O. Pituitary apoplexy. See page 628.

X. Gastrointestinal Complications

A. Mechanisms and predisposing factors

1. Gastrointestinal (GI) complications develop in 1–3% of patients undergoing open-heart surgery. Because they frequently occur in critically ill patients, they are associated with other adverse postoperative complications (usually neurologic, renal, pulmonary, and infectious). The overall mortality rate has averaged around 25% in individual studies, including a 2010 study of over 16,000 patients at the Cleveland Clinic.[234–240] Better results were reported in a 2007 nationwide study in the USA of 2.7 million CABG patients in which the incidence was higher at 4.1%, but the mortality rate was only 12%.[241] The varying results in these studies may be related to different inclusion criteria.

2. The common pathophysiologic mechanism is sympathetic vasoconstriction, hypo-perfusion, and hypoxia of the splanchnic bed.[247,248] This may occur during CPB when there is a regional redistribution of blood flow away from gut mucosa, but may also

result from a postoperative low cardiac output state or hypotension.[248] Inadequate tissue perfusion contributes to mucosal hypoxia with a reduction in absorptive and barrier functions. Numerous changes may occur, including stress ulceration, mucosal atrophy, bacterial overgrowth from stress ulcer prophylaxis, and increased permeability. These changes may potentially lead to bacterial translocation, the systemic inflammatory response syndrome, sepsis, and multisystem organ failure.[247,249]

3. Predictive factors for the development of GI complications have been evaluated in multiple studies and include:[239–251]

   a. **Preoperative comorbidities**: older age, chronic kidney disease, PVD, active smoking, prior GI surgery, use of anticoagulants

   b. **Preoperative cardiac status**: poor LV function or NYHA class IV, urgent or emergent surgery

   c. **Operative**: reoperations, combined valve-CABG cases, long durations of CPB, multiple blood transfusions

   d. **Postoperative:** low cardiac output syndrome (use of inotropes, vasoconstrictors, IABP), bleeding and need for transfusions or exploration, respiratory failure, atrial fibrillation, excessive anticoagulation

   e. Three of the strongest predictors are prolonged mechanical ventilation, acute kidney injury, and sepsis, which together contribute to splanchnic hypoperfusion, hypomotility, and mucosal hypoxia.

4. It has been hypothesized that off-pump surgery might reduce the incidence of GI complications by avoiding the use of CPB. During CPB, there is nonpulsatile perfusion at low mean pressures with a regional distribution of flow away from the splanchnic bed. This can produce splanchnic hypoperfusion, which may be worsened by use of vasoconstrictors. This then produces endothelial dysfunction and a systemic inflammatory response. However, studies have demonstrated that mesenteric hypoperfusion and gastric mucosal hypoxia are present to a similar extent with on- and off-pump surgery.[252,253] Although one study did find a higher incidence of GI complications with on-pump surgery with cardioplegic arrest,[250] several others have not.[240,241,254] GI bleeding has been noted to be more common after off-pump surgery whereas visceral ischemia is more common after on-pump surgery. Thus, the associated mortality rate may arguably be lower after OPCAB.

5. Because of the high mortality rate of GI complications, strict adherence to common principles of perioperative care is important. These include expeditous surgical procedures with good myocardial protection, careful hemostasis to minimize use of blood transfusions, sufficient inotropic support for the low cardiac output syndrome, optimization of renal function, early extubation, mobilization, and other means of preventing infection, and careful anticoagulation when indicated after surgery. Prompt identification and aggressive management are necessary to decrease the mortality associated with GI complications.

B. **Routine care and common complaints.** Most patients have a nasogastric tube inserted in the operating room before heparinization or after its reversal by protamine. This maintains gastric decompression during positive-pressure ventilation, removes gastric contents to minimize the risk of aspiration, decreases gastric acidity, and allows for the administration of oral medications and antacids in the ICU. The tube is usually removed after extubation if bowel sounds are present. An oral diet is then advanced from clear liquids to a regular diet.

1. **Anorexia,** nausea, and a distaste for food are fairly common complaints after surgery and may be attributable to the side effects of medications (narcotics), and possibly to mineral deficiency (especially zinc). Bothersome nausea can be treated by a number of medications which have fairly comparable efficacy.

    a. Metoclopramide (Reglan) 10–20 mg IM qid. This may also stimulate gastro-intestinal motility and decrease the incidence of distention.

    b. The 5-HT$_3$ antagonists are powerful antiemetic medications, although they are significantly more expensive.[255] They may be associated with a proarrhythmic effect from QT interval prolongation. These include:

        i. Ondansetron (Zofran) 4 mg IV

        ii. Dolasetron (Anzemet) 12.5 mg IV

        iii. Granisetron (Kytril) 1 mg IV/PO bid

    c. Droperidol 0.625–2.5 mg IV is very effective, but because it may cause QT prolongation and torsades de pointes, it is best to use the other medications mentioned.

2. **Pharyngeal dysfunction** with dysphagia and difficulty swallowing liquids or solids has been noted in 1–3% of patients undergoing CABG and can lead to silent or overt aspiration pneumonia.[256,257]

    a. Predisposing factors include older age, comorbidities (insulin-dependent diabetes, COPD, and renal dysfunction), CHF, a history of stroke or new perioperative stroke, or perioperative sepsis. Swallowing dysfunction (dysphagia) and pain with swallowing (odynophagia) are more common in patients monitored with intraoperative TEE.[258–260] Because TEE is routine in most institutions, one must be alert to this problem in the early postoperative period if the patient has impaired pharyngeal sensation or coughing at the time of initial oral intake. Dysphagia has been noted in up to 50% of patients who remain intubated more than 48 hours, which results in a delay in resumption of oral feeding and a prolongation of hospital stay.[261]

    b. The occurrence of pharyngeal dysfunction in the absence of common contributing factors (TEE, ventilation) has been ascribed to a new neurologic deficit. Thus, a full neurological evaluation with CT or MRI scanning may be indicated to identify the causative mechanism.

    c. Bedside swallowing tests (usually swallowing 50 mL of water and assessing for a reduction in oxygen saturation by pulse oximetry as well as coughing or choking) can be used as an assessment for aspiration, but have variable sensitivity in detecting silent aspiration.[262–264] A modified barium swallow using videofluoroscopy may be indicated before the patient is allowed to eat.[264,265]

    d. The management of the patient with pharyngeal dysphagia may include dietary modification, postural adjustments, and working with speech therapists on swallowing maneuvers. Persistent dysphagia may require insertion of a feeding tube until satisfactory swallowing can be demonstrated.

3. **Constipation** is a common problem after surgery. Preoperative enemas are usually not given, narcotics are used for analgesia, and elderly patients are often poorly mobilized for several days. Milk of magnesia, bulk laxatives (Metamucil), or stool softeners (Colace) may be helpful in older patients.

C. **Differential diagnosis of acute abdominal pain**

   1. **Manifestations.** The presence of an acute intra-abdominal process can be difficult to detect in a critically ill patient in an ICU setting. It is frequently suspected by the presence of fever, an elevation in WBC count, marked tenderness to abdominal palpation, hemodynamic evidence of sepsis, or a positive blood culture. Arriving at the appropriate diagnosis can be even more challenging, but prompt assessment and management are essential because of the high associated mortality.

   2. **Etiology**

      a. Cholecystitis (acalculous or calculous)

      b. Perforated viscus (gastric or duodenal ulceration, diverticulitis)[266]

      c. Gastritis

      d. Pancreatitis

      e. Ischemic bowel (mesenteric ischemia)

      f. *Clostridium difficile* colitis

      g. Severe paralytic ileus (frequently idiopathic, but occasionally associated with an acute inflammatory process or colitis)

      h. Small bowel or colonic obstruction

      i. Severe constipation

      j. Urinary problems (infection or bladder distention)

      k. Retroperitoneal bleeding

   3. **Evaluation**

      a. Review of preexisting conditions or prior abdominal surgery

      b. Serial abdominal examinations for tenderness or distention, bowel sounds

      c. Laboratory tests: liver function tests, serum amylase and lipase, *C. difficile* titer if diarrhea is present

      d. Radiographic studies

         i. KUB (for obstruction or ileus)

         ii. Semiupright chest x-ray (for free air under the diaphragm)

         iii. An upper abdominal ultrasound or HIDA scan (if biliary tract obstruction is suspected)

         iv. CT scan of the abdomen with contrast

         v. Mesenteric arteriography (if mesenteric ischemia is suspected)

         vi. Diagnostic laparoscopy if other tests are unable to provide a diagnosis[267]

   4. **Treatment.** General surgery consultation should be obtained from the outset because early exploration may reduce the high mortality associated with the development of GI complications. Laparoscopy is very sensitive in evaluating the nature of the problem, but an exploratory laparotomy may be necessary to further assess and potentially treat the problem. Although many patients with these complications are very ill and often septic, they are usually better able to tolerate exploration after cardiac surgery than they had been before.

D. **Paralytic ileus** occasionally persists for several days after surgery. It is frequently a benign, self-limited problem of unclear etiology, but occasionally it may reflect sepsis or a severe intra-abdominal pathologic process. Acute colonic pseudo-obstruction (Ogilvie's syndrome) is a condition of massive colonic dilatation believed to result from autonomic imbalance with either decreased parasympathetic tone or enhanced sympathetic tone.[268] It must be differentiated from mechanical obstruction or toxic megacolon, often related to *C. difficile*.

1. **Contributing factors**
   a. Drugs (early use of catecholamines, narcotic analgesics)
   b. Gastric distention (possibly related to vagal injury)
   c. Congestion of the hepatic or splanchnic bed (from poor venous drainage during surgery or systemic venous hypertension)
   d. Inflammatory processes (e.g., cholecystitis, pancreatitis)
   e. Retroperitoneal bleeding (from groin catheterization, but occasionally spontaneously in an anticoagulated patient)
   f. *Clostridium difficile* colitis
   g. Mesenteric ischemia

2. **Evaluation**
   a. Serial patient examinations for distention, bowel sounds, and tenderness consistent with an inflammatory process (ischemia or perforation).
   b. Laboratory tests: CBC, amylase, liver function tests, *C. difficile* titers if diarrhea.
   c. KUB: colonic dilatation to 9 cm is significant, but the risk of perforation increases when the cecal diameter exceeds 12 cm.
   d. CT scan of the abdomen with contrast.

3. **Management**
   a. Decompression of the bowel is accomplished by keeping the patient NPO with nasogastric suction. This should prevent gastric distention until peristaltic activity returns. A rectal tube may also be beneficial when colonic distention is marked.
   b. Total parenteral nutrition should be started.
   c. Medications that can impair colonic motility must be stopped. These include narcotics, calcium channel blockers and anticholinergic drugs. Although metoclopramide is commonly used to improve GI motility, it has not been shown to be effective in preventing or treating postoperative ileus.[269]
   d. All metabolic disturbances must be corrected and therapy directed at any identifiable precipitating problem.
   e. Because "pseudo-obstruction" may be caused by deficiency of cholinergic tone, use of cholinesterase inhibitors may be beneficial in producing rapid colonic decompression. Neostigmine 2 mg IV has proven effective in this condition, but is not effective in treating a standard postoperative ileus.[268,270]
   f. When colonic distention (>12 cm) persists despite conservative or pharmacologic therapy, decompressive colonoscopy is indicated. If dilatation persists or worsens, urgent surgical intervention, usually by cecostomy or hemicolectomy, is indicated.

E. **Cholecystitis**
   1. **Etiology.** Cholecystitis is a rare late complication of cardiac surgery with an incidence of 0.1–0.3%. It is noted more commonly in older patients, after surgery

requiring prolonged bypass times, and with low cardiac output syndromes requiring inotropes and/or an IABP and continued vasopressor dependence. These risk factors indicate that hypoperfusion is the major mechanism causing cholecystitis, which is more likely to be acalculous than calculous. Other predisposing factors include vascular disease, reexploration for bleeding or multiple transfusions, prolonged mechanical ventilation, bacteremia, and nosocomial infections. Fasting, parenteral nutrition, and narcotics can decrease gallbladder contractility and produce biliary stasis. If surgery is required because of an inadequate response to antibiotics, the mortality rate is significant at 23–43% in three large series.[271–273]

2. **Evaluation**

   a. Serial abdominal examinations may draw attention to an inflammatory process in the right upper quadrant.

   b. Liver function tests (ALT, AST, bilirubin, alkaline phosphatase) may suggest extrahepatic biliary obstruction.

   c. Right upper quadrant ultrasound or HIDA scan can identify a dilated gallbladder and biliary obstruction.

3. **Treatment**

   a. Antibiotic therapy may suffice in patients with acalculous cholecystitis who have no evidence of peritonitis.[272]

   b. If significant clinical improvement does not occur within 24–48 hours, surgical intervention by percutaneous cholecystostomy (especially in critically ill patients) or cholecystectomy (open or laparoscopic) is indicated.

F. Upper GI bleeding

1. **Etiology.** Upper GI bleeding is one of the most common GI complications encountered after both on- and off-pump surgery with an incidence of 0.5–1%. It usually results from stress ulceration from duodenal ulcers and less commonly from gastric ulcers and esophagogastritis.[274,275] The causative mechanism is usually decreased blood flow, mucosal ischemia, and a hypoperfusion/reperfusion injury that may be exacerbated by increased gastric acidity.[276,277] A thorough preoperative history and physical examination (stigmata of liver disease, stool guaiac) may identify patients at increased risk of developing postoperative GI bleeding.

2. **Risk factors**

   a. Preoperative: older age, preexisting gastritis or ulcer disease

   b. Intraoperative: long duration of CPB, valve operations, reoperations

   c. Postoperative: low cardiac output, prolonged mechanical ventilation, coagulopathy or anticoagulation (antiplatelet agents, heparin preparations, warfarin)

3. **Prophylaxis.** Any patient with a history of ulcer disease or gastritis should receive medications in the ICU to prevent stress-related mucosal damage and potentially GI bleeding. In addition, any patient on prolonged ventilatory support, with sepsis, or with a coagulopathy should receive stress ulcer prophylaxis. Although routine prophylaxis may not be necessary in patients at low risk, there is little downside to using sucralfate routinely during the early postoperative period of intubation when the patient may have marginal cardiac output, visceral hypoperfusion, and some degree of coagulopathy.[278]

a. Sucralfate 1 g q6h can be given orally or down a nasogastric tube. It does not raise the gastric pH (which increases gastric bacterial colonization) and may reduce the incidence of nosocomial pneumonia associated with medications that raise the gastric pH.

b. Proton pump inhibitors (PPI) have been shown to be much more effective than H_2 blockers in reducing the incidence of hemorrhagic gastritis and active ulcer formation.[279] Pantoprazole (Protonix) 40 mg can be given IV or PO, whereas other common preparations, such as omeprazole (Prilosec) 20 mg qd, lansoprazole (Prevacid) 15 mg qd, or rabeprazole (Aciphex) 10 mg qd, can be given orally for prophylaxis.

c. Generally, enteric-coated aspirin is recommended for most patients following CABG or tissue valve surgery, although studies have not shown that enteric coating reduces the occurrence of GI bleeding or ulceration.[280]

d. In patients with no known ulcer disease, clopidogrel may cause fewer GI complications than aspirin alone, although, paradoxically, one study suggests this may not be true in patients with prior GI problems.[281] However, combining either clopidogrel or aspirin with a PPI for prophylaxis is considered equally effective.

4. **Manifestations.** Drainage of bright red blood through a nasogastric tube or vomiting of blood is an overt sign of upper GI bleeding. Slow bleeding usually produces melena, but very rapid bleeding may produce bloody stools. Attention should be drawn to potential GI bleeding in the critically ill or heparinized patient with an unexplained fall in hematocrit or progressive tachycardia or hypotension. If GI bleeding cannot be documented, a retroperitoneal bleed should be entertained as a possible diagnosis and evaluated by an abdominal CT scan.

5. **Evaluation and treatment.** Bleeding that persists despite correction of coagulation abnormalities and intensification of a medical regimen requires further evaluation. Bleeding during anticoagulation is commonly associated with some underlying pathology.

a. The PPIs are superior to the H_2 blockers in controlling and preventing recurrent bleeding.[282] A daily 40 mg dose of pantoprazole IV is effective in raising and maintaining the gastric pH >6, which may account for its superiority over the H_2 blockers in maintaining clotting.

b. Ranitidine can be given as a continuous infusion (6.25 mg/h) to maintain the gastric pH >4, but tolerance may develop.

c. Upper GI endoscopy should be performed to identify the site of bleeding and can be used therapeutically with laser bipolar coagulation to control hemorrhage. It can achieve hemostasis in >90% of patients.

d. Somatostatin 250 μg/h for 5 days has been shown to be effective in the treatment severe upper GI bleeding.[283]

6. **Results.** The overall mortality rate for patients developing GI bleeding has improved to about 15–20%, most likely as a result of improved medical and endoscopic therapy. In one series, about 30% of patients required surgery after an initial endoscopic procedure.[275] If the patient requires anticoagulation indefinitely following surgery, e.g., for a mechanical prosthetic valve, a definitive procedure must be performed.

7. Although it is essential to stop all antiplatelet medications or anticoagulants when there is evidence of GI bleeding, it is advisable to resume antiplatelet drugs when feasible for CABG patients and those with tissue valves. Even in patients with a known history of aspirin-induced GI bleeding, resumption of aspirin combined with a PPI was found to be superior to using clopidogrel as an alternative antiplatelet drug.[284] For patients requiring both aspirin and clopidogrel, they can be given safely with a PPI after endoscopic control of a bleeding site.[285]

G. **Lower GI bleeding** may be manifest by bright red blood per rectum, blood-streaked stool, or melena, and can usually be differentiated from upper GI bleeding by passage of a nasogastric tube.

1. **Etiology**

   a. Mesenteric ischemia or ischemic colitis caused by periods of prolonged hypoperfusion

   b. Antibiotic-associated colitis (usually *C. difficile*)

   c. Bleeding from colonic lesions (polyps, tumors, diverticular disease) which may be precipitated by anticoagulation.

   d. Intestinal angiodysplasia. This is termed Heyde's syndrome when associated with aortic stenosis and may be associated with acquired von Willebrand's disease (vWD-IIA). It abates after aortic valve replacement with a tissue valve, which appears to improve the hematologic problem.[286]

2. **Evaluation.** Once an upper GI source has been ruled out, sigmoidoscopy or colonoscopy can be performed. A bleeding scan may identify the bleeding source. Mesenteric arteriography should be considered if bleeding persists.

3. **Treatment** involves correction of any coagulopathy and elimination of precipitating causes. Antibiotics (metronidazole 500 mg PO q8h or vancomycin 125 mg PO qid) can be used for *C. difficile* colitis. Mesenteric angiography with infusion of vasopressin (0.2–0.4 units/min) or selective embolotherapy with injection of autologous clot or Gelfoam into the mesenteric arterial branch may be considered.[287,288] Octreotide (50 μg over 30 minutes) or somatostatin (50 μg bolus followed by an infusion of 250 μg/h) decreases splanchnic blood flow and may be beneficial in patients with GI angiodysplasia.[289] Surgical intervention is rarely required for persistent bleeding.

H. **Mesenteric ischemia** is a rare (0.2–0.4% incidence) but highly lethal complication of cardiac surgery that is usually noted in elderly patients with known generalized atherosclerotic disease. It is often associated with dehydration.[290]

1. **Etiology.** Nonocclusive mesenteric ischemia is the most common etiology, resulting from splanchnic hypoperfusion from a low cardiac output state (after on- or off-pump surgery, but most commonly after a long pump run).[291] Atherosclerotic embolism (usually with use of an IABP) or mesenteric thrombosis (possibly from heparin-induced thrombocytopenia) occur less commonly.[243]

2. **Presentation.** Typical manifestations are a profound ileus or abdominal pain out of proportion to physical findings. The diagnosis can be very difficult to make in the critically ill patient who is frequently ventilated and heavily sedated. Sepsis with hemodynamic instability, lactic acidosis, respiratory distress, GI bleeding, or diarrhea are often present as well. The diagnosis is typically made about 5–10 days after surgery.

3. **Diagnosis** may be suggested by the association of the clinical picture just mentioned with leukocytosis, severe acidosis, an ileus on KUB or evidence of free abdominal fluid. Endoscopy may be helpful in documenting colonic ischemia. Mesenteric CT angiography may show evidence of pneumatosis intestinalis, venous gas, bowel wall thickening, arterial occlusion, or venous thrombosis.[292] Standard mesenteric arteriography may identify thromboembolism, but most commonly demonstrates vasoconstriction of the peripheral mesenteric vessels. Unfortunately, the diagnosis is frequently made at surgery when irreversible changes have occurred. Early suspicion of mesenteric ischemia, based on a persistent paralytic ileus, absent bowel movements for several days despite laxatives, and a borderline or elevated lactate level may allow for earlier successful intervention with a vasodilator infusion, such as papaverine.[293]

4. **Treatment.** Early diagnosis and treatment are essential to lower the mortality rate of mesenteric ischemia, which generally exceeds 65%.[243,290] If mesenteric vasoconstriction is identified, an infusion of papaverine 0.7 mg/kg/h for up to 5 days may be helpful, especially at an earlier stage of ischemia.[293] When ischemia is prolonged, irreversible intestinal necrosis may occur within hours. Emergency abdominal exploration is indicated if bowel necrosis is suspected. Although a limited bowel resection can be performed, a more likely finding is multiple areas of ischemic bowel that prohibit extensive bowel resection. A second-look operation is indicated if the viability of the bowel is in doubt.

I. **Diarrhea** developing in a patient in the ICU setting is often an ominous sign because it may result from bowel ischemia caused by a low flow state. However, it is frequently caused by treatable problems including:

1. Antibiotic usage, which can reduce bowel flora and can lead to diarrhea even in the absence of positive titers for *Clostridium difficile*.

2. *C. difficile* colitis, which has an overall incidence of 0.8% and is usually, but not always, associated with a prolonged duration of antibiotic therapy.[294] The incidence is similar with use of cephaloporins and fluoroquinolones. *C. difficile* is more common in older patients and those receiving multiple blood products. For a patient with persistent diarrhea or with unexplained abdominal pain and a leukocytosis, this diagnosis should be considered, and stool specimens should be sent for *C. difficile* titers. Oral medication may be started immediately upon suspicion of the diagnosis with either metronidazole 500 mg PO q8h or vancomycin 125 mg PO qid for 7–10 days.[295]

3. GI bleeding

4. Intolerance of hyperosmolar tube feedings: dilute with more water and start at a slower infusion rate.

J. **Hepatic dysfunction** manifested by a transient low-grade elevation in liver function tests (LFTs), including ALT, AST, bilirubin, and alkaline phosphatase, is not that uncommon after open-heart surgery. About 25% of patients will develop transient hyperbilirubinemia (total bilirubin >3 mg/dL), but fewer than 1% of patients will have evidence of significant hepatocellular damage that may progress to chronic hepatitis or liver failure.[296,297] The elevated bilirubin may be multifactorial, with increased bilirubin production from hemolysis and impaired liver function contributing to both unconjugated and conjugated hyperbilirubinemia.

1. **Predisposing conditions**

   a. Preexisting liver disease. This may be manifest by elevated LFTs, but occasionally will be associated with normal values. However, impaired synthetic function (low serum albumin, high INR) is a marker for hepatic disease. An elevated bilirubin in patients with CHF is one of the strongest predictors of the occurrence of postoperative hepatic dysfunction.[298]

   b. Comorbidities: CHF, especially right-sided with a high right atrial pressure, may be associated with congestive hepatomegaly; diabetes and hypertension are other risk factors.

   c. Cardiac conditions: patients with preoperative cardiogenic shock (acute MI, papillary muscle rupture, valve thrombosis) often show evidence of a "shock liver" before surgery and are at particularly high risk for developing hepatic and multisystem organ failure after salvage open-heart surgery.

   d. Operative factors: prolonged duration of CPB, complex operations (combined CABG-valve, multiple valves), increasing number of blood transfusions.

   e. Postoperative factors: low cardiac output syndrome, use of multiple inotropes or an IABP.

   f. Medications, including statins and clopidogrel.[299]

2. **Etiology.** Hepatic dysfunction may result from either reduced hepatic perfusion or systemic congestion.

   a. Hepatocellular necrosis

      i. Low cardiac output states usually requiring inotropic and/or vasopressor support

      ii. Right heart failure or severe tricuspid regurgitation (chronic passive congestion)

      iii. Posttransfusion hepatitis C or cytomegalovirus infection (late)

      iv. Drugs (acetaminophen, clopidogrel)

   b. Hyperbilirubinemia

      i. Hemolysis (paravalvular leak, long pump run, sepsis, multiple transfusions, drugs)

      ii. Intrahepatic cholestasis (hepatitis, hepatocellular necrosis, benign postoperative cholestasis, parenteral nutrition, bacterial infections, medications)

      iii. Extrahepatic obstruction (biliary tract obstruction)

3. **Manifestations** depend on the specific diagnosis. Jaundice is a common accompaniment of hepatocellular damage or cholestasis. Severe liver failure may result in a coagulopathy, refractory acidosis, hypoglycemia, renal failure, or encephalopathy.

4. **Evaluation.** The specific LFT abnormalities usually indicate the nature of the problem. Additional tests may include those that detect hemolysis (LDH, reticulocyte count), assess cardiac and valvular function (echocardiography), identify biliary pathology (right upper quadrant ultrasound or HIDA scan), or detect hepatitis (serologies).

5. **Treatment**

   a. An elevated bilirubin is usually a benign and self-limited postoperative occurrence. Bilirubin levels will gradually return to normal when hemodynamics improve unless there is evidence of severe underlying liver pathology. In this situation, progressive and irreversible hepatic dysfunction may result, leading to multisystem organ failure and death.

b. Coagulopathy with "autoanticoagulation" may occur during a period of hepatic dysfunction because of the impaired capacity of the liver to produce clotting factors. In patients requiring anticoagulation, small doses of warfarin should be used to prevent the INR from becoming elevated to dangerous levels. If this occurs, the patient may develop cardiac tamponade or GI bleeding. In addition, the doses of medications that undergo hepatic metabolism must be altered.

c. Stress ulcer prophylaxis should be given using one of the proton pump inhibitors (pantoprazole 40 mg IV/PO qd).

d. Hyperammonemia and encephalopathy can be treated with:[300]

  i. Dietary protein restriction

  ii. Lactulose 30 mL qid with sorbitol

  iii. Oral neomycin 6 g daily

  iv. Zinc sulfate 600 mg qd

e. Blood glucose should be carefully monitored to prevent hypoglycemia.

f. Lactic acidosis may result from impaired lactate metabolism rather than lactate generation from impaired tissue perfusion. Partial correction with sodium bicarbonate or Tris buffer (THAM), if renal function is adequate, should be considered if the base deficit exceeds 10.

K. Hyperamylasemia is noted in a substantial number (35–65%) of patients in the early postbypass period but is associated with clinical pancreatitis in only about 1–3% of patients.[301,302] Isolated hyperamylasemia in the early postoperative period is usually not associated with clinical symptoms or an elevated lipase level, and most commonly arises from a nonpancreatic source, such as the salivary glands, or results from decreased renal excretion. Transient hyperamylasemia has a comparable incidence after on- or off-pump surgery, so it is not directly related to use of CPB.[301] However, some patients with an amylase level >1000 IU/L early after surgery may subsequently develop subclinical pancreatitis about 1 week later.[302] This is suggested by the presence of mild symptoms (anorexia, nausea, ileus) with elevation of serum lipase levels. A brief period of bowel rest may be beneficial for these patients, but no specific treatment is indicated unless there is clinical evidence of overt pancreatitis or GI tract dysfunction.

L. Overt pancreatitis is noted in less than 0.5% of patients undergoing cardiac surgery, but is a serious problem associated with a significant mortality rate.[303] Pancreatic necrosis has been noted in 25% of patients dying from multisystem organ failure after cardiac surgery.[304]

1. Etiology. Pancreatitis usually represents an ischemic, necrotic injury resulting from a low cardiac output state and hypoperfusion. A prolonged duration of CPB may sensitize the pancreas to the subsequent insult of a persistent low output state requiring vasopressors that leads to necrotizing pancreatitis. A history of alcohol abuse is also a risk factor.[302]

2. Presentation is atypical and relatively nonspecific. Fever, elevated WBC, paralytic ileus, and abdominal distention occur first, with abdominal pain, tenderness, and hemodynamic instability representing late manifestations.

3. **Diagnosis** is suggested by the association of abdominal pain with hyperamylasemia, although most patients with fulminant pancreatitis do not have markedly elevated amylase levels. Abdominal ultrasound or CT scan may demonstrate a pancreatic phlegmon or abscess.

4. **Treatment** should begin with nasogastric drainage and antibiotics. Exploratory laparotomy with debridement and drainage is usually performed as a desperation measure, but may be the only hope for survival in patients with aggressive necrotizing pancreatitis.

XI. Nutrition[305]

A. Reversal of the catabolic state with adequate nutrition is important during the early phase of postoperative convalescence. The diet must provide enough calories to allow wounds to heal and to maintain immune competence. Although limitations in salt content, fluids, and cholesterol intake are important, overly strict control should be secondary to providing tasty, high-caloric foods that stimulate the patient's appetite. Too frequently, the combination of anorexia, nausea, and an unpalatable diet prevents the patient from achieving satisfactory nutrition. Oral supplements with low residue, such as Boost (Novartis) or Ensure (Ross) are useful in meeting caloric requirements.

B. Patients requiring ventilatory support, those with swallowing difficulties after extubation, and many patients suffering significant strokes are unable to take oral feedings, but usually have a functional GI tract. Enteral feeding should be initiated as soon as possible, usually at a consistent hourly rate, and increased to goal within a few days. Enteral feeding can be started even with absent bowel sounds, although evidence of distention or high gastric residuals may indicate temporary intolerance to tube feedings. A soft nasogastric feeding tube should be placed and tube feedings initiated after confirming the position of the catheter in the stomach or, preferably, in the small bowel. Use of metoclopramide 20 mg IV along with erythromycin 200 mg IV (in 50 mL NS through a central line or 200 mL NS peripherally) to stimulate gastric motility aids in the placement of these tubes.

C. If the GI tract cannot be used, parenteral nutrition (PN) provided through a central line may be necessary. This should be started within a few days of surgery if the patient cannot tolerate any enteral feedings. When the target goal in calories cannot be met with enteral feeding alone, one should consider adding PN after 7–10 days.

D. Most patients who require tracheostomy for prolonged ventilatory support will benefit from the placement of a feeding tube. If there is no evidence of gastroesophageal reflux, which may increase the risk of aspiration, a percutaneous gastric feeding tube (PEG) can be placed for longer-term feeding. If reflux is present, a feeding jejunostomy tube can be placed at the time of the tracheostomy.

E. Measures to reduce the risk of aspiration in patients on enteral feedings include the following:

1. Elevate the head of the bed 30–45°.

2. Use chlorhexidine mouthwash twice a day to reduce the risk of pneumonia.

3. Use metoclopramide to promote GI motility.

4. Check the gastric residual volume; if it exceeds 500 mL, the tube feeds should be held for 2–4 hours and then restarted as a continuous infusion at a lower rate.

5. Advance the feeding tube into small bowel if necessary.

F. Total caloric intake should be around 25 kcal/kg/day (ideal body weight). In markedly obese patients, only 60–70% of target calories may be provided. General nutritional requirements for adult patients include 1 mL/kg/day of water, 2–5 g/kg/day of glucose, 1.2–2 g/kg/day of protein, and 1.2–1.5 g/kg/day of fat, half of which should be omega-6 polyunsaturated fatty acids. A critically ill patient with multisystem organ failure may require 10–20% more calories with a protein requirement of 2–2.5 g/kg/day.

G. A commonly used tube feeding such as Jevity 1.2 (Ross) will provide 1.2 kcal/mL. Thus, for a 70 kg man, 1500 mL/day will provide 1800 calories or 25 kcal/kg/day.

H. Specific considerations in critically ill patients include the following:

1. Soluble fiber and fibro-oligosaccharides (FOS) should be included in enteral feedings to optimize bowel function and are indicated if the patient develops diarrhea. These are included in standard tube feeds such as Jevity (Ross).

2. Hyperglycemia must be prevented by use of intravenous insulin infusions.

3. Antioxidant vitamins and trace minerals, such as selenium, should be provided to critically ill patients receiving enteral nutrition.

4. Patients with respiratory failure characterized by CO_2 retention might benefit from a feeding that is high-lipid and low-carbohydrate, but this is rarely necessary. If fluid restriction is indicated, a calorie-dense formulation, such as Isosource 1.5 (Nestle Nutrition) or Jevity 1.5 (Ross), which provide 1.5 kcal/mL, can be used. In patients with severe acute lung injury, an anti-inflammatory formula with omega-3 fish oils and antioxidants, such as Impact (Novartis Nutrition) or Oxepa (Ross), may be beneficial.

5. Protein intake should be optimized to promote nitrogen retention while avoiding protein overload. Most patients with acute renal failure can receive standard enteral feedings. Protein intake should be increased to 2.5 g/kg/day for patients on dialysis, which removes about 3–5 g/h of protein. Formulations such as Nova-source Renal (Nestle Nutrition) or Nepro (Abbott) provide high protein, low carbohydrate, and low potassium loads. In patients with chronic kidney disease, protein intake should be reduced to 0.5–0.8 g/kg/day.

6. Monitoring of visceral protein levels (transferrin and prealbumin) may indicate the adequacy of nutrition, but levels have not been shown to correlate with improved outcomes.

XII. Valve-Associated Problems

A. Careful follow-up is required for all patients receiving a prosthetic valve because of the risk of developing valve-related complications, including thromboembolism, endocarditis, anticoagulant-related hemorrhage, and valve degeneration.[306] It has been aptly stated that the use of a prosthetic valve replaces "one disease with another".

B. Thromboembolism. The annual risk of thromboembolism averages 1–2% for aortic valves and 2–4% for mitral valves, with a slightly higher incidence in patients with mechanical valves taking warfarin than in those with bioprosthetic valves taking only aspirin. The recommended regimens for tissue and mechanical valves are summarized in Table 13.3.[65,66]

C. **Valve thrombosis** of a mechanical valve may occur despite therapeutic anticoagulation. It is very rare with a bioprosthetic valve. Suspicion of mechanical valve thrombosis is raised by loss of valve clicks on auscultation and confirmed by fluoroscopy (Figure 2.10, page 101) or two-dimensional echocardiography. Although thrombolytic therapy can be used in selected circumstances, an immediate operation to replace the valve is usually required.

D. **Pregnancy** poses a serious problem for the woman with a prosthetic valve. The incidence of fetal wastage is 60% if warfarin is used during the first trimester, and there is a significant incidence of other congenital defects if pregnancy is completed ("coumadin embryopathy"). Tissue valves have been used for women of child-bearing age, acknowledging the limited durability of valves in this age group. Cryopreserved homograft valves or a pulmonary autograft (Ross procedure) can be considered for young women undergoing aortic valve replacement. One recommended anticoagulation regimen for women with mechanical valves who desire to become pregnant is as follows:[307]

1. Stop warfarin before conception

2. Alternatives during pregnancy

   a. Adjusted-dose UFH (usually 10,000 units SC bid to achieve a PTT of twice control) or LMWH SC bid (to maintain a 4-hour postinjection anti-Xa heparin level >0.5 units/mL) throughout pregnancy.

   b. Either UFH or LMWH as above until the 13th week of pregnancy, then warfarin with a target INR of 2.5–3.0 until the middle of the third trimester, followed by UFH or LMWH (often up to 20,000 units SC q12h) until delivery.

   c. Aspirin may be added to any of these regimens.

3. Before delivery, initiate intravenous heparin

4. With the onset of labor, give heparin 5000 units SC q8h

5. Resume warfarin after delivery

E. **Anticoagulant-related hemorrhage** is a major source of morbidity in patients receiving warfarin, especially in patients over the age of 65. In fact, it has been estimated that more than 20% of patients will experience major or minor bleeding episodes. Patient response to warfarin after surgery is quite variable, and may be related to genetic factors.[308] The use of medications that influence INR levels (most commonly amiodarone and antibiotics) must be taken into consideration when dosing warfarin. It is helpful to use an anticoagulation protocol to initiate warfarin therapy (see Table 13.4 and Appendix 8). **It is absolutely critical that careful follow-up be arranged for any patient discharged on warfarin** to avoid under- or over-anticoagulation. Home self-testing systems make it easier for patients to check their INRs and have been noted to minimize the fluctuation in the INR levels, resulting in less thromboembolism and improved survival.[309,310] In patients whose INRs are hard to regulate, concomitant administration of vitamin K 100–200 μg/day orally helps stabilize the INR.[75,76]

F. **Prosthetic valve endocarditis (PVE)** may develop at any time during the life span of a prosthetic valve with an annual risk of approximately 1–2%. Early endocarditis (within 60 days of surgery) most commonly results from infection with staphylococci (coagulase-negative >*S. aureus*), fungi, Gram-negative organisms, and enterococci. This carries a significantly higher mortality than late PVE. The latter is most commonly caused by coagulase-negative staphylococci and *Streptococcus viridans*. Clinical manifestations may include recurrent fevers, valve dysfunction with regurgitation and heart failure, cerebral or peripheral embolization, and, most ominously, the development of conduction defects resulting from a periannular abscess. The indications for surgery are noted in Chapter 1 (page 39). It is critical that the patient understand the need for prophylactic antibiotics when any dental procedure is performed. The ACC/AHA recommendations detailed in Table 13.5 should be followed.[143]

G. **Hemolysis** usually indicates the development of a paravalvular leak, and is often worse when the leak is smaller due to increased turbulence. It may also result from transvalvular leaks resulting from pannus ingrowth or thrombus formation on a mechanical valve that restricts leaflet movement and may keep one or both leaflets in a partially open fixed position. Subclinical hemolysis is manifest by elevation in the LDH and reticulocyte count. The patient may also develop mild jaundice or persistent anemia necessitating transfusion. Valve re-replacement is indicated for severe hemolysis or a significant paravalvular leak.[311]

H. **Valve failure** is defined as a complication necessitating valve replacement. Mechanical valve failure is usually caused by thrombosis, thromboembolism, endocarditis, or anticoagulation-related bleeding, and rarely by structural failure. In contrast, primary tissue failure is the most common cause of bioprosthetic dysfunction necessitating valve replacement. This occurs more readily in mitral valves, which are subject to more stress than aortic valves. Current-generation tissue valves (porcine or pericardial) generally have some form of anticalcification treatment to hopefully extend their life span. Nonetheless, early failure can occur and constant vigilance and careful follow-up examinations are essential. Bioprosthetic valve failure usually occurs gradually, and surgery can thus be performed on an elective basis at relatively low risk in contrast to the high-risk emergency surgery required for catastrophic mechanical valve failure.

XIII. Discharge Planning

A. As the length of hospital stay continues to decrease, appropriate discharge planning is essential to ensure a smooth convalescence after hospital discharge. Patients requiring additional subacute care may be transferred to rehabilitation hospitals or skilled nursing facilities for several days before going home. Even when patients are well enough to be cared for at home, it is not uncommon for separation anxiety to develop, with both patients and family members experiencing difficulty handling minor problems.

B. Appropriate discharge planning should involve the patient, family members, dietitians, nurses, and physicians. Patients must be given explicit instructions as to how they will feel, how fast they should anticipate recovery, what they must do, what they should look for, and when to contact the surgeon's office or the hospital. Several manuals are available that discuss expectations and the reestablishment of standard routines at home. Phone contact from the doctor's office is very beneficial in allaying patients' fears, answering routine questions, and dealing appropriately with potential problems. Since the definition of operative mortality extends out to 30 days after surgery, it is imperative that patients be contacted at this time to see whether they have been readmitted and see how they are faring. This should be done in order to perform appropriate outcomes analysis and submit accurate data to the Society of Thoracic Surgeons database.

C. Most patients should have an available family member or friend at home for the first week after discharge. This provides reassurance for the patient who may not yet be able to care for him- or herself, and it also provides an objective observer who is able to contact the hospital if serious problems arise.

D. **Medications.** The patient should be provided with a list and schedule of all medications. The reason each medication has been prescribed as well as possible side effects and interactions with other medications should be discussed. If the patient is receiving an anticoagulant such as **warfarin**, it is **absolutely imperative that follow-up be arranged** for prothrombin times (INR) and regulation of drug dosage. The adverse influence of alcohol, other medications, and certain foods on the level of anticoagulation must be emphasized (Appendix 10). The most commonly used medications at the time of discharge include the following:

1. **Aspirin** should be given to all CABG patients, not only to improve graft patency, but also for the secondary prevention of coronary events. Aspirin has been shown to reduce long-term mortality after CABG. It may be used alone for tissue valves or combined with warfarin for patients receiving mechanical valves.

2. **Clopidogrel** should be given in addition to aspirin to patients undergoing CABG for NSTEMIs and to those with recent drug-eluting stents. Platelet aggregometry may be beneficial in patients with stents, in whom platelet inhibition is essential to prevent thrombosis, because clopidogrel unresponsiveness is noted in 30% of patients, primarily due to genetic polymorphisms in the CYP2C19 allele. Medications that reduce the antiplatelet efficacy of clopidogrel include amiodarone and proton pump inhibitors. The latter is less significant with pantoprazole.[312]

3. **Warfarin** is prescribed for patients with atrial fibrillation, mechanical valves, and for some patients receiving tissue valves (see Table 13.3).

4. **Statins** are indicated for all patients with coronary artery disease because of their lipid-lowering and pleiotropic effects. Statins can stabilize plaque, potentially promote plaque regression, mitigate the progression of saphenous vein graft disease, and have been shown to improve the short- and long-term results of CABG and even valve surgery.[313–316] All patients taking statins should have their liver function tests checked at baseline and at 6-month intervals. Although the risk of rhabdomyolysis is low, **the risk is increased in patients taking amiodarone combined with more than 20 mg daily of simvastatin.** This interaction is less significant with atorvastatin (Lipitor) and not seen with rosuvastatin (Crestor) or pravastatin (Pravachol).

5. **β-blockers** are generally prescribed following CABG because of documented survival benefits in postinfarction patients treated medically or undergoing CABG, but they have also been shown to improve long-term survival even in CABG patients with no prior MI or heart failure.[317–319] Carvedilol is often used in patients with impaired LV function. Otherwise, metoprolol is the most commonly

prescribed β-blocker and is benefical for control of hypertension as well. The benefit of continuing β-blockers for AF prophylaxis after discharge is unclear.

6. **Amiodarone** may be continued for prophylaxis of atrial fibrillation, although the optimal duration of therapy is not defined. It can usually be stopped after a couple of weeks if the patient has remained in sinus rhythm. It is recommended for several months following a Maze procedure. Amiodarone can affect hepatic, thyroid, and pulmonary function, so any patient in whom therapy is anticipated beyond one month should have LFTs, thyroid function tests, and pulmonary function tests obtained at baseline. There is a long list of medications that should not be used along with amiodarone available at www.prescribersletter.com.[320] Particular concerns are that amiodarone:

    a. Decreases the metabolism of warfarin, necessitating a 25–50% reduction in warfarin dosing.

    b. Reduces platelet inhibition by clopidogrel.

    c. Increases QT prolongation when used concurrently with fluoroquinolones (ciprofloxacin, levofloxacin), 5-HT_3 antagonists (ondansetron), or haloperidol. These medications are generally contraindicated if amiodarone is being used.

    d. Enhances bradycardia with β-blockers or calcium channel blockers.

7. **ACE inhibitors** are recommended as the preferred antihypertensive drug after surgery, especially in patients with LV dysfunction. Although short-term mortality benefits have not been demonstrated, ACE inhibitors may provide long-term mortality benefits.[319]

E. Prophylactic antibiotics. Any patient who has received prosthetic material (valves or grafts) must be aware of the necessity of prophylactic antibiotics if dental work is contemplated. Patients should be told to inform their physician or dentist accordingly and follow the ACC/AHA guidelines for antibiotic prophylaxis delineated in Table 13.5.[143]

F. Diet. Dieticians should meet with patients before discharge to discuss the particular dietary restrictions for their cardiac disease. This entails discussions of the significance of low-cholesterol or low-salt diets and the provision of appropriate dietary plans.

G. The patient must participate in self-evaluation at home. A daily assessment of pulse rate, oral temperature, and weight should be performed, and all incisions should be inspected for redness, tenderness, or drainage. Visiting nurses are usually recommended for patients discharged home to help with these assessments. Patients should be instructed to contact their physician's office if any abnormalities are noted.

H. Patients should be encouraged to gradually increase their activity as tolerated. Patients with a median sternotomy incision should be discouraged from lifting objects weighing more than 10–15 pounds because it puts strain on the healing sternum. Driving should be avoided for 6 weeks. In contrast, there are few physical limitations on patients who have small thoracotomy incisions for minimally invasive surgery.

I. Lifestyle modification and control of all modifiable risk factors are essential to optimize the long-term results of surgery. These include weight loss, cessation of smoking (with pharmacologic agents initially), and control of dyslipidemias, diabetes, and hypertension. Involvement in cardiac rehabilitation programs is an important aspect of long-term care following surgery.[311,315]

References

1. McGee DC, Gould MK. Preventing complications of central venous catheterization. *N Engl J Med* 2003;348:1123–33.

2. Tripp HF, Bolton JW. Phrenic nerve injury following cardiac surgery: a review. *J Card Surg* 1998;13:218–23.

3. Dimopoulou I, Daganou M, Dafni U, et al. Phrenic nerve dysfunction after cardiac operations. Electrophysiologic evaluation of risk factors. *Chest* 1998;113:8–14.

4. Canbaz S, Turgut N, Halici U, Balci F, Ege T, Duran E. Electrophysiological evaluation of phrenic nerve injury during cardiac surgery – a prospective, controlled, clinical study. *BMC Surg* 2004;4:2.

5. Mills GH, Khan ZP, Moxham J, Desai J, Forsyth A, Ponte J. Effects of temperature on phrenic nerve and diaphragmatic function during cardiac surgery. *Br J Anaesth* 1997;79:726–32.

6. Cassese M, Martinelli G, Nasso G, et al. Topical cooling for myocardial protection: the results of a prospective randomized study of the "shallow technique". *J Card Surg* 2006;21:357–62.

7. Deng Y, Byth K, Paterson HS. Phrenic nerve injury associated with high free right internal mammary artery harvesting. *Ann Thorac Surg* 2003;76:459–63.

8. Merino-Ramirez MA, Juan G, Ramon M, et al. Electrophysiologic evaluation of phrenic nerve and diaphragm function after coronary bypass surgery: prospective study of diabetes and other risk factors. *J Thorac Cardiovasc Surg* 2006;132:530–6.

9. Sharma AD, Parmley CL, Sreeram G, Grocott HP. Peripheral nerve injuries during cardiac surgery: risk factors, diagnosis, prognosis, and prevention. *Anesth Analg* 2000;91:1358–69.

10. Cruz-Martinez A, Armijo A, Fermoso A, Moraleda S, Maté I, Marin M. Phrenic nerve conduction study in demyelinating neuropathies and open-heart surgery. *Clin Neurophysiol* 2000;111:821–5.

11. Katz MG, Katz R, Schachner A, Cohen AJ. Phrenic nerve injury after coronary artery bypass grafting: will it go away? *Ann Thorac Surg* 1998;65:32–5.

12. Elefteriades J, Singh M, Tang P, et al. Unilateral diaphragm paralysis: etiology, impact, and natural history. *J Cardiovasc Surg (Torino)* 2008;49:289–95.

13. Versteegh MI, Braun J, Voigt PG, et al. Diaphragm plication in adult patients with diaphragm paralysis leads to long-term improvement of pulmonary function and level of dyspnea. *Eur J Cardiothorac Surg* 2007;32:449–56.

14. Huttl TP, Wichmann MW, Reichart B, Geiger TK, Schildberg FW, Meyer G. Laparoscopic diaphragmatic plication: long-term results of a novel surgical technique for postoperative phrenic nerve palsy. *Surg Endosc* 2004;18:547–51.

15. Goldhaber SZ, Schoepf UJ. Pulmonary embolism after coronary artery bypass grafting. *Circulation* 2004;109:2712–5.

16. Goldhaber SZ, Hirsch DR, MacDougall RC, Polak JF, Creager MA, Cohn LH. Prevention of venous thrombosis after coronary artery bypass surgery (a randomized trial comparing two mechanical prophylaxis strategies). *Am J Cardiol* 1995;76:993–6.

17. Schwann TA, Kistler L, Engoren MC, Habib RH. Incidence and predictors of postoperative deep vein thrombosis in cardiac surgery in the era of aggressive thromboprophylaxis. *Ann Thorac Surg* 2010;90:760–8.

18. Bednar F, Osmancik P, Hlavicka J, Jedlickova V, Paluch Z, Vanek T. Aspirin is insufficient in inhibition of platelet aggregation and thromboxane formation early after coronary artery bypass surgery. *J Thromb Thrombolysis* 2009;27:394–9.

19. Cartier RE, Robitaille D. Thrombotic complications in beating heart operations. *J Thorac Cardiovasc Surg* 2001;121:920–22.

20. Dunning J, Versteegh M, Fabbri A, et al. Guidelines on antiplatelet and anticoagulation management in cardiac surgery. *Eur J Cardiothorac Surg* 2008;34:73–92.

21. Close VT, Purohit M, Tanos M, Hunter S. Should patients post-cardiac surgery be given low molecular weight heparin for deep-vein thrombosis prophylaxis. *Interact Cardiovasc Thorac Surg* 2006;5:624–9.

22. Geerts WH, Bergqvist D, Pineo GF, et al. Prevention of venous thromboembolism. American College of Chest Physicians evidence-based clinical practice guidelines (8th edition). *Chest* 2008;133:381S–453S.

23. Ramos R, Salem BI, De Pawlikowski MP, Coordes C, Eisenberg S, Leidenfrost R. The efficacy of pneumatic compression stockings in the prevention of pulmonary embolism after cardiac surgery. *Chest* 1996;109:82–5.

24. Ambrosetti M, Ageno W, Salerno M, Pedretti RF. Postoperative pericardial effusion in patients receiving anticoagulants for deep vein thrombosis after coronary artery bypass graft surgery. *J Thromb Haemost* 2005;3:2367–8.

25. Jones HU, Mulestein JB, Jones KW, et al. Early postoperative use of unfractionated heparin or enoxaparin is associated with increased surgical re-exploration for bleeding. *Ann Thorac Surg* 2005;80:519–22.

26. Moores LK, Holley AB. Computed tomography pulmonary angiography and venography: diagnostic and prognostic properties. *Semin Respir Crit Care Med* 2008;29:3–14.

27. Wang F, Fang W, Lv B, et al. Comparison of lung scintigraphy with multi-slice spiral computed tomography in the diagnosis of pulmonary embolism. *Clin Nucl Med* 2009;34:424–7.

28. Kucher N. Catheter embolectomy for acute pulmonary embolism. *Chest* 2007;132:657–63.

29. Eid-Lidt G, Gaspar J, Sandoval J, et al. Combined clot fragmentation and aspiration in patients with acute pulmonary embolism. *Chest* 2008;134:54–60.

30. Digonnet A, Moya-Plana A, Aubert S, et al. Acute pulmonary embolism: a current surgical approach. *Interact Cardiovasc Thorac Surg* 2007;6:27–9.

31. Baerman JM, Kirsh MM, de Buitleir M, et al. Natural history and determinants of conduction defects following coronary artery bypass surgery. *Ann Thorac Surg* 1987;44:150–3.

32. Glikson M, Dearani JA, Hyberger LK, Schaff HV, Hammill SC, Hayes DL. Indications, effectiveness, and long-term dependency on permanent pacing after cardiac surgery. *Am J Cardiol* 1997;80:1309–13.

33. Kimmelstiel CD, Udelson JE, Salem DN, Bojar R, Rastegar H, Konstam MA. Recurrent angina caused by a left internal mammary artery-to-pulmonary artery fistula. *Am Heart J* 1993;125:234–6.

34. Pepi M, Muratori M, Barbier P, et al. Pericardial effusion after cardiac surgery: incidence, site, size, and haemodynamic consequences. *Br Heart J* 1994;72:327–31.

35. Kuvin JT, Harati NA, Pandian NG, Bojar RM, Khabbaz KR. Postoperative cardiac tamponade in the modern surgical era. *Ann Thorac Surg* 2000;74:1148–53.

36. Wessman DE, Stafford CM. The postcardiac surgery syndrome: case report and review of the literature. *South Med J* 2006;99:309–14.

37. Tsang TS, Barnes ME, Hayes SN, et al. Clinical and echocardiographic characteristics of significant pericardial effusions following cardiothoracic surgery and outcomes of echo-guided pericardiocentesis for management: Mayo Clinic experience, 1979–1998. *Chest* 1999;116:322–31.

38. Saito Y, Donohue A, Attai S, et al. The syndrome of cardiac tamponade with "small" pericardial effusion. *Echocardiography* 2008;25:321–7.

39. Imren Y, Tasoglu I, Oktar GL, et al. The importance of transesophageal echocardiography in diagnosis of pericardial tamponade after cardiac surgery. *J Card Surg* 2008;23:450–3.

40. Imazio M. Cecchi E, Demichelis B, et al. Rationale and design of the COPPS trial: a randomised, placebo-controlled, multicentre study on the use of colchicine for the primary prevention of postpericardiotomy syndrome. *J Cardiovasc Med (Hagerstown)* 2007;8:1044–8.

41. Bakhshandeh AR, Salehi M, Radmehr F, Sattarzadeh R, Nasr AR, Sadeghpour AH. Postoperative pericardial effusion and posterior pericardiotomy, related or not? *Heart Surg Forum* 2009;12: E113–5.

42. Horneffer PJ, Miller RH, Pearson TA, Rykiel MF, Reitz BA, Gardner TJ. The effective treatment of postpericardiotomy syndrome after cardiac operations. A randomized placebo-controlled trial. *J Thorac Cardiovasc Surg* 1990;100:292–6.

43. Hoffman M, Fried M, Jabareen F, et al. Anti-heart antibodies in postpericardiotomy syndrome: cause or epiphenomenon? A prospective, longitudinal pilot study. *Autoimmunity* 2002;35:241–5.

44. Kocazeybek B, Erenturk S, Calyk MK, Babacan F. An immunological approach to postpericardiotomy syndrome occurrence and its relation to autoimmunity. *Acta Chir Belg* 1998;98:203–6.

45. Köhler I, Saraiva PJ, Wender OB, Zago AJ. Behavior of inflammatory markers of myocardial injury in cardiac surgery: laboratory correlation with the clinical picture of postpericardiotomy syndrome. *Arq Bras Cardiol* 2003;81:279–90.

46. Kurth T, Glynn RJ, Walker AM, et al. Inhibition of clinical benefits of aspirin on first myocardial infarction by nonsteroidal anti-inflammatory drugs. *Circulation* 2003;108:1191–5.

47. Matsuyama K, Matsumoto M, Sugita T, et al. Clinical characteristics of patients with constrictive pericarditis after coronary bypass surgery. *Jpn Circ J* 2001;65:480–2.

48. Anderson CA, Rodriguez E, Shammas RL, Kypson AP. Early constrictive epicarditis after coronary artery bypass surgery. *Ann Thorac Surg* 2009;87:642–3.

49. Liao P, DeSantis AJ, Schmeltz LR, et al. Insulin resistance following cardiothoracic surgery in patients with and without a preoperative diagnosis of type 2 diabetes during treatment with intravenous insulin therapy for postoperative hyperglycemia. *J Diabetes Complications* 2008;22:229–34.

50. Ascione R, Rogers CA, Rajakaruna C, Angelini GD. Inadequate blood glucose control is associated with in-hospital mortality and morbidity in diabetic and nondiabetic patients undergoing cardiac surgery. *Circulation* 2008;118:113–23.

51. Ouattara A, Lecomte P, Le Manach Y, et al. Poor intraoperative blood glucose control is associated with worsened hospital outcome after cardiac surgery in diabetic patients. *Anesthesiology* 2005;103:687–94.

52. Lazar HL, McDonnell M, Chipkin SR, et al. The Society of Thoracic Surgeons practice guidelines series: blood glucose management during adult cardiac surgery. *Ann Thorac Surg* 2009;87:663–9.

53. Saltzman DJ, Chang JC, Jimenez JC, et al. Postoperative thrombotic thrombocytopenic purpura after open heart operations. *Ann Thorac Surg* 2010;89:119–23.

54. Warkentin TE, Greinacher A, Koster A, Lincoff AM. Treatment and prevention of heparin-induced thrombocytopenia. American College of Chest Physicians evidence-based clinical practice guidelines (8th edition). *Chest* 2008;133:340S–80S.

55. Shantsila E, Lip GYH, Chong BH. Heparin-induced thrombocytopenia. A contemporary clinical approach to diagnosis and management. *Chest* 2009;135:1651–64.

56. Bauer TL, Arepally G, Konkle BA, et al. Prevalence of heparin-associated antibodies without thrombosis in patients undergoing cardiopulmonary bypass surgery. *Circulation* 1997;95:1242–6.

57. Everett BM, Yeh R, Foo SY, et al. Prevalence of heparin/platelet factor 4 antibodies before and after cardiac surgery. *Ann Thorac Surg* 2007;83:592–7.

58. Greinacher A, Levy JH. HIT happens: diagnosing and evaluating the patient with heparin-induced thrombocytopenia. *Anesth Analg* 2008;107:356–8.

59. Pappalardo F, Scandroglio A, Maj G, Zangrillo A, D'Angelo A. Treatment of heparin-induced thrombocytopenia after cardiac surgery: preliminary experience with fondaparinux. *J Thorac Cardiovasc Surg* 2010;139:70–2.

60. Becker RC, Meade TW, Berger PB, et al. The primary and secondary prevention of coronary artery disease. American College of Chest Physicians evidence-based clinical practice guidelines (8th edition). *Chest* 2008;133:776S–814S.

61. Ferraris VA, Ferraris SP, Moliterno DJ, et al. The Society of Thoracic Surgeons practice guideline series: aspirin and other antiplatelet agents during operative coronary revascularization (executive summary). *Ann Thorac Surg* 2005;79:1454–61.

62. Gao C, Ren C, Li D, Li L. Clopidogrel and aspirin versus clopidogrel alone on graft patency after coronary artery bypass grafting. *Ann Thorac Surg* 2009;88:59–63.

63. Kim DH, Daskalakis C, Silvertry SC, et al. Aspirin and clopidogrel use in the early postoperative period following on-pump and off-pump coronary artery bypass grafting. *J Thorac Cardiovasc Surg* 2009;138:1377–84.

64. Lim E, Cornelissen J, Routledge T, et al. Clopidogrel did not inhibit platelet function early after coronary bypass surgery: a prospective randomized trial. *J Thorac Cardiovasc Surg* 2004;128:432–5.

65. Salem DN, O'Gara PT, Madias C, Pauker SP. Valvular and structural heart disease. American College of Chest Physicians evidence-based clinical practice guidelines (8th edition). *Chest* 2008;133:593S–629S.

66. Bonow RO, Carabello BA, Chatterjee K, et al. 2008 focused update incorporated into the ACC/ AHA 2006 guidelines for the management of patients with valvular heart disease. A report of the American College of Cardiology/American Heart Association task force on practice guidelines (Writing committee to revise the 1998 guidelines for the management of patients with valvular heart disease). Endorsed by the Society of Cardiovascular Anesthesiologists, Society for Cardiovascular Angiography and Interventions, and Society of Thoracic Surgeons. *J Am Coll Cardiol* 2008;52:e1–142 (available at acc.org).

67. Oprea D, Memet R, Jovin A, et al. Anticoagulation at discharge after mitral valve repair and long-term mortality. *Circulation* 2006;114:II–734.

68. Asopa S, Patel A, Dunning J. Is short-term anticoagulation necessary after mitral valve repair? *Interact Cardiovasc Thorac Surg* 2006;5:761–5.

69. Kulik A, Rubens FD, Wells PS, et al. Early postoperative anticoagulation after mechanical valve replacement; a systematic review. *Ann Thorac Surg* 2006;81:770–81.

70. Meurin P, Tabet JY, Weber H, Renaud N, Ben Driss A. Low-molecular-weight heparin as a bridging anticoagulant early after mechanical valve replacement. *Circulation* 2006;113:564–9.

71. Steger V, Bail DH, Graf D, Walker T, Rittig K, Ziemer G. A practical approach for bridging anticoagulation after mechanical heart valve replacement. *J Heart Valve Dis* 2008;17:335–42.

72. Ansell J, Hirsh J, Hylek E, Jacobson A, Crowther M, Palareti G. Pharmacology and management of the vitamin K antagonists. American College of Chest Physicians evidence-based clinical practice guidelines (8th edition). *Chest* 2008;133:160S–98S.

73. Johnson SG, Rogers K, Delate T, Witt DM. Outcomes associated with combined antiplatelet and anticoagulant therapy. *Chest* 2008;133:948–54.

74. Schalekamp T, Klungel OH, Souverein PC, de Boer A. Effect of oral antiplatelet agents on major bleeding in users of coumarins. *Thromb Haemostat* 2008;100:1076–83.

75. Reese AM, Farnett LE, Lyons RM, Patel B, Morgan L, Bussey HI. Low-dose vitamin K to augment anticoagulation control. *Pharmacotherapy* 2005;25:1746–51.

76. Sconce E, Avery P, Wynne H, Kamali F. Vitamin K supplementation can improve stability of anticoagulation for patients with unexplained variability in response to warfarin. *Blood* 2007;109:2419–23.

77. Garey KW, Lai D, Dao-Tran TK, Gentry LO, Hwang LY, Davis BR. Interrupted time series analysis of vancomycin compared to cefuroxime for surgical prophylaxis in patients undergoing cardiac surgery. *Antimicrob Agents Chemother* 2008;52:446–51.

78. Engelman RM, Shahian DM, Shemin R, et al. The Society of Thoracic Surgeons practice guidelines series: antibiotic prophylaxis in cardiac surgery, Part II: Antibiotic Choice. *Ann Thorac Surg* 2007;83:1569–76.

79. Edwards FH, Engelman RM, Houck P, Shahian DM, Bridges CR. The Society of Thoracic Surgeons practice guideline series: antibiotic prophylaxis in cardiac surgery, Part I: Duration. *Ann Thorac Surg* 2006;81:397–404.

80. Rosmarakis ES, Prapas SN, Rellos K, Michalopoulos A, Samonis G, Falagas ME. Nosocomial infections after off-pump coronary artery bypass surgery: frequency, characteristics, and risk factors. *Interact Cardiovasc Thorac Surg* 2007;6:759–67.

81. De Santo LS, Bancone C, Santarpino G, et al. Microbiologically documented nosocomial infections after cardiac surgery: an 18-month prospective tertiary care centre report. *Eur J Cardiothorac Surg* 2008;33:666–72.

82. Michalopolous A, Geroulanos S, Rosmarakis ES, Falagas ME. Frequency, characteristics, and predictors of microbiologically documented nosocomial infections after cardiac surgery. *Eur J Cardiothorac Surg* 2006;29:456–60.

83. Pawar M, Mehta Y, Kapoor P, Sharma J, Gupta A, Trehan N. Central venous catheter-related blood stream infections: incidence, risk factors, outcome, and associated pathogens. *J Cardiothorac Vasc Anesth* 2004;18:304–8.

84. Leal-Noval SR, Marquez-Vácaro JA, García-Curiel A, et al. Nosocomial pneumonia in patients undergoing heart surgery. *Crit Care Med* 2000;28:935–40.

85. Fowler VG, O'Brien SM, Muhlbaier LH, Corey GR, Ferguson TB, Peterson ED. Clinical predictors of major infections after cardiac surgery. *Circulation* 2005; 112(9 Suppl):I–358–65.

86. Reddy SL, Grayson AD, Smith G, Warwick R, Chalmers JA. Methicillin resistant Staphylococcus aureus infections following cardiac surgery: incidence, impact and identifying adverse outcome traits. *Eur J Cardiothorac Surg* 2007;32:113–7.

87. Mastoraki A, Kriaras I, Douka E, Mastoraki S, Stravopodis G, Geroulanos S. Methicillin-resistant Staphylococcus aureus preventing strategy in cardiac surgery. *Interact Cardiovasc Thorac Surg* 2008;7:452–6.

88. Muñoz P, Hortal J, Giannella M, et al. Nasal carriage of S. aureus increases the risk of surgical site infection after major heart surgery. *J Hosp Infect* 2008;68:25–31.

89. Jog S, Cunningham R, Cooper S, et al. Impact of preoperative screening for methicillin-resistant Staphylococus aureus by real-time polymerase chain reaction in patients undergoing cardiac surgery. *J Hosp Infect* 2008;69:124–30.

90. Shrestha NK, Banbury MK, Weber M, et al. Safety of targeted perioperative mupirocin treatment for preventing infections after cardiac surgery. *Ann Thorac Surg* 2006;81:2183–8.

91. Tom TSM, Kruse MW, Reichman RT. Update: methicillin-resistant Staphylococcus aureus screening and decolonization in cardiac surgery. *Ann Thorac Surg* 2009;88:695–702.

92. Segers P, Speekenbrink RGH, Ubbink DT, van Ogtrop ML, de Mol BA. Prevention of nosocomial infection in cardiac surgery by decontamination of the nasopharynx and oropharnyx with chlorhexidine gluconate. A randomized controlled trial. *JAMA* 2006;296:2460–6.

93. Tantipong H, Morkchareonpong C, Jaiyindee S, Thamlikitkul V. Randomized controlled trial and meta-analysis of oral decontamination with 2% chlorhexidine solution for the prevention of ventilator-associated pneumonia. *Infect Control Hosp Epidemiol* 2008;29:131–6.

94. Carrel TP, Eisinger E, Vogt M, Turina MI. Pneumonia after cardiac surgery is predictable by tracheal aspirates but cannot be prevented by prolonged antibiotic prophylaxis. *Ann Thorac Surg* 2001;72:143–8.

95. Ferraris VA, Ferraris SP, Saha SP, et al. Perioperative blood transfusion and blood conservation in cardiac surgery: the Society of Thoracic Surgeons and the Society of Cardiovascular Anesthesiologists clinical practice guidelines. *Ann Thorac Surg* 2007;83(5 suppl):S27–86.

96. Russell JA. Management of sepsis. *N Engl J Med* 2006;355:1699–713.

97. Michalopoulos A, Stavridis G, Geroulanos S. Severe sepsis in cardiac surgical patients. *Eur J Surg* 1998;164:217–22.

98. Otero RM, Nguyen HB, Huang DT, et al. Early goal-directed therapy in severe sepsis and septic shock revisited. Concepts, controversies, and contemporary findings. *Chest* 2006;130:1579–95.

99. Dellinger RP. Cardiovascular management of septic shock. *Crit Care Med* 2003;31:946–55.

100. Friedman ND, Bull AL, Russo PL, et al. An alternative scoring system to predict risk for surgical site infection complicating coronary artery bypass graft surgery. *Infect Control Hosp Epidemiol* 2007;28:1162–8.

101. Paul M, Raz A, Leibovici L, Madar H, Holinger R, Rubinovitch B. Sternal wound infection after coronary artery bypass graft surgery: validation of existing risk score. *J Thorac Cardiovasc Surg* 2007;133:397–403.

102. Lu JC, Grayson AD, Jha P, Srinivasan AK, Fabri BM. Risk factors for sternal wound infection and mid-term survival following coronary artery bypass surgery. *Eur J Cardiothorac Surg* 2003;23:943–9.

103. Elenbaas TWO, Hamad MAS, Schönberger JPAM, Martens EJ, van Zundert AAJ, van Straten AHM. Preoperative atrial fibrillation and elevated C-reactive protein levels as predictors of mediastinitis afer coronary artery bypass grafting. *Ann Thorac Surg* 2010;89:704–9.

104. Toumpoulis IK, Anagnostopolous CE, DeRose JJ Jr, Swistel DG. The impact of deep sternal wound infection on long-term survival after coronary artery bypass grafting. *Chest* 2005;127:464–71.

105. Centofani P, Savia F, La Torre M, et al. A prospective study of prevalence of 60-days postoperative wound infections after cardiac surgery. An updated risk factor analysis. *J Cardiovasc Surg (Torino)* 2007;48:641–6.

106. Gummert JF, Barten MJ, Hans C, et al. Mediastinitis and cardiac surgery – an updated risk factor analysis in 10,373 consecutive adult patients. *Thorac Cardiovasc Surg* 2002;50:87–91.

107. Gansera B, Schmidtler F, Gillrath G, et al. Does bilateral ITA grafting increase perioperative complications? Outcome of 4462 patients with bilateral versus 4204 patients with single ITA bypass. *Eur J Cardiothorac Surg* 2006;30:318–23.

108. Nakano J, Okabayashi H, Hanyu M, et al. Risk factors for wound infection after off-pump coronary artery bypass grafting: should bilateral internal thoracic arteries be harvested in patients with diabetes? *J Thorac Cardiovasc Surg* 2008;135:540–5.

109. Baskett RJF, MacDougall CE, Ross DB. Is mediastinitis a preventable complication? A 10-year review. *Ann Thorac Surg* 1999;67:462–5.

110. Steingrímsson S, Gustafsson R, Gudbjartsson T, Mokhtari A, Ingemansson R, Sjögren J. Sternocutaneous fistulas after cardiac surgery: incidence and late outcome during a ten-year follow-up. *Ann Thorac Surg* 2009;88:1910–5.

111. Swenne CL, Lindholm C, Borowiec J, Schnell AE, Carlsson M. Peri-operative glucose control and development of surgical wound infections in patients undergoing coronary artery bypass graft. *J Hosp Infect* 2005;61:201–12.

112. Kühme T, Isaksson B, Dahlin LG. Wound contamination in cardiac surgery. A systematic quantitative and qualitative study of the bacterial growth in sternal wounds in cardiac surgery patients. *APMIS* 2007;115:1001–7.

113. Bouza E, Muñoz P, Alcalá L, et al. Cultures of sternal wound and mediastinitis taken at the end of heart surgery do not predict postsurgical mediastinitis. *Diagn Microbiol Infect Dis* 2006;56:345–9.

114. Dohmen PM, Gabbieri D, Weymann A, Linneweber J, Konertz W. Reduction in surgical site infection in patients treated with microbial sealant prior to coronary artery bypass graft surgery: a case–control study. *J Hosp Infect* 2009;72:119–26.

115. Saso S, James D, Vecht JA, et al. Effect of skeletonization of the internal thoracic artery for coronary revascularization on the incidence of sternal wound infection. *Ann Thorac Surg* 2010;89:661–70.

116. Khalafi RS, Bradford DW, Wilson MG. Topical application of autologous blood products during surgical closure following a coronary artery bypass graft. *Eur J Cardiothorac Surg* 2008;34:360–4.

117. Vander Salm TJ, Okike ON, Pasque MK, et al. Reduction of sternal infection by application of topical vancomycin. *J Thorac Cardiovasc Surg* 1989;98:618–22.

118. Friberg O, Svedjeholm R, Söderquist B, Granfeldt H, Vikerfors T, Källman J. Local gentamicin reduces sternal wound infections after cardiac surgery: a randomized controlled trial. *Ann Thorac Surg* 2005;79:153–62.

119. Tegnell A, Arén C, Öhman L. Coagulase-negative staphylococci and sternal infections after cardiac operation. *Ann Thorac Surg* 2000;69:1104–9.

120. Francel TJ, Kouchoukos NT. A rational approach to wound difficulties after sternotomy: the problem. *Ann Thorac Surg* 2001;72:1411–8.

121. El Oakley RM, Wright JE. Postoperative mediastinitis: classification and management. *Ann Thorac Surg* 1996;61:1030–6.

122. Benlolo S, Matéo J, Raskine L, et al. Sternal puncture allows an early diagnosis of poststernotomy mediastinitis. *J Thorac Cardiovasc Surg* 2003;125:611–7.

123. Misawa Y, Fuse K, Hasegawa T. Infectious mediastinitis after cardiac operations: computed tomographic findings. *Ann Thorac Surg* 1998;65:622–4.

124. Bitkover CY, Gårdlund B, Larsson SA, Åberg B, Jacobsson H. Diagnosing sternal wound infections with 99mTc-labeled monoclonal granulocyte antibody scintigraphy. *Ann Thorac Surg* 1996;62:1412–6.

125. Oates E, Payne DD. Postoperative cardiothoracic infection: diagnostic value of indium-111 white blood cell imaging. *Ann Thorac Surg* 1994;58:1442–6.

126. Poncelet AJ, Lengele B, Delaere B, et al. Algorithm for primary closure in sternal wound infection: a single institution 10-year experience. *Eur J Cardiothorac Surg* 2008;33:232–8.

127. Shrager JB, Wain JC, Wright CD, et al. Omentum is highly effective in the management of complex cardiothoracic surgical problems. *J Thorac Cardiovasc Surg* 2003;125:526–32.

128. Berg HF, Brands WGB, van Geldorp TR, Kluytmans-VandenBergh MFQ, Kluytmans JAJW. Comparison between closed drainage techniques for the treatment of postoperative mediastinitis. *Ann Thorac Surg* 2000;70:924–9.

129. Cartier R, Diaz OS, Carrier M, Leclerc Y, Castonguay Y, Leung TK. Right ventricular rupture. A complication of postoperative mediastinitis. *J Thorac Cardiovasc Surg* 1993;106:1036–9.

130. Roh TS, Lee WJ, Lew DH, Tark KC. Pectoralis major–rectus abdominal bipedicled muscle flap in the treatment of poststernotomy mediastinitis. *J Thorac Cardiovasc Surg* 2008;136:618–22.

131. Immer FF, Durrer M, Muhlemann KS, Erni D, Gahl B, Carrel TP. Deep sternal wound infection after cardiac surgery: modality of treatment and outcome. *Ann Thorac Surg* 2005;80:957–61.

132. Fuchs U, Zittermann A, Stuettgen B, Groening A, Minami K, Koerfer R. Clinical outcome of patients with deep sternal wound infection managed by vacuum-assisted closure compared to conventional therapy with open packing: a retrospective analysis. *Ann Thorac Surg* 2005;79:526–31.

133. Sjögren J, Gustafsson R, Nilsson J, Malmsjö M, Ingemansson R. Clinical outcome after poststernotomy mediastinitis: vacuum-assisted closure versus conventional treatment. *Ann Thorac Surg* 2005;79:2049–55.

134. Moktari A, Petzina R, Gustafsson L, Sjogren J, Malmsjo M, Ingemansson R. Sternal stability at different negative pressures during vacuum-assisted closure therapy. *Ann Thorac Surg* 2006;82:1063–7.

135. Sartipy U, Lockowandt U, Gäbel J, Jidéus L, Dellgren G. Cardiac rupture during vacuum-assisted closure therapy. *Ann Thorac Surg* 2006;82:1110–1.

136. Malmsjo M, Petzina R, Ugander M, et al. Preventing heart injury during negative pressure wound therapy in cardiac surgery: assessment using real-time magnetic resonance imaging. *J Thorac Cardiovasc Surg* 2009;138:712–7.

137. Lepelletier D, Poupelin L, Corvec S, et al. Risk factors for mortality in patients with mediastinitis after cardiac surgery. *Arch Cardiovasc Dis* 2009;102:119–25.

138. Huh J, Bakeen F, Chu D, Wall MJ Jr. Transverse sternal plating in secondary sternal reconstruction. *J Thorac Cardiovasc Surg* 2008;136:1476–8.

139. Plass A, Grünenfelder J, Reuthebuch O, et al. New transverse plate fixation system for complicated sternal wound infection after median sternotomy. *Ann Thorac Surg* 2007;83:1210–2.

140. Reed JF III. Leg wound infections following greater saphenous vein harvesting: minimally invasive vein harvesting versus conventional vein harvesting. *Int J Low Extrem Wounds* 2008;7:210–9.

141. Aziz O, Athanasiou T, Darzi A. Minimally invasive conduit harvesting: a systematic review. *Eur J Cardiothorac Surg* 2006;29:324–33.

142. Allen KB, Fitzgerald EB, Heimansohn DA, Shaar CJ. Management of closed space infections associated with endoscopic vein harvest. *Ann Thorac Surg* 2000;69:960–1.

143. Wilson W, Taubert KA, Gewitz M, et al. Prevention of infective endocarditis: guidelines from the American Heart Association: a guideline from the American Heart Association Rheumatic Fever, Endocarditis, and Kawasaki Disease Committee, Council on Cardiovascular Disease in the Young, and the Council on Clinical Cardiology, Council on Cardiovascular Surgery and Anesthesia, and the Quality of Care and Outcomes Research Interdisciplinary Working Group. *Circulation* 2007;116:1736–54 (available at www.acc.org).

144. Nishimura R, Carabello BA, Faxon DP, et al. ACC/AHA 2008 guideline update on valvular heart disease: focused update on infective endocarditis. A report of the American College of Cardiology/American Heart Association Task Force on practice guidelines. *J Am Coll Cardiol* 2008;52:676–85.

145. Newman MF, Mathew JP, Grocott HP, et al. Central nervous system injury associated with cardiac surgery. *Lancet* 2006;368:694–703.

146. Marasco SF, Sharwood LN, Abramson MJ. No improvement in neurocognitive outcomes after off-pump versus on-pump coronary revascularisation: a meta-analysis. *Eur J Cardiothorac Surg* 2008;33:961–70.

147. Filsoufi F, Rahmanian PB, Castillo JG, Bronster D, Adams DH. Incidence, topography, predictors and long-term survival after stroke in patients undergoing coronary artery bypass grafting. *Ann Thorac Surg* 2008;85:862–71.

148. Bucerius J, Gummert JF, Borger MA, et al. Stroke after cardiac surgery: a risk factor analysis of 16,184 consecutive adult patients. *Ann Thorac Surg* 2003;75:472–8.

149. Nishiyama K, Horiguchi M, Shizuta S, et al. Temporal pattern of strokes after on-pump and off-pump coronary artery bypass graft surgery. *Ann Thorac Surg* 2009;87:1839–4.

150. Charlesworth DC, Likosky DS, Marrin CAS, et al. Development and validation of a prediction model for strokes after coronary artery bypass grafting. *Ann Thorac Surg* 2003;76:436–43.

151. Filsoufi F, Rahmanian PB, Castillo JG, Bronster D, Adams DH. Incidence, imaging analysis, and early and late outcomes of stroke after cardiac valve operation. *Am J Cardiol* 2008;101:1472–8.

152. Aboyans V, Labrousse L, Lacroix P, et al. Predictive factors of stroke in patients undergoing coronary bypass grafting: statins are protective. *Eur J Cardiothorac Surg* 2006;30:300–4.

153. Baker RA, Hallsworth LJ, Knight JL. Stroke after coronary artery bypass grafting. *Ann Thorac Surg* 2005;80:1746–50.

154. Likosky DS, Leavitt BJ, Marrin CAS, et al. Intra- and postoperative predictors of stroke after coronary artery bypass grafting. *Ann Thorac Surg* 2003;76:428–35.

155. Redmond JM, Greene PS, Goldsborough MA, et al. Neurologic injury in cardiac surgical patients with a history of stroke. *Ann Thorac Surg* 1996;61:42–7.

156. Maekawa K, Goto T, Baba T, Yoshitake A, Morishita S, Koshiji T. Abnormalities in the brain before elective cardiac surgery detected by diffusion-weighted magnetic resonance imaging. *Ann Thorac Surg* 2008;86:1563–9.

157. Boivie P, Edström C, Engström KG. Side differences in cerebrovascular accidents after cardiac surgery: a statistical analysis of neurologic symptoms and possible implications for anatomic mechanisms of aortic particle embolization. *J Thorac Cardiovasc Surg* 2005;129:591–8.

158. Kapetanakis EI, Stamou SC, Dullum MKC, et al. The impact of aortic manipulation on neurologic outcomes after coronary artery bypass surgery: a risk-adjusted study. *Ann Thorac Surg* 2004;78:1564–71.

159. Nakamura M, Okamoto F, Nakanishi K, et al. Does intensive management of cerebral hemodynamics and atheromatous aorta reduce stroke after coronary artery surgery? *Ann Thorac Surg* 2008;85:513–9.

160. Clark RE, Brillman J, Davis DA, Lovell MR, Price TRP, Magovern GJ. Microemboli during coronary artery artery bypass grafting. Genesis and effect on outcome. *J Thorac Cardiovasc Surg* 1995;109:249–58.

161. Knipp SC, Matatko N, Wilhelm H, et al. Evaluation of brain injury after coronary artery bypass grafting. A prospective study using neuropsychological assessment and diffusion-weighted magnetic resonance imaging. *Eur J Cardiothorac Surg* 2004;25:791–800.

162. Floyd TF, Shah PN, Price CC, et al. Clinical silent cerebral ischemic events after cardiac surgery: their incidence, regional vascular occurrence, and procedural dependence. *Ann Thorac Surg* 2006;81:2160–6.

163. Spiess BD, Royston D, Levy JH, et al. Platelet transfusions during coronary artery bypass graft surgery are associated with serious adverse outcomes. *Transfusion* 2004;44:1143–8.

164. Sungurtekin H, Boston US, Orszulak TA, Cook DJ. Effect of cerebral embolization on regional autoregulation during cardiopulmonary bypass in dogs. *Ann Thorac Surg* 2000;69:1130–4.

165. Gottesman RF, Sherman PM, Grega MA, et al. Watershed strokes after cardiac surgery: diagnosis, etiology, and outcome. *Stroke* 2006;37:2306–11.

166. Karkouti K, Djaiani G, Borger MA, et al. Low hematocrit during cardiopulmonary bypass is associated with increased risk of perioperative stroke in cardiac surgery. *Ann Thorac Surg* 2005;80:1381–7.

167. Lisle TC, Barrett KM, Gazoni LM, et al. Timing of stroke after cardiopulmonary bypass determines mortality. *Ann Thorac Surg* 2008;85:1556–63.

168. Hogue CW Jr, Murphy SF, Schechtman KB, Davila Roman VG. Risk factors for early or delayed stroke after cardiac surgery. *Circulation* 1999;100:642–7.

169. Kalyani SD, Miller NR, Dong LM, Baumgartner WA, Alejo DE, Gilbert TB. Incidence of and risk factors for perioperative optic neuropathy after cardiac surgery. *Ann Thorac Surg* 2004;78:34–7.

170. Barbut D, Grassineau D, Lis E, Heier L, Hartman GS, Isom OW. Posterior distribution of infarcts in strokes related to cardiac operations. *Ann Thorac Surg* 1998;65:1656–9.

171. Gott JP, Thourani VH, Wright CE, et al. Risk neutralization in cardiac operations: detection and treatment of associated carotid disease. *Ann Thorac Surg* 1999;68:850–7.

172. Timaran CH, Rosero EB, Smith ST, Valentine RJ, Modrall JG, Clagett GP. Trends and outcomes of concurrent carotid revascularization and coronary bypass. *J Vasc Surg* 2008;48:355–60.

173. Versaci F, Reimers B, Del Giudice C, et al. Simultaneous hybrid revascularization by carotid stenting and coronary artery bypass grafting: the SHARP study. *JACC Cardiovasc Interv* 2009;2:393–401.

174. Zacharias A, Schwann TA, Riordan CJ, et al. Operative and 5-year outcomes of combined carotid and coronary revascularization: review of a large contemporary experience. *Ann Thorac Surg* 2002;73:491–8.

175. Katznelson R, Djaiani GM, Borger MA, et al. Preoperative use of statins is associated with reduced early delirium rates after cardiac surgery. *Anesthesiology* 2009;110:67–73.

176. Zingone B, Rauber E, Gatti G, et al. The impact of epiaortic ultrasonographic scanning on the risk of perioperative stroke. *Eur J Cardiothorac Surg* 2006;29:720–8.

177. Rosenberger P, Shernan SK, Löffler M, et al. The influence of epiaortic ultrasonography on intraoperative surgical management in 6051 cardiac surgical patients. *Ann Thorac Surg* 2008;85:548–53.

178. Schachner T, Nagele G, Kacani A, Laufer G, Bonatti J. Factors associated with presence of ascending aortic atherosclerois in CABG patients. *Ann Thorac Surg* 2004;78:2028–32.

179. Hammon JW, Stump DA, Butterworth JR, et al. Coronary artery bypass grafting with single cross-clamp results in fewer persistent neuropsychological deficits than multiple clamp or off-pump coronary artery bypass grafting. *Ann Thorac Surg* 2007;84:1174–9.

180. Martens S, Neumann K, Sodemann C, Deschka H, Wimmer-Greinecker G, Moritz A. Carbon dioxide field flooding reduces neurologic impairment after open heart surgery. *Ann Thorac Surg* 2008;85:543–7.

181. Slater JP, Guarino T, Stack J, et al. Cerebral oxygen desaturation predicts cognitive decline and longer hospital stay after cardiac surgery. *Ann Thorac Surg* 2009;87:36–45.

182. Puskas F, Grocott HP, White WD, Mathew JP, Newman MF, Bar-Yosef S. Intraoperative hyperglycemia and cognitive decline after CABG. *Ann Thorac Surg* 2007;84:1467–73.

183. Salazar JD, Wityk RJ, Grega MA, et al. Stroke after cardiac surgery: short- and long-term outcomes. *Ann Thorac Surg* 2001;72:1195–202.

184. Dacey LJ, Likosky DS, Leavitt BJ, et al. Perioperative stroke and long-term survival after coronary bypass graft surgery. *Ann Thorac Surg* 2005;79:532–7.

185. Koster S, Oosterveld FGJ, Hensens AG, Wijma A, van der Palen J. Delirium after cardiac surgery and predictive validity of a risk checklist. *Ann Thorac Surg* 2008;86:1883–7.

186. Bucerius J, Gummert JF, Borger MA, et al. Predictors of delirium after cardiac surgery: effect of beating-heart (off-pump) surgery. *J Thorac Cardiovasc Surg* 2004;127:57–64.

187. Koster S, Hensens AG, van der Palen J. The long-term cognitive and functional outcomes of postoperative delirium after cardiac surgery. *Ann Thorac Surg* 2009;87:1469–74.

188. Flinn DR, Diehl KM, Seyfried LS, Malani PN. Prevention, diagnosis, and management of postoperative delirium in older adults. *J Am Coll Surg* 2009;209:261–8.

189. Maldonado JR, Wysong A, van der Starre PJ, Block T, Miller C, Reitz BA. Dexmedetomidine and the reduction of postoperative delirium after cardiac surgery. *Psychosomatics* 2009;50:206–17.

190. Reade MC, O'Sullivan K, Bates S, Goldsmith D, Ainslie WR, Bellomo R. Dexmedetomidine vs. haloperidol in delirious, agitated, intubated patients: a randomised open-label trial. *Crit Care* 2009;13:R75.

191. Schrader SL, Wellik KE, Demaerschalk BM, Caselli RJ, Woodruff BK, Wingerchuk DM. Adjunctive haloperidol prophylaxis reduces postoperative delirium severity and duration in at-risk elderly patients. *Neurologist* 2008;14:134–7.

192. Hassaballa HA, Balk RA. Torsade de pointes associated with the administration of intravenous haloperidol: a review of the literature and practical guidelines for use. *Expert Opin Drug Saf* 2003;2:543–7.

193. Skrobik YK, Bergeron N, Dumont M, Gottfried SB. Olanzapine vs haloperidol: treating delirium in a critical care setting. *Intensive Care Med* 2004;30:444–9.

194. Bayindir O, Akpinar B, Can E, Güden M, Sönmez B, Demiroğlu C. The use of the $5-HT_3$-receptor antagonist ondansetron for the treatment of postcardiotomy delirium. *J Cardiothorac Vasc Anesth* 2000;14:288–92.

195. Boettger S, Breitbart W. Atypical antipsychotics in the management of delirium: a review of the empirical literature. *Palliat Support Care* 2005;3:227–37.
196. Kosten TR, O'Connor PG. Management of drug and alcohol withdrawal. *N Engl J Med* 2003;348:1786–95.
197. Rosengart TK, Sweet JJ, Finnin E, et al. Stable cognition after coronary artery bypass grafting: comparisons with percutaneous intervention and normal controls. *Ann Thorac Surg* 2006;82:597–607.
198. Roach GW, Kanchuger M, Mangano CM, et al. Adverse cerebral outcomes after coronary bypass surgery. *N Engl J Med* 1996;335:1857–63.
199. Bar-Yosef S, Anders M, Mackensen GB, et al. Aortic atheroma burden and cognitive dysfunction after coronary artery bypass graft surgery. *Ann Thorac Surg* 2004;78:1556–63.
200. Evered LA, Silbert BS, Scott DA. Postoperative cognitive dysfunction and aortic atheroma. *Ann Thorac Surg* 2010;89:1091–7.
201. Baumgartner WA. Neurocognitive changes after coronary bypass surgery. *Circulation* 2007;116:1879–81.
202. Hernandez F Jr, Brown JR, Likosky DS, et al. Neurocognitive outcomes of off-pump versus on-pump coronary artery bypass: a prospective randomized controlled trial. *Ann Thorac Surg* 2007;84:1897–903.
203. Ernest CS, Worcester MU, Tatoulis J, et al. Neurocognitive outcomes in off-pump versus on-pump bypass surgery: a randomized controlled trial. *Ann Thorac Surg* 2006;81:2105–14.
204. Barber PA, Hach S, Tippett LJ, Ross L, Merry AF, Milsom P. Cerebral ischemic lesions on diffusion-weighted imaging are associated with neurocognitive decline after cardiac surgery. *Stroke* 2008;39:1427–33.
205. Goto T, Baba T, Honma K, et al. Magnetic resonance imaging findings and postoperative neurologic dysfunction in elderly patients undergoing coronary artery bypass grafting. *Ann Thorac Surg* 2001;72:137–42.
206. Knipp SC, Matatko N, Wilhelm H, et al. Cognitive outcomes three years after coronary artery bypass surgery: relation to diffusion-weighted magnetic resonance imaging. *Ann Thorac Surg* 2008;85:872–9.
207. McKhann GM, Borowicz LM, Goldsborough MA, Enger C, Selnes OA. Depression and cognitive decline after coronary artery bypass grafting. *Lancet* 1997;349:1282–4.
208. Ho PM, Arciniegas DB, Grigsby J, et al. Predictors of cognitive decline following coronary artery bypass graft surgery. *Ann Thorac Surg* 2004;77:597–603.
209. Hogue CW Jr, Hershey T, Dixon D, et al. Preexisting cognitive impairment in women before cardiac surgery and its relationship to C-reactive protein concentrations. *Anesth Analg* 2006;102:1602–8.
210. Silbert BS, Scott DA, Evered LA, Lewis MS, Maruff PT. Preexisting cognitive impairment in patients scheduled for elective coronary artery bypass graft surgery. *Anesth Analg* 2007;104:1023–8.
211. McKhann GM, Selnes OA, Grega MA, et al. Subjective memory symptoms in surgical and nonsurgical coronary artery patients: 6-year follow-up. *Ann Thorac Surg* 2009;87:27–35.
212. Selnes OA, Grega MA, Bailey MM, et al. Do management strategies for coronary artery disease influence 6-year cognitive outcomes? *Ann Thorac Surg* 2009;88:445–54.
213. Dajaini G, Fedorko L, Borger MA, et al. Continuous-flow cell saver reduces cognitive decline in elderly patients after coronary bypass surgery. *Circulation* 2007;116:1888–9.
214. Motallebzadeh R, Bland JM, Markus HS, Kaski JC, Jahangiri M. Neurocognitive function and cerebral emboli: randomized study of on-pump verus off-pump coronary artery bypass surgery. *Ann Thorac Surg* 2007;83:475–82.
215. Lund C, Hol PK, Lundblad R, et al. Comparison of cerebral embolization during off-pump and on-pump coronary artery bypass surgery. *Ann Thorac Surg* 2003;76:765–70.
216. Selnes OA, Goldsborough MA, Borowicz LM Jr, Enger C, Quaskey SA, McKhann GM. Determinants of cognitive change after coronary artery bypass surgery: a multifactorial problem. *Ann Thorac Surg* 1999;67:1669–76.
217. Hong SW, Shim JK, Choi YS, Kim DH, Chang BC, Kwak YL. Prediction of cognitive dysfunction and patient's outcome following valvular heart surgery and the role of cerebral oximetry. *Eur J Cardiothorac Sug* 2008;33:560–5.

218. Newman MF, Kirschner JL, Phillips-Bute B, et al. Longitudinal assessment of neurocognitive function after coronary-artery bypass surgery. *N Engl J Med* 2001;344:395–402.

219. Rothenhäusler HB, Grieser B, Nollert G, Reichart B, Schelling G, Kapfhammer HP. Psychiatric and psychosocial outcome of cardiac surgery with cardiopulmonary bypass: a prospective 12-month follow-up study. *Gen Hosp Psychiatry* 2005;27:18–28.

220. Pignay-Demaria V, Lespérance F, Demaria RG, Frasure-Smith N, Perrault LP. Depression and anxiety and outcomes of coronary artery bypass surgery. *Ann Thorac Surg* 2003;75:314–21.

221. Ho PM, Masoudi FA, Spertus JA, et al. Depression predicts mortality following cardiac valve surgery. *Ann Thorac Surg* 2005;79:1255–9.

222. Freedland KE, Skala JA, Carney RM, et al. Treatment of depression afer coronary artery bypass surgery: a randomized controlled trial. *Arch Gen Psychiatry* 2009;66:387–96.

223. Schweickert WD, Hall J. ICU-acquired weakness. *Chest* 2007;131:1541–9.

224. Thiele TI, Jakob H, Hund E, Genzwuerker H, Herold U, Schweiger P, Hagl S. Critical illness polyneuropathy: a new iatrogenically induced syndrome after cardiac surgery? *Eur J Cardiothorac Surg* 1997;12:826–35.

225. Unlü Y, Velioğlu Y, Koçak H, Becit N, Ceviz M. Brachial plexus injury following median sternotomy. *Interact Cardiovasc Thorac Surg* 2007;6:235–7.

226. Canbaz S, Turgut N, Halici U, Sunar H, Balci K, Duran E. Brachial plexus injury during open heart surgery – controlled prospective trial. *Thorac Cardiovasc Surg* 2005;53:295–9.

227. Thomas NJ, Harvey AT. Paraplegia after coronary bypass operations: relationship to severe hypertension and vascular disease. *J Thorac Cardiovasc Surg* 1999;117:834–6.

228. Geyer TE, Naik MJ, Pillai R. Anterior spinal artery syndrome after elective coronary artery bypass grafting. *Ann Thorac Surg* 2002;73:1971–3.

229. Vazquez-Jimenez JF, Krebs G, Schiefer J, et al. Injury of the common peroneal nerve after cardiothoracic operations. *Ann Thorac Surg* 2002;73:119–22.

230. James T, Friedman SG, Scher L, Hall M. Lower extremity compartment syndrome after coronary artery bypass. *J Vasc Surg* 2002;36:1069–70.

231. Papas TT, Mikroulis D, Papanas N, Lazarides MK, Bougioukas G. Lower extremity compartment syndrome following coronary artery bypass. *J Cardiovasc Surg (Torino)* 2007;48:249–52.

232. Kolli A, Au JT, Lee DC, Klinoff N, Ko W. Compartment syndrome afer endoscopic harvest of the great saphenous vein during coronary artery bypass grafting. *Ann Thorac Surg* 2010;89:271–3.

233. Alameddine AK. Lower limb ischemia with compartment syndrome related to femoral artery cannulas. *Ann Thorac Surg* 1997;64:884–5.

234. Vander Salm TJ. Prevention of lower extremity ischemia during cardiopulmonary bypass via femoral cannulation. *Ann Thorac Surg* 1997;63:251–2.

235. Hendrickson SC, Glower DD. A method for perfusion of the leg during cardiopulmonary bypass via femoral cannulation. *Ann Thorac Surg* 1998;65:1807–8.

236. Bleiziffer S, Hettich I, Eisenhauer B, et al. Neurologic sequelae of the donor arm after endoscopic versus conventional radial artery harvesting. *J Thorac Cardiovasc Surg* 2008;136:681–7.

237. Hamdan AL, Moukarbel RV, Farhat F, Obeid M. Vocal cord paralysis after open-heart surgery. *Eur J Cardiothorac Surg* 2002;21:671–4.

238. Itagaki T, Kikura M, Sato S. Incidence and risk factors of postoperative vocal cord paralysis in 987 patients after cardiovascular surgery. *Ann Thorac Surg* 2007;83:2147–52.

239. Recht MH, Smith JM, Woods SE, Engel AM, Hiratzka LF. Predictors and outcomes of gastrointestinal complications in patients undergoing coronary artery bypass graft surgery: a prospective, nested case–control study. *J Am Coll Surg* 2004;198:742–7.

240. Sanisoglu I, Guden M, Bayramoglu Z, et al. Does off-pump CABG reduce gastrointestinal complications? *Ann Thorac Surg* 2004;77:619–25.

241. Musleh GS, Patel NC, Grayson AD, et al. Off-pump coronary artery bypass surgery does not reduce gastrointestinal complications. *Eur J Cardiothorac Surg* 2003;23:170–4.

242. D'Ancona G, Baillot R, Poirier B, et al. Determinants of gastrointestinal complications in cardiac surgery. *Tex Heart Inst J* 2003;30:280–5.

243. Mangi AA, Christison-Lagay ER, Torchiana DF, Warshaw AL, Berger DL. Gastrointestinal complications in patients undergoing heart operation: an analysis of 8709 consecutive cardiac surgical patients. *Ann Surg* 2005;241:895–901.

244. Díaz-Gómez JL, Nutter B, Xu M, et al. The effect of postoperative gastrointestinal complications in patients undergoing coronary artery bypass surgery. *Ann Thorac Surg* 2010;90:109–16.

245. Filsoufi F, Rahmanian PB, Castillo JG, Scurlock C, Legnani PE, Adams DH. Predictors and outcome of gastrointestinal complications in patients undergoing cardiac surgery. *Ann Surg* 2007;246:323–9.

246. Rodriguez F, Nguyen TC, Galanko JA, Morton J. Gastrointestinal complications after coronary artery bypass grafting: a national study of morbidity and mortality predictors. *J Am Coll Surg* 2007;205:741–7.

247. McSwenney ME, Garwood S, Levin J, et al. Adverse gastrointestinal complications after cardiopulmonary bypass: can outcome be predicted from preoperative risk factors? *Anesth Analg* 2004;98:1610–7.

248. Ohri SK, Velissaris T. Gastrointestinal dysfunction following cardiac surgery. *Perfusion* 2006;21:215–23.

249. Baue AE. The role of the gut in the development of multiple organ dysfunction in cardiothoracic patients. *Ann Thorac Surg* 1993;55:822–9.

250. Raja SG, Haider Z, Ahmad M. Predictors of gastrointestinal complications after conventional and beating heart coronary surgery. *Surgeon* 2003;1:221–8.

251. Andersson B, Nilsson J, Brandt J, Höglund P, Andersson R. Gastrointestinal complications after cardiac surgery. *Br J Surg* 2005;92:326–33.

252. Velissaris T, Tang A, Murray M, El-Minshawy A, Hett D, Ohri S. A prospective randomized study to evaluate splanchnic hypoxia during beating-heart and conventional coronary revascularization. *Eur J Cardiothorac Surg* 2003;23:917–24.

253. Fiore G, Brienza N, Cicala P, et al. Superior mesenteric artery blood flow modifications during off-pump coronary surgery. *Ann Thorac Surg* 2006;82:62–7.

254. Croome KP, Kiaii B, Fox S, Quantz M, McKenzie N, Novick RJ. Comparison of gastrointestinal complications in on-pump versus off-pump coronary artery bypass grafting. *Can J Surg* 2009;52:125–8.

255. Hill RP, Lubarsky DA, Phillips-Bute B, et al. Cost-effectiveness of prophylactic antiemetic therapy with ondansetron, droperidol, or placebo. *Anesthesiology* 2000;92:958–67.

256. Ferraris VA, Ferraris SP, Moritz DM, Welch S. Oropharyngeal dysphagia after cardiac operations. *Ann Thorac Surg* 2001;71:1792–6.

257. Harrington OB, Duckworth JK, Starnes CL, et al. Silent aspiration after coronary artery bypass grafting. *Ann Thorac Surg* 1998;65:1599–603.

258. Hogue CW Jr, Lappas GD, Creswell LL, et al. Swallowing dysfunction after cardiac operations. Associated adverse outcomes and risk factors including intraoperative transesophageal echocardiography. *J Thorac Cardiovasc Surg* 1995;110:517–22.

259. Kallmeyer IJ, Collard CD, Fox JA, Body SC, Shernan SK. The safety of intraoperative transesophageal echocardiography: a case series of 7200 cardiac surgical patients. *Anesth Analg* 2001;92:1126–30.

260. Rousou JA, Tighe DA, Garb JL, et al. Risk of dysphagia after transesophageal echocardiography during cardiac operations. *Ann Thorac Surg* 2000;69:486–9.

261. Barker J, Martino R, Reichardt B, Hickey EJ, Ralph-Edwards A. Incidence and impact of dysphagia in patients receiving prolonged endotracheal intubation after cardiac surgery. *Can J Surg* 2009;52:119–24.

262. Ramsey DJ, Smithard DG, Kalra L. Early assessments of dysphagia and aspiration risk in acute stroke patients. *Stroke* 2003;34:1252–7.

263. Kagaya H, Okada S, Saitoh E, Baba M, Yokoyama M, Takahashi H. Simple swallowing provocation test has limited applicability as a screening tool for detecting aspiration, silent aspiration, or penetration. *Dysphagia* 2010;25:6–10.

264. Bours GJ, Speyer R, Lemmens J, Limburg M, de Wit R. Bedside screening tests vs. videofluoroscopy or fiberoptic endoscopic evaluation of swallowing to detect dysphagia in patients with neurological disorders: a systematic review. *J Adv Nurs* 2009;65:477–93.

265. Partik BL, Scharitzer M, Schueller G, et al. Videofluoroscopy of swallowing abnormalities in 22 symptomatic patients after cardiovascular surgery. *Am J Roentgenol* 2003;180:987–92.

266. Alebouyeh N, Toefigh M, Ghasemzadeh N, Mirheydari S, Azargashb E. Predictors of gastrointestinal perforation in patients undergoing coronary artery bypass graft (CABG) surgery in Tehran, Iran. *Ann Thorac Cardiovasc Surg* 2007;13:251–3.

267. Hackert T, Keinle P, Weitz J, et al. Accuracy of diagnostic laparoscopy for early diagnosis of abdominal complications after cardiac surgery. *Surg Endosc* 2003;17:1671–4.

268. Saunders MD. Acute colonic pseudo-obstruction. *Best Pract Res Clin Gastroenterol* 2007;21:671–87.

269. Gannon RH. Current strategies for preventing or ameliorating postoperative ileus: a multimodal approach. *Am J Health Syst Pharm* 2007;64(20 Suppl 13):S8–12.

270. Ponec RJ, Saunders MD, Kimmey MB. Neostigmine for the treatment of acute colonic pseudo-obstruction. *N Engl J Med* 1999;341:137–41.

271. Rady MY, Kodavatiganti R, Ryan T. Perioperative predictors of acute cholecystitis after cardiovascular surgery. *Chest* 1998;114:76–84.

272. Passage J, Joshi P, Mullany DV. Acute cholecystitis complicating cardiac surgery: case series involving more than 16,000 patients. *Ann Thorac Surg* 2007;83:1096–101.

273. Mastoraki A, Mastoraki S, Kriaras I, Douka E, Geroulanos S. Complications involving gall bladder and biliary tract in cardiovascular surgery. *Hepatogastroenterology* 2008;55:1233–7.

274. Norton ID, Pokorny CS, Baird DK, Selby WS. Upper gastrointestinal haemorrhage following coronary artery bypass grafting. *Aust N Z J Med* 1995;25:297–301.

275. Jayaprakash A, McGrath C, McCullagh E, Smith F, Angelini G, Probert C. Upper gastrointestinal haemorrhage following cardiac surgery: a comparative study with vascular surgery patients from a single centre. *Eur J Gastroenterol Hepatol* 2004;16:191–4.

276. Steinberg KP. Stress-related mucosal disease in the critically ill patient: risk factors and strategies to prevent stress-related bleeding in the intensive care unit. *Crit Care Med* 2002;30(suppl):S362–4.

277. Ali T, Harty RF. Stress-induced ulcer bleeding in critically ill patients. *Gastroenterol Clin North Am* 2009;38:245–65.

278. Van der Voort PH, Zandstra DF. Pathogenesis, risk factors, and incidence of upper gastrointestinal bleeding after cardiac surgery: is specific prophylaxis in routine bypass procedures needed? *J Cardiothorac Vasc Anesth* 2000;14:293–9.

279. Hata M, Shiono M, Sekino H, et al. Prospective randomized trial for optimal prophylactic treatment of the upper gastrointestinal complications after open heart surgery. *Circ J* 2005;69:331–4.

280. Walker J, Robinson J, Stewart J, Jacob S. Does enteric-coated aspirin result in a lower incidence of gastrointestinal complications compared to normal aspirin? *Interact Cardiovasc Thorac Surg* 2007;6:519–22.

281. Ziegelin M, Hoschtitzky A, Dunning J, Hooper T. Does clopidogrel rather than aspirin plus a proton-pump inhibitor reduce the frequency of gastrointestinal complications after cardiac surgery? *Interact Cardiovasc Thorac Surg* 2007;6:534–7.

282. Huggins RM, Scates AC, Latour JK. Intravenous proton-pump inhibitors versus H2-antagonists for treatment of GI bleeding. *Ann Pharmacother* 2003;37:433–7.

283. Torres AJ, Landa I, Hernandez F, et al. Somatostatin in the treatment of severe upper gastrointestinal bleeding: a multicentre controlled trial. *Br J Surg* 2005;73:786–9.

284. Chan FK, Ching JY, Hung LC, et al. Clopidogrel versus aspirin and esomeprazole to prevent recurrent ulcer bleeding. *N Engl J Med* 2005;352:238–44.

285. Ng FH, Chan P, Kwanchung CP, et al. Management and outcome of peptic ulcers or erosions in patients receiving a combination of aspirin plus clopidogrel. *J Gastroenterol* 2008;43:679–86.

286. Pate GE, Chandavimol M, Naiman SC, Webb JG. Heyde's syndrome: a review. *J Heart Valve Dis* 2004;13:701–12.

287. Darcy M. Treatment of lower gastrointestinal bleeding: vasopressin infusion versus embolization. *J Vasc Interv Radiol* 2003;14:535–43.

288. Kosmoliaptsis V, Singhal V, Vohrah A, Dimitri W. Selective embolotherapy as a treatment option for lower gastrointestinal haemorrhage following open-heart surgery. *Interact Cardiovasc Thorac Surg* 2007;6:558–60.

289. Junquera F, Saperas E, Videla S, et al. Long-term efficacy of octreotide in the prevention of recurrent bleeding from gastrointestinal angiodysplasia. *Am J Gastroenterol* 2007;102:254–60.

290. Schütz A, Eichinger W, Breuer M, Gansera B, Kemkes BM. Acute mesenteric ischemia after open heart surgery. *Angiology* 1998;49:267–73.

291. Katz MG, Schachner A, Ezri T, et al. Nonocclusive mesenteric ischemia after off-pump coronary artery bypass surgery: a word of caution. *Am Surg* 2006;72:228–31.

292. Kirkpatrick ID, Kroeker MA, Greenberg HM. Biphasic CT with mesenteric CT angiography in the evaluation of acute mesenteric ischemia: initial experience. *Radiology* 2003;229:91–8.

293. Klotz S, Vestring T, Rötker J, Schmidt C, Scheld HH, Schmid C. Diagnosis and treatment of nonocclusive mesenteric ischemia after open heart surgery. *Ann Thorac Surg* 2001;72:1583–6.

294. Crabtree T, Aitchison D, Meyers BF, et al. Clostridium difficile in cardiac surgery: risk factors and impact on postoperative outcome. *Ann Thorac Surg* 2007;83:1396–402.

295. Kelly CP, LaMont JT. Clostridium difficile: more difficult than ever. *N Engl J Med* 2008;359:1932–40.

296. An Y, Xiao YB, Zhong QJ. Hyperbilirubinemia after extracorporeal circulation surgery: a recent and prospective study. *World J Gastroenterol* 2006;12:6722–6.

297. Mastoraki A, Karatzis E, Mastoraki S, Kriaras I, Sfirakis P, Geroulanos S. Postoperative jaundice after cardiac surgery. *Hepatobiliary Pancreat Dis Int* 2007;6:383–7.

298. Nishi H, Takahashi T, Ichikawa H, Matsumiya G, Matsuda H, Sawa Y. Prediction of postoperative hepatic dysfunction after cardiac surgery in patients with chronic congestive heart failure. *Gen Thorac Cardiovasc Surg* 2009;57:357–62.

299. Goyal RK, Srivastava D, Lessnau KD. Clopidogrel-induced hepatocellular injury and cholestatic jaundice in an elderly patient: case report and review of the literature. *Pharmacotherapy* 2009;29:608–12.

300. Riordan SM, Williams R. Treatment of hepatic encephalopathy. *N Engl J Med* 1997;337:473–9.

301. Wan S, Arifi AA, Chan CS, et al. Is hyperamylasemia after cardiac surgery due to cardiopulmonary bypass? *Asian Cardiovasc Thorac Ann* 2002;10:115–8.

302. Ihaya A, Muraoka R, Chiba Y, et al. Hyperamylasemia and subclinical pancreatitis after cardiac surgery. *World J Surg* 2001;25:862–4.

303. Perez A, Ito H, Farivar RS, et al. Risk factors and outcomes of pancreatitis after open heart surgery. *Am J Surg* 2005;190:401–5.

304. Lonardo A, Grisendi A, Bonilauri S, Rambaldi M, Selmi I, Tondelli E. Ischaemic necrotizing pancreatitis after cardiac surgery. A case report and review of the literature. *Int J Gastroenterol Hepatol* 1999;31:872–5.

305. Martindale RG, McClave SA, Vanek VW, et al. Guidelines for the provision and assessment of nutrition support therapy in the adult critically ill patient: Society of Critical Care Medicine and American Society for Parenteral and Enteral Nutrition: executive summary. *Crit Care Med* 2009;37:1757–61.

306. Akins CW, Miller DC, Turina MI, et al. Guidelines for reporting mortality and morbidity after cardiac valve interventions. *Ann Thorac Surg* 2008;85:1490–5.

307. Bates SM, Greer IA, Pabinger I, Sofaer S, Hirsh J. Venous thromboembolism, thrombophilia, antithrombotic therapy, and pregnancy. American College of Chest Physicians evidence-based clinical practice guidelines (8th edition). *Chest* 2008;133:844S–86S.

308. Epstein RS, Moyer TP, Aubert RE, et al. Warfarin genotyping reduces hospitalization rates. Results from the MM-WES (Medco-Mayo Warfarin Effectiveness Study). *J Am Coll Cardiol* 2010;55:2804–12.

309. Eitz T, Schenk S, Fritzsche D, et al. International normalized raioin self-management lowers the risk of thromboembolic events after prosthetic heart valver replacement. *Ann Thorac Surg* 2008;85:949–55.

310. Koertke H, Zittermann A, Wagner O, Koerfer R. Self-management of oral anticoagulation therapy improves long-term survival in patients with mechanical heart valve replacement. *Ann Thorac Surg* 2007;83:24–9.

311. Shapira Y, Vaturi M, Sagie A. Hemolysis associated with prosthetic heart valves: a review. *Cardiol Rev* 2009;17:121–4.

312. Juurlink DN, Gomes T, Ko DT, et al. A population-based study of the drug interaction between proton pump inhibitors and clopidogrel. *CMAJ* 2009;180:713–8.

313. Lazar HL. Role of statin therapy in the coronary bypass patient. *Ann Thorac Surg* 2004;78:730–40.

314. Hata M, Takayama T, Sezai A, Yoshitake I, Hirayama A, Minami K. Efficacy of aggressive lipid controlling therapy for preventing saphenous vein graft disease. *Ann Thorac Surg* 2009;88:1440–4.

315. Paraskevas KI. Applications of statins in cardiothoracic surgery: more than just lipid-lowering. *Eur J Cardiothorac Surg* 2008;33:377–90.

316. Fedoruk LM, Wang H, Conaway MR, Kron IL, Johnston KC. Statin therapy improves outcomes after valvular heart surgery. *Ann Thorac Surg* 2008;85:1521–6.

317. Okrainec K, Platt R, Pilotte L, Eisenberg MJ. Cardiac medical therapy in patients undergoing coronary artery bypass graft surgery. A review of randomized controlled trials. *J Am Coll Cardiol* 2005;45:177–84.

318. Charlson ME, Isom OW. Care after coronary-artery bypass surgery. *N Engl J Med* 2003;348:1456–63.

319. Chan AYM, McAlister FA, Norris CM, et al. Effect of β-blocker use on outcomes after discharge in patients who underwent cardiac surgery. *J Thorac Cardiovasc Surg* 2010;140:182–7.

320. Prescriber's letter 2009;16:250812 (available at www.prescribersletter.com).

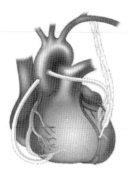

APPENDICES

 **1A** American College of Cardiology Classes of Recommendation and Levels of Evidence

Class I   Benefit greatly exceeds the risk and the procedure/treatment should be performed/administered (is effective)

Class IIa   Benefit exceeds the risk and it is reasonable to perform procedure or administer treatment (most likely effective)

Class IIb   Benefit probably exceeds the risk and the procedure/treatment may be considered (usefulness/efficacy less well-established)

Class III   The risk may exceed the benefit and the procedure/treatment should not be performed/administered (not recommended)

Level A   Evidence from multiple randomized trials or meta-analyses

Level B   Limited evidence from single randomized trials or nonrandomized studies with some conflicting evidence of benefit

Level C   Expert opinions or case studies

These are general summations of the recommendations for treatment.

1B New York Heart Association Functional Classification

I   No limitation of physical activity.

II   Slight limitation of physical activity. Ordinary activity results in fatigue, palpitations, dyspnea, or angina pain.

III   Marked limitation of physical activity. Less than ordinary activity causes fatigue, palpitations, dyspnea, or angina pain.

IV   Inability to carry out any physical activity without discomfort. Symptoms may be present even at rest.

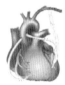

2 Typical Preoperative Order Sheet

1. Admit to: _____
2. Surgery date: _____
3. Planned procedure: _____
4. Diagnostic Studies
   - ☐ CBC with differential
   - ☐ PT/INR   ☐ PTT
   - ☐ Electrolytes, BUN, creatinine, blood glucose
   - ☐ Liver function tests (bilirubin, AST, ALT, alkaline phosphatase, albumin)
   - ☐ TSH level
   - ☐ Lipid profile
   - ☐ Hemoglobin A1c level
   - ☐ Urinalysis and urine culture, if indicated
   - ☐ Electrocardiogram
   - ☐ Chest x-ray PA and lateral
   - ☐ Room air oxygen saturation by pulse oximetry; obtain arterial blood gas if < 90%
   - ☐ Antibody screen   ☐ Crossmatch: __ units PRBC
   - ☐ Carotid duplex studies
   - ☐ Bilateral digital radial artery studies
   - ☐ Bilateral venous mapping
   - ☐ Pulmonary function tests
   - ☐ Other: _____
5. Treatments/Assessments
   - ☐ Admission vital signs
   - ☐ Measure height and weight
   - ☐ NPO after midnight except sips of water with meds
   - ☐ Surgical clippers to remove hair at 5 AM morning of surgery from chest, legs and both groins
   - ☐ Hibiclens scrub to chest and legs night before and AM of surgery
   - ☐ Incentive spirometry teaching
6. Medications
   - ☐ Mupirocin 2% (Bactroban ointment): apply Q-tip nasal swabs the evening before and the morning of surgery
   - ☐ Chlorhexidine 0.12% (Peridex) gargle on-call to OR
   - ☐ Cefazolin   ☐ 1 g IV   ☐ 2 g IV – send to OR with patient
   - ☐ Vancomycin 15–20 mg/kg = _____ g IV – send to OR with patient
   - ☐ Discontinue clopidogrel immediately
   - ☐ Reduce aspirin to 81 mg daily if patient on a higher dose
   - ☐ Discontinue heparin at _____
   - ☐ Continue heparin drip into OR
   - ☐ Discontinue low-molecular-weight heparin after AM/PM dose on _____
   - ☐ Discontinue IIb/IIIa inhibitor at 3 AM prior to surgery
   - ☐ Other: _____

3 Typical Orders for Admission to the ICU

1. Admit to ICU on _____ MD service
2. Procedure:_____
3. Vital signs q15 minutes until stable, then q30 min or per protocol
4. Continuous ECG, arterial, PA tracings, SaO_2 on bedside monitor
5. Cardiac output q15 min × 1 hour, then q1h × 4 hours, then q2–4h when stable
6. IABP 1 : 1; check distal pulses manually or with Doppler q1h
7. Chest tubes to chest drainage system with −20 cm H_2O suction; record hourly until <30 mL/h, then q8h
8. Bair Hugger warming system if core temperature < 35 °C
9. Urinary catheter to gravity drainage and record hourly
10. Elevate head of bed 30°
11. Hourly I & O
12. Daily weights
13. Advance activity after extubation (dangle, OOB to chair)
14. VTE prophylaxis
    - ☐ T.E.D. elastic stockings (apply on POD #1)
    - ☐ Sequential compression devices
    - ☐ Heparin 5000 units SC bid starting on POD #_____
    - ☐ Low-molecular-weight heparin (Lovenox) 40 mg SC daily starting on POD #_____
15. GI/Nutrition: ☐ NPO while intubated
    - ☐ Nasogastric tube to low suction
    - ☐ Clear liquids as tolerated 1h after extubation and removal of NG tube
16. Ventilator settings
    FIO_2: ____in SIMV mode
    IMV rate: _____breaths/min
    Tidal volume: _____ mL
    PEEP: ____cm H_2O
    Pressure support: _____ cm H_2O
17. Respiratory care
    - ☐ Endotracheal suction q4h, then prn
    - ☐ Wean ventilator to extubate per protocol (see Tables 10.3–10.5, pages 400–402)
    - ☐ O2 via face mask with FIO_2 0.6–1.0 per protocol
    - ☐ O2 via nasal prongs @ 2–6 liters/min to keep SaO_2 >95%
    - ☐ Incentive spirometer q1h when awake
    - ☐ Cough pillow at bedside
    - ☐ Albuterol 0.5 mL of 0.5% solution (2.5 mg) in 3 mL normal saline q6h via nebulizer or metered dose inhaler 6 puffs via endotracheal tube (90 µg/inhalation)

(continued)

(Continued)

18. Laboratory tests
  - ☐ On arrival: STAT ABGs, CBC, electrolytes, glucose
    STAT PT, PTT, platelet count if chest tube output >100/h
    (thromboelastogram, if available)
    STAT chest x-ray (if not done in operating room)
    STAT ECG
  - ☐ 4 and 8 hours after arrival and prn: potassium, hematocrit, ABGs (respiratory distress)
  - ☐ ABGs per protocol (prior to weaning and prior to extubation)
  - ☐ 3 AM on POD #1: CBC, lytes, BUN, creatinine, blood glucose, ECG, CXR, INR (if patient to receive warfarin after valve procedure)
19. Pacemaker settings: Mode: ☐ Atrial   ☐ VVI   ☐ DVI   ☐ DDD
    Atrial output: _____ mA   Ventricular output ___ mA
    Rate: _____/min   AV interval: ____ msec
    Sensitivity: ☐ Asynchronous   ☐ Demand
    ☐ Pacer off but attached
20. Cardiac Rehab consult
21. Notify MD/PA for:
    a. Systolic blood pressure <90 or >140 mm Hg
    b. Cardiac index <2.0 L/min/m^2
    c. Urine output <30 mL/h for 2 hours
    d. Chest tube drainage >100 mL/h
    e. Temperature >38.5 °C
22. IV Drips/Medications (with suggested ranges)
    Allergies_____
    a. IV drips:
      - ☐ Dextrose 5% in 0.45 NS 250 mL via Cordis/triple lumen to KVO
      - ☐ Arterial line and distal Swan-Ganz port: NS flushes at 3 mL/h
      - ☐ Epinephrine 1 mg/250 mL D5W: _____ μg/min to maintain cardiac index >2.0 (0.01–0.06 μg/kg/min or 1–4 μg/min)
      - ☐ Milrinone 20 mg/100 mL D5W: _____ μg/kg/min (0.375–0.625 μg/kg/min)
      - ☐ Dopamine 400 mg/250 D5W: _____ μg/kg/min (2–20 μg/kg/min)
      - ☐ Dobutamine 250 mg/250 D5W: _____ μg/kg/min (5–20 μg/kg/min)
      - ☐ Norepinephrine 4–8 mg/250 mL D5W: _____ μg/min to keep systolic BP > 100 (0.01–1.0 μg/kg/min)
      - ☐ Phenylephrine 20 mg/250 mL NS: _____μg/min to keep systolic BP >100 (0.1–3.0 μg/kg/min)
      - ☐ Vasopressin 15 units/150 mL D5W: _____ units/min (0.01–0.07 units/min)
      - ☐ Nitroprusside 50 mg/250 mL D5W: _____ μg/kg/min to keep systolic BP < 130 (0.1–5 μg/kg/min)
      - ☐ Clevidipine 50 mg/100 mL D5W: _____mg/h to keep systolic BP <130 (2–5 mg/h)
      - ☐ Nicardipine 25 mg/250 mL D5W: _____ mg/h to keep BP <130 (5–15 mg/h)
      - ☐ Nitroglycerin 50 mg/250 mL D5W: _____ μg/kg/min (0.1–2.0 μg/kg/min)
      - ☐ Diltiazem: 100 mg/100 mL D5W: _____mg/h (for radial artery prophylaxis)
      - ☐ Esmolol 2.5 g/250 NS: _____ μg/kg/min (25–100 μg/kg/min)
      - ☐ Amiodarone: after initial IV load in OR, 900 mg/500 D5W: 1 mg/min × 6 hours, then decrease to 0.5 mg/min × 18 hours
      - ☐ Lidocaine 2 g/250 mL D5W: _____ mg/min IV; wean off at 06:00 POD #1
      - ☐ Nesiritide: 1.5 mg/100 ml: _____ μg/min (0.01–0.03 μg/kg/min)
      - ☐ Fenoldopam: 10 mg/250 D5W: 0.1 μg/kg/min

b. Antibiotics
- [ ] Cefazolin 1 g IV q8h for 6 doses
- [ ] Vancomycin 1 g IV q12h for 4 doses

c. Sedatives/analgesics
- [ ] Propofol infusion 10 mg/mL: 25–50 µg/kg/min; wean to off per protocol
- [ ] Dexmedetomidine: 400 µg (2 vials of 2 mL of 100 µg/mL solution)/100 mL NS: bolus dose of ____ (1 µg/kg) over 10 minutes, then maintenance infusion of ____ (0.2–0.7 µg/kg/h)
- [ ] Midazolam 2 mg IV q2h prn agitation; stop after extubation
- [ ] Morphine sulfate ____ mg IV q2h prn for pain (while intubated)
- [ ] Meperidine 25–50 mg IV prn shivering
- [ ] Ketorolac 30–60 mg IV q6h prn for moderate-to-severe pain (4–10 on pain scale); stop after 72 hours
- [ ] Percocet 5/325 mg 1–2 tablets PO q4h prn for pain after extubation; start with 1 tablet for mild pain (1–3 on pain scale); give additional tablet 60 minutes later if no change in pain. Give 2 tablets for moderate-to-severe pain (4–10 on pain scale)

d. Other medications
- [ ] β-blocker starting at 08:00 on POD #1, then q12h; hold for HR <60 or SBP <100
  - [ ] Metoprolol 25 mg PO/per NG tube bid
  - [ ] Carvedilol 3.125 mg PO/per NG tube bid
- [ ] Amiodarone 400 mg PO bid to start after amiodarone infusion discontinued
- [ ] Magnesium sulfate 2 g in 50 mL NS IV over 2 hours on POD #1 in AM
- [ ] Sucralfate 1 g per NG tube q6h until NG tube removed
- [ ] Pantoprazole (Protonix) 40 mg IV/PO qd
- [ ] Aspirin   [ ] 81 mg   [ ] 325 mg PO qd (starting 8 hours after arrival); hold for platelet count < 75,000 or chest tube drainage >50 mL/h
- [ ] Warfarin ____ mg starting _____; check with HO for daily dose (use warfarin protocol) - see Appendix 8
- [ ] Nitroglycerin 100 mg/250 mL D5W at 10–15 µg/min until taking PO (radial artery prophylaxis); then convert to:
  - [ ] Amlodipine 5 mg PO qd
  - [ ] Amlodipine 10 mg PO qd
  - [ ] Isosorbide mononitrate sustained release (Imdur) 20 mg PO qd
- [ ] Simvastatin ____ mg qd hs (no more than 20 mg if on amiodarone)
- [ ] Mupirocin 2% (Bactroban ointment) via Q-tip nasal swab the evening after surgery and bid × 3 days
- [ ] Chlorhexidine 0.12% oral wash (Peridex) 15 mL with brushing q12 hr (at 0900 and 2100 while intubated)

e. PRN medications
- [ ] Acetaminophen 650 mg PO/PR q4h prn temp >38.5 °C
- [ ] Metoclopramide 10 mg IV/PO q6h prn nausea
- [ ] Ondansetron 4 mg IV q4h prn nausea
- [ ] KCl 80 mEq/250 mL D5W via central line to keep K^+ > 4.5 mEq/L:
  - [ ] K^+ 4.0–4.5 KCl 10 mEq over 30 min
  - [ ] K^+ 3.5–3.9 KCl 20 mEq over 60 min
  - [ ] K^+ <3.5   KCl 40 mEq over 90 min
- [ ] Initiate hyperglycemia protocol if blood glucose >150 mg/dL on admission or any time within the first 48 hours (see Appendix 6)
- [ ] Other

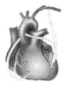

4 Typical Transfer Orders from the ICU

ALLERGIES: _____

1. Transfer to: _____
2. Procedure: _____
3. Condition: _____
4. NURSING
    - ☐ Vital signs q4h × 2 days, then q shift
    - ☐ ECG telemetry
    - ☐ I & O q 8 hours
    - ☐ Daily weights
    - ☐ Foley catheter to gravity drainage; D/C on __/__ at __; due to void in 8 h
    - ☐ Chest tubes to −20 cm H_2O suction
    - ☐ Ambulate in hall with cardiac rehab
    - ☐ T.E.D. stockings
    - ☐ SpO_2 q8h and 1 time before and after ambulation
    - ☐ Wire and wound care per protocol
    - ☐ Wean oxygen via nasal prongs from 6 L/min to 2 L/min to keep $SpO_2 > 92\%$
    - ☐ Incentive spirometry q1h when awake
    - ☐ Glucose via fingerstick/glucometer AC and qhs in diabetics
    - ☐ Notify housestaff for heart rate > 110 or systolic blood pressure > 150 mm Hg
    - ☐ Saline lock, flush q8h and prn
5. Diet
    - ☐ NPO
    - ☐ Clear liquids/no added salt (NAS)
    - ☐ Full liquids/NAS
    - ☐ NAS, low fat, low cholesterol diet
    - ☐ _____ cal ADA, NAS low cholesterol diet, if diabetic
    - ☐ Fluid restriction ___ mL per 24 hours (IV + PO)
6. Temporary pacemaker settings
    - ☐ Pacemaker on: Mode: ☐ Atrial ☐ VVI ☐ DVI ☐ DDD
      Atrial output ____ mA Ventricular output ____ mA
      Rate ____ /min AV interval ____ msec
    - ☐ Pacer attached but off
    - ☐ Detach pacer but keep at bedside
7. Laboratory studies
    - ☐ Chest x-ray after chest tube removal
    - ☐ In AM after transfer: CBC, lytes, BUN, creat, blood glucose
    - ☐ Daily PT/INR if on warfarin
    - ☐ Daily PTT and platelet count if on heparin (see Appendix 7)
    - ☐ Fingerstick blood glucose at 4 AM on POD #2 (___/___); if >150 mg/dL, treat per insulin sliding scale protocol and repeat fingerstick at 5:30 AM
    - ☐ On day prior to discharge: chest x-ray, ECG, CBC, electrolytes, BUN, creatinine

8. Consults
   - ☐ Cardiac rehabilitation
   - ☐ Social services
   - ☐ Physical therapy
   - ☐ Occupational therapy
   - ☐ Nutrition
9. Medications
   a. Antibiotics
   - ☐ Cefazolin 1 g IV q8h for___ more doses (6 doses total); last dose on ___/___ at ___ hours
   - ☐ Vancomycin 1g IV q12h for ___ more doses (4 doses total); last dose on ___/___ at ___ hours
   - ☐ Mupirocin 2% (Bactroban ointment) via Q-tip nasal swab the evening after surgery and bid × 3 days total
   - ☐ Chlorhexidine 0.12% oral wash (Peridex) 15 mL with brushing q12h
   b. Cardiovascular medications
   - ☐ Metoprolol ___ mg PO q12h. Hold for HR < 60 or SBP < 100
   - ☐ Carvedilol ___ mg PO q12h. Hold for HR < 60 or SBP < 100
   - ☐ Amiodarone ___ mg PO q12h
   - ☐ Lisinopril ___ mg PO qd
   - ☐ Diltiazem 30 mg PO q6h (radial artery grafts)
   - ☐ Amlodipine 5 mg PO qd (radial artery grafts)
   - ☐ Imdur (sustained release) 20 mg PO qd (radial artery grafts)
   - ☐ Simvastatin ___ mg qd hs (no more than 20 mg if on amiodarone)
   c. Anticoagulants/antiplatelet agents
   - ☐ Enteric-coated aspirin ☐ 81 mg ☐ 325 mg PO qd (hold for platelet count < 75,000)
   - ☐ Clopidogrel 75 mg PO qd
   - ☐ Low-molecular-weight heparin (Lovenox) ___ mg SC ___
   - ☐ Heparin 5000 units SC bid
   - ☐ Heparin 25,000 units/500 mL D5W at ___units/h starting on _____ (per protocol – see Appendix 7)
   - ☐ Warfarin ___mg PO qd starting on _____; daily dose check with HO (per protocol – see page 672 and Appendix 8)
   d. Pain medications
   - ☐ Morphine sulfate via PCA pump or 10 mg IM q3h prn severe pain
   - ☐ Ketorolac 15–30 mg IV q6h prn moderate-to-severe pain (4–10 on pain scale); D/C after 72 hours
   - ☐ Acetaminophen with oxycodone (Percocet) 1–2 tabs PO q4h prn pain (start with one tablet for moderate pain (4–6 pain scale); give additional tablet after 1 hour if no change in pain; give 2 tablets for severe pain (7–10 pain scale)
   - ☐ Acetaminophen with codeine (Tylenol #3) 1–2 tabs PO q4h prn mild pain (1–3 pain scale)
   - ☐ Acetaminophen 650 mg PO q4h prn mild pain (1–3 pain scale)
   e. GI medications
   - ☐ Pantoprazole (Protonix) 40 mg PO qd
   - ☐ For nausea:
     - ☐ Metoclopramide 10 mg IV/PO q6h prn
     - ☐ Ondansetron 4–8 mg q4h IV/PO prn
     - ☐ Prochlorperazine 10 mg PO/IM/IV q6h prn
   - ☐ Milk of magnesia 30 mL PO qhs prn

(continued)

(continued)

      ☐ Docusate (Colace) 100 mg PO bid
      ☐ Bisacodyl (Dulcolax) 10 mg suppository prn constipation
  f. Diabetes medications
      ☐ Oral hypoglycemic: _____
      ☐ ___ units regular insulin (Novolin R or Humulin R) SC ___ qAM ___ qPM
      ☐ ___ units NPH insulin (Novolin N or Humulin N) SC ___ qAM ___ qPM
      ☐ Sliding scale: treat fingerstick/glucometer glucose according to the following
        scale at 06:00, 11:00, 15:00, and 20:00:
          140–160, give 2 units regular insulin SC (Novolin R or Humulin R)
          161–200, give 4 units regular insulin SC
          201–250, give 6 units regular insulin SC
          251–300, give 8 units regular insulin SC
          301–350, give 10 units regular insulin SC
          > 350, call house officer
  g. Other medications
      ☐ Acetaminophen 650 mg PO q3h prn temp > 38.5 °C
      ☐ Chloral hydrate 0.5–1.0 g PO qhs prn sleep
      ☐ Furosemide ___ mg IV/PO q __ h
      ☐ Potassium chloride ___ mEq PO bid (while on furosemide)
      ☐ Albuterol 2.5 mg/5 mL NS via nebulizer q4h prn
      ☐ Levalbuterol (Xopenex) 0.63 mg in 3 mL NS q8h via nebulizer or two inha-
        lations q4–6h through a pressured MDI
      ☐ Duoneb inhaler q6h

      ☐ Other: _____

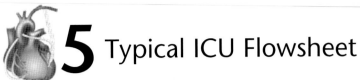

5 Typical ICU Flowsheet

ADULT CARDIOTHORACIC ICU
PATIENT CARE RECORD

DATE: _____ / _____ / _____   SURGEON: _____
POD #: _____   PROCEDURE: _____
PAGE #: _____

TIME	VITAL SIGNS												
	T	RHY/RATE	BP	CVP	PAD/PCW	CO	CI	SVR/SV Ratio	IABP	RIKER	PAIN	
1													
2													
3													
4													
5													

IV INFUSIONS

mL	DOSE	DOSE	DOSE	mL	DOSE	DOSE	DOSE

IV INFUSIONS

mL	DOSE	DOSE	mL	DOSE	DOSE	mL

MEDICATIONS
NAME/DOSE ROUTE

COMMENTS

COLLOID
TYPE   AMOUNT

FEEDS

URINE	NG	OTHER	CHEST TUBES						PULSES				VENTILATION					BLOOD GASES				OTHER		HEMATOLOGY/CHEMISTRY							
									LEFT	RIGHT	OTHER																					
AMT			AMT	AMT	AMT				DP	PT	DP	PT	DP	PT	Vent Mode	FIO2 PEEP	TV Rate	Pt's Rate	Press Supp	pH	pCO2	pO2	HCO3	O2 Sat	Hct Hgb	Plts WBC	PT PTT	INR	Na K	BUN Cr	BS	iCa TCa	Mg phos	OTHER
TOTAL			TOTAL	TOTAL	TOTAL																										

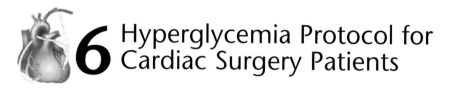

6 Hyperglycemia Protocol for Cardiac Surgery Patients

Goal: to maintain blood sugar (BS) between 110 and 150 mg/dL after surgery

- ☐ Check glucometer BS q1h
- ☐ Decrease to q4h if no changes in insulin drip rate for 6 h and serum BS <130 on three consecutive measurements.
- ☐ Correlate glucometer BS to serum BS daily
- ☐ Maintain serum potassium between 4.0 and 4.5 mEq/L
- ☐ Page house officer for BS <90 or >320
- ☐ Initiate protocol for BS >150 mg/dL on admission or at any subsequent time

Blood Sugar	Regular Insulin IV Bolus	Infusion Rate
151–200	No bolus	2 units/h
201–240	4 units	2 units/h
241–280	6 units	4 units/h
281–320	10 units	6 units/h

IV Insulin Adjustment Protocol

Blood Sugar	Insulin IV Bolus and Infusion Rate
<90	IV bolus with 1/2 amp 50% dextrose and stop infusion
91–110	Stop infusion; restart at 50% of previous rate once BS is <150
111–150	No change in infusion rate
151–200	Increase infusion rate by 2 units/h
201–240	IV bolus with 4 units and increase infusion by 2 units/h
241–280	IV bolus with 6 units and increase infusion by 2 unit/h
281–320	IV bolus with 10 units and increase infusion by 4 units/h
>320	Page house officer

Transition to Subcutaneous Insulin

1. Take hourly requirement for insulin (units/h) over the past 4 hours and multiply × 24 hours for total daily dose of insulin (e.g. 1 unit/h × 24 = 24 units/day)
2. Downtitrate by 80% for total daily dose of SC insulin (e.g. 24 units becomes 20 units/day)
3. Give 50% of total daily dose as basal insulin glargine (Lantus) and 50% as very-fast acting insulin (Novolog) divided into three daily doses with first dose 30 minutes before stopping insulin infusion. Subsequent requirements may be adjusted based upon response to these initial doses.
4. In this example, with 20 units/day, the patient would receive 10 units of Lantus and approximately 4 units of Novolog tid.

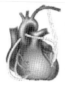

7 Heparinization Protocol for Cardiac Surgery Patients

1. Patient weight: ___ kg
2. PT, PTT, CBC, and platelet count before starting heparin
3. Initial PTT 6 h after starting infusion (4 h if a bolus is given)
4. Recheck PTT after changing infusion rate
5. Daily PTT in AM
6. Check platelet count daily if <100,000 and qod if >100,000 while on heparin
7. Guaiac all stools
8. Notify house officer for any bleeding, PTT <35 or >100 seconds
9. Discontinue all previous heparin orders. Do not administer for 12 h after last dose of low-molecular-weight heparin
10. Heparin bolus
    ☐ No bolus
    ☐ Give IV bolus of 80 units/kg = ___ units (round to nearest 100)
11. Heparin infusion 25,000/250 mL 0.45% NS @ ___ units/h (usually 15–18 units/kg)
    ☐ 40–60 kg   600 units/hour
    ☐ 61–70 kg   800 units/hour
    ☐ 71–80 kg   1000 units/hour
    ☐ 81–90 kg   1100 units/hour
    ☐ 91–100 kg 1200 units/hour
    ☐ >100 kg   1500 units/hour
12. Heparin adjustment schedule

PTT (sec)	Infusion Rate	Recheck PTT in
<45	Increase by 4 units/kg/h	4h
46–55	Increase by 2 units/kg/h	4h
56–65	No change	8h
66–75	Reduce by 1 unit/kg/h	6h
76–90	Reduce by 2 units/kg/h	4h
91–100	Stop for 1h & reduce by 3 units/kg/h	4h
>100	Stop for 2h & reduce by 4 units/kg/h	4h

8 Protocol for Initiating Warfarin

Assess whether patient is at greater risk for sensitivity to warfarin – if so, use low-dose protocol

a. Small, elderly females

b. Over age 75

c. Renal (creatinine >1.5 mg/dL) or hepatic dysfunction

d. Interacting medications (amiodarone, antibiotics)

Day	INR	Standard	Low-dose
1	WNL	5 mg	2.5 mg
2	<1.5	5 mg	2.5 mg
	1.5–1.9	2.5 mg	1.25 mg
	≥2	HOLD*	HOLD*
3	<1.5	7.5 mg	5 mg
	1.5–1.9	5 mg	2.5 mg
	2–3	2.5 mg	HOLD*
	>3	HOLD*	HOLD*
4	<1.5	10 mg	7.5 mg
	1.5–1.9	7.5 mg	5 mg
	2–3	5 mg	HOLD*
	>3	HOLD*	HOLD*
5	<1.5	10 mg	10 mg
	1.5–1.9	10 mg	5 mg
	2–3	5 mg	HOLD*
	>3	HOLD*	HOLD*
6	<1.5	12.5 mg	10 mg
	1.5–1.9	10 mg	7.5 mg
	2–3	5 mg	2.5 mg
	>3	HOLD*	HOLD*

*Restart warfarin when INR is less than 3

9 INR Reversal Protocol

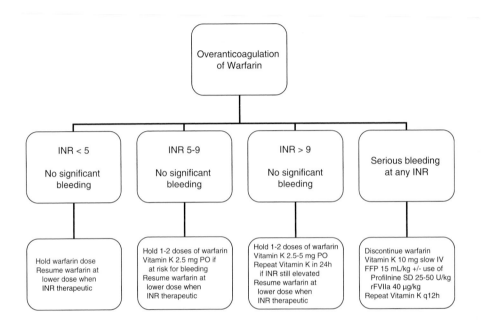

10 Drug, Food, and Dietary Supplement Interactions with Warfarin

Potentiation (increase INR)	Inhibition (decrease INR)	No Effect
Acetaminophen	Azathioprine	Alcohol (if no liver disease)
Alcohol (if liver disease)	Barbiturates	Antacids
Amiodarone	Bosentan	Atenolol
Anabolic steroids	Carbamazepine	Cefazolin
Aspirin	Chlordiazepoxide	Famotidine
Azithromycin	Cholestyramine	Furosemide
Chloral hydrate	Cyclosporine	Ibuprofen
Citalopram	Dicloxacillin	Ketorolac
Clofibrate	Nafcillin	Metoprolol
Diltiazem	Rifampin	Nizatidine
Fenofibrate	Sucralfate	Ranitidine
Floxin-antibiotics		Vancomycin
Fluvastatin		
Gemfibrozil		
Lovastatin		
Metronidazole		
Omeprazole		
Phenytoin		
Propafenone		
Propranolol		
Sertraline		
Simvastatin		
Tramadol		
Foods and herbal supplements		
Fish oils	Avocado	Green tea
Grapefruit	Ginseng	
Mango	Green leafy vegetables	
	Multivitamins with vitamin K	
	Soy milk	

This is partial list of the some of the more commonly used drugs in cardiac surgical patients. (Adapted in part from Ansell et al., Chest 2008;133:160S–198S.)

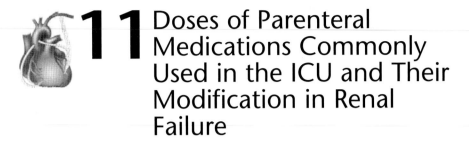

11 Doses of Parenteral Medications Commonly Used in the ICU and Their Modification in Renal Failure

Drug Class	Usual Dosage	Route of Elimination	Adjustment in Moderate Renal Failure
Analgesics			
Fentanyl	50–100 µg IV → 50–200 µg/h	H	no change
Hydromorphone (Dilaudid)	1–2 mg IV/IM q4–6h	H	no change
Ketorolac (Toradol)	15–30 mg IV q6h (×72 h)	R	reduce
Meperidine (Demerol)	50–100 mg IM q3h	H	use with caution
Morphine	2–10 mg IV/IM q2–4h	H	no change
Antacids			
Pantoprazole (Protonix)	40 mg IV over 15 min	H	no change
Ranitidine (Zantac)	50 mg IV q8h or 6.25 mg/h	R	reduce
Antianginals			
Esmolol	0.25–0.5 mg/kg IV → 0.05–0.2 mg/kg/min IV	M	no change
Metoprolol (Lopressor)	15 mg IV q15 min × 3	H	no change

Drug Class	Usual Dosage	Route of Elimination	Adjustment in Moderate Renal Failure
Antiarrhythmics			
Amiodarone (Cordarone)	150 mg IV → 1 mg/min × 6h → 0.5 mg/min × 18 h, then 1 g/day	H	no change
Lidocaine	1 mg/kg IV → 1–4 mg/min	H	no change
Antibiotics (prophylactic doses)			
Cefazolin (Ancef, Kefzol)	1–2 g IV → 1 g IV q8h	R	reduce
Cefuroxime (Zinacef)	1.5 IV → 1.5 g IV q8h	R	reduce
Vancomycin	15–20 mg/kg → 1g IV q8h	R	reduce
Antiemetics			
Dolasetron (Anzemet)	12.5 mg IV	H/R	no change
Droperidol (Inapsine)	0.625–1.25 mg IV	H	no change
Metoclopramide (Reglan)	10–20 mg IM/IV qid	R > H	reduce
Ondansetron (Zofran)	4–8 mg IV	H	no change
Prochlorperazine (Compazine)	5–10 mg IM q4h	H	no change
Antihypertensives (see Table 11.8, page 497)			
Diuretics			
Acetazolamide (Diamox)	250–500 mg IV q6h	R	use with caution
Bumetanide (Bumex)	1–5 mg IV q12h or 0.5–2 mg/h drip	R > H	use with caution

Drug Class	Usual Dosage	Route of Elimination	Adjustment in Moderate Renal Failure
Chlorothiazide (Diuril)	500 mg IV qd	R	use with caution
Ethacrynic acid (Edecrin)	50–100 mg IV q6h	H > R	use with caution
Furosemide (Lasix)	10–200 mg IV q6h or 5–40 mg/h drip	R > H	use with caution
Inotropic agents (see Table 11.6, page 460)			
Paralytic agents (see also Table 4.3, page 196)			
Atracurium (Tracrium)	0.3 mg/kg IV → 0.2–0.4 mg/kg/h	M	no change
Doxacurium (Nuromax)	0.06 mg/kg → 0.005 mg/kg q30 min	R	reduce
Pancuronium (Pavulon)	0.1 mg/kg IV → 0.01 mg/kg q1h or 2–4 mg/h	R > H	no change
Rocuronium (Zemuron)	0.6–1.2 mg/kg IV → 10 µg/kg/min	H	no change
Vecuronium (Norcuron)	0.1 mg/kg IV → 0.01 mg/kg q30–45 min or 2–6 mg/h	H	no change
Psychotropics/Sedatives			
Dexmedetomidine (Precedex)	1 µg/kg load, then 0.2–0.7 µg/kg/h	H	no change
Haloperidol (Haldol)	1–10 mg IM/IV q4–6h	H	no change
Lorazepam (Ativan)	1–2 mg IV/2–4 mg IM q6h	H	no change
Midazolam (Versed)	2.5–5 mg IV q1–2h	H	no change
Propofol (Diprivan)	25–50 µg/kg/min	M	no change

Drug Class	Usual Dosage	Route of Elimination	Adjustment in Moderate Renal Failure
Other			
Aminophylline	5 mg/kg IV load → 0.2–0.9 mg/kg/h	H	no change
Flumazenil	0.2 mg q30 sec, then 0.3 mg, then 0.5 mg up to 3 mg max/h	H	no change
Naloxone	0.4–2 mg IV	H	no change

Medications metabolized by the liver do not require reduction in dosage for renal failure; medications metabolized by the kidneys must be adjusted according to the serum creatinine, or more precisely by the glomerular filtration rate. The reader should refer to the *Physician's Desk Reference* for complete prescribing information. H, hepatic metabolism; R, renal elimination; M, metabolized in the bloodstream.

12 Doses of Nonparenteral Drugs Commonly Used After Heart Surgery and Their Modifications in Renal Failure

Drug Class	Usual Dosage	Route of Elimination	Adjustment in Moderate Renal Failure
Analgesics			
Acetaminophen	650 mg PO q4h	R	reduce
Hydromorphone (Dilaudid)	2–4 mg q4–6h	H	no change
Ketorolac (Toradol)	20 mg PO → 10 mg q4–6h	R	reduce
Ibuprofen	400–800 mg PO tid	R	reduce
Oxycodone[a]	4.5 mg PO q6h	H	no change
Hydrocodone[a]	5 mg PO q4–6h	H	no change
[a] usually given with acetaminophen 325 mg (Vicodin or Percocet)			
Antacids/antireflux medications			
Sucralfate (Carafate)	1 g PO qid	R	reduce
H_2 blocker			
Famotidine (Pepcid)	20–40 mg PO qhs	R > M	reduce
Nizatidine (Axid)	150 mg PO bid or 300 qhs	R	reduce
Ranitidine (Zantac)	150 mg PO bid	R	reduce

Drug Class	Usual Dosage	Route of Elimination	Adjustment in Moderate Renal Failure
Proton pump inhibitors			
Lansoprazole (Prevacid)	15 mg PO qd	H	no change
Omeprazole (Prilosec)	20 mg PO qd	H	no change
Pantoprazole (Protonix)	40 mg PO qd	H	no change
Antianginals			
Beta-blockers			
Atenolol (Tenormin)	25–50 mg PO qd	R	reduce
Bisoprolol (Zebeta)	2.5–20 mg PO qd	H	no change
Metoprolol (Lopressor)	25–100 mg PO bid	H	no change
Calcium channel blockers			
Diltiazem	30–60 mg PO tid 180–360 qd of long–acting	H	no change
Nicardipine	20–40 mg PO tid	H	no change
Nifedipine	10–30 mg PO/SL tid	H	no change
Verapamil	80–160 mg PO tid	H	no change
Nitrates			
Isosorbide dinitrate (Isordil)	5–40 mg PO tid	H	no change
Isosorbide mononitrate (Imdur, Ismo)	20 mg PO qd	–	no change
Nitropaste	1–3" q4h	H	no change
Antiarrhythmics			
Amiodarone	400 mg PO tid weaned to 200 mg qd	H	no change
Digoxin	0.125–0.25 mg PO qd	R	reduce
Sotalol	80 mg PO bid	R	reduce

Drug Class	Usual Dosage	Route of Elimination	Adjustment in Moderate Renal Failure
Antibiotics			
Cephalexin	500 mg PO qid	R	reduce
Ciprofloxacin	500 mg PO bid	R	reduce
Antidiabetic drugs (oral hypoglycemics)			
Chlorpropamide (Diabinese)	250 mg PO qd	R	avoid
Glipizide (Glucotrol)	5 mg PO qAM	H	no change
Glyburide (Micronase, Diabeta)	2.5–5 mg PO qAM	H = R	use with caution
Metformin (Glucophage)	500 mg PO bid	R	avoid
Pioglitazone (Actos)	15–30 mg PO qd	H	no change
Rosiglitazone (Avandia)	4–8 mg PO qd	H	no change
Antiemetics			
Dolasetron (Anzemet)	100 mg PO	H/R	no change
Metoclopramide (Reglan)	10–20 mg PO qid	R > H	reduce
Ondansetron (Zofran)	8–16 mg PO	H	no change
Prochlorperazine (Compazine)	5–10 mg PO q6h	H	no change
Antihypertensives			
Angiotensin-converting enzyme (ACE) inhibitors			
Captopril (Capoten)	6.25–50 mg PO bid	R	avoid
Enalapril (Vasotec)	2.5–5 mg PO qd	R	avoid
Lisinopril (Zestril)	5–20 mg PO qd	R	avoid
Quinapril (Accupril)	10 mg PO qd	R	avoid
Ramipril (Altace)	2.5 mg PO qd	R > H	reduce

Drug Class	Usual Dosage	Route of Elimination	Adjustment in Moderate Renal Failure
Angiotensin II receptor blockers (ARBs)			
Candesartan (Atacand)	8–32 mg PO qd or in 2 divided doses	H	no change
Irbesartan (Avapro)	150–300 mg PO qd	H	no change
Losartan (Cozaar)	25–100 mg PO qd or in 2 divided doses	H	no change
Valsartan (Diovan)	80–160 mg PO qd	H	no change
Beta-blockers *(see also antianginals)*			
Carvedilol (Coreg)	3.125–25 mg PO bid	H	reduce
Labetalol (Trandate, Normodyne)	100–400 mg PO qid	H	no change
Nevibolol (Bystolic)	5–40 mg PO qd	H	no change
Calcium channel blockers *(see also antianginals)*			
Amlodipine (Norvasc)	2.5–10 mg PO qd	H	no change
Nicardipine (Cardene)	20–40 mg PO tid	H	no change
Others			
Clonidine (Catapres)	0.1–0.3 mg PO bid	R	reduce
Doxazosin (Cardura)	1.0–8 mg PO qd	H	no change
Prazosin (Minipress)	1.0–7.5 mg PO bid	H	no change
Cholesterol-lowering medications			
Atorvastatin (Lipitor)	10–80 mg PO qd	H	no change
Ezetimibe (Zetia)	10 mg PO qd	–	no change
Fluvastatin (Lescol)	40–80 mg PO qd	H	no change
Lovastatin (Mevacor)	10–80 mg PO qd	H	no change
Niacin (Niaspan)	500–1000 mg PO qd	H	reduce
Pravastatin (Pravachol)	40–80 mg PO qd	H	no change
Rosuvastatin (Crestor)	10–20 mg PO qd	–	no change
Simvastatin (Zocor)	10–80 mg PO qd	H	no change

Drug Class	Usual Dosage	Route of Elimination	Adjustment in Moderate Renal Failure
Diuretics			
Acetazolamide (Diamox)	250–500 mg PO qid	R	reduce
Furosemide (Lasix)	10–100 mg PO bid	R > H	no change
Hydrochlorothiazide (Hydrodiuril)	50–100 mg PO qd	R	no change
Metolazone (Zaroxolyn)	5–20 mg PO qd	R	no change
Diuretics (potassium-sparing)			
Amiloride (Midador)	5–10 mg PO qd	R	avoid
Eplerenone (Inspra)	50 mg PO qd	H	no change
Spironolactone (Aldactone)	25 mg PO qd	R	avoid
Psychotropics/Sedatives/Antidepressants			
Alprazolam (Xanax)	0.25–0.5 mg PO tid	H, R	reduce
Bupropion (Wellbutrin, Zyban)	100 mg PO bid	H	no change
Buspirone (Buspar)	7.5 mg PO bid	–	no change
Citalopram (Celexa)	20 mg PO qd	H	no change
Chlordiazepoxide (Librium)	5–25 mg PO tid	H	no change
Fluoxetine (Prozac)	20–40 mg PO qd	H	no change
Haloperidol (Haldol)	0.5–2.5 mg PO tid	H	no change
Lorazepam (Ativan)	1–2 mg PO bid or hs	H	no change
Olanzepine (Zyprexa)	5–10 mg PO qd	H	no change
Paroxetine (Paxil)	20–50 mg PO qd	H/R	reduce
Quetiapine (Seroquel)	25–100 mg PO bid	H	no change
Risperidone (Risperdal)	2 mg PO qd	H	no change
Sertraline (Zoloft)	50–200 mg PO qd	H	no change
Venlafaxine (Effexor)	25 mg PO bid or tid	R	reduce

Drug Class	Usual Dosage	Route of Elimination	Adjustment in Moderate Renal Failure
Sleep medications			
Chloral hydrate	500–1000 mg PO hs	H	no change
Diphenhydramine (Benadryl)	25–50 mg PO hs	H	no change
Temazepam (Restoril)	15–30 mg PO hs	H	no change
Triazolam (Halcion)	0.125–0.25 mg PO hs	H	no change
Zaleplon (Sonata)	5–10 mg PO hs	H	no change
Zolpidem (Ambien)	10 mg PO hs	H	no change
Others			
Amitriptyline (Elavil)	10–20 mg PO qhs or bid	H	no change
Carbamazepine (Tegretol)	200 mg PO bid	H	no change
Gabapentin (Neurontin)	300 mg PO qd–600 mg tid	R	reduce
Theophylline (Theodur)	300 mg PO bid	H	no change
Varenicline (Chantix)	0.5–1.0 mg PO qd	–	no change

Antianginal medications given four times a day (qid) are usually taken 4 hours apart during the daytime. Other medications should generally be taken at equally spaced intervals.

Medications metabolized by the liver do not require reduction in dosage for renal failure; medications metabolized by the kidneys must be adjusted according to the serum creatinine, or more precisely, by the glomerular filtration rate. The reader should refer to the *Physician's Desk Reference* for complete prescribing information

H, hepatic metabolism; R, renal elimination; M, metabolized in the bloodstream.

13 Definitions from the STS Data Specifications (Version 2.7 2011)

Preoperative conditions

1. **Chronic lung disease**
   a. Mild: FEV_1 60–75% of predicted, and/or chronic inhaled or oral bronchodilators
   b. Moderate: FEV_1 50–59% of predicted, and/or on chronic steroid therapy aimed at lung disease
   c. Severe: FEV_1 <50% of predicted, and/or room air PO_2 <60 torr or PCO_2 >50 torr

2. **Peripheral arterial disease**
   a. Claudication either with exertion or at rest
   b. Amputation for arterial vascular insufficiency
   c. Vascular reconstruction, bypass surgery, or percutaneous intervention to the extremities
   d. Documented abdominal aneurysm with or without repair
   e. Positive noninvasive test (ankle brachial index $\leq$ 0.9, ultrasound, MRA, CTA of >50% in any peripheral artery) or angiographic imaging
   f. Does not include carotid disease

3. **Neurologic condition**
   a. Unresponsive neurologic state within 24 hours of surgery
   b. Cerebrovascular disease
      i. CVA symptoms >24 hours after onset (remote >2 weeks, recent within 2 weeks)
      ii. Transient ischemic attack (TIA) with recovery within 24 hours
      iii. Noninvasive carotid test >79% diameter stenosis
      iv. Prior carotid surgery or stenting

4. **Diabetes mellitus:** history of diabetes with one of the following:
   a. HbA1c >6.5%
   b. Fasting plasma glucose >126 mg/dL
   c. Two-hour plasma glucose >200 mg/dL during oral glucose tolerance test
   d. Random plasma glucose >200 mg/dL in patient with classic symptoms of hyperglycemia

5. **Renal failure** on dialysis (serum creatinine should be noted for all patients)

6. **Dyslipidemia:** known history of dyslipidemia with:
   a. Total cholesterol >200 mg/dL
   b. LDL $\geq$130 mg/dL or treatment initiated for LDL >100 mg/dL in patients with known CAD
   c. HDL <40 mg/dL

7. **Hypertension**
   a. BP >140 mm Hg systolic or >90 mm Hg diastolic in patients without diabetes or chronic kidney disease
   b. BP >130 mm Hg systolic or >80 mm Hg diastolic on at least two occasions in patients with diabetes or chronic kidney disease
   c. History of hypertension treated with medication, diet, and/or exercise

8. **Congestive heart failure:** evidence in the 2 preceding of symptoms of CHF, including unusual dyspnea on light exertion, recurrent dyspnea occurring in the supine position, fluid retention; or the description of rales, jugular venous distention, pulmonary edema on physical examination, or pulmonary edema on chest x-ray presumed to be cardiac dysfunction.

9. **Stable angina:** angina without a change in frequency or pattern for 6 weeks prior to surgery; pain controlled with rest and/or oral or transcutaneous medications

10. **Unstable angina**
    a. Rest angina
    b. New onset of angina within 2 months of surgery
    c. Increasing angina (intensity, duration, and/or frequency)

11. **Non-ST-elevation myocardial infarction (NSTEMI)** with hospitalization
    a. Cardiac biomarkers > upper limit of normal (ULN) with a clinical presentation consistent with or suggestive of ischemia; ECG changes and/or ischemic symptoms may or may not be present.
    b. Absence of ECG changes of an ST-elevation infarction

12. **ST-elevation MI (STEMI)**
    a. Cardiac biomarkers >ULN
    b. New >0.1 mV ST segment elevation in two contiguous leads or new left bundle branch block

13. **Cardiogenic shock:** clinical state of end-organ hypoperfusion due to cardiac failure at the time of the procedure with:
    a. Persistent hypotension (systolic BP < 80–90 mm Hg or mean arterial pressure 30 mm Hg lower than baseline) ***and***
    b. Severe reduction in cardiac index (<1.8 L/min/m^2 without support or < 2.2 L/min/m^2 with support)

14. **Resuscitation:** CPR required within 1 hour before the start of the operative procedure which includes the institution of anesthetic management

15. **Urgency**
    a. Elective: the patient's cardiac function has been stable in the days or weeks prior to the operation. The procedure could be deferred without an increased risk of compromised cardiac outcome.
    b. Urgent: procedure required during same hospitalization in order to minimize chance of further clinical deterioration. This includes, but is not limited to, worsening sudden chest pain, CHF, an acute MI, threatening coronary anatomy, IABP, unstable angina requiring IV NTG, or rest angina
    c. Emergent: surgery is indicated without delay for ongoing, refractory, or unrelenting cardiac compromise, with or without hemodynamic instability,

and not responsive to any form of therapy except cardiac surgery. Conditions include:

  i. Shock with or without circulatory support

  ii. Pulmonary edema requiring intubation

  iii. Acute evolving MI within 24h before surgery

  iv. Ongoing ischemia including rest pain despite maximal medical therapy and/or IABP

d. Emergent salvage: patient is undergoing CPR en route to the operating room or prior to anesthesia induction

Postoperative complications

1. **Operative mortality:** death occurring during the hospitalization in which the surgery was performed (even if after 30 days) or death occurring after hospital discharge, but within 30 days, unless clearly unrelated to the operation

2. **Neurologic deficits**

   a. Permanent stroke: neurologic deficit of abrupt onset caused by disturbance in blood supply to the brain persisting > 24 h

   b. Transient ischemic attack: loss of neurologic function that was abrupt in onset but with complete return of function within 24 h

   c. Coma/encephalopathy

   d. Paralysis, paraparesis, or paraplegia related to spinal cord ischemia

3. **Renal failure:** acute or worsening renal function resulting in one or both more of the following:

   a. Increase of serum creatinine to > 2 mg/dL and to $2 \times$ the most recent preoperative creatinine

   b. New requirement for dialysis

4. **Prolonged ventilation:** prolonged postoperative mechanical ventilatory support for >24 h

5. **Myocardial infarction**: elevation of biomarkers (CK-MB or troponin) to more than 5 times the 99th percentile of the normal reference range during the first 72h after a CABG **plus**:

   a. New pathologic Q waves or LBBB **or**

   b. Angiographically documented new graft or native coronary artery occlusion **or**

   c. Imaging evidence of new loss of viable myocardium

6. **Deep sternal wound infection:** infection involving the muscle, bone, and/or mediastinum occurring within 30 days of surgery requiring operative intervention with all of the following:

   a. Wound opened with excision of tissue or reexploration of mediastinum

   b. Positive culture unless patient on antibiotics at time of culture or no culture obtained

   c. Treatment with antibiotics beyond perioperative prophylaxis

14 Body Surface Area Nomogram

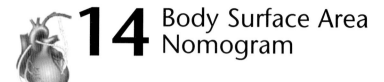

Height	Body Surface Area	Weight

cm 200 — 79 in
78
195 — 77
76
190 — 75
74
185 — 73
72
180 — 71
70
175 — 69
68
170 — 67
66
165 — 65
64
160 — 63
62
155 — 61
60
150 — 59
58
145 — 57
56
140 — 55
54
135 — 53
52
130 — 51
50
125 — 49
48
120 — 47
46
115 — 45
44
110 — 43
42
105 — 41
40
cm 100 — 39 in

2.80 m²
2.70
2.60
2.50
2.40
2.30
2.20
2.10
2.00
1.95
1.90
1.85
1.80
1.75
1.70
1.65
1.60
1.55
1.50
1.45
1.40
1.35
1.30
1.25
1.20
1.15
1.10
1.05
1.00
0.95
0.90
0.86 m²

kg 150 — 330 lb
145 — 320
140 — 310
135 — 300
— 290
130 — 280
125 — 270
120 — 260
115 — 250
110 — 240
105 — 230
100 — 220
95 — 210
90 — 200
— 190
85 — 180
80 —
75 — 170
— 160
70 — 150
65 — 140
60 — 130
55 — 120
50 — 110
— 105
45 — 100
— 95
40 — 90
— 85
35 — 80
— 75
— 70
kg 30 — 66 lb

15 Body Mass Index Chart

Weight (in Pounds)

Height (in Inches)	120	130	140	150	160	170	180	190	200	210	220	230	240	250	260
82	13	14	15	16	17	18	19	20	21	22	23	24	25	26	27
80	13	14	15	16	18	19	20	21	22	23	24	25	26	27	29
78	14	15	16	17	18	20	21	22	23	24	25	27	28	29	30
76	15	16	17	18	19	21	22	23	24	26	27	28	29	30	32
74	15	17	18	19	21	22	23	24	26	27	28	30	31	32	33
72	16	18	19	20	22	23	24	26	27	28	30	31	33	34	35
70	17	19	20	22	23	24	26	27	29	30	32	33	34	36	37
68	18	20	21	23	24	26	27	29	30	32	33	35	36	38	40
66	19	21	23	24	26	27	29	31	32	34	36	37	39	40	42
64	21	22	24	26	27	29	31	33	34	36	38	39	41	43	45
62	22	24	26	27	29	31	33	35	37	38	40	42	44	46	48
60	23	25	27	29	31	33	35	37	39	41	43	45	47	49	51
58	25	27	29	31	33	36	38	40	42	44	46	48	50	52	54
56	27	29	31	34	36	38	40	43	45	47	49	52	54	56	58
54	29	31	34	36	39	41	43	46	48	51	53	55	58	60	63

Normal   Overweight   Obese

Weight (in Kilograms)

Height (in Inches)	60	65	70	75	80	85	90	95	100	105	110	115	120	125	130
2.15	13	14	15	16	17	18	19	21	22	23	24	25	26	27	28
2.10	14	15	16	17	18	19	20	22	23	24	25	26	27	28	29
2.05	14	15	17	18	19	20	21	23	24	25	26	27	29	30	31
2.00	15	16	18	19	20	21	23	24	25	26	28	29	30	31	33
1.95	16	17	18	20	21	22	24	25	26	28	29	30	32	33	34
1.90	17	18	19	21	22	24	25	26	28	29	30	32	33	35	36
1.85	18	19	20	22	23	25	26	28	29	31	32	34	35	37	38
1.80	19	20	22	23	25	26	28	29	31	32	34	35	37	39	40
1.75	20	21	23	24	26	28	29	31	33	34	36	38	39	41	42
1.70	21	22	24	26	28	29	31	33	35	36	38	40	42	43	45
1.65	22	24	26	28	29	31	33	35	37	39	40	42	44	46	48
1.60	23	25	27	29	31	33	35	37	39	41	43	45	47	49	51
1.55	25	27	29	31	33	35	37	40	42	44	46	48	50	52	54
1.50	27	29	31	33	36	38	40	42	44	47	49	51	53	56	58
1.45	29	31	33	36	38	40	43	45	48	50	52	55	57	59	62

16 Technique of Thoracentesis

A. The level of the fluid should be determined on chest x-ray and confirmed by dullness to percussion. The skin is prepped and draped. One percent lidocaine is used for local anesthesia of the skin. A 22 gauge needle is passed to the upper border of the rib and the periosteum is anesthetized. The needle is then passed over the rib into the pleural space.

B. When the pleural space has been entered, fluid should be aspirated to confirm that the effusion has been located. A larger "intracatheter" needle is then passed into the pleural cavity, the plastic catheter advanced, and the metal needle withdrawn to prevent injury to the lung as it expands to appose the parietal pleura. The fluid is then aspirated into collection bottles.

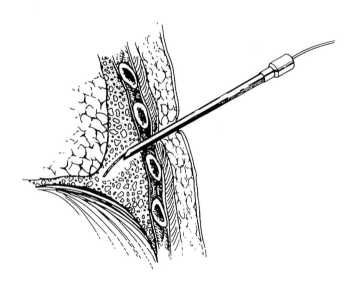

17 Technique for Tube Thoracostomy

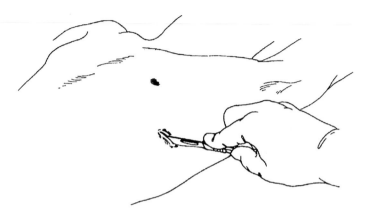

1. Skin incision. One percent lidocaine is used for local anesthesia. A subcutaneous wheal is raised over the fifth or sixth intercostal space in the mid-axillary line. The needle is passed to the upper border of the rib and the periosteum is anesthetized. Fluid should be aspirated from an effusion to confirm its location. A 1 cm incision is then made.

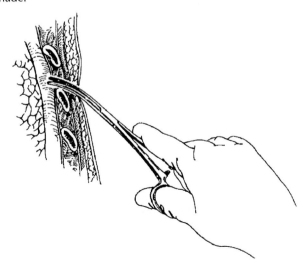

2. Pleural entry. The dissection is carried down to and through the intercostal muscles with a Kelly clamp, the parietal pleura is penetrated, and the pleural cavity is entered. Finger dissection should be used only if loculations are known to be present.

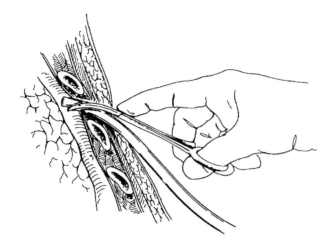

3. Chest tube placement. The chest tube is inserted and directed towards the apex for air and posteriorly for fluid. The tube should be clamped during insertion if fluid is being drained. The tube is then secured with a 2-0 silk suture. A trocar should **never** be used to penetrate the pleura.

18 Technique of Insertion of Percutaneous Tracheostomy Tube

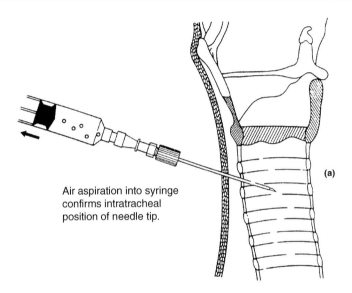

Air aspiration into syringe
confirms intratracheal
position of needle tip.

(a)

This procedure should be performed with the assistance of an individual trained in airway management and bronchoscopy. The diagrams represent an overview of the procedure derived from the package insert for the Ciaglia percutaneous tracheostomy set (Cook Medical).

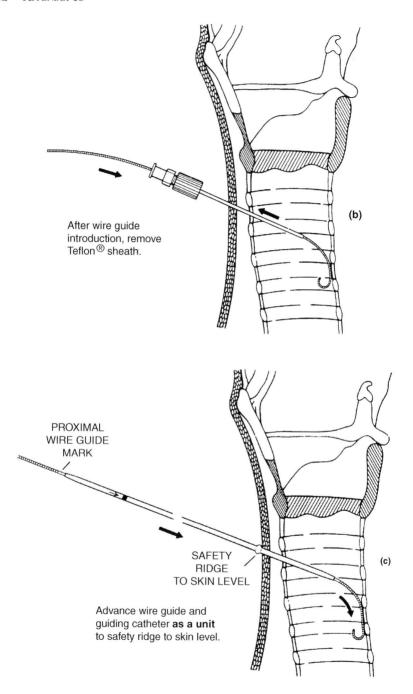

After wire guide
introduction, remove
Teflon® sheath.

(b)

PROXIMAL
WIRE GUIDE
MARK

SAFETY
RIDGE
TO SKIN LEVEL

(c)

Advance wire guide and
guiding catheter **as a unit**
to safety ridge to skin level.

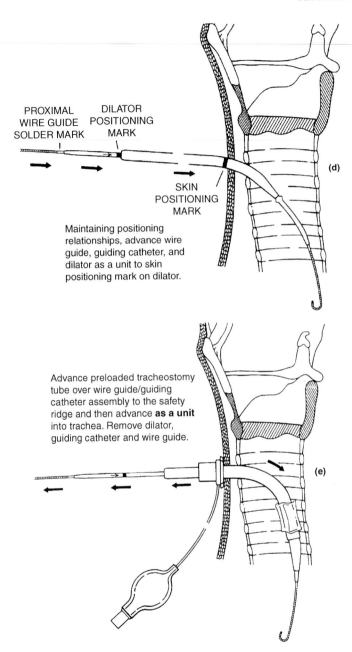

PROXIMAL   DILATOR
WIRE GUIDE   POSITIONING
SOLDER MARK   MARK

SKIN
POSITIONING
MARK

(d)

Maintaining positioning
relationships, advance wire
guide, guiding catheter, and
dilator as a unit to skin
positioning mark on dilator.

Advance preloaded tracheostomy
tube over wire guide/guiding
catheter assembly to the safety
ridge and then advance **as a unit**
into trachea. Remove dilator,
guiding catheter and wire guide.

(e)

Index

Note: page numbers with an *f* indicates figures; those with a *t*, tables; those with an *a*, appendix